Physical Therapist Assistant Exam Review Guide

Mark Dutton, PT

Allegheny General Hospital
Pittsburgh, Pennsylvania

WITHDRAWN

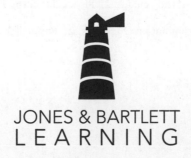

JONES & BARTLETT
L E A R N I N G

World Headquarters
Jones & Bartlett Learning
40 Tall Pine Drive
Sudbury, MA 01776
978-443-5000
info@jblearning.com
www.jblearning.com

Jones & Bartlett Learning
Canada
6339 Ormindale Way
Mississauga, Ontario L5V 1J2
Canada

Jones & Bartlett Learning
International
Barb House, Barb Mews
London W6 7PA
United Kingdom

Jones & Bartlett Learning books and products are available through most bookstores and online booksellers. To contact Jones & Bartlett Learning directly, call 800-832-0034, fax 978-443-8000, or visit our website, www.jblearning.com.

Substantial discounts on bulk quantities of Jones & Bartlett Learning publications are available to corporations, professional associations, and other qualified organizations. For details and specific discount information, contact the special sales department at Jones & Bartlett Learning via the above contact information or send an email to specialsales@jblearning.com.

The author, editor, and publisher have made every effort to provide accurate information. However, they are not responsible for errors, omissions, or for any outcomes related to the use of the contents of this book and take no responsibility for the use of the products and procedures described. Treatments and side effects described in this book may not be applicable to all people; likewise, some people may require a dose or experience a side effect that is not described herein. Drugs and medical devices are discussed that may have limited availability controlled by the Food and Drug Administration (FDA) for use only in a research study or clinical trial. Research, clinical practice, and government regulations often change the accepted standard in this field. When consideration is being given to use of any drug in the clinical setting, the health care provider or reader is responsible for determining FDA status of the drug, reading the package insert, and reviewing prescribing information for the most up-to-date recommendations on dose, precautions, and contraindications, and determining the appropriate usage for the product. This is especially important in the case of drugs that are new or seldom used.

Production Credits
Publisher: David D. Cella
Acquisitions Editor: Katey Birtcher
Associate Editor: Maro Gartside
Production Manager: Julie Champagne Bolduc
Production Editor: Jessica Steele Newfell
Marketing Manager: Grace Richards
Manufacturing and Inventory Control Supervisor: Amy Bacus
Composition: Glyph International
Cover Design: Kate Ternullo
Rights and Permissions Supervisor: Christine Myaskovsky
Assistant Photo Researcher: Elise Gilbert
Printing and Binding: Courier Kendallville
Cover Printing: Courier Kendallville

Photo Credits
All chapter and section openers © Patrick Hermans/ShutterStock, Inc.; **10-4** © Dr. P. Marazzi/Photo Researchers, Inc.

To order this product, use ISBN: 978-1-4496-2850-5

Library of Congress Cataloging-in-Publication Data
Dutton, Mark.
 Physical therapist assistant exam review guide / Mark Dutton.
   p. ; cm.
 Includes bibliographical references and index.
 ISBN 978-0-7637-9757-7 (pbk. : alk. paper)
 1. Physical therapy assistants—Examinations—Study guides. 2. Physical therapy assistants—Examinations, questions, etc.
 I. Title.
 [DNLM: 1. Physical Therapy Modalities—Examination Questions. 2. Physical Therapy (Specialty)—Examination Questions.
WB 18.2]
 RM701.6.P552 2012
 615.8'2076—dc22
                              2010052509

6048
Printed in the United States of America
15 14 13 12 11   10 9 8 7 6 5 4 3 2 1

Brief Contents

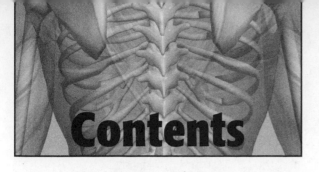

Contents

CHAPTER 11 Geriatric Physical Therapy **407**

SECTION III Therapeutic Procedures **429**

CHAPTER 12 Therapeutic Exercise **431**

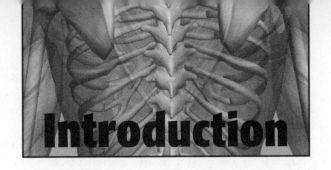

Introduction

The purpose of the *Physical Therapist Assistant Exam Review Guide* is to help physical therapist assistant (PTA) candidates prepare for the National Physical Therapy Examination (NPTE) for Physical Therapist Assistants. All jurisdictions that license PTAs require the candidate to successfully complete the NPTE. These requirements may differ from state to state or within the same state. Licensure of healthcare practitioners by the states and other jurisdictions of the United States is a means by which the public is protected from incompetent or immoral practitioners. The Federation of State Boards of Physical Therapy (FSBPT) develops, maintains, and administers the National Physical Therapy Examinations (NPTE) for physical therapists (PTs) and PTAs.

The NPTE for PTAs is offered on the computer at over 300 Prometric Testing Centers within the United States. The exam content is divided into three large groups of questions. The largest portion of the examination content, approximately 73%, falls into the actual delivery of physical therapy interventions to patients throughout the life span and affecting different body systems. Of the remainder of the examination, approximately 15% involves understanding and use of equipment and devices and the application of therapeutic modalities while the other 12% focuses on safety and professional roles, teaching/learning, and evidence-based practice. In terms of emphasis placed on the various systems, the FSBPT 2010 Candidate Handbook provides the following information: musculoskeletal (21.33%), neuromuscular (20%), cardiovascular/pulmonary (12.67%), integumentary (6%), other systems (12.67%), and non-systems (27.33%).

To sit for the NPTE for PTAs, the candidate must contact the state or jurisdiction in which he or she plans to apply for a license. Once the completed application has been returned to the appropriate agency, along with all necessary monies and documentation, the state forwards this paperwork to the Federation of State Boards of Physical Therapy (FSBPT), which then sends an authorization-to-test letter providing a timeline for taking the examination.

The NPTE for PTAs is a 200-question (50 pretest with 150 scored), multiple-choice examination designed to determine if a candidate possesses the minimal competency necessary to practice as a physical therapist assistant. The 200 questions, each with four possible choices, are administered to candidates in four sections consisting of 50 questions each, with each section containing pretest items and scored items. The questions are designed to test a candidate's knowledge, comprehension, application, and analysis of a variety of clinical scenarios.

Candidates have four hours to complete the four sections, which are not timed individually, so candidates must effectively manage the allotted time. Therefore, time management is critical. Candidates are unable to return to previously completed sections once a new section is initiated. Candidates have the opportunity to take one scheduled break at the conclusion of section 2, immediately prior to beginning section 3. Additional unscheduled breaks can be taken at the conclusion of a given section; however, the elapsed time will not stop. It is important to complete all of the questions, even if educated guesses must be used for some of the questions. Given the importance of this test, every effort must be made to obtain a successful passing score—some states limit the number of times one may take the NPTE for PTAs. Three times per 12-month period is the limit for sitting for the examination, with some states allowing only three opportunities to take the NPTE for PTAs in total.

Physical Therapist Assistant Exam Review Guide is designed to equip candidates with excellent study tools intended to review the required level of didactic information and to prepare the candidate for the examination by focusing on the key topic areas. The NPTE for PTAs is aimed to test a candidate's ability to apply the didactic knowledge in clinical situations, so without this knowledge the candidate will find the examination extremely difficult. The candidate is faced with wondering how much time should be spent on studying, and whether he or she is sufficiently prepared to take the examination. Usually, 4 to 6 weeks of independent, structured review is adequate.

Included in this book is the essential information of each subject area in an easy-to-study design. Illustrations, Key Point boxes, and tables are provided to help retain information. The information presented in this study guide is intended to be all-inclusive so candidates do not have to use a number of texts to study for the exam. While it is hoped that the majority of information presented is familiar to candidates, some areas may require additional study prior to the examination. In addition to the chapters covering musculoskeletal, neuromuscular, cardiovascular, pulmonary, pediatric, geriatric, and integumentary physical therapy, there are also chapters on special topics such as administration, research, pharmacology, orthotics/prosthetics, therapeutic modalities, gait and functional training, therapeutic exercise, pediatrics, geriatrics, and cardiovascular, pulmonary, integumentary, and pathological/psychological conditions. Given the important roles that therapeutic exercise and both the musculoskeletal and neurologic systems play in the field of physical therapy, greater emphasis is placed on these subject areas, as reflected in the relative size of their respective chapters.

The questions at the end of each chapter are designed to assess the reader's theoretical knowledge. Ideally, the end-of-chapter questions should be attempted prior to taking the sample simulated NPTE for PTAs examination provided online.

The online simulated exam questions are designed to determine if the candidate has sufficient mastery of a particular content area and is able to apply it accurately to the clinical situation described in the question. The software is designed so the candidate has the ability to revisit questions he or she would like to view again. At the end of the examination, the software can help diagnose the strengths and vulnerabilities of the candidate's academic and clinical backgrounds by providing a performance analysis, which offers feedback with regard to areas of vulnerability and strength, emphasizing those areas that require additional study.

It is hoped that the contents of *Physical Therapist Assistant Exam Review Guide* and the online examination will help the reader organize and focus his or her study in the most efficient and effective manner.

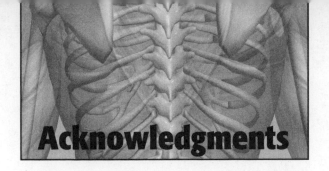

Acknowledgments

I would like to thank the following, who in their own way, helped bring this book to fruition:

- My family, who provided me with the necessary space and time to complete this project.
- The team at Jones & Bartlett Learning: David Cella for his confidence in this project and Maro Gartside for her patience, guidance, and support.
- The staff of Human Motion Rehabilitation, Allegheny General Hospital.

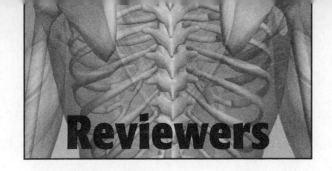

Reviewers

Clarence Chan, PT, DPT
Associate Professor
LaGuardia Community College, City University of New York

Stephanie Russell, PTA, MA
Academic Coordinator of Clinical Education, Instructor
PTA Program
Pennsylvania State University

Kelli Walsingham, PTA, BSSFM
Assistant Coordinator
PTA Program
Gulf Coast Community College

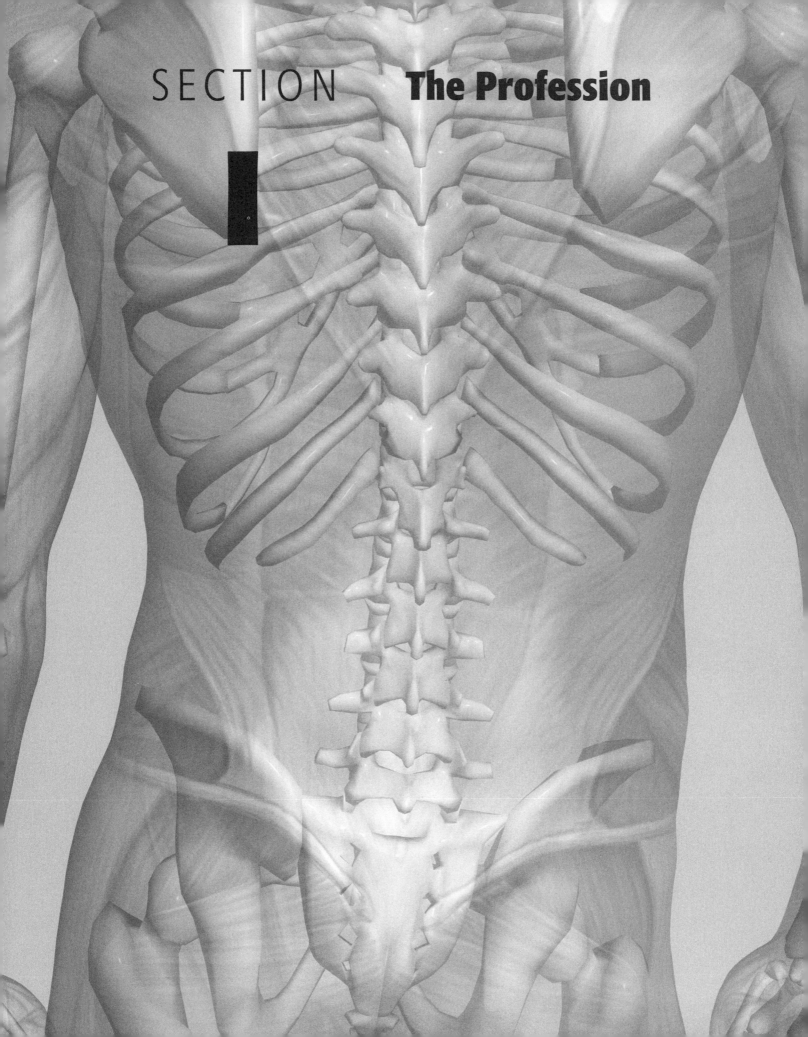

SECTION **The Profession**

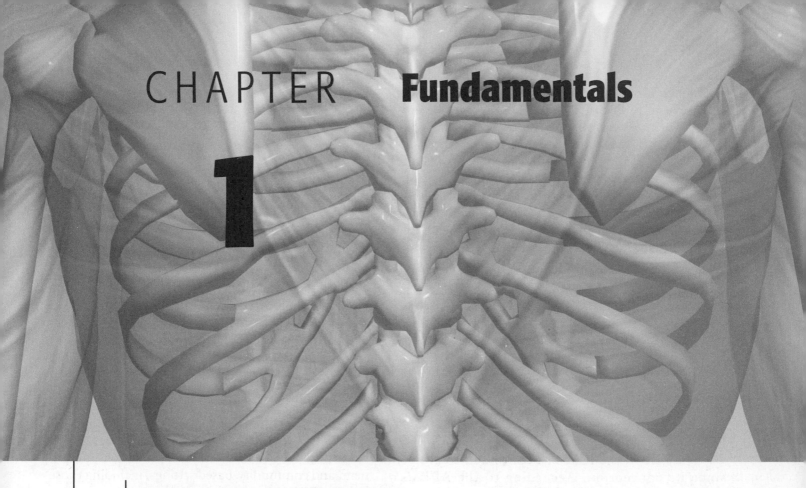

CHAPTER Fundamentals

1

The Guide to Physical Therapist Practice

The Guide to Physical Therapist Practice[1] was developed by the American Physical Therapy Association (APTA) "to encourage a uniform approach to physical therapist practice and to explain to the world the nature of that practice."[1] *The Guide for Conduct of the Physical Therapist Assistant, The Standards of Practice for Physical Therapy,* and *The Standards of Ethical Conduct for the Physical Therapist Assistant* are provided in the appendices.

> **● Key Point** The *Guide*[1] has defined physical therapy as follows: "Physical therapy includes diagnosis and management of movement dysfunction and enhancement of physical and functional abilities; restoration, maintenance, and promotion of optimal physical function, optimal fitness and wellness, and optimal quality of life as it relates to movement and health; and prevention of the onset, symptoms, and progression of impairments, functional limitations, and disabilities that may result from diseases, disorders, conditions, or injuries."

The Guide to Physical Therapist Practice[1] is divided into two parts:

- Part 1 delineates the physical therapist's scope of practice and describes patient management.
- Part 2 describes each of the diagnostic preferred practice patterns of patients typically treated.

Within the *Guide*, physical therapy is defined as the care and services provided by or under the direction and supervision of a physical therapist. *Physical therapists* are the only professionals who provide physical therapy. It is the function of the physical therapist to examine the patient; evaluate the data and identify problems; determine the diagnosis, the prognosis, and the plan of care (POC), and implement the POC (intervention).[2] *Physical therapist assistants* (PTAs), who are under the direction and supervision of the physical therapist (PT), are the only paraprofessionals who assist in the provision of physical therapy interventions. It is the sole responsibility of the physical therapist to determine the most appropriate utilization of the physical therapist assistant that will ensure delivery of service that is safe, effective, and efficient.[1]

● **Key Point** The American Physical Therapy Association (APTA) House of Delegates (HOD) first authorized the training of physical therapist assistants at its 1967 annual conference by adopting *The Policy Statement on Training and Utilization of the Physical Therapist Assistant*. In 1977, the Commission on Accreditation in Education (CAE), the precursor to the Commission on Accreditation in Physical Therapy Education (CAPTE), was established and recognized by the U.S. Department of Education and by the Council on Postsecondary Accreditation. The activities of the CAE included accreditation of programs for the physical therapist assistant.

The role of the PTA has continued to evolve since its conception. According to the APTA's HOD (HOD 06-96-39 and HOD 06-00-16-27), the PTA is specifically defined as "a technically educated health care provider who assists the physical therapist in the provision of physical therapy.... In the contemporary provision of physical therapy services, the physical therapist is considered the professional practitioner of physical therapy, while the physical therapist assistant, educated at the technical level, is considered the paraprofessional. The core function of the PTA is to implement the plan of treatment established by the supervising physical therapist."

The PTA is governed by a number of factors, including:

■ APTA standards.
■ Individual state and federal laws regulating practice acts, including administrative rules for practice. Supervision of the PTA may be spelled out separately from other support personnel, or the PTA may be included in language that defines supervision for all support personnel. When the state laws do not delineate supervision requirements, PTs should rely on the APTA guidelines. State regulations always supersede the APTA guidelines.

■ Specifications of entitlement programs such as Medicare.

● **Key Point** The efficient and effective function of the PTA relies on strong interpersonal communication skills between patient and physical therapist, keen observation, and sound clinical decision-making. Much about becoming an effective clinician relates to an ability to communicate with the patient, the patient's family, and the other members of the healthcare team.

Members of the Healthcare Team

The physical therapist assistant (PTA) is only one vital member of the rehabilitation team and is responsible and accountable to the other members of the team (**Table 1-1**).[3] The responsibility for patient care is shared by the entire rehabilitation team and by the patient.

Practice Settings

PTAs practice in a broad range of inpatient, outpatient, and community-based settings, including those listed in **Table 1-2**.

Models of Disablement

A disablement model is designed to detail the functional consequences and relationships of disease, impairment, and functional limitations of the patient (**Table 1-3**). The PTA's understanding of the process of disablement, and the factors that affect its development, is crucial to achieving the goal of restoring or improving function and reducing disability in the individual. *The Guide to Physical Therapist Practice*[2] employs terminology from the Nagi disablement model,[4] but also describes its framework as being consistent with other disablement models.[5] In 1980 the Executive Board of the World Health Organization published a document for trial purposes, the International Classification of Functioning, Disability and Health (ICFDH-I or ICF) (refer to Table 1-3). In 2001, a revised edition was published (ICFDH-II) that emphasized "components of health" rather than "consequences of disease" (i.e., participation rather than disability) and environmental and personal factors as important determinants of health.[6]

TABLE 1-1	Potential Key Members of the Orthopedic Rehabilitation Team
Personnel	**Description**
Orthopedic surgeon	The orthopedic surgeon performs surgery for conditions involving the musculoskeletal system. Orthopedic surgeons use both surgical and nonsurgical approaches to treat musculoskeletal trauma, sports injuries, degenerative diseases, infections, tumors, and congenital disorders.
Physiatrist	A physiatrist is a physician specializing in physical medicine and rehabilitation who has been certified by the American Board of Physical Medicine and Rehabilitation. The primary role of the physiatrist is to diagnose and treat patients with disabilities involving musculoskeletal, neurological, cardiovascular, or other body systems.
Primary care physician (PCP)	The primary care physician, usually an internist, general practitioner, or family medicine physician, provides primary care services and manages routine healthcare needs. Most PCPs serve as gatekeepers for the managed-care health organizations—provide authorization for referrals to other specialty physicians or services, including physical therapy.
Chiropractor (DC)	A chiropractor is a doctor trained in the science, art, and philosophy of chiropractic. A chiropractic evaluation and treatment is directed at providing a structural analysis of the musculoskeletal and neurologic systems of the body. According to chiropractic doctrine, abnormal function of these two systems may affect function of other systems in the body. In order to practice, chiropractors are usually licensed by a state board.
Physical therapy director	A physical therapy director: • Is typically a physical therapist who has demonstrated qualifications based on education and experience in the field of physical therapy and who has accepted the inherent responsibilities of the role • Establishes guidelines and procedures that will delineate the functions and responsibilities of all levels of physical therapy personnel in the service and the supervisory relationships inherent to the functions of the service and the organization • Ensures that the objectives of the service are efficiently and effectively achieved within the framework of the stated purpose of the organization and in accordance with safe physical therapist practice • Interprets administrative policies • Acts as a liaison between line staff and administration • Fosters the professional growth of the staff
Staff physical therapist (PT)	The staff physical therapist: • Is responsible for the examination, evaluation, diagnosis, prognosis, and intervention of patients • Assists in the supervision of physical therapy personnel in the service All states require physical therapists to obtain a license to practice.
Physical therapist assistant (PTA)	The physical therapist assistant: • Works under the supervision of a physical therapist • Provides care such as teaching patients/clients exercise for mobility, strength, and coordination; training for activities such as walking with crutches, canes, or walkers; and implementing adjunctive interventions • May modify an intervention only in accordance with changes in patient status and within the established plan of care developed by the physical therapist • Typically has an associate's degree from an accredited PTA program and is licensed, certified, or registered in most states
Physical therapist/occupational therapist (PT/OT) aide	The physical therapist/occupational therapist aide: • May be involved in support services directed by PTs and PTAs • Receives on-the-job training and is permitted to function only with continuous on-site supervision by a physical therapist or in some cases a physical therapist assistant • Is limited to performing methods and techniques that do not require clinical decision-making or clinical problem-solving by a physical therapist or a physical therapist assistant

(continued)

TABLE 1-1

Potential Key Members of the Orthopedic Rehabilitation Team (continued)

Personnel	Description
PT and PTA student	The PT or PTA student can perform duties commensurate with his or her level of education. The PT clinical instructor (CI) is responsible for all actions and duties of the affiliating student, and can supervise both physical therapy and physical therapist assistant students (a PTA may only supervise a PTA student—not a PT student).
Volunteer	A volunteer is a member of the community who has an interest in assisting with rehab departmental activities. Responsibilities include taking phone messages, and basic nonclinical/secretarial duties. Volunteers may not provide or setup patient treatment, transfer patients, clean whirlpools, or maintain equipment.
Occupational therapist (OT)	An occupational therapist assesses functioning in activities of everyday living, including dressing, bathing, grooming, meal preparation, writing, and driving, which are essential for independent living. The minimum educational requirements for the registered occupational therapist are described in the current *Essentials and Guidelines of an Accredited Educational Program for the Occupational Therapist* (AOTA, 1991a). All states require an OT to obtain a license to practice.
Certified OT assistant (COTA)	A certified OT assistant: • Works under the direction of an occupational therapist • Performs a variety of rehabilitative activities and exercises as outlined in an established treatment plan The minimum educational requirements for the COTA are described in the current *Essentials and Guidelines of an Accredited Educational Program for the Occupational Therapy Assistant* (AOTA, 1991b)
Certified orthotist (CO)	A certified orthotist designs, fabricates, and fits orthoses (braces, splints, collars, corsets), prescribed by physicians, to patients with disabling conditions of the limbs and spine. A CO must have successfully completed the examination of the American Orthotist and Prosthetic Association.
Certified prosthetist (CP)	A certified prosthetist designs, fabricates, and fits prostheses for patients with partial or total absence of a limb. A CP must have successfully completed the examination of the American Orthotist and Prosthetic Association.
Physician's assistant (PA)	A physician's assistant is a medically trained professional who can provide many of the health care services traditionally performed by a physician, such as taking medical histories and doing physical examinations, making a diagnosis, and prescribing and administering therapies.
Nurse practitioner (NP)	A nurse practitioner is registered nurse with additional specialized graduate-level training who performs physical exams and diagnostic tests, counsels patients, and develops treatment programs.
Athletic trainer (ATC)	A certified athletic trainer is a professional specializing in athletic health care. In cooperation with the physician and other allied health personnel, the athletic trainer functions as an integral member of the athletic health care team in secondary schools, colleges and universities, sports medicine clinics, professional sports programs, and other athletic healthcare settings. Certified athletic trainers have, at minimum, a bachelor's degree, usually in athletic training, health, physical education, or exercise science.

TABLE 1-2   Practice Settings

Setting	Characteristics
Hospital	An institution whose primary function is to provide inpatient diagnostic and therapeutic services for a wide variety of medical, surgical, and nonsurgical conditions. In addition, most hospitals provide some outpatient services, particularly emergency care. Hospitals may be classified in a number of ways, including by: • Length of stay (short-term or long-term) • Teaching or nonteaching • Major types of services: psychiatric, tuberculosis, general, and other specialties, such as maternity, pediatric, or ear, nose, and throat (ENT) • Type of ownership or control: federal, state, or local government; for-profit and nonprofit
Primary care	Basic or entry-level of health care that includes diagnostic, therapeutic, or preventive services. Care is provided on an outpatient basis by primary-care physicians, including family practice physicians, internists, and pediatricians.
Secondary care	Services provided by medical specialists, such as cardiologists, urologists, and dermatologists, who generally do not have first contact with the patients. This level of care may require inpatient hospitalization or ambulatory same-day surgery.
Tertiary care (tertiary health care)	Highly specialized care that is given to patients in a hospital setting who are in danger of disability or death (organ transplants, major surgical procedures). Services provided often require sophisticated technologies (e.g., neurosurgeons or intensive care units). Specialized care is usually provided because of a referral from primary or secondary medical care personnel.
Transitional care unit	Non-medically based facility, which may be in group home or part of a continuum of rehabilitation center. The typical stay is 4 to 8 months. A greater focus placed on compensation versus restoration.
Skilled nursing facility (SNF)	A freestanding facility, or part of a hospital, that is licensed and approved by the state (Medicare certified) where eligible individuals receive skilled nursing care and appropriate rehabilitative and restorative services. Sometimes referred to as an *extended care facility*. An SNF accepts patients in need of rehabilitation and medical care that is of a lesser intensity than that received in the acute care setting of a hospital and provides skilled nursing, rehabilitation, and various other health services on a daily basis. Medicare defines *daily* as seven days a week of skilled nursing care and five days a week of skilled therapy. Physician orders must be rewritten every 60 days.
Acute rehabilitation facility	Usually based in a medical setting. An acute rehabilitation facility provides early rehabilitation, social, and vocational services as soon as the patient is medically stable. Primary emphasis is to provide intensive physical and cognitive restorative services in the early months to disabled persons to facilitate their return to maximum functional capacity. Typical stay is 3 to 4 months (short term).
Chronic care facility	Long-term care facility that is facility- or community-based. Sometimes referred to as *extended rehabilitation*. Designed for patients with permanent or residual disabilities caused by a non-reversible pathological health condition. Chronic care facilities are also used for patients who demonstrate slower than expected progress. Used as a placement facility—stays can be 60 days or longer, but not permanent.
Comprehensive outpatient rehabilitation facility (CORF)	CORFs must provide coordinated outpatient diagnostic, therapeutic, and restorative services, at a single fixed location, to outpatients for the rehabilitation of injured, disabled, or sick individuals. CORFs are surveyed every six years at a minimum.
Custodial care facility	Provides medical or nonmedical services that do not seek to cure, but which are necessary for the patient who is unable to care for him- or herself. Custodial care facilities provide care during periods when the medical condition of the patient is not changing and care for patients who do not require the continued administration of medical care by qualified medical personnel. This type of care is not usually covered under managed-care plans.

(continued)

TABLE
1-2

Practice Settings (continued)

Setting	Characteristics
Hospice care	A facility or program that is licensed, certified, or otherwise authorized by law that provides supportive care for the terminally ill. Hospice care focuses on the physical, spiritual, emotional, psychological, financial, and legal needs of the dying patient and the family. Services provided by an interdisciplinary team of professionals and perhaps volunteers in a variety of settings, including hospitals, freestanding facilities, and at home. Medicare and Medicaid require that at least 80% of hospice care is provided at home. Eligibility for reimbursement includes: • Medicare eligibility • Certification of terminal illness (less than or equal to six months of life) by physician
Personal care	Optional Medicaid benefit that allows a state to provide services to assist functionally impaired individuals in performing the activities of daily living (e.g., bathing, dressing, feeding, grooming).
Ambulatory care (outpatient care)	Includes outpatient preventative, diagnostic, and treatment services that are provided at medical offices, surgery centers, or outpatient clinics (including private practice physical therapy clinics, outpatient satellites of institutions or hospitals). Outpatient care is designed for patients who do not require overnight hospitalization. More cost effective than inpatient care, and therefore favored by managed-care plans.

TABLE
1-3

Disablement Model Comparisons

WHO/The International Classification of Functioning, Disability and Health (ICFDH-I)	NAGI Scheme	WHO/The International Classification of Functioning, Disability and Health (ICFDH-II)
Disease The intrinsic pathology or disorder	*Pathology/Pathophysiology* Interruption or interference with normal processes and efforts of an organism to regain normal state	*Health Condition* Dysfunction of a body function and/or structure
Impairment Loss or abnormality of psychological, physiologic, or anatomic structure or function	*Impairment* Anatomic, physiologic, mental or emotional abnormalities or loss	*Impairment* Problems in body function or structure such as a significant deviation or loss
Disability Restriction or lack of ability to perform an activity in a normal manner	*Functional Limitation* Limitation in performance at the level of the whole organism or person	*Activity Limitation* Limitation in execution of a task or action by an individual
Handicap Disadvantage or disability that limits or prevents fulfillment of a normal role (depends on age, sex, sociocultural factors for the person)	*Disability* Limitation in performance of socially defined roles and tasks within a socio-cultural and physical environment	*Participation Restriction* Prevents fulfillment of involvement in a life situation

Abbreviation: WHO: World Health Organization.

- *Impairment:* Loss or abnormality of anatomic, physiologic, or psychologic structure or function. Not all impairments are modifiable by physical therapy, and not all impairments cause activity limitations and participation restrictions.[1]
- *Primary impairment:* An impairment resulting from active pathology or disease. Primary impairment can create secondary impairments and can lead to secondary pathology. Examples include loss of sensation, loss of strength.
- *Secondary impairment:* An impairment that originates from primary impairment and pathology.[1] Examples include pressure sores, contractures, and cardiovascular deconditioning. When an impairment is the result of multiple underlying causes and arises from a combination of primary or secondary impairments, the term *composite impairment* is sometimes used.[7] For example, a patient who sustained a fracture of the tibial plateau and whose knee was immobilized for several weeks is likely to exhibit a balance impairment of the involved lower extremity after the immobilization has been removed. It is important to be able to recognize functionally relevant impairments, as not all impairments are necessarily linked to functional limitations or disability.
- *Functional limitation:* A restriction of the ability to perform, at the level of the whole person, a physical action, activity, or task in an efficient, typically expected, or competent manner.[1]

> **● Key Point**   An example using the above definitions:

- *Pathology/pathophysiology:* Osteoarthritis of the hip. *Impairment:* Loss of range of motion at the hip; muscle weakness in the lower extremity.
- *Related functional limitation:* Slow, painful gait; inability to ambulate 20 feet in 9 seconds; inability to rise from chair; inability to ascend/descend 10 steps.
- *Disability:* Patient is unable to leave house.

The Five Elements of Patient/Client Management

> **● Key Point**   Note the following definitions:

- *Patient:* Person with diagnosed impairments or functional limitations.
- *Client:* Person who is not necessarily diagnosed with impairments or functional limitations, but seeks services for prevention or promotion of health, wellness, and fitness.

The PTA must be aware of the sequence, organization, and administration of an examination performed by the PT. This awareness increases the PTA's understanding of the rationale for the decision-making and plan of care. The five elements of patient/client management include:[2]

1. Examination of the patient
2. Evaluation of the data and identification of problems
3. Determination of the diagnosis
4. Determination of the prognosis and plan of care (POC)
5. Implementation of the POC (intervention)

Throughout the patient's plan of care, the PTA must communicate changes in the patient status relative to data from the initial examination and make safe and appropriate modifications to the existing program based on consultation with the supervising PT.

Examination

The examination is an ongoing process that begins with the patient referral or initial entry and continues throughout the course of the rehabilitation program. The process of examination includes gathering information from the chart, other caregivers, the patient, the patient's family, caretakers, and friends in order to identify and define the patient's problem(s).[8] The examination consists of three components of equal importance—patient history, systems review, and tests and measures.[2] These components are closely related in that they often occur concurrently. One further element, observation, occurs throughout.

> **● Key Point**   A continual assessment with each treatment session by the PTA allows the PT to evaluate progress and modify interventions as appropriate.[2] It is not unusual for patients to neglect to provide the PT with information pertinent to their condition during the examination, often because they feel it is irrelevant. If such information is provided to the PTA, the PTA must decide whether the information needs to be communicated to the PT.

Patient History

Obtaining the patient history involves the gathering of information from the review of the medical records and interviews with the patient, family members, caregiver, and other interested persons about the patient's history and current functional and health status.[9]

> **● Key Point**   It is estimated that 80% of the information needed to explain the presenting patient problem can be obtained through a thorough history.[10]

Systems Review

The systems review is a brief or limited examination that provides additional information about the general health and the continuum of patient/client care throughout the lifespan.

Tests and Measures

The tests and measures portion of the examination involves the physical examination of the patient and provides the PT with objective data to accurately determine the degree of specific function and dysfunction.[9] A number of recognized tests and measures are commonly performed, but not all are used every time—the physical examination may be modified by the PT based on the patient history and the systems review.

Numerous special tests exist for each area of the body. These tests are performed by the PT only if there is some indication that they would be helpful in confirming or implicating a particular structure or providing information as to the degree of tissue damage.

> **● Key Point** In the joints of the spine, examples of special tests include directional stress tests (posterior–anterior pressures and anterior, posterior, and rotational stressing), joint quadrant testing, vascular tests, and repeated movement testing. Examples of special tests in the peripheral joints include ligament stress tests (i.e., Lachman for the anterior cruciate ligament), articular stress testing (valgus stress applied at the elbow), and rotator cuff impingement tests.

It is important to remember that the interpretation of the findings from the special tests depends on the sensitivity and specificity of the test, the skill and experience of the PT, as well as the PT's degree of familiarity with the tests.

Evaluation

Following the history, systems review, and the tests and measures, the PT makes an evaluation based on an analysis and organization of the collected data and information.[3] An evaluation uses judgment to make sense of the findings in order to identify a relationship between the symptoms reported and the signs of disturbed function.[11] The evaluation process may also identify possible problems that require consultation with, or referral to, another provider.

Diagnosis

Diagnosis, as performed by a PT, refers to a cluster of signs and symptoms, syndromes, or categories. It is used to guide the PT in determining the most appropriate intervention strategy for each patient.[12] A physical therapy diagnosis includes a prioritization of the identified impairments, functional limitations, and disabilities.

Prognosis and Plan of Care

The prognosis, determined by the PT, is the predicted level of optimum function that the patient will attain and an identification of the barriers that may impact the achievement of optimal improvement (age,

medications, socioeconomic status, comorbidities, cognitive status, nutrition, social support, medical prognosis, and environment) within a certain time frame.[3] This prediction helps guide the intensity, duration, frequency, and type of the intervention, in addition to providing justifications for the intervention. Knowledge of the severity of an injury, the age, physical and health status of a patient, and the healing processes of the various tissues involved are among the factors used by the PT in determining the prognosis. The plan of care (POC), which outlines anticipated patient management, involves the setting of goals, coordination of care, progression of care, and discharge (**Table 1-4**). The POC:[12]

- Is based on the examination, evaluation, diagnosis, and prognosis, including the predicted level of optimal improvement
- Includes statements that identify anticipated goals and the expected outcomes
- Describes the specific interventions to be used, and the proposed frequency and duration of the interventions that are required to reach the anticipated goals and expected outcomes
- Includes documentation that is dated and appropriately authenticated by the PT who established the plan of care
- Includes patient and family (as appropriate) goals, and a focus on patient education
- Includes plans for discharge of the patient/client, taking into consideration achievement of anticipated goals and expected outcomes, and provides for appropriate follow-up or referral

> **● Key Point** Communication between clinician and patient begins when the clinician first meets the patient, continues throughout any additional sessions, and involves *interacting with the patient* using terms he or she can understand.

> **● Key Point** From the patient's point of view, there is no substitute for interest, acceptance, and especially empathy on the part of the clinician.[12] Empathy is the capability to share and understand another human being's emotions and feelings.

Intervention

According to the *Guide to Physical Therapist Practice*,[3] an intervention is "the purposeful and skilled interaction of the PT and the patient/client and, when appropriate, with other individuals involved in the patient/client care, using various physical therapy procedures and techniques to produce changes in the condition consistent with the

| TABLE |
| 1-4 |

TABLE 1-4 Essential Data Collection Skills for Carrying Out a Plan of Care

Aerobic Capacity and Endurance
Measures standard vital signs
Recognizes and monitors responses to positional changes and activities
Observes and monitors thoracoabdominal movements and breathing patterns with activity

Anthropometrical Characteristics
Measures height, weight, length, and girth

Arousal, Mentation, and Cognition
Recognizes changes in the direction and magnitude of patient's state of arousal, mentation, and cognition

Assistive, Adaptive, Orthotic, Protective, Supportive, and Prosthetic Devices
Identifies the individual's and caregiver's ability to care for the device
Recognizes changes in skin condition while using devices and equipment
Recognizes safety factors while using the device

Gait, Locomotion, and Balance
Describes the safety, status, and progression of patients while engaged in gait, locomotion, and balance

Integumentary Integrity
Recognizes absent or altered sensation
Recognizes normal and abnormal integumentary changes

Joint Integrity and Mobility
Recognizes normal and abnormal joint movement

Muscle Performance
Measures muscle strength by manual muscle testing
Observes the presence or absence of muscle mass
Recognizes normal and abnormal muscle length
Recognizes changes in muscle tone

Pain
Administers standardized questionnaires, graphs, behavioral scales, or visual analog scales for pain
Recognizes activities, positioning, and postures that aggravate or relieve pain or altered sensations

Posture
Describes resting posture in any position
Recognizes alignment of trunk and extremities at rest and during activities

Range of Motion
Measures functional range of motion
Measures range of motion using a goniometer

Applicable Standards
3.3.2.9.   Adjusts interventions within the plan of care established by the physical therapist in response to patient clinical indications and reports this to the supervising physical therapist.
3.3.2.10. Recognizes when intervention should not be provided due to changes in the patient's status and reports this to the supervising physical therapist.
3.3.2.11. Reports any changes in the patient's status to the supervising physical therapist.
3.3.2.12. Recognizes when the direction to perform an intervention is beyond that which is appropriate for a physical therapist assistant and initiates clarification with the physical therapist.
3.3.2.13. Participates in educating patients and caregivers as directed by the supervising physical therapist.
3.3.2.14. Provides patient-related instruction to patients, family members, and caregivers to achieve patient outcomes based on the plan of care established by the physical therapist.
3.3.2.15. Takes appropriate action in an emergency situation.
3.3.2.16. Completes thorough, accurate, logical, concise, timely, and legible documentation that follows guidelines and specific documentation formats required by state practice acts, the practice setting, and other regulatory agencies.
3.3.2.17. Participates in discharge planning and follow-up as directed by the supervising physical therapist.
3.3.2.18. Reads and understands the healthcare literature.

Data from Accreditation Handbook PTA Criteria Appendix A-32.

diagnosis and prognosis." The purpose of a rehabilitative intervention is to improve the tolerance of a healing tissue to tension and stress, and to ensure that the tissue has the capacity to tolerate the various stresses that will be placed on it. As an example, with contractile tissues, such as the muscles, this can be accomplished through measured rest, rehabilitative exercise, high-voltage electrical stimulation, central (cardiovascular) aerobics, general conditioning, and absence from overuse.[13]

> **● Key Point** Three components make up the physical therapy intervention:[3]
>
> 1. Coordination, communication, and documentation. Many interventions involve other healthcare disciplines:
>   - *Multidisciplinary approach:* Each discipline involved retains its methodologies and assumptions without change or development from other disciplines within the multidisciplinary relationship. An example would be a team meeting that includes the physician, case manager, PT, occupational therapist (OT), and nurse to discuss a patient's care and progress.
>   - *Interdisciplinary approach:* This approach blends the practices and assumptions of each discipline involved. An example would be a patient being co-treated in physical and occupational therapy.
>   - *Transdisciplinary approach:* This approach crosses many disciplinary boundaries to create a holistic approach. Under this approach, the role differentiation between disciplines is defined by the needs of the situation rather than by discipline-specific characteristics. An example would be addressing the variety of needs in a patient with cerebral palsy (CP).
> 2. Patient/client-related instruction.
> 3. Direct interventions (e.g., manual therapy techniques, therapeutic exercise). Procedural interventions can be broadly classified into three main groups:[7,9]
>   - *Restorative interventions:* These interventions are directed toward remediating or improving the patient's status in terms of impairments, functional limitations, and recovery of function.
>   - *Compensatory interventions:* These interventions are directed toward promoting optimal function using residual abilities.
>   - *Preventative interventions:* These interventions are directed toward minimizing potential impairments, functional limitations, and disabilities and maintaining health.

The inert structures, such as ligaments and menisci, rely more on the level of tension and force placed on them for their recovery, which stimulates the fibroblasts to produce fiber and glycosaminoglycans.[14] Thus, the intervention chosen for these structures must involve the repetitive application of modified tension in the line of stress based on the stress of daily activities, or sporting activity.[14]

> **● Key Point** The most successful intervention programs are those that are custom designed from a blend of clinical experience and scientific data. The level of improvement achieved is related to accurate goal setting and the attainment of those goals.

The therapeutic strategy is determined solely from the responses obtained from tissue loading and the effect that loading has on symptoms. Once these responses have been determined, the focus of the intervention is to provide sound and effective self-management strategies for patients that avoid harmful tissue loading.[15]

Interventions are typically aimed at addressing short- and long-term goals, both of which are dynamic in nature, being altered as the patient's condition changes, by designing strategies with which to achieve those goals. Intervention strategies can be subdivided into active (direct) or passive (indirect), with the goal being to make the intervention as active as possible at the earliest opportunity.

Cultural Influences

It is important that clinicians are sensitive to cultural issues in their interactions with patients. Cultural influences shape the framework within which people view the world, define and organize reality, and function in their everyday life. In many cases individuals group themselves on the basis of cultural similarities, and, as a result, form cultural groups.

> **● Key Point** Ethnocentrism is the tendency to believe that one's ethnic or cultural group is centrally important, and that all other groups are measured in relation to one's own. The ethnocentric individual will judge other groups relative to his or her own particular ethnic group or culture, especially with concern to language, behavior, customs, and religion. An example would be a patient believing he or she would receive a better level of care from a clinician of the same race and religion.

Cultural groups share behavioral patterns, symbols, values, beliefs, and other characteristics that distinguish them from other groups. At the group level, cultural differences are generally variations of differing emphasis or value placed on particular practices. Whenever possible, the PTA should use any available resource, such as an interpreter.

Patient Education

Patient education is an important component of the plan of care. According to the *Accreditation Handbook*, PTA Criteria, Appendix A-3, the PTA:

> 3.3.2.19. *Under the direction and supervision of the physical therapist, instructs other members of the health care team using established*

techniques, programs, and instructional materials commensurate with the learning characteristics of the audience.

3.3.2.20. Educates others about the role of the physical therapist assistant.

Motivation

PTAs should keep in mind that for patients, motivation plays a critical role; success is more motivating than is failure. Basic principles of motivation are applicable to learning in any situation:

- The environment can be used to focus the patient's attention on what needs to be learned.
- Interesting visual aids, such as booklets, posters, or practice equipment, motivate learners by capturing their attention and curiosity.
- Incentives, including privileges and receiving praise from the educator, motivate learning. Both affiliation and approval are strong motivators.
- Internal motivation is longer lasting and more self-directive than is external motivation, which must be repeatedly reinforced by praise or concrete rewards. However, some individuals have little capacity for internal motivation and must be guided and reinforced constantly.
- Learning is most effective when an individual is ready to learn—that is, when one wants to know something.

Maslow's Hierarchy of Needs

Another helpful framework to consider in relation to patient education is Abraham Maslow's hierarchy of needs. This concept is based on a hierarchy of biogenic and psychogenic needs that humans must progress through. Maslow hypothesizes that the higher needs in this hierarchy come into focus only when all the needs that are lower down in the pyramid are mainly or entirely satisfied. Maslow's hierarchy is often depicted as a pyramid consisting of five levels (Figure 1-1). The lower levels (physiological and safety needs) are referred to as *deficiency needs*, and the top three levels (love/belonging, status, and self-actualization needs) are referred to as *being needs*. According to Maslow, in order for an individual to progress up the hierarchy to the being needs, his or her deficiency needs must be met. Growth forces create upward movement in the hierarchy, whereas regressive forces push predominant needs further down the hierarchy.

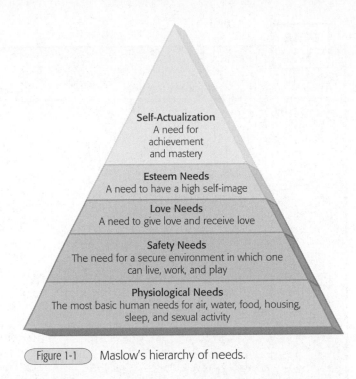

Self-Actualization
A need for achievement and mastery

Esteem Needs
A need to have a high self-image

Love Needs
A need to give love and receive love

Safety Needs
The need for a secure environment in which one can live, work, and play

Physiological Needs
The most basic human needs for air, water, food, housing, sleep, and sexual activity

Figure 1-1   Maslow's hierarchy of needs.

● **Key Point**   Various studies have found that compliance with physical therapy programs is approximately 40%.[16] Compliance can be improved by:[17–19]

- Involving the patient in the intervention planning and goal setting
- Setting realistic goals for both the short and the long term
- Promoting high expectations regarding final outcome
- Promoting perceived benefits
- Projecting a positive attitude
- Providing clear instructions and demonstrations with appropriate feedback
- Keeping the exercises pain-free or with a low level of pain
- Encouraging patient problem solving

Theories of Learning

A vast array of learning theories have been developed over the years. **Table 1-5** outlines some of the more common theories of learning.

Domains of Learning

Bloom[20] identified three domains of learning:

- *Cognitive:* Primarily concerned with knowledge and the development of intellectual skills, including the recall or recognition of specific facts, procedural patterns, and concepts that serve in the development of intellectual abilities and skills. There are six major categories (knowledge, comprehension, application, analysis, synthesis, and evaluation) starting from the simplest behavior and moving to the most complex. The simplest

TABLE 1-5   Learning Theories

Theory	Principal Elements	Strategies
Androgeny (Adult Learning)	Adults need to know why they need to learn something. Adults need to learn experientially. Adults approach learning as problem-solving. Adults learn best when the topic is of immediate value.	There is a need to explain why specific things are being taught (e.g., certain commands, functions, operations). Instruction should be task-oriented instead of memorization—learning activities should be in the context of common tasks to be performed. Instruction should take into account the wide range of different backgrounds of learners; learning materials and activities should allow for different levels/types of previous experience with computers. Since adults are self-directed, instruction should allow learners to discover things for themselves, providing guidance and help when mistakes are made.
Behaviorist (Stimulus–Response Theory)—Operant Conditioning	Learning is a function of a change in overt behavior. Changes in behavior are the result of an individual's response to events (stimuli) and their consequences that occur in the environment. The response of one behavior becomes the stimulus for the next response. Learning occurs when an individual engages in specific behaviors in order to receive certain consequences (learned association). Behavior can be controlled or shaped by operant conditioning.	Desired or correct behaviors are identified so that frequent and scheduled reinforcements (positive reinforcement) can be given to reinforce the desired behaviors. Negative behaviors are ignored (negative reinforcement) so that these behaviors become weakened to the point where they disappear (extinction). Negative consequences are administered to individuals who perform undesirable behaviors (punishment). Reinforcement frequency and schedules: • *Continuous reinforcement:* A behavior is reinforced every time it occurs. • *Partial reinforcement:* A behavior is reinforced intermittently. • *Fixed interval:* The period of time between the occurrences of each instance of reinforcement is fixed or set. • *Variable interval:* The period of time between the occurrences of each instance of reinforcement varies around a constant average.
Experiential Learning	Two types of learning: 1. *Cognitive (meaningless):* academic knowledge such as learning vocabulary or multiplication tables. 2. *Experiential (significant):* applied knowledge such as personal change and growth.	Significant learning takes place when the subject matter is relevant to the personal interests of the student. Learning that is threatening to the self (e.g., new attitudes or perspectives) are more easily assimilated when external threats are at a minimum. Learning proceeds faster when the threat to the self is low. Self-initiated learning is the most lasting and pervasive.

ones must be mastered first before progressing to the more complicated ones.

- *Affective:* Primarily concerned with emotions, values, and attitudes, including feelings, values, appreciation, enthusiasms, and motivations. There are five specific levels (receiving, responding, valuing, organization, and characterization).
- *Psychomotor:* Primarily concerned with physical action and motor skills, including coordination. The seven major categories of this domain include perception, set, guided response, mechanism, complex overt response, affectation, and origination.

Types of Learners

Litzinger and Osif[21] organized individuals into four main types of learners, based on instructional strategies:

- *Accommodators:* Look for the significance of the learning experience. These learners enjoy being active participants in their learning and will ask many questions, such as, "What if?" and "Why not?"
- *Divergers:* Motivated to discover the relevancy of a given situation and prefer to have information presented in a detailed, systematic, and reasoned manner.

- *Assimilators:* Motivated to answer the question, "What is there to know?" These learners like accurate, organized delivery of information, and they tend to respect the knowledge of the expert. They are perhaps less instructor-intensive than some other types of learners and will carefully follow prescribed exercises, provided a resource person is clearly available and able to answer questions.
- *Convergers:* Motivated to discover the relevancy, or "how," of a situation. The instructions given to this type of learner should be interactive, not passive.

Other learning styles include:

- *Visual:* Assimilate information by observation, using visual cues and information such as pictures, anatomic models, and physical demonstrations.
- *Auditory:* Prefer to learn by having things explained to them verbally.
- *Tactile:* Learn through touch and interaction; is the most difficult of the three groups to teach. Close supervision is required with this group until they have demonstrated to the clinician that they can perform the exercises correctly, and independently. Proprioceptive neuromuscular facilitation (PNF) techniques, with the emphasis on physical and tactile cues, often work well with this group.

Practice and Feedback

Behavioral psychology emphasizes practice variables in sensory-motor skills such as massed (concentrated—concentrating the learning or practice in a short period of time) versus spaced (distributed—spreading out the learning or practice over a longer period of time) practice, part versus whole task learning (learning parts of a skill versus the whole skill), and feedback/reinforcement schedules.

Long-term retention of motor skills depends upon regular practice. Learning and retention of sensory-motor skills is improved by both the quantity and quality of feedback (knowledge of results) during training. Two ways in which learning/teaching of motor skills can be facilitated include:

1. Slowing down the rate at which the information is presented
2. Reducing the amount of information that needs to processed

Some form of guided learning seems most appropriate when high proficiency on a new skill is involved. In contrast, if the task is to be recalled and transferred to a new situation, then some type of problem-solving strategy may be better. Guided learning may be most effective in early training, while learning through trial and error is important in advanced training.

There is evidence that mental rehearsal, especially involving imagery, facilitates performance. This may be because it allows additional memory processing related to physical tasks (e.g., the formation of schema) or because it maintains arousal or motivation for an activity. Many forms of sensory-motor behavior are learned by imitation, especially complex movements such as dance, crafts, or manual therapy techniques.

Education

The strengths and weaknesses of various presentation methods are outlined in **Table 1-6**. A number of guidelines when using visual aids are outlined in **Table 1-7**.

Specific Approaches for Education

The various patient types encountered by the PTA respond differently to teaching methods:

- *Infants/children:* Sessions need to be short and interactive, and they should include structured play and frequent breaks.
- *Adolescents:* It is important to establish whether the adolescent patient is comfortable in the presence of a parent/guardian during therapy sessions.
- *Adults:* Adults need to learn experientially. They generally approach learning as problem-solving, and they learn best when the topic is of immediate value.
- *Elderly:* Special attention is required to identify any signs of visual or hearing loss. Group sessions are often more beneficial than one-on-one sessions.

Documentation

Documentation of the assessment and intervention processes is an important part of any therapeutic regimen. Documentation in health care includes any entry made in the patient/client record. As a record of client care, documentation provides useful information for the clinician, other members of the healthcare team, and third-party payers. The APTA is committed to developing and improving

TABLE 1-6 Teaching Methods

Teaching Method	Strengths	Weaknesses	Preparation
Lecture	Presents factual material in direct, logical manner Contains experience that inspires Useful for large groups	Experts are not always good teachers Audience is passive Learning is difficult to gauge Communication is one way	Needs clear introduction and summary Needs time and content limit to be effective Should include examples, anecdotes
Videotapes/slides	Entertaining way of teaching content (colorful) and raising issues Keeps group's attention Looks professional Stimulates discussion Demonstrates three-dimensional movement	Can raise too many issues to have a focused discussion Discussion may not have full participation Only as effective as following discussion Can be expensive	Need to set up equipment Effective only if facilitator prepares questions to discuss after the show
Discussion	Pools ideas and experiences from group Effective after a presentation, film, or experience that needs to be analyzed Allows everyone to participate in an active process	Not practical with more that 20 people Few people can dominate Others may not participate Time consuming Can get off the track	Requires careful planning by facilitator to guide discussion Requires question outline

Data from Dutton M: McGraw-Hill's National Physical Therapy Examination (ed 1). New York, McGraw-Hill, 2009

TABLE 1-7 Guidelines for the Use of Visual Aids

Flip Charts	Slides
Choose a chart size that is appropriate for the design, your height, and the size of the audience.	Slides should be used instead of flip charts if the group is large.
Draw the art to fit the vertical shape of the chart.	Design the visuals for continuous viewing and as notes.
Make the lettering dark enough and large enough to be read by everyone in the audience.	Maintain continuity—have all slides horizontal or vertical, not mixed.
During preparation, leave several blank pages between each one to allow for corrections and additions. For the final presentation, remove all but one blank page at the beginning so that you can turn to that blank page when there is no relevant visual.	Allow sufficient production time. Place no more than 15 words per slide. Use black or blue background with bright colors. Check the position and order of the slide in the carousel tray or PowerPoint.
Securely attach the chart to the easel and adjust the easel height for the presentation.	Use a conventional pointer.
When writing on the flip chart, don't speak to the chart.	Keep as many lights on as possible.

Data from Dutton M: McGraw-Hill's National Physical Therapy Examination (ed 1). New York, McGraw-Hill, 2009

the art and science of physical therapy, including practice, education, and research. To help meet these responsibilities, the APTA Board of Directors has approved a number of guidelines for physical therapy documentation. These guidelines are intended as a foundation for the development of more specific guidelines in specialty areas, while at the same time providing guidance across all practice settings. In all instances, it is the position of the APTA that the physical therapy examination, evaluation, diagnosis, prognosis, and intervention shall be documented, dated, and authenticated by the PT or PTA as appropriate. The APTA's Documentation Guidelines are as follows:

- The documentation must be consistent with the APTA's Standards of Practice.
- All documentation must be legible and use medically approved abbreviations or symbols.
- All documentation must be written in black or blue ink, and the mistakes must be crossed out with a single line through the error, initialed, and dated by the PTA.
- Each intervention session must be documented. The patient's name and identification number must be on each page of the documentation record.
- Informed consent for the interventions must be signed by a competent adult. If the adult is not competent, the consent must be signed by the patient/client's legal guardian. If the patient is a minor, the consent must be signed by the parent or an appointed guardian.
- Each document must be dated and signed by the PT/PTA using the first and the last name and the professional designation; professional license number may be included but can be optional.
- All communications with other healthcare providers or healthcare professionals must be recorded.
- The PTA student's notes should be cosigned by the PTA (clinical instructor) or by the PT (clinical instructor).
- Nonlicensed personnel notes should be cosigned by the PT.

● Key Point Medical records must be properly stored and be accessed only by the appropriate staff. If the patient is present and has the capacity to make healthcare decisions, a healthcare provider may discuss the patient's health information with a family member, friend, or other person if the patient agrees or, when given the opportunity, does not object. However, a healthcare provider may not discuss a patient's condition with a patient's family member if the patient has stated he or she does not want the family to know about his or her condition.

The SOAP (Subjective, Objective, Assessment, Plan) note format has traditionally been used to document the examination and intervention process.

- *Subjective:* Information about the condition from patient or family member.
- *Objective:* Measurement a clinician obtains during the physical examination.

- *Assessment:* Analysis of problem, including the long- and short-term goals.
- *Plan:* A specific intervention plan for the identified problem.

More recently, the Patient/Client Management format is being used by clinicians familiar with the *Guide to Physical Therapist Practice.*[8] The Patient/Client Management model described in the *Guide to Physical Therapist Practice* has the following components:

- *History:* Information gathered about the patient's history.
- *Systems review:* Information gathered from performing a brief examination or screening of the patient's major systems addressed by physical therapy; also includes information gathered about the patient's communication, affect, cognition, learning style, and education needs.
- *Tests and measures:* Results from specific tests and measures performed by the PT.
- *Diagnosis:* Includes a discussion of the relationship of the patient's functional deficits to the patient's impairments and/or disability as determined by the PT, as well as a discussion of other healthcare professionals to which the PT has referred the patient or believes the patient should be referred.
- *Prognosis:* Includes the predicted level of improvement that the patient will be able to achieve according to the PT and the predicted amount of time to achieve that level of improvement. The prognosis should also include the PT's professional opinion of the patient's rehabilitation potential.
- *Plan of care:* Includes the Expected Outcomes (Long-Term Goals), Anticipated Goals (Short-Term Goals), and Interventions, including an Education Plan for the patient or the patient's care givers or significant others.

The purposes of documentation are as follows:[8]

- To document what the clinician does to manage the individual patient's case.
- To record examination findings, patient status, intervention provided, and the patient's response to treatment.
- To communicate with all other members of the healthcare team; this helps provide consistency among the services provided and includes communication between the PT and the PTA.

- To provide information to third-party payers, such as Medicare and other insurance companies who make decisions about reimbursement based on the quality and completeness of the physical therapy note.
- To be used for quality assurance and improvement purposes and for issues such as discharge planning.
- To serve as a source of data for quality assurance, peer and utilization review, and research.

> **• Key Point** The physical therapy documentation is considered a legal document, and it becomes a part of the patient's medical record.

The PTA reads the initial documentation of the examination, evaluation, diagnosis, prognosis, anticipated outcomes and goals, and intervention plan, and is expected to follow the POC as outlined by the PT in the initial patient note.[8] After the patient has been seen by the PTA for a period of time (the time varies according to the policies of each facility or healthcare system and state law), the PTA must write a progress note documenting any changes in the patient's status that have occurred since the PT's initial note was written.[8] Also, after a discussion about the diagnosis and prognosis with the PT, expected outcomes, anticipated goals, and interventions, the PTA rewrites or responds to the previously written expected outcomes and documents the revised POC accordingly.[8] In many facilities (according to the policies of each facility or healthcare system and state law), the PT then cosigns the PTA's notes, indicating agreement with what is documented.[8]

> **• Key Point** Students in PT or PTA programs may document when the record is additionally authenticated by the PT or, when permissible by law, documentation by a PTA student may be authenticated by a PTA.

Infection Control

Infection is a process in which an organism establishes a parasitic relationship with its host.[22] This invasion and multiplication of microorganisms produces an immune response and subsequent signs and symptoms.

Common signs and symptoms of infectious disease include:

- Fever, chills, and malaise
- Nausea, vomiting
- Headache
- Confusion
- Tachycardia
- Joint effusion andmyalgia
- Cough and sore throat

> **• Key Point** A great variety of micro-organisms are responsible for infectious diseases, including fungi (yeast and molds), helminths (e.g., tapeworms), mycobacteria, viruses, mycoplasmas, bacteria, rickettsiae, chlamydiae, protozoa, and prions.

Nosocomial (those that originate or occur in a hospital or hospital-like setting) infections can be caused by infections from the:

- Central nervous system
- Surgical site
- Urinary tract
- Respiratory tract
- Bloodstream
- Intestinal tract

Clinicians can help prevent transmission of nosocomial infections from themselves to others, from client to client, and from client to self by following procedures, standard precautions, and proper hand-washing techniques (**Table 1-8**), infection control, and isolation procedures (**Table 1-9** and **Table 1-10**).

> **• Key Point** Do not confuse infection and inflammation. *Infection* is the harmful colonization of a host by an infecting organism. *Inflammation* is the complex biological response of vascular tissues to harmful stimuli while initiating the healing process for the tissue.

Various terms are used to describe asepsis techniques:

- *Sterilization:* Destroys all viable microorganisms
- *Disinfection:* Reduces microorganisms
- *Antisepsis:* Inhibits or destroys microorganisms

> **• Key Point** Methods of antisepsis include the use of:
> - Antiseptic solutions, such as alcohol and iodine
> - Germicidal soaps
> - Mercurial
> - Quaternary ammonia
> - Antibacterial additives

The more common infectious diseases are outlined in **Table 1-11**.

TABLE 1-8   Standard Precautions

Hand Washing

1. Wash hands after touching blood, body fluids, secretions, excretions, and contaminated items, whether or not gloves are worn.
2. Wash hands immediately after removing gloves, between patient contacts, and when otherwise indicated to reduce transmission of microorganisms.
3. Wash hands between tasks and procedures on the same patient to prevent cross-contamination of different body sites.
4. Use plain (nonantimicrobial) for routine hand washing.
5. An antimicrobial agent or a waterless antiseptic agent may be used for specific circumstances (hyperendemic infections) as defined by infection control.

**Hand washing should be performed using water after removing all jewelry. The hands should be washed with soap for at least 30 seconds while avoiding touching any contaminated surface. Rinse thoroughly, using a paper towel barrier when turning off the water.

Gloves

1. Wear gloves (clean, unsterile gloves are adequate) when touching blood, body fluids, secretions, excretions, and contaminated items; put on clean gloves just before touching mucous membranes and nonintact skin.
2. Change gloves between tasks and procedures on the same patient after contact with materials that may contain high concentrations of microorganisms.
3. Remove gloves promptly after use, before touching uncontaminated items and environmental surfaces, and before going on to another patient; wash hands immediately after glove removal to avoid transfer of microorganisms to other patients or environments.

Mask and Eye Protection or Face Shield

1. Wear mask and eye protection or a stay shield to protect mucous membranes of the eyes and nose during procedures and patient care activities that are likely to generate splashes or sprays of blood, body fluids, secretions, and excretions.

Gown

1. Wear a gown (a clean, unsterile gown is adequate) to protect skin and prevent soiling of clothing during procedures and patient care activities that are likely to generate splashes or sprays of blood, body fluids, secretions, and excretions.
2. Select a gown that is appropriate for the activity and the amount of fluid likely to be encountered.
3. Remove a soiled gown as soon as possible and wash hands to avoid transfer of microorganisms to other patients or environments.

Patient Care Equipment

1. Handle used patient care equipment soiled with blood, body fluids, secretions, and excretion in a manner that prevents skin and mucous membrane exposures, contamination of clothing, and transfer of microorganisms to other patients or environments.
2. Ensure that reusable equipment is not used for the care of another patient until it has been cleaned and reprocessed appropriately.
3. Ensure that single use items are discarded properly.

Environmental Control

1. Follow hospital procedures for the routine care, cleaning, and disinfection of environmental surfaces, beds, bed rails, bedside equipment, and other frequently touched surfaces.

Linen

1. Handle, transport, and process used linen soiled with blood, body fluids, secretions, and excretion in a manner that prevents skin and mucous membrane exposures and contamination of clothing, and avoids transfer of microorganisms to other patients or environments.

Occupational Health and Blood-Borne Pathogens

1. Prevent injuries when using needles, scalpels, and other sharp instruments or devices; when handling sharp instruments and procedures; when cleaning used instruments; and when disposing of used needles.
2. Never recap used needles, or otherwise manipulate them using both hands, or use any other technique that involves directing the point of the needle toward any part of the body; rather, use either a one-handed "scoop" technique or mechanical device designed for holding the needle sheath.
3. Do not remove used needles from disposable syringes by hand, and do not bend, break, or otherwise manipulate used needles by hand.
4. Place used disposable syringes and needles, scalpel blades, or other sharp items in appropriate puncture-resistant container for transport to the reprocessing area.
5. Use mouthpieces, resuscitation bags, or other ventilation devices as an alternative to mouth-to-mouth resuscitation.

Patient Placement

1. Use a private room for a patient who may contaminate the environment or who does not (or cannot be expected to) assist in maintaining appropriate hygiene or environmental control.
2. Consult Infection Control if private room is not available.

Data from Centers for Disease Control and Prevention, Hospital Infection Control Practices Advisory Committee. Part II: Recommendations for Isolation Precautions in Hospitals, February 1997

<table>

TABLE 1-9	Airborne, Droplet, and Contact Precautions

Airborne Precautions

In addition to Standard Precautions, use Airborne Precautions, or the equivalent, with all patients known or suspected to be infected with serious illness transmitted by airborne droplet nuclei (small-particle residue) that remain suspended in the air and that can be dispersed widely by air currents within a room or over a long distance (for example, Mycobacterium tuberculosis, measles virus, chickenpox virus).

1. Use a respiratory isolation room.
2. Wear respiratory protection (mask) when entering room.
3. Limit movement and transport of patient to essential purposes only. Mask patient when transporting out of area.

**Personal protective equipment (PPE) includes items (e.g., gowns, masks, gloves, mouthpieces) that are used as barriers to protect against a patient with a potentially infectious disease.

Droplet Precautions

In addition to Standard Precautions, use Droplet Precautions, or the equivalent, for patients known or suspected to be infected with serious illness microorganisms (e.g., mumps, rubella, pertussis, influenza) transmitted by large-particle droplets that can be generated by the patient during coughing, sneezing, talking, or the performance of procedures.

1. Use isolation room.
2. Wear respiratory protection (mask) when entering room.
3. Limit movement and transport of patient to essential purposes only. Mask patient when transporting out of area.

Contact Precautions

In addition to Standard Precautions, use Contact Precautions, or the equivalent, for specified patients known or suspected to be infected or colonized with serious illness transmitted by direct patient contact (and or skin to skin contact) or contact with items in patient environment.

1. Use isolation room.
2. Wear gloves when entering room; change gloves after having contact with infective material; remove gloves before leaving patient's room; wash hands immediately with an antimicrobial agent or waterless antiseptic agent. After glove removal and hand washing, ensure that hands do not touch contaminated environmental items.
3. Wear a gown when entering room if you anticipate your clothing will have substantial contact with the patient, environmental surfaces, or items in the patient's room, or if the patient is incontinent or has diarrhea, ileostomy, colostomy, or wound drainage not contained by dressing. Remove gown before leaving patient's room; after gown removal, ensure that clothing does not contact potentially contaminated environmental surfaces.
4. Use single-patient-use equipment.
5. Limit movement and transport of patient for essential purposes only. Use precautions when transporting patient to minimize risk of transmission of microorganisms to other patients and contamination of environmental surfaces or equipment.

Data from Guidelines for isolation precautions in hospitals. Part II. Recommendations for isolation precautions in hospitals. Hospital Infection Control Practices Advisory Committee. Am J Infect Control 24:32–52, 1996

<table>

TABLE 1-10	Creating and Maintaining a Sterile Field

Creating Generally, creating a sterile field involves a sequence of procedures:

1. *Gowning* (putting on sterile, surgical gown). The gown is held firmly away from the sterile field and then shaken so that it unfolds while keeping the hands above waist level. Only the inside of the gown should be touched as both arms are placed into the sleeves up to the sleeve cuffs. The gown is then tied in the back.
2. *Gloving* (putting on sterile, surgical gloves). Using the gown sleeve cuffs as mittens, the glove package is opened. Still using the sleeve cuff as a mitten, the right glove is grasped with the left hand and pulled on over the open end of the gown sleeve. Then, the first three fingers of the right hand reach under the fold of the left glove (touching the sterile portion of the left glove) and hold the glove while the left hand is positioned inside the glove. Once both gloves are donned, the left glove is used to unfold the right glove's cuff.
3. *Applying cap and mask.* Contact with the hair should be avoided while applying the cap, and all hair should be contained within the cap. The mask is applied by first positioning it over the bridge of the nose and securing it using the upper ties behind the head and the lower ties behind the neck.

**A properly gloved and gowned provider's sterile area extends from the chest to the level of the sterile field. Sleeves are sterile from 5 centimeters above the elbow to the cuff.

**Areas below the level of the draped client are considered nonsterile.

TABLE 1-10 Creating and Maintaining a Sterile Field (continued)

Maintaining	Place only sterile items within the sterile field (only the top surface of the table or sterile drape is considered sterile; the outer 1 inch of the field is considered nonsterile).
	Open, dispense, and transfer items without contaminating them (the edges of all packaging of sterile items become nonsterile once the package is opened).
	Do not allow unsterile personnel to reach across the sterile field or to touch sterile items.
	Avoid talking, coughing, or sneezing.
	A sterile barrier that has been wet, cut, or torn, should be considered contaminated.
	Do not place sterile items near open windows or doors.
	The sterile field should never be left unattended.
	When in doubt about whether something is sterile, consider it contaminated.

TABLE 1-11 Common Infectious Diseases

Disease	Description	Mode of Transmission	Prevention
Tuberculosis	A highly contagious bacterial infection caused by *Mycobacterium tuberculosis (M. tuberculosis)*. The lungs are primarily involved, but the infection can spread to other organs.	Tuberculosis can develop after inhaling droplets sprayed into the air from a cough or sneeze by someone infected with *M. tuberculosis.*	Isolation of infected individuals until cleared from the contagious stage. Despite improved methods of detection and management, tuberculosis remains a worldwide health problem.
Hepatitis	An inflammation of the liver. Several different viruses cause viral hepatitis. They are named the hepatitis A, B, C, D, and E viruses. Some cases of viral hepatitis cannot be attributed to the hepatitis A, B, C, D, or E viruses. These types are called non-A–E hepatitis.	Hepatitis A is transmitted through fecal–oral transmission, contaminated food or water, and infected food handlers. Hepatitis B and C is transmitted through contact with infected body fluids or tissues via oral or sexual contact, blood and blood products exposure, maternal–fetal transmission, and contaminated needles. Hepatitis D spreads through contact with infected blood. This disease occurs only in people who are already infected with hepatitis B. Hepatitis E spreads through contaminated food or water (by feces from an infected person), but it is uncommon in the United States.	Hepatitis A (HAV) can be prevented with good hygiene, washing after using the toilet, sanitation, and immunization. Hepatitis B (HBV) and C (HCV) can be prevented through vaccine, education, lifestyle changes, and healthy habits. There is no cure for HBV.
Acquired immunodeficiency syndrome (AIDS)	The HIV retrovirus chiefly infects human T4 (helper) lymphocytes, the major regulators of the immune response, and destroys or inactivates them. AIDS can result in an increase in opportunistic infections, neurologic dysfunction, and unusual cancers.	The HIV retrovirus is transmitted by body fluids exchange (in particular blood and semen), which is associated with high-risk behaviors (e.g., unprotected sexual contact, needle sharing).	Prevention involves avoidance from high-risk behaviors. AIDS is now considered a chronic rather than a terminal illness.

(continued)

TABLE 1-11	Common Infectious Diseases (continued)		
Disease	Description	Mode of Transmission	Prevention
Influenza	One of the most contagious airborne communicable diseases. Results from contamination with 1 of 3 key types of virus, A, B, or C.	Transmitted person-to-person by direct deposition of virus-laden large droplets onto the mucosa of the upper respiratory tract of an immunologically liable person.	All healthcare workers must follow the guidelines for isolation precautions both for themselves and their patients. This is especially important for the clinician treating aged, immunocompromised, or, chronically ill individuals.

● **Key Point** It is very important for the PTA to be able to recognize the signs and symptoms of infection so that the PT and the patient's physician can be notified immediately. An infection may cause redness, warmth, and inflammation around the affected area, and the area may become stiff, drain pus, and begin to lose range of motion.

Patient Safety

It is extremely important for the PTA to detect malfunctions of the various systems, often referred to as *red flags*, through observation and subjective complaints. Any of the following should cause immediate concern for the PTA, who must consult with the supervising PT or medical personnel:[23]

- *Fatigue:* Complaints of feeling tired or run down are extremely common and therefore are significant only if the patient reports that tiredness interferes with the ability to carry out typical daily activities and when the fatigue has lasted for 2 to 4 weeks or longer. Many serious illnesses can cause fatigue.
- *Malaise:* Malaise is a sense of uneasiness or general discomfort that is often associated with conditions that generate fever.
- *Fever/chills/sweats:* These are signs and symptoms that are most often associated with systemic illnesses such as cancer, infections, and connective tissue disorders such as rheumatoid arthritis. To qualify as a red flag, the fever should have some longevity (2 weeks or longer).
- *Unexpected weight change:* A change in weight is a sensitive but nonspecific finding that can be a normal physiologic response, but it may also be associated with depression, cancer, or gastrointestinal disease.
- *Nausea/vomiting:* Persistent vomiting is not usually reported to a PT; patients generally tell their physician. However, the PTA should be aware that a low-grade nausea can be caused by systemic illness or an adverse drug reaction.
- *Dizziness/lightheadedness:* Dizziness (vertigo) is a nonspecific neurologic symptom that requires a careful diagnostic workup. A report of vertigo, although potentially problematic, is not a contraindication to the continuation of the examination. Differential diagnosis includes primary central nervous system diseases, vestibular and ocular involvement, and, more rarely, metabolic disorders.[24] Careful questioning can help in the differentiation of central and peripheral causes of vertigo. Dizziness provoked by head movements or head positions could indicate an inner ear dysfunction. Dizziness provoked by certain cervical motions, particularly extension or rotation, also may indicate vertebral artery compromise.
- *Paresthesia/numbness/weakness:* Changes in mentation or cognition can be a manifestation of multiple disorders, including delirium, dementia, head injury, stroke, infection, fever, and adverse drug reactions. The clinician notes whether the patient's communication level is age appropriate, whether the patient is oriented to person, place, and time, and whether his or her emotional and behavioral responses appear to be appropriate to the circumstances.

● Key Point Indications of domestic abuse include:

- Unexplained bruises or abrasions
- Noncompliance and frequent missing of appointments
- Lack of independent transportation or inability to communicate by phone
- Abusers often accompany their victims to all appointments and refuse to allow the victim to be interviewed alone

Vital Signs

The four so-called *vital* signs, which are standard in most medical settings, are temperature, heart rate, blood pressure, and respiratory rate. Pain is often referred to as the fifth vital sign.

Temperature

Body temperature is one indication of the metabolic state of an individual; measurements provide information concerning basal metabolic state, possible presence or absence of infection, and metabolic response to exercise.[25]

● Key Point

- "Normal" body temperature of the adult is 98.6°F (37°C). However, temperatures in the range of 96.5°F (35.8°C) to 99.4°F (37.4°C) are not at all uncommon. Fever or pyrexia is a temperature exceeding 100°F (37.7°C).[26] At this point, physical therapy should be discontinued.
- Hyperpyrexia refers to extreme elevation of temperature (above 41.1°C or 106°F).[25]
- Hypothermia refers to an abnormally low temperature (below 35°C or 95°F).
- Normal temperature of an infant is 98.2°F.
- Normal temperature of a child is 98.6°F.
- Normal temperature of an adolescent is 98.6°F.
- In adults over 75 years of age and in those who are immune-compromised (e.g., transplant recipients, corticosteroid users, persons with chronic renal insufficiency, anyone taking excessive antipyretic medications), The fever response may be blunted or absent.[25]

● Key Point Caution should be used when prescribing exercises for a patient who has a fever. Exercise should not be attempted if the patient has a temperature of 99.5°F or above, due to the increased stresses placed on the cardiopulmonary and immune systems.

Heart Rate

In most people, the pulse is an accurate measure of heart rate. The heart rate or pulse is taken to obtain information about the resting state of the cardiovascular system and the system's response to activity or exercise and recovery.[25] It is also used to assess patency of the specific arteries palpated and the presence of any irregularities in the rhythm.[25]

● Key Point

- "Normal" resting adult heart rate (HR): 70 beats per minute (bpm) (range = 60–100).
- Bradycardia: Less than 60 bpm. At <60 bpm, the supervising PT should be informed and the patient should be monitored carefully.
- Tachycardia: More than 100 bpm. At 110 bpm, the supervising PT should be informed and the patient should be monitored carefully.
- Normal HR for an infant: 120 bpm (range = 70–170).
- Normal HR for a child: 125 bpm (range = 75–140).
- Normal HR for an adolescent: 85 bpm (range = 50–100).

Respiratory Rate

The normal chest expansion difference in adults between the resting position and the fully inhaled position is 2 to 4 centimeters (females > males). As per the PT's instructions, the PTA should compare measurements of both the anterior–posterior diameter and the transverse diameter during rest and at full inhalation.

● Key Point The following are normal respiratory rates (RR) at rest:

- Adult: 12–18 breaths per minute; at 30 breaths per minute, the supervising PT should be informed and the patient should be monitored carefully
- Infant: 30–50 breaths per minute
- Child: 20–40 breaths per minute
- Adolescent: 15–22 breaths per minute

Blood Pressure

Blood pressure is a measure of vascular resistance to blood flow.[25] Arterial blood pressure (BP) is measured by:

- *Systolic pressure:* The pressure exerted on the brachial artery when the heart is contracting.[25]
- *Diastolic pressure:* The pressure exerted on the brachial artery during the relaxation phase of the heart contraction.[25]

● Key Point The values for resting blood pressure in adults are:

- *Normal:* systolic blood pressure <120 mm Hg and diastolic blood pressure <80 mm Hg
- *Prehypertension:* Systolic blood pressure 120–139 mm Hg or diastolic blood pressure 80–90 mm Hg
- *Stage 1 hypertension:* Systolic blood pressure 140–159 mm Hg or diastolic blood pressure 90–99 mm Hg
- *Stage 2 hypertension:* Systolic blood pressure ≥ 160 mm Hg or diastolic blood pressure ≥ 100 mm Hg

The normal values for resting blood pressure in children are:

- *Systolic:* Birth to 1 month, 60–90; up to 3 years of age, 75–130; over 3 years of age, 90–140
- *Diastolic:* Birth to 1 month, 30–60; up to 3 years of age, 45–90; over 3 years of age, 50–80

Pain

Concomitant with most soft tissue injuries are pain, inflammation, and edema. Pain serves as a protective mechanism, allowing an individual to be aware of a situation's potential for producing tissue damage, thus minimizing further damage. Pain may be constant, variable, or intermittent. Variable pain is perpetual but varies in intensity. Variable pain usually indicates the involvement of both a chemical and a mechanical source.

First Aid

Life- or limb-threatening emergencies require rapid assessment, intervention, and transportation to definitive care. Although such events are thankfully uncommon, the clinician must be able to recognize such events and act accordingly. In addition to a working knowledge of basic life support/cardiopulmonary resuscitation (CPR) (see Chapter 6), the clinician should be comfortable with the application of first aid until the local emergency medical services (EMS) or other medical assistance arrives. **Table 1-12** outlines some of the more common situations that require first aid and the appropriate actions to take.

Laboratory Tests and Values

The PTA needs to understand laboratory test values, their variations, their interpretations, and their implications when treating a patient. It is important to remember that false negatives and false positives are associated with laboratory testing, and that the more tests are ordered, the greater the chance that some tests will be false. Many laboratory values can reveal potential precautions for, or contraindications to, therapy, particularly exercise. For example, a patient with diabetes mellitus requires careful monitoring of glucose levels before, during, and after exercise. The purposes of laboratory tests are:

1. To screen for disease or system imbalance (**Table 1-13** and **Table 1-14**)
2. To monitor progress of a disease

Some of the more common laboratory tests, their related physiology, and reference ranges are outlined in **Table 1-15**.

TABLE 1-12	Situations That Require First Aid and Appropriate Action	
Situation	**Description**	**Appropriate Action**
Anaphylaxis	A life-threatening allergic reaction that can cause shock, a sudden drop in blood pressure, and trouble breathing.	Immediately call 911 or facility's emergency number.
		Ask the person if he or she is carrying an epinephrine autoinjector to treat an allergic attack.
		Have the person lie still on his or her back, then loosen tight clothing and cover the person with a blanket. Don't give the person anything to drink.
		If there's vomiting or bleeding from the mouth, turn the person on his or her side to prevent choking. If there are no signs of breathing, coughing, or movement, begin cardiopulmonary resuscitation (CPR).
Burn, including chemical burn	The severity of the burn depends on the extent of damage to body tissues (see Chapter 8).	For minor burns, including first-degree burns and second-degree burns limited to an area no larger than 3 inches (7.6 centimeters) in diameter, cool the burn by holding the burned area under cool (not cold) running water for 10 or 15 minutes or until the pain subsides. If this is impractical, immerse the burn in cool water or cool it with cold compresses. Cooling the burn reduces swelling by conducting heat away from the skin. Don't put ice on the burn. Next, cover the burn with a sterile gauze bandage. Wrap the gauze loosely to avoid putting pressure on burned skin.
		For major burns (third-degree), call 911 or the facility's emergency number. Until an emergency unit arrives, don't remove burned clothing, but make sure the victim is no longer in contact with smoldering materials or exposed to electricity, smoke, or heat. Do not immerse large severe burns in cold water as this can cause a drop in body temperature (hypothermia) and deterioration of blood pressure and circulation (shock). Cover the area of the burn. Use a cool, moist, sterile bandage; clean, moist cloth; or moist towels. When possible, elevate the burned body part or parts above heart level. Check for signs of circulation (breathing, coughing, or movement). If there is no breathing or other sign of circulation, begin CPR.
Chemical splash in the eye	A number of chemicals used in the clinic can be very corrosive.	Immediately flush the eye with water. Use clean, lukewarm tap water for at least 20 minutes, and use whichever of these approaches is quickest:
		Get into a shower and, while holding the affected eye or eyes open, aim a gentle stream of lukewarm water on the forehead over the affected eye, or direct the stream on the bridge of the nose if both eyes are affected. Hold your affected eye or eyes open.
		Placed the head down and turn it to the side. Then ask the person to hold the affected eye open under a gently running faucet.
Choking	Occurs when a foreign object gets lodged in the throat or esophagus, blocking the flow of air.	To confirm that choking is occurring, determine whether the individual is demonstrating an inability to talk, difficulty breathing, or an inability to cough forcefully or whether the skin, lips, and nails are turning blue or dusky.
		If choking is occurring, first deliver five back blows between the person's shoulder blades with the heel of your hand. Next, perform five abdominal thrusts (Heimlich maneuver). The Heimlich maneuver is performed by standing behind the person and wrapping your arms around his or her waist. Tip the person forward slightly. Making a fist your hand, position it slightly above the person's navel and, while grasping the fist with the other hand, press it hard into the abdomen with a quick, upward thrust (as if trying to lift the person up). Alternate between five back blows and five abdominal thrusts until the blockage is dislodged. If the person becomes unconscious, attempt to remove the blockage and perform CPR.

(continued)

TABLE 1-12	Situations That Require First Aid and Appropriate Action (continued)	
Situation	Description	Appropriate Action
Fainting	Occurs when the blood supply to the brain is momentarily inadequate, resulting in a temporary loss of consciousness.	Position the person on his or her back. If the person is breathing, restore blood flow to the brain by raising the person's legs above heart level—about 12 inches (30 centimeters)—if possible. Loosen belts, collars, or other constrictive clothing. If the person doesn't regain consciousness within one minute, call 911 or your local emergency number. In addition, check the person's airway to be sure it's clear. If vomiting occurs, turn the patient on his or her side. Check for signs of circulation (breathing, coughing, or movement). If absent, begin CPR. Call 911 or your local emergency number. Continue CPR until help arrives or the person responds and begins to breathe.
Cardiac arrest	Occurs when an artery supplying the heart with blood and oxygen becomes partially or completely blocked. A heart attack generally causes chest pain for more than 15 minutes, but it can also have no symptoms at all.	Call 911 or your local emergency medical assistance number. If possible, have the person chew and swallow an aspirin, unless he or she is allergic to aspirin. Begin CPR.
Heatstroke	The most severe of the heat-related problems, often resulting from exercise or heavy work in hot environments combined with inadequate fluid intake.	Move the person out of the sun and into a shady or air-conditioned space. Call 911 or emergency medical help. Cool the person by covering him or her with damp sheets or by spraying with cool water. Direct air onto the person with a fan or newspaper. Have the person drink cool water or other nonalcoholic beverage without caffeine, if he or she is able.

TABLE 1-13	Acid–Base Disorders		
Type	Findings	Causes	Signs and Symptoms
Respiratory acidosis	High P_{CO_2} levels	Alveolar hypoventilation (e.g., COPD, head injury, drug overdose, lung disease, pain)	Early signs and symptoms include anxiety, restlessness, dyspnea/cyanosis, disorientation, and headache. Late signs and symptoms include confusion, somnolence, and coma.
Metabolic alkalosis	High H_{CO_3} levels	Loss of hydrogen ions; vomiting or nasogastric (NG) suction generates metabolic alkalosis by the loss of gastric secretions, which are rich in hydrochloric acid (HCl). Renal losses of hydrogen ions occur whenever the distal delivery of sodium increases in the presence of excess aldosterone (hypokalemia). Alkali administration: Administration of sodium bicarbonate in amounts that exceed the capacity of the kidneys to excrete this excess bicarbonate may cause metabolic alkalosis. Contraction alkalosis: Loss of bicarbonate-poor, chloride-rich extracellular fluid, as observed with thiazide diuretic or loop diuretic therapy or chloride diarrhea concentration.	Vague symptoms of weakness, irritability, and mental changes.

TABLE 1-13 Acid–Base Disorders (continued)

Type	Findings	Causes	Signs and Symptoms
Respiratory alkalosis	Low P_{CO_2} levels	Alveolar hyperventilation: Central nervous system disorder (pain, anxiety, fear, cerebrovascular accident, meningitis). Hypoxemia (e.g., high altitudes, severe anemia), mechanical ventilation.	Tachypnea, numbness and tingling, blurred vision, diaphoresis, dizziness, arrhythmia syncope, and early tetany.
Metabolic acidosis	Low H_{CO_3} levels	Inability to excrete the dietary H^+ load (chronic renal disease, hypoaldosteronism); ketoacidosis (diabetes, alcoholism, and starvation). Lactic acidosis (circulatory failure, drugs and toxins, and hereditary causes). GI $H_{CO_3}^-$ loss (diarrhea).	An increase in alveolar ventilation (Kussmaul's breathing), which results in a compensatory respiratory alkalosis. In addition, nausea and vomiting, cardiac dysrhythmias, lethargy, and coma can occur.

Data from Dutton M: McGraw-Hill's National Physical therapy Examination (ed 1). New York, McGraw-Hill, 2009

TABLE 1-14 Signs and Symptoms of Electrolyte Disturbances

Disturbance	Definition and Possible Causes	Signs and Symptoms
Hyperkalemia	High blood level of potassium. Possible causes include kidney failure, Addison disease, muscle trauma, and high-potassium diet.	Muscle weakness and/or flaccid paralysis Diarrhea and/or abdominal cramps Bradycardia and/or arrhythmia
Hypokalemia	Low blood level of potassium. Possible causes include decreased food intake/poor nutrition, Cushing disease, kidney disease, and diuretic medications.	Muscle fatigue and/or cramp Diarrhea and/or vomiting Dizziness and/or arrhythmia Irritability and/or confusion Slow reflex and/or orthostatic hypotension
Hypernatremia	High blood level of sodium. Possible causes include kidney disease, dehydration, decreased fluid intake, Cushing disease, and salt water ingestion.	Restlessness and/or convulsions Tachycardia and/or agitation Weight gain and/or pitting edema Pulmonary edema and/or hypertension
Hyponatremia	Low blood level of sodium. Possible causes include excessive fluid loss and Addison disease.	Muscle weakness and/or muscle twitching Hypotension and/or tachycardia Restlessness and/or convulsions Anxiety and/or headache
Hypercalcemia	High blood level of calcium. Possible causes include bone atrophy, bone cancer, and hyperparathyroidism.	Generalized weakness and/or decreased muscle tone Hypertension and/or cardiac arrest Drowsiness and/or lethargy Weight loss and/or anorexia
Hypocalcemia	Low blood levels of calcium. Possible causes include renal disease/failure, decreased gastrointestinal absorption of calcium, decreased vitamin D.	Muscle cramps and spasms Arrhythmia Convulsions and/or hypotension Numbness and tingling

	TABLE 1-15	Laboratory Values

Test	Related Physiology	Reference Range Example
Arterial PO_2	Reflects the dissolved oxygen level based on the pressure it exerts on the bloodstream.	80–100 mm Hg
Arterial P_{CO_2}	Reflect the dissolved carbon dioxide level based on the pressure it exerts on the bloodstream.	36–44 mm Hg
Arterial pH	Reflects the free hydrogen on and concentration; collectively, this test and the arterial PO_2 and arterial PCO_2 tests help reveal the acid-based status and how well oxygen is being delivered to the body.	7.35–7.45
Oxygen saturation	Usually a bedside technique (pulse oximetry) to indicate the level of oxygen transport.	95%–100%
Creatine phosphokinase (CPK)	An enzyme found predominantly in the heart, brain, and skeletal muscle. Aids in protein catabolism. Can be separated into subunits or isoenzymes, each derived from a specific tissue, CPK-BB = brain CPK-MB = cardiac CPK-MM = skeletal muscle	Total CPK: Less than 30
Lactate dehydrogenase (LDH)	Present in all body tissues and abundant in red blood cells. Acts as a marker for hemolysis. Isoenzymes are LDH 1–5.	105–333 IU/L (international units per liter)
Alkaline phosphate	An enzyme most active at pH 9.1. Associated with bone metabolism/calcification and lipid transport.	Adults: 13–39 IU/L Infants–Adolescents: Up to 104 IU/L
Sodium (Na)	Major extracellular cation; serves to regulate serum osmolality, fluid, and acid-base balance; maintains transmembrane electric potential for neuromuscular functioning.	136–145 mmol/L
Potassium (K)	Major intracellular cation; maintains normal hydration and osmotic pressure.	3.5–5.5 mmol/L
Chloride (Cl)	Extracellular anion; maintains electrical neutrality of extracellular fluid.	96–106 mmol/L
Carbon dioxide	Reflects body's ability to control pH; important in bicarbonate–carbonic acid blood buffer system.	24–30 mmol/L
Anion gap (sodium minus the sum of chloride and carbon dioxide)	Calculated value helpful in evaluating metabolic acidosis.	3–11 mmol/L
Calcium (Ca)	Transmission of nerve impulses, muscle contractility; cofactor in enzyme reactions and blood coagulation.	8.5–10.8 mg/dL; inversely related to phosphorus level
Phosphorous (PO_4)	Integral to structure of nucleic acids, in adenosine triphosphate energy transferred, and in phospholipid function. Phosphate helps to regulate calcium levels, metabolism, base balance, and bone metabolism.	2.6–4.5 mg/dL; inversely related to calcium level
Blood urea nitrogen (BUN); measures renal function and protein intake	Amino acid metabolism in the liver produces urea as waste; urea is filtered by the kidney with the portion passively reabsorbed being measured in the plasma.	Adult range: 8–22 mg/dL
Creatinine (a measure of renal function)	Muscle creatine degradation produces creatinine, which in turn is excreted by the kidneys.	Adult range: 0.7–1.4 mg/dL
BUN/creatinine ratio	Assessment of kidney and liver function.	Adult range: 6–25 mg/dL

TABLE 1-15	Laboratory Values (continued)	
Test	**Related Physiology**	**Reference Range Example**
Alanine aminotransferase (ALT)	Enzyme released in cytolysis and necrosis of liver cells.	1–21 units/L
Aspartate aminotransferase (AST)	Enzyme released in cytolysis and necrosis of liver cells; also in heart and skeletal muscle tissues.	7–27 units/L
Alkaline phosphatase (ALP)	Enzyme released in cytolysis and necrosis of liver cells; also in bone.	13–39 units/L
γ-Glutamyltransferase	Enzyme released in cytolysis and necrosis of liver cells; also in kidney tissue.	5–38 units/L
Albumin	Index of liver synthetic capacity.	3.5–5.0 g/dL
Bilirubin, total	Bilirubin is the predominant pigment in bile, and the major metabolite of hemoglobin.	0.2–1.0 mg/dL; direct: 0–0.2 mg/dL; indirect: 0.2–1.0 mg/dL
Ammonium	Liver converts ammonia from blood to urea.	12–55 μmol/L
WBC count (measures mature and immature WBCs in 1 μL of whole blood—used in conjunction with WBC differential)	Produced in bone marrow; WBCs provide defense against foreign agents/organisms.	4000–10,000 WBCs/μL
WBC differential (visual or computer observation and count of different types of WBCs)	Differentiation of white blood cell types by relative percentages. Cell types usually seen (in descending order): neutrophils (PMN), lymphocytes, monocytes, eosinophils, basophils.	All components totaled equal 100%
Segmented neutrophils	Phagocytize.	~37%–77%
Band neutrophils	Phagocytize; less mature neutrophil.	~0%–11%
Lymphocytes	B-cells produce immunoglobulins; T-cells provide regulatory and effector functions in immunity.	~10%–44%
Monocytes	Phagocytize and contribute to cellular and humoral immunity in association with T-lymphocytes.	~2%–10%
Eosinophils	Also function as phagocytes, somewhat less effectively than neutrophils.	~0%–7%
Basophils	Also function as phagocytes; synthesize and store histamine.	~0%–2%
Red blood cell (RBC)/ erythrocyte count (measures the number of RBCs in 1 μL of blood)	Produced in bone marrow, carry oxygen to tissues.	$4.2–6.2 \times 10^6$ μL
Hemoglobin	Reflects concentration of hemoglobin in blood.	12–16 g/dL (values of 8–10 g/dL typically result in decreased exercise tolerance, increased fatigue, and tachycardia, condition that may contraindicate aggressive therapeutic measures, including strength and endurance training)
Hematocrit	Measure of the ratio of packed red blood cells to whole blood. By dividing the hematocrit level by 3, one can approximate the hemoglobin level.	36%–54% (approximately 3 times hemoglobin)

(continued)

TABLE 1-15	Laboratory Values (continued)	
Test	**Related Physiology**	**Reference Range Example**
Indices: Mean cell volume (MCV)	Measure of average size of RBCs—the ratio of hematocrit to red blood cell count.	80–100 fl
Indices: Mean cell hemoglobin concentration (MCHC)	Indicates the average concentration of hemoglobin to hematocrit, and manages the percentage of hemoglobin in 100 mL of blood.	32–36 g/dL; cannot exceed 37 g/dL
Indices: Mean cell hemoglobin (MCH)	Indicates average weight of hemoglobin per RBC.	28–32 picograms (pg)
RBC distribution width	Standard deviation of MCV; measure of degree of uniformity in size of RBCs.	11.7%–14.2%
Erythrocyte sedimentation rate (ESR)	Nonspecific indicator of inflammation or tissue damage.	0–20 mm/1 hour
Platelet count	Reflects potential to address injury to vessel walls, thus regulating homeostasis.	140,000–450,000 µL

Data from Wall LJ: Laboratory tests and values, in Boissonnault WG (ed): Primary Care for the Physical Therapist: Examination and Triage. St. Louis, Elsevier Saunders, 2005, pp 348–367; and Lotspeich-Steinger CA, Stiene-Martin AE, Koepke JA: Clinical hematology; principles, procedures, correlations. Philadelphia, J. B. Lippincott, 1992

Pharmacology

A drug is any substance that can be used to modify a chemical process or processes in the body—for example, to treat an illness, relieve a symptom, enhance a performance or ability, or alter states of mind. Drug therapy (see Chapter 15) is one of the mainstays of modern treatments, and PTAs often encounter patients who are taking various medications.

Abbreviations

Medical abbreviations are used throughout the various disciplines in health care to document client status or progression. It is important to remember that before using abbreviations The PTA must ensure that they are approved for use by the facility to avoid miscommunication. **Table 1-16** outlines some of the more common abbreviations used by physical therapy professionals.

Imaging Studies

For healthcare professionals involved in the primary management of neuromusculoskeletal disorders, diagnostic imaging is an essential tool. The availability of diagnostic images varies greatly depending on the practice setting. Although the interpretation of diagnostic images is always the responsibility of the radiologist, it is important for the clinician to know what importance to attach to these reports, and the strengths and weaknesses of the various techniques that image bone and soft tissues, such as muscle, fat, tendon, cartilage, and ligament. In general, imaging tests have a high sensitivity (few false negatives) but low specificity (high false-positive rate), so they are not used in isolation.

Conventional (Plain Film) Radiography

Tissues of greater density allow less penetration of the x-rays and therefore appear lighter on the film. The following structures are listed in order of descending density: metal, bone, soft tissue, water or body fluid, fat, and air. Because air is the least dense material in the body, it absorbs the least amount of x-ray particles, resulting in the darkest portion of the film. In contrast, bone absorbs the greatest amount and therefore appears white. When studying radiographs, a systematic approach such as the mnemonic ABCS is recommended:[29]

- *A: Architecture or alignment.* The entire radiograph is scanned from top to bottom, side to side, and in each corner to check for the normal shape and alignment of each bone. The outline of each bone should be smooth and continuous.

TABLE
1-16

Commonly Used Abbreviations

AAROM	Active assistive range of motion	ER	External rotation or emergency room
abd	Abduction	E-stim	Electrical stimulation
ACL	Anterior cruciate ligament	ex	Exercise
add	Adduction	ext	Extension
ADL	Activities of daily living	FES	Functional electrical stimulation
Ad lib.	As desired	Flex	Flexion
AE	Above elbow	FWB	Full weight-bearing
AFO	Ankle foot orthosis	Fx	Fracture
AK	Above knee	HEP	Home exercise program
amb	Ambulation	HNP	Herniated nucleus pulposus
ANS	Autonomic nervous system	HP	Hot pack
A-P	Anterior–posterior	HR	Heart rate or hold-relax
AROM	Active range of motion	Hx	History
ASIS	Anterior superior iliac spine	ICU	Intensive care unit
BE	Below elbow	Ind	Independent
bid	Twice a day	IR	Internal rotation
BK	Below knee	JRA	Juvenile rheumatoid arthritis
BP	Blood pressure	Jt	Joint
bpm	Beats per minute	KAFO	Knee–ankle-foot orthosis
CC	Chief complaint	LBP	Low back pain
CGA	Contact guard assist	LCL	Lateral collateral ligament
c/o	Complains of	LE	Lower extremity
CPM	Continuous passive motion	LOB	Loss of balance
CR	Contract–relax	LTG	Long-term goal
CTLSO	Cervical–thoracic–lumbar–sacral orthosis	MCL	Medial collateral ligament
CTR	Carpal tunnel release	MCP	Metacarpophalangeal
d/c	Discontinued or discharged	MMT	Manual muscle test
DDD	Degenerative disk disease	MVA	Motor vehicle accident
DF	Dorsiflexion	N/A	Not applicable
DIP	Distal interphalangeal	NWB	Nonweight-bearing
DJD	Degenerative joint disease	OOB	Out of bed
DOB	Date of birth	OP	Outpatient
DOE	Dyspnea on exertion	OR	Operating room
DTR	Deep tendon reflexes	ORIF	Open reduction and internal fixation
DVT	Deep vein thrombosis	OT	Occupational therapy
Dx	Diagnosis	PCL	Posterior cruciate ligament
EMG	Electromyography	PF	Plantarflexion

(continued)

| TABLE 1-16 | Commonly Used Abbreviations (continued) |

PIP	Proximal interphalangeal	TBI	Traumatic brain injury
PMH	Past medical history	TDWB	Touchdown weight-bearing
PNF	Proprioceptive neuromuscular facilitation	TENS	Transcutaneous electrical nerve stimulation
Post op	Postoperative	THA	Total hip arthroplasty
PRE	Progressive resistive exercises	Tid	Three times a day
Prn	As needed	TKA	Total knee arthroplasty
PROM	Passive range of motion	TKE	Terminal knee extension
PWB	Partial weight-bearing	TMJ	Temporomandibular joint
qid	Four times a day	TTWB	Toe touch weight-bearing
RA	Rheumatoid arthritis	Tx	Traction
r/o	Rule out	UE	Upper extremity
ROM	Range of motion	US	Ultrasound
RTC	Rotator cuff	WB	Weight-bearing
Rx	Treatment	WBAT	Weight-bearing as tolerated
SCI	Spinal cord injury	WFL	Within functional limits
SLR	Straight leg raise	WNL	Within normal limits
SOB	Short of breath	y/o	Year(s) old
STG	Short-term goal		

Breaks in continuity usually represent fractures. Malalignments may indicate subluxations or dislocations, or in the case of the spine, scoliosis. Malalignment in a trauma setting must be considered traumatic rather than degenerative until proven otherwise.[30]

- *B: Bone density.* The clinician should assess both general bone density and local bone density. The cortex of the bone should appear denser than the remainder of the bone. Subchondral bone becomes sclerosed in the presence of stress in accordance with Wolff's law[31] and increases its density. This is a radiographic hallmark of osteoarthritis.
- *C: Cartilage spaces.* Each joint should have a well-preserved joint space between the articulating surfaces. A decreased joint space typically indicates that the articular cartilage is thinned from a degenerative process such as osteoarthritis.
- *S: Soft tissue evaluation.* Trauma to soft tissues produces abnormal images resulting from effusion, bleeding, and distension.

Arthrography

Arthrography is the study of structures within an encapsulated joint using a contrast medium with or without air that is injected into the joint space. The contrast medium distends the joint capsule. This type of radiograph is called an *arthrogram*. An arthrogram outlines the soft tissue structures of a joint that would not be visible with a plain-film radiograph. This procedure is commonly performed on patients with injuries involving the shoulder or the knee.

Myelography

Myelography is the radiographic study of the spinal cord, nerve roots, dura mater, and spinal canal. The contrast medium is injected into the subarachnoid space, and a radiograph is taken. This type of radiograph is called a *myelogram*. Myelography is used frequently to diagnose intervertebral disk herniations, spinal cord compression, stenosis, nerve root injury, or tumors. The nerve root and its sleeve can be observed clearly on direct myelograms.

Discography

Discography is the radiographic study of the intervertebral disc. A radiopaque dye is injected into the disc space between two vertebrae. A radiograph is then taken. This type of radiograph is called a *discogram*. An abnormal dye pattern between the intervertebral discs indicates a rupture of the disc.

Angiography

Angiography is the radiographic study of the vascular system. A water-soluble radiopaque dye is injected either intra-arterially (arteriogram) or intravenously (venogram). A rapid series of radiographs is then taken to follow the course of the contrast medium as it travels through the blood vessels. Angiography is used to help detect injury to or partial blockage of blood vessels.

Computed Tomography

A computed tomography (CT) scanner system, also known as computerized axial tomography (CAT) and computerized transaxial tomography (CTI), consists of a scanning gantry that holds the x-ray tube and detectors (moving parts), a moving table or couch for the patient, an x-ray generator, computer processing unit, and a display console or workstation.[32] Images are obtained in the transverse (axial) plane of the patient's body by rotating the x-ray tube 360 degrees. The x-rays are absorbed in part by the patient's body. The amount of x-rays transmitted through the body is detected in the opposite side of the gantry by an array of detectors. Image quality in CT imaging depends on a variety of factors that are mostly selected by the operator. Two parameters are used to define the image quality of a given system:[32]

- *Spatial resolution:* Spatial resolution is defined as the ability of the system to distinguish between two closely spaced objects. For improvement of spatial resolution, the operator selects a small matrix size (256 × 256), small field of view, and thin slices. Special reconstruction algorithms can also be chosen to improve spatial resolutions.
- *Contrast resolution:* Contrast resolution is defined as the ability of the system to discriminate between two adjacent areas with different attenuation values. The contrast resolution of CT is dramatically better than conventional radiography (approximately 100 times), and the images provide greater soft tissue detail than do plain films.[30]

As with plain radiographs, air appears as the darkest portion of the film, and bone appears white.

CT Myelogram

A CT myelogram (CTM) is a diagnostic tool that uses radiographic contrast media (dye) that is injected into the subarachnoid space (cerebrospinal fluid; CSF). After the dye is injected, the contrast medium serves to illuminate the spinal canal, cord, and nerve roots during imaging. The low viscosity of the water-soluble contrast permits filling of the nerve roots and better visualization.[30]

Magnetic Resonance Imaging

Unlike CT, which depends upon multiple thin slices of radiation that are "backplotted" through Fourier transformers, magnetic resonance imaging (MRI) is the result of the interaction between magnetic fields, radiofrequency (RF) waves, and complex image reconstruction techniques. Normally, the axes of protons in the body have a random orientation. However, if the body or body part is placed within a high magnetic field, the protons align themselves parallel with or perpendicular to the direction of the magnetic field. The protons, now spinning synchronously at an angle within the magnetic field, induce a current in a nearby transmitter–receiver coil or antenna. This small nuclear signal is then recorded, amplified, measured, and localized (linked to the exact location in the body where the MRI signal is coming from), producing a high-contrast, clinically useful MR image.

Radionucleotide Scanning

Radionucleotide scanning involves the introduction of bone-seeking isotopes that are administered to the patient orally or intravenously and allowed to localize to the skeleton. The photon energy emitted by the isotopes is then recorded using a gamma camera 2 to 4 hours later. The pathophysiologic basis of the technique is complex but depends on localized differences in blood flow, capillary permeability, and metabolic activity that accompany any injury, infection, repair process, or growth of bone tissue.[33] The most common radionucleotide scanning test is the bone scan. This test is used to detect particular areas of abnormal metabolic activity within a bone. The abnormality shows up as a so-called hot spot that is darker in appearance than normal tissue.

REVIEW Questions

1. What was/were developed to "encourage a uniform approach to physical therapist practice and to explain to the world the nature of that practice"?
   a. State licensure laws
   b. *The Guide to Physical Therapist Practice*
   c. The National Physical Therapy Examination
   d. The Medicare Act of 1973

2. True or false: Physical therapists are the only professionals who provide physical therapy.

3. What is the function of the Commission on Accreditation in Physical Therapy Education (CAPTE)?
   a. To design policies and procedures with regard to physical therapy
   b. To make autonomous decisions concerning the accreditation status of continuing education programs for the physical therapists and physical therapist assistants
   c. To design questions for the National Physical Therapy Examination
   d. To oversee state licensing laws

4. The purpose of clinical education is to provide student clinicians with opportunities to:
   a. Observe and work with a variety of patients under professional supervision and in diverse professional settings and to integrate knowledge and skills at progressively higher levels of performance and responsibility
   b. Provide a student with the opportunity to take a break from school work
   c. Develop clinical reasoning skills and management skills, as well as to master techniques that develop competence at the level of a beginning practitioner
   d. a and c.

5. A loss or abnormality of anatomic, physiologic, or psychologic structure or function in a description of which category of the disablement model?
   a. Impairment
   b. Functional limitation
   c. Disability
   d. None of the above

6. Which element of the patient/client management includes gathering information from the chart, other caregivers, the patient, the patient's family, caretakers, and friends in order to identify and define the patient's problem(s)?
   a. Evaluation
   b. Intervention
   c. Examination
   d. Tests and measures

7. What is the purpose of the re-examination?
   a. To allow the clinician to evaluate progress and modify interventions as appropriate
   b. To provide the insurance companies with justification for payment
   c. All of the above
   d. None of the above

8. Which component of the examination includes an analysis of posture, structural alignment or deformity, scars, crepitus, color changes, swelling, muscle atrophy, and the presence of any asymmetry?
   a. Palpation
   b. Observation
   c. Patient history
   d. None of the above

9. What are anthropometrics?
   a. Measurable physiological characteristics, including height and weight
   b. Studies involving the history of man
   c. A form of laboratory test
   d. None of the above

10. Which of the elements of patient/client management attempts to identify a relationship between the symptoms reported and the signs of disturbed function?
    a. Test and measures
    b. Patient history
    c. Examination
    d. None of the above

11. Which of the elements of patient/client management determines the predicted level of function that the patient will attain and an identification of the barriers that may impact the achievement of optimal improvement (age, medication(s), socioeconomic status, comorbidities, cognitive status, nutrition, social support, and environment) within a certain time frame?
    a. Evaluation
    b. Examination
    c. Prognosis
    d. Diagnosis

12. Which of the following statements is/are true about the plan of care?
    a. It is based on the examination, evaluation, diagnosis, and prognosis, including the predicted level of optimal improvement.
    b. It describes the specific interventions to be used, and the proposed frequency and duration of the interventions that are required to reach the anticipated goals and expected outcomes.
    c. It includes plans for discharge of the patient/client taking into consideration achievement of anticipated goals and expected outcomes, and provides for appropriate follow-up or referral.
    d. All of the above
13. Which of the elements of patient/client management can be defined as "the purposeful and skilled interaction of the clinician and the patient/client and, when appropriate, with other individuals involved in the patient/client care, using various physical therapy procedures and techniques to produce changes in the condition consistent with the diagnosis and prognosis"?
    a. Examination
    b. Prognosis
    c. Intervention
    d. Evaluation
14. What is the major difference between a client and a patient?
15. What are the four components of the traditional SOAP note?
16. True or false: Correction fluid/tape can be used to correct text in the medical records.
17. Which of the following patient attributes would not impact the clinician's choice of an intervention?
    a. Comorbidities
    b. Physiological impairments
    c. Anatomic impairments
    d. Race
18. In a typical physical therapy department, which staff member ensures that the objectives of the service are efficiently and effectively achieved within the framework of the stated purpose of the organization?
    a. Staff physical therapist
    b. Physical therapy director
    c. Department secretary
    d. None of the above
19. True or false: A PTA may modify and intervention only in accordance with changes in patient status and within the established plan of care developed by the physical therapist.
20. The following are all job responsibilities of the PT volunteer, except:
    a. Taking phone messages
    b. Cleaning the whirlpool
    c. Performing secretarial functions
    d. All of the above are job responsibilities of the PT volunteer
21. Which of the following is/are included in the APTA Code of Ethics?
    a. A physical therapist shall exercise sound professional judgment
    b. A physical therapist shall achieve and maintain professional competence
    c. A physical therapist shall respect the rights and dignity of all individuals and shall provide compassionate care
    d. a and c
    e. All of the above
22. You are a PTA assigned a PTA student who is performing his first clinical internship. Which of the following would be the most appropriate goals for this physical therapy student?
    a. To be able to perform an orthopedic examination on all patients
    b. To perform all aspects of treatment using correct body mechanics
    c. To correctly reassess all patient problems
    d. To perform all patient care duties assigned
23. Which of the following duties cannot be performed legally by a PTA?
    a. Call a physician about a patient's status
    b. Add 3 pounds to a patient's current exercise protocol
    c. Allow a patient to increase in frequency from 2 times/week to 3 times/week
    d. Perform ultrasound on a patient
24. CORF is an abbreviation for which of the following?
    a. Certified Owner of a Rehabilitation Facility
    b. Certified Outpatient Rehabilitation Facility
    c. Control Organization for Rehabilitation Facilities
    d. None of the above
25. A PTA is performing a chart review and discovers that lab results reveal that the patient has malignant cancer. When treating the patient, the PTA is asked by the patient, "Did my lab results come back?" The appropriate response for the PTA is:

a. To inform the patient about the results and contact the social worker to assist in consultation of the family

b. To inform the patient that it would be inappropriate for him or her to comment on the lab results before the physician has assessed the lab results and spoken to the patient

c. To inform the patient that he or she has a malignant cancer

d. To tell the patient the results are in, but that physical therapists are not allowed to comment on the results

26. A PTA is instructing a PTA student in documentation using a SOAP note. Where should the following phrase be placed in a SOAP note: "The patient reports wanting to return to playing soccer in 5 weeks"?

a. Subjective

b. Objective

c. Assessment

d. Plan

27. True or false: The PTA is frequently called upon to modify or adjust therapeutic interventions in consultation with the supervising physical therapist, based on a variety of physiologic responses from the patient. These responses include, but are not limited to, changes in a patient's signs and symptoms, range of motion (ROM), strength, endurance, function, balance, and coordination.

References

1. Guide to Physical Therapist Practice (ed 2). American Physical Therapy Association. Phys Ther 81:1–746, 2001

2. Guide to Physical Therapist Practice: Revisions. American Physical Therapy Association. Phys Ther 79, 2001

3. Guide to Physical Therapist Practice (ed 2). Phys Ther 81:S13–S95, 2001

4. Nagi S: Disability concepts revisited: implications for prevention, in Pope A, Tartov A (eds): Disability in America: Toward a National Agenda for Prevention. Washington, DC, National Academy Press, 1991, pp 309–327

5. Brandt EN Jr, Pope AM: Enabling America: Assessing the role of rehabilitation science and engineering. Washington, DC: Institute of Medicine, National Academy Press, 1997

6. Palisano RJ, Campbell SK, Harris SR: Evidence-based decision-making in pediatric physical therapy, in Campbell SK, Vander Linden DW, Palisano RJ (eds): Physical Therapy for Children. St. Louis, Saunders, 2006, pp 3–32

7. Schenkman M, Butler RB: A model for multisystem evaluation, interpretation, and treatment of individuals with neurologic dysfunction. Phys Ther 69:538–547, 1989

8. Kettenbach G: Background information, in Kettenbach G (ed): Writing SOAP Notes with Patient/Client Management Formats (ed 3). Philadelphia, F. A. Davis, 2004, pp 1–5

9. O'Sullivan SB: Clinical decision-making, in O'Sullivan SB, Schmitz TJ (eds): Physical Rehabilitation (ed 5). Philadelphia, F. A. Davis, 2007, pp 3–24

10. Goodman CC, Snyder TK: Introduction to the interviewing process, in Goodman CC, Snyder TK (eds): Differential Diagnosis in Physical Therapy. Philadelphia, Saunders, 1990, pp 7–42

11. Grieve GP: Common Vertebral Joint Problems. New York, Churchill Livingstone, 1981

12. Guide to Physical Therapist Practice (ed 2). American Physical Therapy Association. Phys Ther 81:9–746, 2001

13. Nirschl RP: Prevention and treatment of elbow and shoulder injuries in the tennis player. Clin Sports Med 7:289–308, 1988

14. Grimsby O, Power B: Manual therapy approach to knee ligament rehabilitation, in Ellenbecker TS (ed): Knee Ligament Rehabilitation. Philadelphia, Churchill Livingstone, 2000, pp 236–251

15. McKenzie R, May S: Introduction, in McKenzie R, May S (eds): The Human Extremities: Mechanical Diagnosis and Therapy. Waikanae, New Zealand, Spinal Publications New Zealand Ltd, 2000, pp 1–5

16. Deyo RA: Compliance with therapeutic regimens in arthritis: Issues, current status, and a future agenda. Sem Arthritis Rheum 12:233–244, 1982

17. Blanpied P: Why won't patients do their home exercise programs? J Orthop Sports Phys Ther 25:101–102, 1997

18. Chen CY, Neufeld PS, Feely CA, et al: Factors influencing compliance with home exercise programs among patients with upper extremity impairment. Am J Occup Ther 53:171–180, 1999

19. Friedrich M, Cermak T, Madebacher P: The effect of brochure use versus therapist teaching on patients performing therapeutic exercise and on changes in impairment status. Phys Ther 76:1082–1088, 1996

20. Bloom BS: Taxonomy of Educational Objectives, Handbook I: The Cognitive Domain. New York, David McKay, 1956

21. Litzinger ME, Osif B: Accommodating diverse learning styles: Designing instruction for electronic information sources, in Shirato L (ed): What Is Good Instruction Now? Library Instruction for the 90s. Ann Arbor, MI, Pierian Press, 1993

22. Goodman CC, Kelly Snyder TE: Infectious disease, in Goodman CC, Boissonnault WG, Fuller KS (eds): Pathology: Implications for the Physical Therapist (ed 2). Philadelphia, Saunders, 2003, pp 194–235

23. Boissonnault WG: Review of systems, in Boissonnault WG (ed): Primary Care for the Physical Therapist: Examination and Triage. St. Louis, Elsevier Saunders, 2005, pp 87–104

24. Mohn A, di Ricco L, Magnelli A, et al: Celiac disease—associated vertigo and nystagmus. J Pediatr Gastroenterol Nutr 34:317–318, 2002

25. Bailey MK: Physical examination procedures to screen for serious disorders of the low back and lower quarter, in Wilmarth MA (ed): Medical screening for the physical therapist. Orthopaedic Section Independent Study Course 14.1.1 La Crosse, Wisconsin, Orthopaedic Section, APTA, 2003, pp 1–35

26. Judge RD, Zuidema GD, Fitzgerald FT: Vital Signs, in Judge RD, Zuidema GD, Fitzgerald FT (eds): Clinical Diagnosis (ed 4). Boston, Little, Brown and Company, 1982, pp 49–58

27. Huskisson EC: Measurement of pain. Lancet 2:127, 1974

28. Halle JS: Neuromusculoskeletal scan examination with selected related topics, in Flynn TW (ed): The Thoracic Spine and Rib Cage: Musculoskeletal Evaluation and Treatment. Boston, Butterworth-Heinemann, 1996, pp 121–146

29. Swain JH: An introduction to radiology of the lumbar spine, in Wadsworth C (ed): Orthopedic Physical Therapy Home Study Course. La Crosse, WI, Orthopedic Section, APTA, 1994

30. Iwasaki T, Zheng M: Sensory feedback mechanism underlying entrainment of central pattern generator to mechanical resonance. Biol Cybern 94:245-61. Epub Jan 10, 2006

31. Wolff J: The Law of Remodeling (Maquet P, Furlong R, (trans)). Berlin, Springer-Verlag, 1986 (1892)

32. Yamaguchi T: The central pattern generator for forelimb locomotion in the cat. Prog Brain Res 143:115–122, 2004

33. Norris BJ, Weaver AL, Morris LG, et al: A central pattern generator producing alternative outputs: temporal pattern of premotor activity. J Neurophysiol 96:309–326. Epub Apr 12, 2006

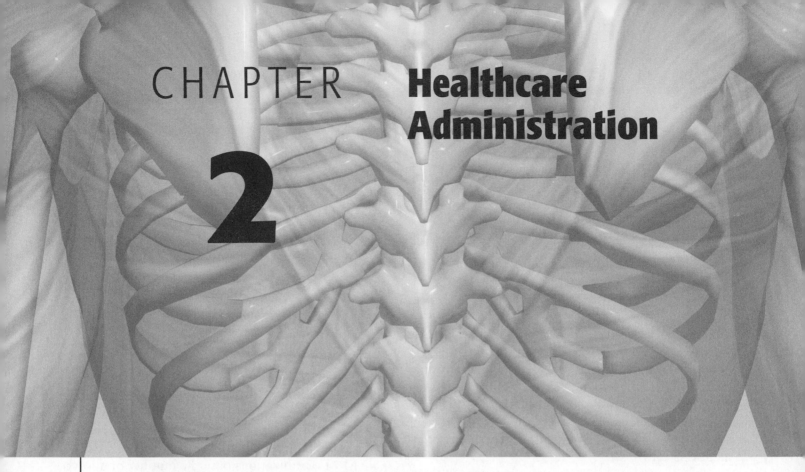

CHAPTER 2

Healthcare Administration

Administration, according to the *Guide to Physical Therapist Practice*, is "the planning, directing, organizing, and managing of human, technical, environmental, and financial resources effectively and efficiently."[1] Nowadays, the United States has several types of privately and publicly funded health insurance plans that provide healthcare services:

- Private health insurance companies
- Independent health plans
- Government health insurance
- Consumer-driven healthcare programs

Private Health Insurance

In the private health insurance industry within the United States, there are three types of firms:

- *Commercial stock companies:* Private stockholder-owned corporations that operate in the national marketplace. Examples include Aetna, Travelers, and Connecticut General.
- *Mutual companies:* Also operate in the national marketplace and have private holders, but differ because the policyholders are also the owners. Examples include Mutual of Omaha, Prudential, and Metropolitan Life.
- *Nonprofit insurance plans:* Are granted exclusive franchises to geographical areas and to a particular line of insurance. Examples include Blue Cross and Blue Shield and Delta Dental.

These plans can include commercial insurance, fee-for-service, or traditional indemnity plans, or they can be for employers who are self-insured. They have the following characteristics:

- Preauthorization may not be needed.
- Patients have the freedom to choose their own providers.
- The number of physical therapy visits allowed should be usual, customary, and reasonable; this is often contractually defined in the insurance policy.

Independent Health Plans

These are organized programs by third-party payers ("gatekeepers") that are designed to control access (usually through the primary care physician) to inpatient and ambulatory health services by directing patients to certain providers. The independent health plans include managed care plans, preferred provider organizations (PPOs), and health maintenance organizations (HMOs).

Managed Care Plans

Managed care plans are designed to ensure the medical necessity of the proposed service and the delivery of the service (pre-admission or pre-treatment certification, surgical opinion programs, concurrent reviews, individual/large case management, financial incentives, or penalties). Failure to comply with managed care requirements or decisions usually reduces health benefit coverage for claims. The penalties may affect both patients and providers. Managed care is essential to the structure of alternative delivery and financing systems, such as HMO and PPO arrangements.

Preferred Provider Organizations

A preferred provider organization is a group of providers, usually hospitals or physicians, that offers healthcare services as an entity to employers at a negotiated, often discounted, price. PPOs have the following characteristics:

- Patients are not locked into PPO providers, but they receive financial incentives to use services within the PPO network.
- Preauthorization is needed before services can be provided.
- Most plans limit the number of physical therapy visits, depending on the diagnosis.
- An employer can offer employees a traditional healthcare plan, HMO, or PPO.

Health Maintenance Organizations

A health maintenance organization is a form of managed care that offers prepaid, comprehensive health coverage for both hospital and physician services with specific healthcare providers using a fixed structure or capitated rates. HMOs have the following characteristics:

- Employers contract for health services as a benefit to their employees.
- Employees are locked into using the system of member healthcare providers and affiliated facilities.
- Some of these organizations allow patients to seek care "out of network" but at a higher, or additional, cost to the patient.
- Employees may have to pay a small fee to visit (copay), such as $10 per visit.
- The primary care physicians (PCPs) act as gatekeepers for any medical care required beyond their scope of practice. For example, a PCP must authorize physical therapy services before they can be provided.
- Most organizations base the number of allowed physical therapy visits on the diagnosis.

● **Key Point** A point-of-service (POS) plan, also known as an open-ended HMO, is an insurance plan in which members need not choose how to receive services until the time they need them.

● **Key Point** A *point-of-purchase plan* is a benefit plan that expands enrollee options to choose providers. It usually consists of two or more delivery and financing options, including an alternative delivery system, such as an HMO or PPO, and another plan such as traditional fee-for-service coverage. The participant is not locked in, but may change coverage options each time care is obtained. The scope of benefits and payment provisions are structured to provide incentives for greater use of the alternative delivery system option.

The *primary care network plan* is similar to an HMO that provides health services for a fixed price, relying on participating primary care physicians to serve as "gatekeepers" to control patient access to institutional services and specialty care. The PCP determines the patient's need for specialty care and any resulting referrals.

Consolidated Omnibus Budget Reconciliation Act (COBRA)

COBRA is a law passed by the U.S. Congress on a reconciliation basis and signed by President Ronald Reagan in 1985 that, among other things, requires employers to allow an employee to continue health insurance coverage for a period of time after leaving employment, death of a spouse, a decrease in hours, or a divorce.

Government Health Insurance

Medicare, Medicaid, and the Federal Employees Health Benefit Plans are the U.S. government health plans.

Medicare

Created in 1965 through the extension of title XVII of the Social Security Act, Medicare insures people over 65, the disabled, and renal dialysis and transplant patients without regard to income level. Medicare is administered by the Center for Medicare and Medicaid Services (CMS), an agency within the U.S. Department of Health and Human Services. **Table 2-1** provides a list of common Medicare terminology. Medicare is funded by a special payroll tax under the Federal Insurance Contributions Act (FICA). Beneficiaries must pay premiums, deductibles, and coinsurance. **Table 2-2** gives the details for each Medicare plan.

Medicaid

A joint state and federal program mandated by title XIX of the Social Security Act, Medicaid pays for medical and other services on behalf of certain low-income groups (the poor, elderly, and disabled who do not receive Medicare, regardless of age):

- State governments set the rules for Medicaid, which means that the individual states determine the eligibility, scope, duration, and amount of services provided, and these are subject to change.
- Preauthorization is needed by a physician before treatment can begin (according to the Medicaid managed care option under section 1915(b) of the Social Security Act).

TABLE 2-1 Medicare Terminology

Term	Description
Balanced Budget Act of 1997 (BBA)	This law made sweeping changes in the Medicare and Medicaid programs. Several of the significant provisions of the BBA were payment reductions to healthcare providers, new prospective payment systems for healthcare providers, and reduction of coverage of healthcare services by the Medicare and Medicaid programs.
Health Care Financing Administration (HCFA)	Previous name for Center for Medicare and Medicaid Services (CMS).
Medicare Bonus Payment	An additional 10% payment to the physician above the allowed charge for services delivered to Medicare Beneficiaries in designated Health Professional Shortage Areas.
Medicare Cost HMO or Contract	Prospective payment for acute and primary healthcare (monthly fee per patient with settlement annually based on actual costs). Primarily used in rural areas where full capitation is not feasible.
Medicare Cost Report (MCR)	An annual report required of all institutions participating in the Medicare program. The MCR records each institution's total costs and charges associated with providing services to all patients, the portion of those costs and charges allocated to Medicare patients, and the Medicare payments received.
Medicare Insured Group (MIG)	Employer (or union) groups receiving a capitated rate from Medicare in exchange for integrating Medicare-covered services into the employer's own traditional retiree health plan.
Medicare Payment Advisory Commission (MedPAC)	A nonpartisan congressional advisory body charged with providing policy advice and technical assistance concerning the Medicare program and other aspects of the health system. It conducts independent research, analyzes legislation, and makes recommendations to Congress. The Physician Payment Review Commission (PPRC) has been merged with the Prospective Payment Assessment Commission (ProPAC) to create MedPAC.
Medicare Provider Analysis and Review File (MedPAR)	An HCFA data file that contains charge data and clinical characteristics, such as diagnoses and procedures, for every hospital inpatient bill submitted to Medicare for payment.

(continued)

| TABLE 2-1 | Medicare Terminology (continued) |

Medicare Risk Contract	A contract between Medicare and a health plan under which the plan receives monthly capitated payments to provide Medicare-covered services for enrollees, and thereby assumes insurance risk for those enrollees. A plan is eligible for a risk contract if it is a federally qualified HMO or a competitive medical plan.
Medicare Secondary Payer	Is implemented when rates are set higher than actual costs to recover *unreimbursed* costs from government, uninsured, underinsured, and other payers.
Medigap	A policy guaranteeing to pay a Medicare beneficiary's co-insurance, deductible, and co-payments and one that will provide additional health plan or nonMedicare coverage for services up to a predefined benefit limit. In essence, the product pays for the portion of the cost of services not covered by Medicare.
Medicare Select	A form of Medigap insurance that allows insurers to experiment with the provision of supplemental benefits through a network of providers. Coverage is often limited to those services furnished by the participating network providers and emergency out-of-area care.
Medicare Self Referral Option	A Medicare + Choice (Part C) point-of-service option that allows enrollees in a Medicare-risk HMO to go out of plan at a higher cost.
Medicare Supplement Policy	See Medigap.
Medicare Waiver (222)	Section of the Social Security Amendments of 1972 allowing the federal government to waive Medicare payment rules and allow alternative payment methods, including capitation.

TABLE 2-2	Types of Medicare Insurance

Part A Medicare hospital insurance that helps pay for medically necessary inpatient hospital care (with a limit on the number of hospital days), and, after a hospital stay and limited inpatient care in a skilled nursing facility, for limited home healthcare (Medicare pays 80%) or hospice care	Provides basic protection against the cost of health care. Does not cover all medical expenses or the cost of long-term care. Provides coverage for patients who have been on Social Security disability for 24 months. Requires annual deductible fees to be paid by the patient.
Part B Medicare medical insurance	Helps pay for: • Medically necessary physician services. • Outpatient hospital services and supplies that are not covered by the hospital insurance (laboratory tests and x-rays). • Ambulance transportation. • Outpatient physical and occupational therapy services (hospital and private practice). • Home healthcare provided by a physical therapist in independent practice. • Durable medical equipment (e.g., wheelchairs, canes, walkers) that is determined to be "medically necessary" by the physician. • Medical supplies that the hospital insurance does not cover. Each patient must pay a monthly premium. Physical therapy treatment does not need to be given on a daily basis. The physician responsible for the care of the patient referred for physical therapy must certify the plan of care minimally every 30 days.
Part C Medicare + Choice	A Medicare program under which eligible Medicare enrollees can elect to receive benefits through a managed care program that places providers at risk for those benefits.

- Many states have adopted HMO-like models to manage their Medicaid programs.
- Payments are sent directly to the healthcare providers, not the patient.
- The patient may be responsible for a copayment for some services.

● Key Point Medicaid ranks second only to education as an expense at the state level, and it is expected to grow four times faster than any other area of expense in the coming years. Because of the growing expense, states that once had generous policies are cutting back and in some cases capping the number of people served by a program.

● Key Point Medicaid waivers are an exception to the usual requirements of Medicaid granted to a state by CMS. States may:

- Waive provisions of Medicaid law to test new concepts that are consistent with the goals of the Medicaid program. System-wide changes are possible under this provision. These waivers are frequently used to establish Medicaid managed care programs.
- Waive freedom of choice. States may require that beneficiaries enroll in HMOs or other managed care programs, or select a physician to serve as their primary care case manager.
- Waive various Medicaid requirements to establish alternative, community-based services for (a) individuals who would otherwise require the level of care provided in a hospital or skilled nursing facility, and/or (b) people already in such facilities who need assistance returning to the community. Target populations for 1915(c) waivers include older adults, people with disabilities, people with mental retardation, people with chronic mental illness, and people with AIDS.
- Limit expenditures for nursing facility and home and community-based services for people 65 years and older so that they do not exceed a projected amount. The amount is determined by taking the base year expenditure (the last year before the waiver) and adjusting for inflation. This eliminates requirements that programs be statewide and be comparable for all target populations. Income rules for eligibility can also be waived.

Although the number of uninsured people is high, the uninsured have some recourse to emergency treatment:

- Hospital emergency rooms (those that receive tax exemption, federal Hill–Burton grants, or loans) are not allowed to turn away patients because of inability to pay. However, care is limited to emergency care only and does not include routine care.
- The costs incurred by this population are covered by a surcharge on insurance payments.

HCFA Common Procedural Coding System

The HCFA Common Procedural Coding System (HCPCS) is a federal coding system for medical procedures. HCPCS includes CPT (Current Procedural Terminology) codes, national alphanumeric codes, and local alphanumeric codes. The national codes are developed by the CMS to supplement CPT codes. They include physician services not included in CPT as well as non-physician services, such as ambulance service, physical therapy, and durable medical equipment. The local codes are developed by local Medicare carriers to supplement the national codes. HCPCS codes are five-digit codes made up of a letter followed by four numbers. HCPCS codes beginning with A through V are national; those beginning with W through Z are local.

● Key Point The majority of codes used in physical therapy billing are in the CPT 97000 series.

International Classification of Disease Codes

The International Classification of Disease (ICD) coding has been selected as part of the code standard under HIPAA to describe diseases and other health problems in electronic transactions using 17 categories based on etiology and affected anatomical systems.

● Key Point ICD codes were originally developed to classify and code mortality data, such as from death certificates. In its expanded "clinical modification" (ICD-CM), it has come to be used for morbidity (illness and disease) data in a broad range of settings, such as inpatient and outpatient clinic records, physician offices, and other surveys.

ICD is divided into categories based on a five-digit code (which limits the size of the vocabulary). The first three digits represent the basic diagnosis, and the last two digits add more specific information. For example, 710 is used to represent *diffuse diseases of connective tissue*, whereas 710.1 is used for *systemic sclerosis*.

● Key Point CPT/HCPCS procedural coding must match the ICD-9 diagnostic coding to determine appropriateness of procedures.

Fee-for-Service

Fee-for-service plans have the following characteristics:

- There is no "defined population" for which the insurance company is responsible.
- Contacts with the system are initiated by patients.
- Neither physicians nor insurance companies are responsible for providing care beyond what is indicated when patients seek care.

- The insurance company has no managerial control over the providers, and there is no capacity for centralized decision making.

The disadvantages cited for this type of plan are:

- The insurance company is not responsible for the overall health of its subscribers or for the quality of care delivered by individual physicians.
- Physicians alone decide what care their patients should receive.
- Where there is uncertainty about the appropriate level of care, physicians have a financial incentive to overuse care.

> ● **Key Point** In fee-for-service plans, physicians have income incentives to maximize the services they deliver to patients, whereas administrators have market incentives to keep premiums low.

Workers' Compensation

Workers' compensation programs were established and are regulated by state law to provide medical benefits and compensation for injuries and diseases that occur in the course of employment. Workers' compensation is financed by covered employers that are insured or self-insured under property and casualty lines and is mandatory for employers in almost all states. All large employers (10 or more employees) or high-risk employers must contribute to workers' compensation.

Some states limit the number of visits to obtain a diagnosis and/or require a preapproval process be followed for reimbursement. Other states require the total number of visits or total number of weeks (duration) and the number of treatments per week (frequency) to be usual, customary, and reasonable.

> ● **Key Point** An estimated 34 million Americans do not have health insurance. Of these, 56% are workers, 28% are children, and 16.5% are nonworking adults. Eighty-three percent of workers have private health insurance. Individuals who cannot pay for health care can receive pro bono or free care through philanthropic donations and services.
> The federal Hill–Burton Act was enacted in 1947 to support the construction and modernization of healthcare institutions. Hospitals that receive Hill–Burton funds must provide specific levels of charity care.

Consumer-Driven Healthcare Programs

Consumer-driven health (CDH) care is a new paradigm for healthcare delivery. Defined narrowly, CDH care refers to health plans in which individuals have a personal health savings account (HSA) or a health reimbursement arrangement (HRA) from which they pay medical expenses directly while a high-deductible health insurance policy protects them from catastrophic medical expenses. High-deductible policies cost less, but the user pays routine medical claims using a pre-funded spending account, often with a special debit card provided by a bank or insurance plan. The main characterisitics of CDH care include:

- Those who opt for plans with high benefit levels may have to contribute a significant amount of their own money in addition to an employer's contribution, whereas those with more basic coverage contribute less of their own money.
- More choice and greater control over one's health plan are characteristics of a consumer-driven healthcare marketplace. Members have economic incentives to better manage their own care—they realize economic rewards for making good decisions and bear economic penalties for making ill-advised ones.

Controlling Quality of Care

In the United States, healthcare regulation is undertaken to improve performance and quality through an enormous variety of different governmental and nongovernmental agencies. These entities have varying statutory authority, scope and remit, approaches and outcomes, resulting in a complex, overlapping, duplicative, and sometimes contradictory regulatory environment.

Fiscal Regulations

Regulatory controls within the U.S. healthcare system include the fraud and abuse provisions included in the Health Insurance Portability and Accountability Act (HIPAA) of 1996 and the 1997 Balanced Budget Act.

Certificate of Need Regulations

Certificate of need (CON) laws are intended to regulate major capital expenditures, which may adversely impact the cost of healthcare services, to prevent the unnecessary expansion of healthcare facilities, and to encourage the appropriate allocation of resources for healthcare purposes. CON laws became part of almost every state by 1978 after the 1974 National Health Act was passed.

Patient Self-Determination Act

The Patient Self-Determination Act (PSDA) of 1990 requires many Medicare and Medicaid providers (hospitals, nursing homes, hospice programs, home health agencies, and HMOs) to give adult individuals, at the time of inpatient admission or enrollment, certain information about their rights under state laws governing advance directives, including:

1. The right to participate in and direct their own healthcare decisions
2. The right to accept or refuse medical or surgical treatment
3. The right to prepare an advance directive
4. Information on the provider's policies that govern the utilization of these rights

The act also prohibits institutions from discriminating against a patient who does not have an advance directive.

● **Key Point**   An advance directive is a written instruction, such as a living will or a durable power of attorney for health care, that provides instructions for the provision of medical treatment *in anticipation* of those times when the individual executing the document no longer has decision-making capacity.

Accreditation

A number of regulations exist within the U.S. healthcare system that attempt to ensure quality of care. These include:

- Hospital accreditation and licensure, which includes Medicare conditions of participation (COP), and The Joint Commission (TJC) (see "Voluntary Accreditation" section)
- State accreditation and licensure, including the Department of Health
- Nursing home accreditation and licensure (including TJC; COP; the Nursing Home Reform Act, part of the Omnibus Budget Reconciliation Act of 1987; and state regulations)

● **Key Point**   The goal of the Occupational Safety and Health Administration (OSHA) is to create a safe and healthful working environment for employees. Employers must provide a working environment that is free from recognized hazards, and employees must adhere to health and safety standards. The National Institute for Safety and Health (NIOSH) is the research arm of OSHA. NIOSH has developed *Elements of Ergonomics Programs*, a primer based on workplace evaluations of musculoskeletal disorders that is useful in developing ergonomics programs.

Health Professionals Regulation

Under the federal system of government in the United States, each state regulates health care professionals' practice. Health professional practice acts are statutory laws that establish licensing or regulatory agencies or boards to generate rules that regulate medical practice. State licensing statutes establish the minimum level of education and experience required to practice, define the functions of the profession, and limit the performance of these functions to licensed persons.

Health Insurance Regulation

Health insurance regulation occurs at both the federal and state levels. Such regulations cover the gamut, regulating Blue Cross and Blue Shield carriers (which, if not for-profit, are often regulated somewhat differently than their commercial counterparts), commercial insurance companies, self-insured plans, and various flavors of managed care, including HMOs and PPOs. These entities write group coverage for employers, associations, or similar groups, as well as provide individual coverage.

Access-Related Insurance Regulations

A number of regulations monitor the accessibility of health care. These include:

- The Health Maintenance Organization Act of 1973
- Antidiscrimination restrictions (including the Rehabilitation Act of 1973, Pregnancy Discrimination Act of 1978, Americans with Disabilities Act of 1990, and Child Abuse Prevention and Treatment Act Amendments of 1984)
- Continuation of coverage requirements (including the Consolidated Omnibus Reconciliation Act of 1986 and state rules)
- Mandated health benefits (including mandated standards of care such as bone marrow transplants)

There are three federally mandated health insurance benefits:

- Mental Health Parity Act of 1996
- Newborns' and Mothers' Protection Health Act of 1996
- Women's Health and Cancer Rights Act of 1998

Voluntary Accreditation

Accreditation of healthcare institutions is a voluntary process by which an authorized agency or organization evaluates and recognizes health services according to a set of standards describing the structures and processes that contribute to desirable patient outcomes. Accreditation is not new to the health system. The first initiative toward accreditation was taken in the United States as early as 1910.

Voluntary Accrediting Agencies

Outpatient centers for comprehensive rehabilitation can be accredited by TJC, AC-MRDD, and/or CARF.

The Joint Commission

The Joint Commision (TJC) is a private organization created in 1951 to provide voluntary accreditation to hospitals. Many states rely on TJC accreditation as a substitute for their own inspection programs. In 1964, the TJC began charging hospitals for the surveys it performed. TJC has high standards of quality assurance and rigorous process of evaluation, which makes it a much-esteemed agency for accreditation. Health services certified by TJC are given "deemed status" (in 1965, Congress passed amendments to the Social Security Act stating that hospitals accredited by TJC are "deemed" to be in compliance with most of Medicare's "Conditions of Participation for Hospitals" and therefore are able to participate in Medicare and Medicaid and are eligible for millions of federal healthcare dollars.)

> ● **Key Point** The Joint Commission requires that all electrical equipment in hospitals be inspected every 12 months.

Over a period of time, after several experiments, TJC established itself as an esteemed accreditation body by 1987. In the 1990s, TJC revised its standards to reflect the changing functions of hospitals, seeking to move away from departments toward patient experience of hospital systems. Recently, TJC has moved toward trying to find standards that reflect the integration of hospital services rather than examining them in isolation. It also has begun to examine outcome measures instead of simple process standards for good practice. TJC accredits more than 80% of the nation's hospitals. It also accredits skilled nursing facilities, hospices, health plans, and other care organizations that provide home care, mental health care, laboratory, ambulatory care, and long-term services.

The Joint Commission does have some disadvantages:

- Hospitals pay for TJC surveys, and more than 70% of TJC's revenue comes directly from the organizations it is supposed to inspect.

- Hospitals and other healthcare providers are notified weeks or months in advance that a TJC survey team will be arriving–giving the provider plenty of time to make cosmetic changes, prepare staff to answer questions, update patient and personnel records, and increase staff levels.
- Although TJC encourages workers to speak with survey takers, most workers do not have legal protection from retaliation if they do so.

> ● **Key Point** The Joint Commission evaluates hospitals every three years.

Accreditation Council for Services for Mentally Retarded and Other Developmentally Disabled Persons

The Accreditation Council for Services for Mentally Retarded and Other Developmentally Disabled Persons (AC-MRDD) is a voluntary agency that accredits programs or agencies that serve people with developmental disabilities.

Commission on Accreditation of Rehabilitation Facilities

The Commission on Accreditation of Rehabilitation Facilities (CARF) is a nonprofit organization designed to recognize standards of excellence in rehabilitation programs across the nation. CARF accreditation standards were developed with the input of consumers, rehabilitation professionals, state and national organizations, and third-party purchasers. It is designed to establish standards of quality for freestanding rehabilitation facilities and the rehabilitative programs of larger hospital systems in the areas of behavioral health, employment (work hardening programs) and community support services, and medical rehabilitation (spinal cord injury, chronic pain), and to determine how well an organization is serving its patients, consumers, and the community. Programs accredited by CARF have demonstrated that they meet the national standards for rehabilitation programs.

Comprehensive Outpatient Rehabilitation Facility

A comprehensive outpatient rehabilitation facility (CORF) is a nonresidential facility established and operated exclusively for the purpose of providing diagnostic, therapeutic, and restorative services for the rehabilitation of injured, disabled, or sick people, at a single fixed location, by or under the supervision of a physician. At minimum, these facilities must provide physician services, physical therapy, and social or psychological services. With the exception of physical therapy, speech pathology, and occupational therapy, services must be provided on the facility's premises. However, one visit to the patient's home is covered to evaluate the home environment in relation to the patient's treatment plan. A CORF must have only one location. If other institutions, such as hospitals, establish a comprehensive outpatient rehabilitation facility, it must be functionally and operationally independent. The CORF accreditation group conducts certification surveys for compliance with federal and state regulations and investigates any complaints filed against one of these providers. Certification is achieved by adherence to federal requirements, including:

- Submission of a complete application
- Required documentation
- Successful completion of a survey

In accordance with federal directives, up to 16.6% of CORFs are surveyed annually. Each CORF must be surveyed for certification as directed by the Centers for Medicare and Medicaid Services (CMS). An application for certification includes submission of a completed application, required documentation, and successful completion of a survey. There are no fees and no renewal applications required for certification. There are no state licensing requirements imposed by the agency.

The typical accreditation process involves several steps:

1. The organization submits an application for review.
2. A survey is conducted by the accrediting agency.
3. The organization conducts a self-study or self-assessment to examine itself based on the accrediting agency standards.
4. An individual reviewer or surveyor, or a team visiting the organization, conducts an on-site review.
5. The whole staff of the organization is involved in the accreditation and reaccreditation process. Tasks include document preparation, hosting the site visit team, and participating in interviews with the accreditors.
6. The accreditation surveyor or team issues a report granting or denying accreditation.

If accredited, the organization undergoes periodic review, typically every three years. Some accrediting bodies may perform unannounced or unscheduled site surveys to ensure ongoing compliance.

Health Insurance and Portability Accountability Act

The purpose of the Health Insurance and Portability Accountability Act (HIPAA) is to provide a mechanism to spread the risk of unforeseen medical expenditures across a broad base to protect the individual from personal expenditures. The 1996 federal legislation makes long-term care insurance premiums tax deductible if nonreimbursable medical expenses, including part or all of long-term care premiums, exceed 7.5% of an individual's gross income. HIPAA also excludes long-term care insurance benefits from taxable income. Not all long-term care insurance coverage qualifies for this benefit.

HIPAA Privacy Rule

The U.S. Department of Health and Human Services (HHS) issued the Privacy Rule to implement the requirement of the HIPAA Act of 1996.

- The Privacy Rule standards address the use and disclosure of individuals' health information (protected health information [PHI]) by organizations subject to the Privacy Rule ("covered entities") as well as standards for individuals' rights to understand and control how their health information is used.
- A major goal of the Privacy Rule is to ensure that individuals' health information is properly protected while allowing the flow of health information needed to provide and promote high quality health care and to protect the public's health and well-being.
- The Privacy Rule applies to those who transmit health information in electronic form in connection with transactions.
- The Privacy Rule protects all "individually identifiable health information" (PHI) held or transmitted by a covered entity (health plans, healthcare clearinghouses, and any healthcare provider) or its business associate (limited to legal, actuarial, accounting, consulting, data aggregation, management, administrative, accreditation, or financial services), in any form or media, whether electronic, paper, or oral.

Ethical Issues

Ethics, also known as moral philosophy, is a branch of philosophy that addresses questions about morality, justice, right versus wrong, free will, and honesty.

Malpractice

Malpractice can be defined as a dereliction from professional duty or a failure to exercise an accepted degree of professional skill or learning by one rendering professional services that results in injury, loss, or damage. Malpractice also encompasses an injurious, negligent, or improper practice. PTAs

are personally responsible for negligence and other acts that result in harm to a patient through professional/patient relationships. *Negligence* is defined as failure to do what reasonably competent practitioners would have done under similar circumstances. To find a practitioner negligent, harm must have occurred to the patient. Examples include:

- Causing a burn with a hot pack
- Using defective equipment that leads to injury
- Failing to prevent a patient from falling
- Causing an injury to a patient through improper prescription of exercises
- Performing any action or inaction that is inconsistent with the Code of Ethics or the Standards of Practice (see Chapter 1)

Sexual Harassment

Sexual harassment is bullying, intimidation, or coercion of a sexual or gender-based nature, or the unwelcome or inappropriate promise of rewards in exchange for sexual favors. Often, but not always, the harasser is in a position of power or authority over the victim (due to differences in age, or social, political, educational, or employment relationships). Sexual harassment in the workplace involves the following:

- Submission to the conduct is made either explicitly or implicitly a term or condition of an individual's employment
- Submission to or rejection of the conduct by an individual is used as a basis for employment decisions affecting such individual
- The conduct has the purpose or effect of unreasonably interfering with an individual's work performance or creating an intimidating, hostile, or offensive working environment

Informed Consent

Informed consent is the process by which a fully informed individual can participate in choices about his or her health care. It originates from the legal and ethical right the patient has to direct what happens to his or her body and from the ethical duty of the physician to involve the patient in his or her health care. The most important goal of informed consent is that the patient must have an opportunity to be an informed participant in his or her healthcare decisions. Basic consent entails letting the patient know what you would like to do and asking the person if that will be all right. The more formal process should include cover the following elements:

- The nature of the decision/procedure
- Reasonable alternatives to the proposed intervention
- Relevant risks, benefits, and uncertainties related to each alternative
- Assessment of patient understanding
- The acceptance of the intervention by the patient

Americans with Disabilities Act

The Americans with Disabilities Act (ADA) of 1989[2] marked the first explicit national goal of achieving equal opportunity, independent living, and economic self-sufficiency for individuals with disabilities.[3] To qualify as a person with disability, the individual must have a physical or mental impairment that substantially limits the performance of one or more major life activities (**Table 2-3**).

The ADA secures equal opportunity for individuals with disabilities in employment, public

TABLE 2-3	**ADA Major Life Activities**

Social/Emotional

Interaction with others (e.g., speech difficulties such as pressured speech, lack of clarity, withdrawal, or responding with difficulty or too quickly; self-absorption; inability to relate to or listen to others, including inability to relate due to paranoia, delusions, hallucinations, obsessive–compulsive ideation, negativity; inability to regulate mood and anxiety; inability to maintain appropriate distance from others)

Forming and maintaining relationships with others

Communication with others (e.g., answering questions, following directions, using intelligible speech, recognizing and expressing emotions appropriately, expressing needs, following a sequence)

Cognitive

Concentration (as a major life activity itself and also resulting in limitations on other major life activities, such as interaction with others, self-care)

Making decisions

Complex thinking (e.g., planning, reconciling perceptions from different senses such as seeing and hearing, sorting relevant from irrelevant details, problem solving, changing from one task to another)

Abstract thinking (e.g., generalizing or transferring learning from one setting to another, such as transferring skill of cooking in one kitchen to another kitchen)

Memory (long- or short-term)

Attention

Perception

Distinguishing real from unreal events

Initiating and completing actions

Processing information

Physical

Taking care of personal needs, such as eating, dressing, toileting, bathing, hygiene, household chores, managing money, following medication or treatment regimens, following safety precautions

Eating (e.g., regulating amounts appropriately, maintaining appropriate diet, need for strict eating schedule)

Sleeping (e.g., ability to fall asleep, obtain restful sleep, or sleep without interruption; avoiding excessive sleeping)

Reproduction

Sexual activity

Traveling

accommodations, transportation, state and local government services, and telecommunications. Title III of the ADA applies to entities that are open to the public (**Table 2-4**). Some examples of public accommodations are as follows:

- Restaurants
- Hotels
- Theaters
- Retail stores and shopping centers
- Grocery stores
- Parks that are not owned by the government
- Hospitals, doctor's offices, and outpatient clinics
- Law offices

Public accommodations must make reasonable modifications in policies, practices, and procedures that deny equal access to individuals with disabilities. However, a public accommodation does not have

TABLE 2-4	ADA Accessibility Requirements	
Structure	**Requirement**
Doorways	Minimum width of 32 inches
	Maximum depth of 24 inches
Thresholds	Less than ¾ inch for sliding doors
	Less than ½ inch for other doors
Ramps	Minimum width of 36 inches
	Must have hand rails on both sides
	12 inches of length for each inch of vertical rise
	Handrails required for a rise of 6 inches or more or for horizontal runs of 72 inches or more
	Grade ≤ 8.3%
Carpet	Requires ½-inch pile or less
Hallway clearance	36-inch width
Wheelchair turning radius (U-turn)	60-inch width
	78-inch length
Forward reach in wheelchair	Low reach 15 inches
	High reach 48 inches
Side reach in wheelchair	Reach over obstruction to 24 inches
Bathroom sink	Not less than 29 inches in height
	Not greater than 40 inches from floor to bottom of mirror or paper dispenser 17 inches minimum depth under sink to back wall
Bathroom toilet	17–19 inches from floor to top of toilet
	Not less than 36-inch grab bars
	Grab bars should be 1¼–1½ inches in diameter
	1½-inch spacing between grab bars and wall
	Grab bar placement 33 to 36 inches up from floor level
Hotels	Approximately 2% of total rooms must be accessible
Parking spaces	96 inches wide
	240 inches in length
	Adjacent aisle must be 60 by 240 inches.
	Approximately 2% of the total spaces in a parking lot must be accessible

to modify a policy if it would greatly alter its goods, services, or operations. Other impacts of the ADA include:

- Employers may not ask job applicants about medical information or require a physical examination prior to offering employment.
- After employment is offered, an employer can ask for a medical examination only if it is required of all employees holding similar jobs.
- If an individual is turned down for work based on the results of a medical examination, the employer must prove that it is physically impossible for the person to do the work required.

Statutory Laws

Statutes are defined as laws that are passed by Congress and the various state legislatures. These statutes are the basis for statutory law. The legislature passes statutes that are later put into the federal code of laws or pertinent state code of laws. Statutory law consists of the acts of legislatures declaring, commanding or prohibiting something; a particular law established by the will of the legislative department of government. A number of statutory laws impact physical therapy.

The Individuals with Disabilities Education Act

The Individuals with Disabilities Education Act (IDEA) is a federal law that governs how states and public agencies provide early intervention, special education, and related services to children with disabilities. Under the requirements of the IDEA, the educational needs of children with disabilities from birth to age 21 are addressed in cases that involve 13 specified categories of disability. This provision is based on an individualized plan (see Chapter 10).

Licensure

Professional licensing laws are enacted by all states. These laws are designed to protect the consumer against professional incompetence and exploitation by opportunists. They also make a determination as to the minimal standards of education. In the case of physical therapy, the minimal licensing requirements include:

- Graduation from an accredited program or its equivalent in physical therapy.
- Successful completion of a national licensing examination. Licensure examination and related

activities are the responsibility of the Federation of State Boards of Physical Therapy. All states belong to this association.

- Ethical and legal standards relating to continuing practice of physical therapy.
- All PTAs must have a license to practice. Each state determines criteria to practice and issue a license.

Workers' Compensation Acts

The rules and regulations of individual states' workers' compensation systems are the primary factors influencing the provision of physical therapy services for patients with work-related injuries. Workers' compensation laws are designed to ensure that employees who are injured or disabled on the job are provided with fixed monetary awards, eliminating the need for litigation. The laws provide a no-fault system that pays all medical benefits and replaces salary (usually at 66%) until recovery occurs. In turn, employees forfeit the right to sue their employers for damages. The laws vary from state to state, but most states identify four types of disability:

- *Temporary partial:* The injured worker is able to do some work but is still recuperating from the effects of the injury and is, thus, temporarily limited in the amount or type of work that can be performed compared with the pre-injury work.
- *Temporary total:* The injured worker is unable to work during a period when he or she is under active medical care and has not yet reached what is called "maximum medical improvement."
- *Permanent partial:* The injured worker is capable of employment but is not able to return to the former job. Benefits are usually paid according to a prescribed schedule for a fixed number of weeks.
- *Permanent total:* The injured worker cannot return to any gainful employment. Lifetime benefits are provided to the employee.

REVIEW Questions

1. What is HMO an acronym for?
2. In an HMO setup, which individual serves as a gatekeeper for the insurance company by being responsible for the authorization of specialty

services, and who receives bonuses based on how much they conserve medical resources?

3. True or false: Medicare and Medicaid are government-funded programs.

4. True or false: Medicare is funded by special contributions by members of the U.S. Senate.

5. What is the State Children's Health Insurance Program (SCHIP)?

6. Who does the Ryan White Act provide funds for to cover the cost of medications?

7. What is the purpose of the Certificate of Need (CON) laws?

8. What is an advance directive?

9. Which act secures equal opportunity for individuals with disabilities in employment, public accommodations, transportation, state and local government services, and telecommunications?

10. The WorkAgain Center, specializing in work hardening and conditioning, is scheduled for an accreditation survey. The appropriate agency to conduct this program is:
    a. The Commission on Accreditation of Rehabilitation Facilities (CARF)
    b. The Joint Commission (TJC)
    c. The Occupational Safety and Health Administration (OSHA)
    d. The Department of Health and Human Services

11. How often does The Joint Commission (TJC) survey hospitals?
    a. Once per year
    b. Every 2 years
    c. Every 3 years
    d. Every 5 years

12. Which of the following is a correct statement about Medicare?
    a. Medicare Part A is only for patients over 85 years old.
    b. Medicare Part B is only for patients 65–84 years old.
    c. Medicare Part A is only for inpatient treatment.
    d. Medicare Part B is only for use in long-term facilities.

13. Under what part of Medicare are outpatient physical therapy services reimbursed for?
    a. Part A
    b. Part B
    c. Part C
    d. Part D

14. Which act resulted in payment reductions to healthcare providers, new prospective payment systems for healthcare providers, and reduction of coverage of healthcare services by the Medicare and Medicaid programs?

15. What was the purpose of the Health Insurance and Portability Accountability Act (HIPAA)?

16. True or false: A major goal of HIPAA's Privacy Rule is to ensure that individuals' health information is properly protected while allowing the flow of health information needed to provide and promote high-quality health care and to protect the public's health and well-being.

17. Which type of health insurance plan allows individuals to have a personal health account, such as a health savings account (HSA) or a health reimbursement arrangement (HRA), from which they pay medical expenses directly?

18. Define malpractice.

19. True or false: Every individual (PT, PTA, student PT, or student PTA) is liable for his or her own negligence.

20. How often does The Joint Commission (TJC) require that all electrical equipment in hospitals be inspected?
    a. Every 3 months
    b. Every 6 months
    c. Every 12 months
    d. Every 3 years

21. A 50-year-old steelworker, who is married with four children, has been laid off his job for the last year. The family is currently on welfare. While cutting his grass he has a stroke and is admitted to the hospital. In this case, the third-party payer that would provide assistance is:
    a. Medicaid
    b. Workers' Compensation
    c. Medicare Part A
    d. Social Security

22. When billing Medicare, Medicaid, and many other third-party payers, providers are required to use the appropriate:
    a. CPT and Common Procedural Coding System procedure codes
    b. Current Procedural Terminology (CPT) procedure codes
    c. Common Procedural Coding System of Center for Medicare and Medicaid Services (CMS)
    d. Resource Based Relative Value Scale (RBRVS)

23. True or false: The PTA must obtain informed consent from the patient before an intervention is rendered.

References

1. Guide to Physical Therapist Practice (ed 2). Phys Ther 81:S13–S95, 2001
2. Americans with Disabilities Act of 1989: 104 Stat 327.101–336, 42 USC 12101 s2 (a) (8), 1989
3. Waddell G, Waddell H: A review of social influences on neck and back pain disability, in Nachemson AL, Jonsson E (eds): Neck and Back Pain: The Scientific Evidence of Causes, Diagnosis, and Treatment. Philadelphia, Lippincott Williams and Wilkins, 2000, pp 13–55

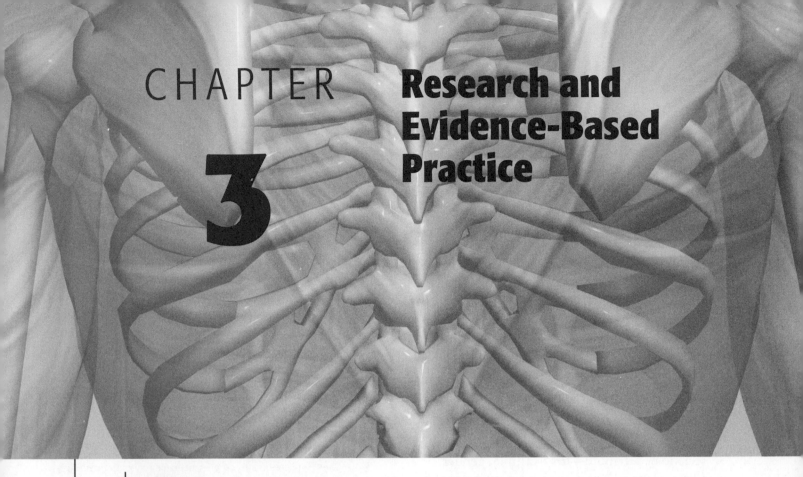

CHAPTER 3

Research and Evidence-Based Practice

Research

Research involves a controlled, systematic approach to obtain an answer to a question.[1] Three research types are recognized:

- *Experimental:* Involves the careful manipulation of a variable and measuring the effects of this manipulation.[1]
- *Historical:* The process of systematically examining past events to discover generalizations.[1]
- *Descriptive* (also known as *statistical research*): Describes data and characteristics about the population or phenomenon being studied by answering the questions who, what, where, when, and how.

Statistics is a branch of applied mathematics concerned with finding patterns in data and inferring connections between events.[2]

- *Descriptive statistics* describe what is or what the data shows. Descriptive statistics include the collection, organization, summarization, and presentation of data.[2]
- *Inferential statistics*, based on probability theory, are used to try to reach conclusions that extend beyond the immediate data alone.[2]

● **Key Point** Much of the initial groundwork in statistics concerns making an accurate guess, or hypothesis.

● **Key Point** A *population* consists of all subjects (human or otherwise) that are being studied. A *sample* is a group of subjects selected from a population. A *statistic* is a characteristic or measure obtained by using all the data values from a sample.

A valid informed consent for research purposes must include all of the following elements:

- An understandable explanation of the purpose and procedures to be used
- All reasonable and foreseeable risks and discomforts
- All potential benefits of participation

Variables

A *variable* is a measurement of phenomena that can assume more than one value or more than one category.[1] Two traits of a variable should always be achieved:

- Each variable should be *exhaustive*; it should include all possible answerable responses.
- Each variable should be *mutually exclusive*; no respondent should be able to have two attributes simultaneously.

Variables can be classified as:

- *Qualitative:* A variable that can be placed into a distinct category according to some characteristic or attribute—for example, gender.
- *Quantitative:* A variable that is numeric and can be ordered or ranked—for example, age, height, and weight.

Quantitative variables can be further classified into two groups:[2]

- *Discrete:* A variable that can assume only certain values that are countable—for example, number of children in a family.
- *Continuous:* A variable that can assume an infinite number of possible values in an interval between any two specific values—for example, temperature.

> **● Key Point** Dependency refers to the "role" of the variable in the experiment or study. The *independent variable* is manipulated by the researcher; independent variables are controlled or fixed in order to observe their effect on dependent variables—for example, a treatment or program or cause. The *dependent variable* is measured by the researcher. For example, if a study examines the effects of ice on pain levels, the ice is the independent variable and the measurement of pain levels is the dependent variable.

Levels of Measurement

The four classic scales (or levels) of measurement are:[2]

- *Nominal (Classificatory; Categorical):* Classifies data into mutually exclusive, exhaustive categories in which no order or ranking can be imposed. Examples include arbitrary labels, such as zip codes, religion, and marital status. This is the weakest level of measurement.
- *Ordinal (Ranking):* Classifies data into categories that can be ranked, although precise differences between the ranks do not exist. Examples include letter grades (e.g., A, B, C) and body builds (e.g., small, medium, large).
- *Interval:* Ranks data. Precise differences between units of measure do exist, although there is no meaningful zero. Examples include temperature (degrees centigrade, degrees Fahrenheit), IQ, and calendar dates.
- *Ratio:* Possesses all the characteristics of interval measurement, and there exists a true zero. Examples include height, weight, age, and salary.

Data Collection and Sampling Techniques

Researchers use samples to produce a representative sample of the target population.

> **● Key Point** *Bias* or *systematic error* refers to the tendency to consistently underestimate or overestimate a true value. *Probability* can be defined as the chance of an event occurring. The classic theory of probability states that the chance of a particular outcome occurring is determined by the ratio of the number of favorable outcomes (or successes) to the total number of outcomes.

Probability Sampling

Probability sampling is any method of sampling that utilizes some form of *random selection* and uses a process or procedure that ensures that the different units in the population have equal probabilities of being chosen. Four basic methods of probability sampling are employed:

- *Simple random sampling:* All items have some chance of selection that can be calculated, thereby minimizing sampling bias.
- *Systematic sampling:* Sometimes referred to as interval sampling, this means that there is a gap, or interval, between each selection (e.g., every 20th person).
- *Stratified random sampling:* Involves dividing the population into homogeneous subgroups called strata and then taking a simple random sample in each subgroup. Stratified sampling ensures that the overall population will be represented, as well as key subgroups of the population.
- *Cluster sampling:* Involves dividing the population into groups or clusters (such as geographic boundaries) and then randomly selecting

sample clusters and using all members of the selected clusters as subjects of the samples.

Nonprobability Sampling

Nonprobability sampling is any sampling method where some elements of the population have no chance of selection, or where the probability of selection cannot be accurately determined. This type of sampling is often utilized in physical therapy. Nonprobability sampling includes:

- *Accidental/convenience sampling:* Involves the sample being drawn from that part of the population that is close to hand.
- *Quota sampling:* The population is first segmented into mutually exclusive subgroups, and then a judgment is used to select the subjects or units from each segment based on a specified proportion (a sample of 200 females and 300 males between the ages of 45 and 60).
- *Purposive sampling:* The researcher chooses the sample based on who he or she thinks would be appropriate for the study. This method is used primarily when there is a limited number of people that have expertise in the area being researched.
- *Case study:* The research is limited to one group, often with a similar characteristic or of small size.

Measures of Central Tendency

When populations are small, it is not necessary to use samples because the entire population can be used to gain information. Measures found by using all the data values in the population are called *parameters*. Measures of central tendency are measures of the location of the middle or the center of a distribution where data tend to cluster. Multiple metrics are used to describe this clustering:

- *Mean:* The arithmetic mean is what is commonly called the average. When the word *mean* is used without a modifier, it can be assumed that it refers to the arithmetic mean. The mean of a sample is typically denoted as $\bar{x}$. The mean is the sum of all the scores divided by the number of scores.
- *Median:* The median is the middle of a distribution: half the scores are above the median and half are below the median. The median is less

sensitive to extreme scores than the mean, and this makes it a better measure than the mean for highly skewed distributions.

- *Mode:* The mode is the most frequently occurring score in a distribution. The advantage of the mode as a measure of central tendency is that its meaning is obvious. Further, it is the only measure of central tendency that can be used with nominal data.

Measures of Variation

Although measures of central tendency locate only the center of a distribution, other measures, such as a determination of the spread of a group of scores, are often needed to describe data. To examine the spread or variability of a data set, three measures are commonly used:[3]

- *Range:* The most elementary measure of variation, defined as the difference between the highest and lowest values (the highest value minus the lowest value).
- *Variance:* The average of the squares of the distance that each value is from the mean.
- *Standard deviation* (σ; SD): A determination of the spread of a group of scores; the average deviation of values around the mean. The SD is based on the distance of sample values from the mean and provides information about how tightly all the various examples are clustered around the mean in a set of data. When the examples are tightly bunched together and the bell-shaped curve is steep, the SD is small. When the examples are spread apart and the bell curve is relatively flat, the SD is relatively large. Mathematically, the standard deviation equals the square root of the mean of the square deviation, or the square root of the variance. The range can be used to approximate the standard deviation by dividing the range value by 4.

Measures of Position

In addition to measures of central tendency and measures of variation, measures of position are used to locate the relative position of a data value in the data set.[3] One of the most common measures of position is the percentile. Percentiles divide the data set into 100 equal groups. The Nth percentile is defined as the value such that N% of the value lies below it. For example, a score in the 95th percentile represents the top 5% of scores.

- The lower quartile is defined as the 25th percentile; 75% of the measures are above the lower quartile.
- The middle quartile is defined as the 50th percentile, which is the median of all the measures.
- The upper quartile is defined as the 75th percentile; 25% of the measures are above the upper quartile.

The Normal Distribution

Normal distributions are a family of distributions that have a symmetrical and general shape.

● **Key Point** The standard normal distribution is a normal distribution with a mean of 0 and a standard deviation of 1.

The mean, median, and mode of a normal distribution have the same value due to the symmetry of the bell-shaped distribution. The curve has no boundaries, and only a small fraction of the values fall outside of three standard deviations (a measure of how spread out a distribution is) above or below the mean:

- One standard deviation away from the mean in either direction on the horizontal axis accounts for approximately 68% of the people in the group.
- Two standard deviations away from the mean account for approximately 95% of the people.
- Three standard deviations account for about 99% of the people.

● **Key Point** The z value is actually the number of standard deviations that a particular x value is away from the mean.

● **Key Point** *Skewness* is a measure of the degree of asymmetry of a distribution.

- If the left tail (the tail at the small end of the distribution) is more pronounced than the right tail (the tail at the large end of the distribution), the mean and median are to the left of the mode and the distribution is said to have negative or left skewness.
- If the right tail is more pronounced that the left tail, the mean and median are to the right of the mode and the distribution has positive or right skewness.
- If the two halves of the curve are symmetrical (mirror images), the mean, the median, and the mode are all at the same point and the data distribution has zero skewness.

Evidence-Based Practice

Evidence-based practice (EBP), the integration of three key elements—best research evidence, clinical expertise, and patient values—is having an increasing impact on the profession of physical therapy.

● **Key Point** Sackett and colleagues[4] define *best evidence* as:

- Clinically relevant research, often from the basic sciences, but especially from patient-centered clinical research
- The accuracy and precision of diagnostic tests
- The power of prognostic markers
- The efficacy and safety of therapeutic, rehabilitative, and preventative regimens

Determining whether an approach is evidence-based involves a six-step process:

1. A clinical problem is identified and an answerable research question is formulated.
2. A systematic literature review is conducted and evidence collected.
3. The research evidence is summarized and critically analyzed.
4. The research evidence is synthesized and applied to clinical practice.
5. The outcomes of the selected action are assessed.
6. The findings are summarized for future reference.

Hierarchy of Evidence

When integrating evidence into clinical decision-making, an understanding of how to appraise the quality of the evidence offered by clinical studies is important. Judging the strength of the evidence becomes an important part of the decision-making process.

● **Key Point** Clinical prediction rules (CPRs) are tools designed to assist clinicians in decision-making when caring for patients. However, although there is a growing trend to produce a number of CPRs in the field of physical therapy, few CPRs currently exist.

A hierarchy of evidence reflects the relative authority of various types of research. Although there is no single, universally accepted hierarchy of evidence, there is broad agreement on the relative strength of the principal types of research.

Systematic Review

A *systematic review* is a comprehensive literature review focused on a single question that tries to identify, appraise, select, and synthesize all high-quality research evidence relevant to that question. Selection of the articles for inclusion is usually performed by reviewing the titles and abstracts of the articles identified and excluding those that do not meet the eligibility criteria. The aim of the systematic review is to minimize bias by using an objective and transparent approach for research synthesis. The best-known source of systematic reviews for healthcare is the Cochrane Database of Systematic Reviews section of the Cochrane Library.

Meta-Analysis

A *meta-analysis* combines the results of several randomized controlled studies that address a set of related research hypotheses. The advantages of meta-analysis include the ability both to control for between-study variation and to minimize the problem of small sample size. The disadvantages of using meta-analysis are that the sources of bias are not controlled by the method (a meta-analysis is a statistical examination of scientific studies, not an actual scientific study) and that it relies heavily on published studies, which may create exaggerated outcomes.

Randomized Controlled Trial

A *randomized controlled trial* (RCT) is a study in which people are allocated at random (by chance alone) to receive one of several clinical interventions. One of these interventions is the standard of comparison or control. The control may be a standard practice, a placebo ("sugar pill"), or no intervention at all. The most important advantage of proper randomization is that it eliminates selection bias, balancing both known and unknown prognostic factors, in the assignment of treatments.

> ● **Key Point** Randomized controlled trials (RCTs) provide the strongest, most relevant evidence to inform practice. Some evidence hierarchies place systematic review and meta-analysis above RCTs, since these often combine data from multiple RCTs, and possibly from other study types as well.

Cohort Study

A *cohort study* is an observational study of subjects who share a common characteristic or experience within a defined period. The study groups are observed over a period of time and compared with another group that is not affected by the condition under investigation. The advantages of cohort study data are the longitudinal observation of the individual through time and the collection of data at regular intervals, which reduces recall error. However, cohort studies are expensive to conduct, can be influenced by other lifestyle variables, and have a long follow-up time to generate useful data.

Case Control Study

Case control is a type of epidemiological study design that is used to identify factors that may contribute to a medical condition by comparing subjects who have that condition (the "cases") with patients who do not have the condition but are otherwise similar (the "controls"). Case-control studies are relatively inexpensive and frequently used, but their retrospective, nonrandomized nature limits the conclusions that can be drawn from them.

Cross-Sectional Study

Cross-sectional studies involve data collected at a single point in time (snapshot) in which groups can be compared at different ages with respect to independent variables (e.g., looking at a particular group to see if a substance or activity is related to the health effect being investigated). Cross-sectional research takes a "slice" of its target group and bases its overall finding on the views or behaviors of those targeted, assuming them to be typical of the whole group. This type of data is often used to assess the prevalence of acute or chronic conditions in a population.

Case Series

A *case series*, which can be either retrospective or prospective, is a study that tracks patients with a known exposure given similar treatment or examines their medical records for exposure and outcome. Case series may be confounded by selection bias, which limits the authority on the causality of correlations observed.

Case Report

A *case report* is a detailed report of the symptoms, signs, diagnosis, treatment, and follow-up of an individual patient. The most common use for a case report is to record and alert other health care professionals to rare occurrences. Because a case report is a type of anecdotal evidence, the findings are less scientifically rigorous than controlled clinical data.

Outcome Measurement Tools

The trend toward using outcome measures in the decision-making process is consistent with the evidence-based approach and represents the final step in the evaluation of clinical performance.[5,6] Outcome measurement is a process that describes a systematic method to gauge the effectiveness and efficiency of an intervention in daily clinical practice.[7] Effectiveness in this context refers to the validity and reliability of the tool. The efficiency of an intervention is a function of utilization (number of outpatient visits, length of inpatient stay) and the costs of care and outcome.

Outcome measurement tools can be divided into those that assess cognition, endurance, pain, balance, and mobility, and those that measure the performance of basic and instrumental activities of daily living (BADLs and IADLs).

Cognition Assessment Tools

The Mini Mental State Examination

The Mini Mental State Examination (MMSE) or Folstein test is a brief 30-point questionnaire that is commonly used to assess the severity of cognitive impairment at a given point in time and to follow the course of cognitive changes in an individual over time, thus making it an effective way to document an individual's response to treatment. The MMSE test includes simple questions and problems in a number of areas: the time and place of the test, the ability to repeat lists of words, arithmetic skills, language use and comprehension, and basic motor skills. Any score greater than or equal to 25 points (out of 30) is effectively normal (intact). Below this, scores can indicate severe ($\leq$ 9 points), moderate (10–20 points), or mild (21–24 points) impairment.

The Short Portable Mental Status Questionnaire

The Short Portable Mental Status Questionnaire (SPMSQ) is a 10-item screening tool used to detect the presence of intellectual impairment and to determine its degree, particularly in the elderly population. The maximum score is 10, and the following scoring system is used:

0–2 errors	normal mental functioning
3–4 errors	mild cognitive impairment
5–7 errors	moderate cognitive impairment
8 or more errors	severe cognitive impairment

The Instrumental Activities of Daily Living Scale

The Instrumental Activities of Daily Living (IADL) scale measures the functional impact of emotional and cognitive impairments by assessing a person's ability to perform tasks such as using a telephone, doing laundry, handling finances, and taking responsibility for medication intake. Measuring eight domains, the test can be administered in 10 to 15 minutes. The scale may provide an early warning of functional decline or signal the need for further assessment.

The Clock Drawing Test

This simple test is used as a part of a neurological test or as a screening tool for Alzheimer disease, general cognitive processing, and adaptive functioning such as memory. The person undergoing testing is asked to draw a clock, put in all the numbers, and then set the hands at 11:10. There are a number of scoring systems for this test. The Alzheimer disease cooperative scoring system is based on a score of 5 points:

1 point for the clock circle
1 point for all the numbers in the correct order
1 point for the numbers in the proper special order
1 point for the two hands of the clock
1 point for the correct time

A normal score is 4 or 5 points.

The Time and Change Test

The Time and Change (T&C) test is an easy and time-saving test validated for the detection of dementia. The T&C test is designed to assess how well a patient understands time and the ability of the patient to calculate using money. The "time" component of the T&C test evaluates the ability of a subject to comprehend that the hands of a clock indicate 11:10 while being timed. In the "change" component of the T&C test, the subject is required to provide change for a dollar using a variety of coins while being timed.

Endurance Assessment Tools

Visual Analog Scale

The Visual Analog Scale (VAS) relies upon an individual's self-report to measure dyspnea and is one of the easiest scales to use. It features a horizontal 10-centimeter line with descriptive phrases indicating minimal and maximal extremes of breathlessness at each end. The patient marks a point on the line that corresponds with his or her perception of the severity of the sensation. The interval is measured in millimeters along the line. Changes in perception of dyspnea are noted as moving toward less or more shortness of breath.

Baseline Dyspnea Index

The Baseline Dyspnea Index (BDI) is a scale designed to assess dyspnea using a multidimensional format to measure the associated effort and resultant impairment. The BDI rates the severity of dyspnea at a single point in time, and the transition dyspnea index (TDI) is used to note changes from the baseline assessment. Each index rates three different categories: magnitude of task, magnitude of effort, and functional impairment. Each category has five grades, ranging from severe to unimpaired.

Ventilatory Response Index

Previously referred to as the Dyspnea Index, the Ventilatory Response Index (VRI) was developed by physical therapists at Rancho Los Amigos Hospital in the late 1970s. The VRI is measured on a scale of 0 to 4 points. The individual inhales with a normal breath and then is instructed to try to count to 15 out loud over a period of 7.5 to 8 seconds. The number of additional breaths taken to complete the count of 15 correlates to a patient's level of intensity of exercise.

The Six-Minute Walk Test

The Six-Minute Walk Test (6MWT) is a useful instrument to assess a patient's functional exercise capacity. It requires a 100-foot hallway but no exercise equipment or advanced training, and its results are highly correlated with those of cycle ergometer–based or treadmill-based exercise tests. The 6MWT measures the distance that a patient can quickly walk on a flat, hard surface in 6 minutes and provides an assessment of the global and integrated responses of all the systems involved during exercise, including the pulmonary and cardiovascular systems, systemic circulation, peripheral circulation, blood, neuromuscular units, and muscle metabolism.

Borg Rating of Perceived Exertion Scale

An individual's perception of effort (relative perceived exertion) is closely related to the level of physiological effort.[9,10] A high correlation exists between a person's rating of perceived exertion (RPE) multiplied by 10 and his or her actual heart rate. For example, if a person's RPE is 12, $12 \times 10 = 120$, so the heart rate should be approximately 120 beats per minute. The original scale introduced by Borg[10] rated exertion on a scale of 6 to 20, but a more recent one designed by Borg included a category (C) ratio (R) scale, the Borg CR10 Scale® (**Table 3-1**). Note that this calculation is only an approximation of heart rate; the actual heart rate can vary quite a bit depending on age and physical condition. It is important, therefore, to closely monitor the patient's response to exercise.

Pain Assessment Tools

Brief Pain Inventory

The Brief Pain Inventory (BPI), based on the Wisconsin Brief Pain Questionnaire, is designed to provide information on the intensity of pain (the sensory dimension) as well as the degree to which pain interferes with function (the reactive dimension). The BPI

TABLE 3-1	Borg Rating of Perceived Exertion		
Traditional Scale	**Verbal Rating**	**Revised 10-Grade Scale**	**Verbal Rating**
6		0	Nothing at all
7	Very, very light	0.5	Very, very weak
8		1.0	Very weak
9	Very light	2.0	Weak (light)
10		3.0	Moderate
11	Fairly light	4.0	Somewhat strong
12		5.0	Strong (heavy)
13	Somewhat hard	6.0	
14		7.0	Very strong
15	Hard	8.0	
16		9.0	
17	Very hard	10.0	Very, very strong (almost maximum)
18			
19	Very, very hard		Maximal

Data from Borg GAV: Psychophysical basis of perceived exertion. Med Sci Sports Exerc 14:377–381, 1992

also asks questions about pain relief, pain quality, and the patient's perception of the cause of pain. For simplicity and lack of ambiguity, the BPI uses numeric rating scales (NRS) of 0 to 10. Since pain can be variable over a day, the BPI asks patients to rate their pain at the time of responding to the questionnaire (pain now), and also at its worst, least, and average over the previous week. The ratings can also be made for the past 24 hours.

McGill Pain Questionnaire

The McGill Pain Questionnaire (MPQ) is a self-report inventory of 78 pain descriptors distributed across 20 subcategories (with six additional descriptors in the present pain index). The subcategories are further grouped into three broad categories, termed sensory, affective, and evaluative, in addition to a miscellaneous category. The implication is that each word reflects a particular sensory quality of pain.

The patient is asked to indicate on a body diagram the location of the pain and to rate his or her symptoms based on the 20 categories of verbal descriptors of pain. The 20 categories are ranked according to severity. The patient is then asked to describe how the pain changes with time (continuous, rhythmic, or brief) and how strong the pain is (mild, discomforting, distressing, horrible, or excruciating). The most commonly reported measure from the MPQ instrument, the pain-rating index total, provides an estimate of overall pain intensity. This measure, obtained by summing all the descriptors selected from the 20 subclasses, has a possible range of 0 to78. Separate scores for each class can also be obtained.

Faces Pain Scale

The Faces Pain Scale (FPS) is a self-report measure used to assess the intensity of children's pain from age 4 or 5 onward. The FPS uses six different faces, from happy to tearful, to demonstrate how a person might be feeling. The person is asked to choose the face that best describes how he or she is feeling.

Balance and Mobility

Timed "Up & Go"

The timed "Up & Go" test evaluates gait and balance. The patient gets up out of a standard armchair (seat height of approximately 46 centimeters [18.4 inches]), walks a distance of 3 meters (10 feet), turns, walks back to the chair and sits down again. The patient wears regular footwear and, if applicable, uses any customary walking aid (e.g., cane, walker). No physical assistance is given. The clinician uses a stopwatch or a wristwatch with a secondhand to time this activity. A score of 30 seconds or greater indicates that the patient has impaired mobility and requires assistance (i.e., has a high risk of falling). This test has been shown to be as valid as sophisticated gait testing. A simpler alternative is the "Get Up and Go" test. In this test, the patient is seated in an armless chair placed 3 meters (10 feet) from a wall. The patient stands, walks toward the wall (using a walking aid if one is typically employed), turns without touching the wall, returns to the chair, turns, and sits down. This activity does not need to be timed. Instead, the clinician observes the patient and makes note of any balance or gait problems.

Berg Balance Scale

The Berg Balance Scale (BBS) was developed to measure balance among older people with impairment in balance function by assessing the performance of functional tasks. It is a valid instrument used for evaluation of the effectiveness of interventions and for quantitative descriptions of function in clinical practice and research. There are 14 tasks, each scored on a five-point ordinal scale from 0 to 4. Zero indicates the lowest level of function, and 4 the highest level of function. The maximum score is 56, with a score less than 45 indicating an increased risk for falling. A change of eight (8) BBS points is required to reveal a genuine change in function between two assessments among older people who are dependent in activities of daily living (ADL) and living in residential care facilities.

Tinetti Performance-Oriented Mobility Assessment

The Tinetti Performance-Oriented Mobility Assessment (POMA), also known as the Tinetti Gait and Balance Instrument or simply the Tinetti assessment tool, is an easily administered task-oriented test that measures an older adult's gait and balance abilities. The POMA is designed to determine an elder's risk for falls within the next year. It takes about 8 to 10 minutes to complete. The higher the score, the better the performance. Scoring is done on a three-point scale with a range on each item of 0 to 2, with 0 representing the most impairment. Individual scores are then combined to form three scales: a Gait Scale, a Balance Scale, and overall Gait and Balance Scale. The maximum score for Gait is 12 points, while the maximum for Balance is 16 points, with a total maximum for the overall Tinetti Instrument of 28 points. A score of less than 19 indicates a high risk for falls, and a score between 19 and 24 indicates a risk for falls.

Elderly Mobility Scale

Seven scale items assess the participant's bed and chair mobility, gait including timed walk, and balance including functional reach. The maximum score is 20, with higher scores indicating greater independence.

BADL and IADL Assessment Tools

Physical Performance Test

The Physical Performance Test (PPT)[11] is a performance-based measure of both BADL and IADL that has been used to describe and monitor physical performance. The PPT takes about 10 minutes to administer. Scoring is based on the time taken to complete a series of usual daily tasks such as writing a sentence, eating, donning and doffing a jacket, turning 360 degrees when standing, lifting a book, picking up a penny from the floor, and walking 50 feet.

Functional Status Questionnaire

The Functional Status Questionnaire (FSQ)[12] is a self-report measure of physical, psychological, and social role functions in patients who are ambulatory. The test takes about 15 minutes and has been found to have both construct (the test developed from a theory actually measures what the theory intended) and convergent (the scores correlate with the scores of other tests designed to measure the same criteria) reliability.[12]

Sickness Impact Profile

The Sickness Impact Profile (SIP)[13] is a widely used health status measure. It measures both physical and psychosocial outcomes from the patient's perspective. The SIP is composed of 136 items that address the following areas: ambulation, mobility, body care and movement, social interaction, communication, alertness, emotional behavior, sleep and rest, eating, work, home management, and recreation and pastime activities. The SIP questionnaire has been extensively and successfully tested for its internal consistency, external validity, responsiveness to changes over time, and test-retest reliability in a wide range of clinical situations.[14]

Functional Rating Index

The Functional Rating Index (FRI)[15] is an instrument specifically designed to quantitatively measure the subjective perception of function and pain of the spinal musculoskeletal system. The FRI consists of 10 items that measure both pain and function of the neck and back. Of these 10 items, eight refer to activities of daily living that might be adversely affected by a spinal condition, and the two refer to two different attributes of pain. Using a five-point scale for each item, the patient ranks his or her perceived ability to perform a function and/or the quantity of pain at the present time.[15] When all 10 items are completed, the FRI score is calculated as follows: (total score divided by 40) × 100%.

Patient-Specific Functional Scale

The Patient-Specific Functional Scale (PSFS)[16] is a patient-specific outcome measure that investigates functional status by asking the patient to name activities that are difficult to perform based on his or her condition and to rate the level of limitation with each activity.[17] The PSFS has been shown to be valid and responsive to change for patients with various clinical conditions, including knee pain,[18] low back pain,[16] neck pain,[19] and cervical radiculopathy.[17]

Short Musculoskeletal Function Assessment

The Short Musculoskeletal Function Assessment (SMFA)[20] is a 46-item questionnaire. The first 34 items refer to activities of daily living. The patient ranks his or her perceived difficulty or problems with these tasks to provide a dysfunction index. The 12 remaining items are ranked according to how much they bother the patient and provide the clinician with a "bother" index.

FIM™

For over 15 years, FIM was an acronym for "Functional Independence Measure." It is still often cited as this in the literature. The current owners of the FIM™ instrument (Uniform Data System for Medical Rehabilitation, a division of UB Foundation Activities, Inc.) have decided that the acronym FIM no longer stands for anything and should be referred to only as FIM™. The FIM™ is the most widely accepted functional assessment measure in use in the rehabilitation community. The FIM™ was developed to resolve the long-standing problem of lack of uniform measurement and data on disability and rehabilitation outcomes. FIM™ scores range from 1 to 7: an FIM™ item score of 7 is categorized as "complete independence," while a score of 1 is "total assist" (performs less than 25% of task). Scores below 6 indicate that another person is required for supervision or assistance. The FIM™ measures independent performance in self-care, sphincter control, transfers (e.g., bed to chair), locomotion, communication, and social cognition. By adding the points for each item, the possible total score ranges from 18 (lowest) to 126 (highest) for level of independence.

Barthel Index

The Barthel scale or Barthel ADL index is used to measure performance in basic activities of daily living. It uses 10 variables describing ADLs and mobility. The items include feeding, moving from wheelchair to bed and return, grooming, transferring to and from a toilet, bathing, walking on a level surface, going up and down stairs, dressing, and maintaining continence of bowel and bladder. The person receives a score based on whether they have received help while doing each task. The scores for each of the items are summed to create a total score. The higher the score, the more independent the person is. A higher number is associated with a greater likelihood of being able to live at home with a degree of independence following discharge from hospital.

REVIEW **Questions**

1. Explain the differences between a sample and a population.
2. In the following statement, determine whether a descriptive or inferential statistic has been used. In the year 2010, 148 million Americans will be enrolled in a health maintenance organization (HMO).
3. In the following statement, determine whether a descriptive or inferential statistic has been used. The national average annual medicine expenditure per person is $1,058.
4. Classify each of the following as nominal-level, ordinal-level, interval-level, or ratio-level measurements: Pages in the city of Pittsburgh telephone book, weights of air humidifiers, ages of students in a classroom.
5. Which of the following variables is qualitative?
   a. Number of cars sold in one year by a local dealer
   b. Times it takes to perform an ultrasound
   c. Colors of theraband in a PT department
   d. Capacity in cubic feet of a Hubbard tank
6. Which of the following variables is continuous?
   a. Water temperatures of three whirlpools in the PT Department
   b. Number of ultrasound treatments provided each day by the physical therapy department
7. Name the four basic sampling methods.

8. In the following example which type of sampling is being used: Every seventh patient entering a physical therapy department.
9. True or false: Probability is used as a basis for inferential statistics.
10. The number of absences per year that a worker has is an example of what type of data?
11. A researcher divided subject into two groups according to gender and then selected members from each group for his sample. What sampling method was the researcher using?
12. For the situation where the most typical case is desired, which measure of central tendency—mean, median, or mode—should be used?
13. If the mean of five values is 64, find the sum of the values.
14. Find the mean of 10, 20, 30, 40, and 50.
15. What is the relationship between the variance and the standard deviation?
16. True or false: In a data set, the mode will always be unique.
17. Why is the standard normal distribution important in statistical analysis?
18. What is the total area under the standard normal distribution curve?
19. What percentage of the area falls below the mean? Above the mean?
20. About what percentage of the area under the normal distribution curve falls within one standard deviation above and below the mean?
21. You decide to use a group of healthy, college student volunteers to study the effects of BAPS board exercises on ankle ROM and balance scores. Twenty volunteers participate in the 20-minute exercise sessions three times a week for 6 weeks. Measurements are taken at the beginning and end of the sessions. At the conclusion of the study, significant differences were found in both sets of scores. Based on this research design, you conclude:
   a. The validity of the study was threatened with the introduction of sampling bias.
   b. BAPS board exercises are an effective intervention to improve ankle stability following chronic ankle sprain.
   c. The reliability of the study was threatened with the introduction of systematic error of measurement.
   d. The Hawthorne effect may have influenced the outcomes of the study.

22. A valid informed consent for research purposes must include all of the following elements except:

    a. A statement ensuring the subject's commitment to participate for the duration of the study.

    b. An understandable explanation of the purpose and procedures to be used.

    c. All reasonable and foreseeable risks and discomforts.

    d. All potential benefits of participation.

23. A study of the local population was necessary to determine the need for a new physical therapy center in the area. The researchers performing the study divided the population by sex and selected a random sample from each group. This is an example of what type of random sample?

    a. Systematic random sample

    b. Random cluster sample

    c. One-stage cluster sample

    d. Stratified random sample

24. You read a clinical study investigating the relationship between ratings of perceived exertion (RPE) and type of exercise: arm isokinetics versus leg isokinetics. The study reports a correlation of 0.55 with the arm isokinetics and a correlation of 0.80 with the leg isokinetics. From these findings, you could determine:

    a. Leg isokinetic exercises are highly correlated with RPE, while arm isokinetic exercises are only moderately correlated.

    b. Both arm and leg isokinetic exercises are only moderately correlated with RPE.

    c. Both arm and leg isokinetic exercises are highly correlated with RPE.

    d. The common variance of both types of testing is only 25%.

References

1. Underwood FB: Clinical research and data analysis, in Placzek JD, Boyce DA (eds): Orthopaedic Physical Therapy Secrets. Philadelphia, Hanley & Belfus, 2001, pp 130–139

2. Bluman AG: The nature of probability and statistics, in Bluman AG (ed): Elementary Statistics: A Step by Step Approach (ed 4). New York, McGraw-Hill, 2008, pp 1–32

3. Bluman AG: Measures of central tendency, in Bluman AG (ed): Elementary Statistics: A Step by Step Approach (ed 4). New York, McGraw-Hill, 2008, pp 101–176

4. Sackett DL, Strauss SE, Richardson WS, et al: Evidence Based Medicine: How to Practice and Teach EBM (ed 2). Edinburgh, Scotland, Churchill Livingstone, 2000

5. Guide to Physical Therapist Practice (ed 2). Phys Ther 81:S13–S95, 2001

6. Jette AM, Keysor JJ: Uses of evidence in disability outcomes and effectiveness research. Milbank Quarterly 80:325–345, 2002

7. Salive ME, Mayfield JA, Weissman NW: Patient outcomes research teams and the agency for health care policy and research. Health Serv Res 25:697–708, 1990

8. Blair SJ, McCormick E, Bear-Lehman J, et al: Evaluation of impairment of the upper extremity. Clin Orthop 221:42–58, 1987

9. Borg GAV: Psychophysical basis of perceived exertion. Med Sci Sports Exerc 14:377–381, 1992

10. Borg GAV: Perceived exertion as an indicator of somatic stress. Scand J Rehabil Med 2:92–98, 1970

11. Reuben DB, Siu AL: Measuring physical function in community dwelling older persons: A comparison of self admimistered, interviewer administered, and performance-based measures. J Am Geriatr Soc 43:17–23, 1995

12. Tager IB, Swanson A, Satariano WA: Reliability of physical performance and self-reported functional measures in an older population. J Gerontol 53:M295–M300, 1998

13. de Bruin AF, de Witte LP, Stevens F, et al: Sickness Impact Profile: The state of the art of a generic functional status measure. Soc Sci Med 35:1003–1014, 1992

14. Bergner M, Bobbitt RA, Carter WB, et al: The Sickness Impact Profile: Development and final revision of a health status measure. Med Care 19:787, 1981

15. Feise RJ, Michael Menke J: Functional rating index: A new valid and reliable instrument to measure the magnitude of clinical change in spinal conditions. Spine 26:78–86; discussion 87, 2001

16. Stratford P, Gill C, Westaway M, et al: Assessing disability and change on individual patients: a report of a patient specific measure Physiotherapy Canada 47:258–263, 1995

17. Cleland JA, Fritz JM, Whitman JM, et al: The reliability and construct validity of the Neck Disability Index and patient specific functional scale in patients with cervical radiculopathy. Spine. 31:598–602, 2006

18. Chatman AB, Hyams SP, Neel JM, et al: The Patient-Specific Functional Scale: measurement properties in patients with knee dysfunction. Phys Ther 77:820–829, 1997

19. Westaway MD, Stratford PW, Binkley JM: The patient-specific functional scale: Validation of its use in persons with neck dysfunction. J Orthop Sports Phys Ther. 27:331–338, 1998

20. Swiontkowski MF, Engelberg R, Martin DP, et al: Short musculoskeletal function assessment questionnaire: Validity, reliability, and responsiveness. J Bone Joint Surg 81A:1256–1258, 1999

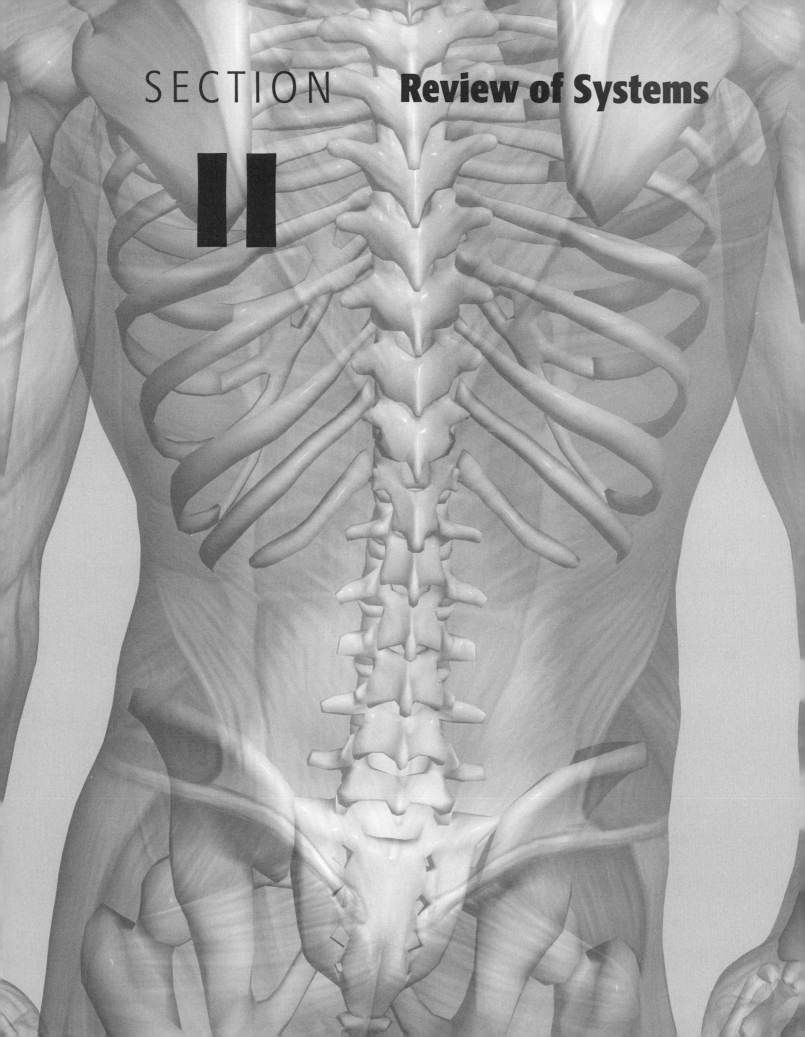

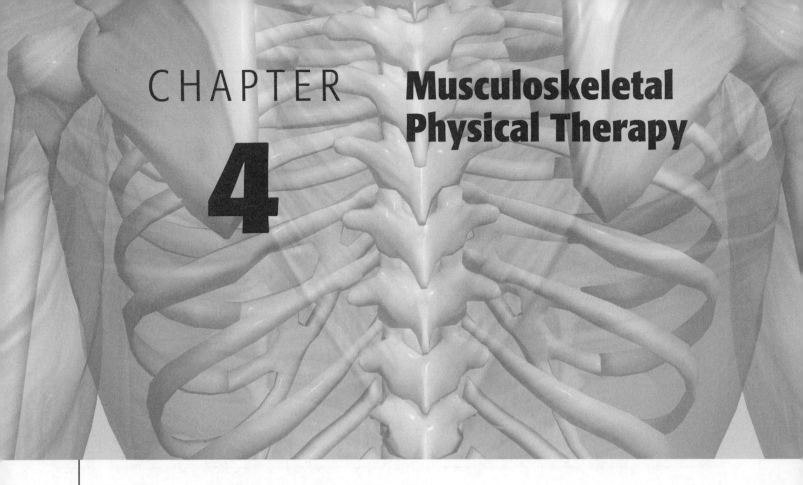

Components of the Musculoskeletal System

The musculoskeletal system includes bones, fascia, muscles with their related tendons and synovial sheaths, bursa, and joint structures such as cartilage, menisci, capsules, and ligaments.

Bone

Bone is a highly vascular and metabolically active form of connective tissue, composed of collagen, calcium phosphate, water, amorphous proteins, and cells (**Table 4-1**). There are approximately 206 bones in the body.

> ● **Key Point** Note the following definitions:
> • *Periosteum:* A thin, tough membrane that covers each long bone and helps secure the attachments of muscles and ligaments to bone.
> • *Medullary canal:* The central hollow tube within the diaphysis of a long bone, which is important for storing bone marrow and provides a passageway for nutrient-carrying arteries.

The function of a bone is to provide support, enhance leverage, protect vital structures, provide attachments for both tendons and ligaments, and store minerals, particularly calcium.

Fascia

Fascia is a continuous laminated sheet of connective tissue that extends without interruption from the top of the head to the tips of the toes, surrounding and permeating every tissue and organ of the body, including nerves, vessels, tendons, aponeuroses, ligaments, capsules, and the intrinsic components of muscle.[1,2]

TABLE 4-1	General Structure of Bone	
Site	**Description**
Epiphysis	The region between the growth plate or growth plate scar and the expanded end of bone, covered by articular cartilage
	The location of secondary ossification centers during development
	Forms bone ends
Physis (a.k.a. epiphyseal plate)	The region that separates the epiphysis from the metaphysis
	The zone of endochondral ossification in an actively growing bone or the epiphyseal scar in a fully grown bone
	Vulnerable prior to growth spurt and mechanically weak
Metaphysis	The junctional region between the growth plate and the diaphysis
	Contains abundant cancellous (trabecular) bone, which heals rapidly, but the cortical bone thins here relative to the diaphysis
	Common site for many primary bone tumors and similar lesions (osteomyelitis)
Diaphysis	Forms shaft of bone
	Large surface for muscle origin
	Composed mainly of cortical (compact) bone
	The medullary canal contains marrow and a small amount of trabecular bone

Tendon

A tendon is a cordlike structure that attaches muscle to bone. The site where the muscle and tendon meet is called the *myotendinous junction* (MTJ). The MTJ is very vulnerable to tensile failure; it is the location of most common muscle strains caused by tensile forces in a normal muscle–tendon unit.[3,4]

● **Key Point** A tendency for a tear near the MTJ has been reported in the biceps and triceps brachii, rotator cuff muscles, flexor pollicis longus, fibularis (peroneus) longus, medial head of the gastrocnemius, rectus femoris, adductor longus, iliopsoas, pectoralis major, semimembranosus, and the entire hamstring group.[5–7]

Ligaments

Skeletal ligaments connect bones across joints and contribute to the stability of joint function by preventing excessive motion,[8] acting as guides to direct motion, and providing proprioceptive information for joint function (**Table 4-2** and **Table 4-3**).[9,10]

● **Key Point** Ligaments have a rich sensory innervation through specialized mechanoreceptors and free nerve endings that provide information about proprioception and pain, respectively.

Muscle

A single muscle cell is called a *muscle fiber* or *myofiber*. There are approximately 430 skeletal muscles in the body, each of which can be considered anatomically as a separate organ. Each muscle cell contains many structural components called *myofilaments*, which run parallel to the myofibril axis. The myofilaments are made up of two protein filaments: actin (thin) and myosin (thick). Structures called *myosin cross-bridges* serve to connect the actin and myosin filaments. During contraction, the cross-bridges attach. During relaxation, the cross-bridges detach. The regulation of cross-bridge attachment and detachment is a function of two proteins found in the actin filaments: tropomyosin and troponin. Tropomyosin attaches directly to the actin filament, whereas troponin is attached to the tropomyosin rather than directly to the actin filament.

● **Key Point** Tropomyosin and troponin function as the switch for muscle contraction and relaxation. In a relaxed state, the tropomyosin physically blocks the cross-bridges from binding to the actin. For contraction to take place, the tropomyosin must be moved.

TABLE
4-2

Major Ligaments of the Upper Quadrant

Joint	Ligament(s)	Function
Shoulder complex	Coracoclavicular	Fixes the clavicle to the coracoid process
	Costoclavicular	Fixes the clavicle to the costal cartilage of the first rib
	Coracohumera	Reinforces the upper portion of the joint capsule
	Glenohumeral ("Z")	Reinforces the anterior and inferior aspect of the joint capsule
	Coracoacromial	Protects the superior aspect of the joint
Elbow and forearm	Annular	Maintains the relationship between the head of the radius and the humerus and ulna
	Ulnar (medial) collateral	Provides stability against valgus (medial) stress, particularly in the range of 20° to 130° of flexion and extension
	Radial (lateral) collateral	Provides stability against varus (lateral) stress and functions to maintain the ulnohumeral and radiohumeral joints in a reduced position when the elbow is loaded in supination
	The interosseous membrane of the forearm	Divides the forearm into anterior and posterior compartments, serves as a site of attachment for muscles of the forearm, and transfers forces from the radius, to the ulna, to the humerus
Wrist	Extrinsic palmar	Provide the majority of the wrist stability
	Intrinsic	Serve as rotational restraints, binding the proximal carpal row into a unit of rotational stability
	Interosseous	Binds the carpal bones together
	Triangular fibrocartilage complex (TFCC)	Suspends the distal radius and ulnar carpus from the distal ulna
		Provides a continuous gliding surface across the entire distal face of the radius and ulna for flexion/extension and translational movements
		Provides a flexible mechanism for stable rotational movements of the radiocarpal unit around the ulnar axis
		Cushions the forces transmitted through the ulnocarpal axis
Fingers	Volar and collateral interphalangeal	Prevent displacement of the interphalangeal joints

TABLE
4-3

Major Ligaments of the Spine and Lower Quadrant

Joint	Ligament	Function
Spine	Anterior longitudinal ligament	Functions as a minor assistant in limiting anterior translation and vertical separation of the vertebral body
	Posterior longitudinal ligament	Limits hyperextension of the spine
	Ligamentum flavum	Resists vertebral distraction of the vertebral body
	Interspinous	Resists posterior shearing of the vertebral body
	Intratransverse	Acts to limit flexion over a number of segments
	Iliolumbar (lower lumbar)	Provides some protection against intervertebral disc protrusions
	Nuchal (represents the supraspinal ligaments of the lower vertebrae)	Resists separation of the lamina during flexion
		Resists shear forces and separation of the spinous processes during flexion
		Prevents excessive rotation
		Resists side bending of the spine and helps in preventing rotation
		Resists flexion, extension, axial rotation, and side bending of L5 on S1
		Resists cervical flexion

(continued)

Joint	Ligament	Function
Sacroiliac	Sacrospinous	Resists forward tilting of the sacrum on the hip bone during weight bearing of the vertebral column
	Sacrotuberous	Resists forward tilting (nutation) of the sacrum on the hip bone during weight bearing of the vertebral column
	Interosseous	Resists anterior and inferior movement of the sacrum
	Posterior (dorsal) sacroiliac	Resists backward tilting (counternutation) of the sacrum on the hip bone during weight bearing of the vertebral column
	Anterior (ventral) sacroiliac	Consists of numerous thin bands
		Is a capsular ligament
Hip	Ligamentum teres	Transports nutrient vessels to the femoral head
	Iliofemoral (Y ligament)	Is the strongest of the hip ligaments
	Ischiofemoral	Limits hip extension
	Pubofemoral	Limits anterior displacement of the femoral head and internal rotation of the hip
		Limits hip extension and abduction of the hip
Knee	Medial collateral	Stabilizes medial aspect of tibiofemoral joint against valgus stress
	Lateral collateral	Stabilizes lateral aspect of tibiofemoral joint against varus stress
	Anterior cruciate	Resists anterior translation of the tibia and posterior translation of the femur
	Posterior cruciate	Resists posterior translation of the tibia and anterior translation of the femur
Ankle	Medial collaterals (Deltoid)	Include the tibionavicular, calcaneotibial, anterior talotibial, and the posterior talotibial ligaments
	Lateral collaterals	Provide stability between the medial malleollus, navicular, talus, and calcaneus against eversion
		Include the anterior talofibular, calcaneofibular, talocalcaneal, posterior talocalcaneal, and the posterior talofibular ligaments
		Are static stabilizers of the lateral ankle, especially against inversion
Foot	Long plantar	Provides indirect plantar support to the calcaneocuboid joint by limiting the amount of flattening of the lateral longitudinal arch of the foot
	Bifurcate	Supports the medial and lateral aspects of the foot when weight bearing in a plantar flexed position
	Calcaneocuboid	Provides plantar support to the calcaneocuboid joint and possibly helps to limit flattening of the lateral longitudinal arch

Each muscle fiber is innervated by a somatic motor neuron. One neuron and the muscle fibers it innervates constitute a motor unit or functional unit of the muscle. Each motor neuron branches as it enters the muscle to innervate a number of muscle fibers. Activation of varying numbers of motor neurons results in gradations in the strength of muscle contraction. Whenever a somatic motor neuron is activated, all of the muscle fibers that it innervates are stimulated and contract with *all-or-none* twitches. Although the muscle fibers produce all-or-none contractions, muscles are capable of a wide variety of responses, ranging from activities requiring a high level of precision to activities requiring high tension.

● **Key Point**   The graded contractions of whole muscles occur because the number of fibers participating in the contraction varies. An increase in the force of movement is achieved by recruiting more cells into cooperative action.

Cartilage

Cartilage, as it relates to the musculoskeletal system, comes in two major forms:

- *Hyaline:* Hyaline cartilage covers the ends of long bones and, along with the synovial fluid that bathes it, provides a smooth, almost frictionless, articulating surface.[11]

> ● **Key Point** Hyaline cartilage is the most abundant cartilage within the body. The patella has the thickest articular cartilage in the body.

- *Fibrocartilage:* Fibrocartilage is found in the pubic symphysis, the annulus fibrosus of the intervertebral disc, the meniscus, and the joint surfaces of the temporomandibular joint (TMJ).

Joint

A joint represents the junction between two or more bones. Joints are regions where bones are capped and surrounded by connective tissues that hold the bones together and determine the type and degree of movement between them.[12] Arthrology is the study of the classification, structure, and function of joints. Joints may be classified as synovial, fibrous, or cartilaginous (**Table 4-4**).

> ● **Key Point** An *amphiarthrosis*, a type of joint that is formed primarily by fibrocartilage and hyaline cartilage, plays an important role in shock absorption. One example is the intervertebral body joints of the spine.

Synovial joints can be broadly classified according to structure or analogy into the following categories:[13]

- *Spheroid:* As the name suggests, a spheroid joint is a freely moving joint in which a sphere on the head of one bone fits into a rounded cavity in the other bone. Spheroid (ball-and-socket) joints allow motions in three planes (see "Kinesiology"). Examples of a spheroid joint surface include the heads of the femur and humerus.
- *Trochoid:* The trochoid (pivot) joint is characterized by a pivot-like process turning within a ring, or a ring on a pivot, the ring being formed partly of bone, partly of ligament. Trochoid joints permit only rotation. Examples of a trochoid joint include the proximal radioulnar joint and the atlantoaxial joint.
- *Condyloid:* The condyloid joint is characterized by an ovoid articular surface, or condyle. One bone may articulate with another by one surface

TABLE 4-4	Joint Types		
Type	**Characteristics**	**Examples**	
Synovial			
Diarthrosis	Fibroelastic joint capsule filled with a lubricating substance called *synovial fluid*	Hip, knee, shoulder, and elbow joints	
Fibrous	United by bone tissue, ligament or membrane		
Synarthrosis (eventual fusion is termed a synostosis)	Immovable joint	Sagittal suture of the skull	
Syndesmosis	Joined together by a dense fibrous membrane	The interosseous membrane between the tibia and fibular	
Gomphosis	Very little motion	The teeth and corresponding sockets are the only gomphosis joints in the body	
	Bony surfaces connected like a peg in a hole (the periodontal membrane is the fibrous component)		
Cartilaginous			
Synchondrosis	Joined by either hyaline or fibrocartilage	The epiphyseal plates of growing bones and the articulations between the first rib and the sternum	
	May ossify to a synostosis once growth is completed		
Symphysis	Generally located at the midline of the body	The symphysis pubis	
	Two bones covered with hyaline cartilage and connective by fibrocartilage		

or by two, but never more than two. If two distinct surfaces are present, the joint is called *condylar* or *bicondylar*. The elliptical cavity of the joint is designed in such a manner as to permit the motions of flexion, extension, adduction, abduction, and circumduction, but no axial rotation (see "Kinesiology"). The wrist joint is an example of this form of articulation.

- *Ginglymoid:* A ginglymoid (hinge) is characterized by a spool-like surface and a concave surface. An example of a ginglymoid joint is the humeroulnar joint.
- *Ellipsoid:* Ellipsoid joints are similar to spheroid joints in that they allow the same type of movement, albeit to a lesser magnitude. The ellipsoid joint allows movement in two planes (flexion/extension, abduction/adduction) and is biaxial. Examples of this joint are the radiocarpal articulation at the wrist and the metacarpophalangeal articulation in the phalanges.
- *Planar:* As its name suggests, a planar (gliding) joint is characterized by two flat surfaces that slide over each other. Movement at this type of joint does not occur about an axis and is termed *nonaxial*. Examples of a planar joint include the intermetatarsal joints and some intercarpal joints.
- *Sellar:* The other major type of articular surface is the sellar (saddle) joint.[14] Sellar joints are characterized by a convex surface in one cross-sectional plane and a concave surface in the plane perpendicular to it. Examples of a sellar joint include the carpometacarpal joint of the thumb, the humeroulnar joint, and the calcaneocuboid joints.

Although the above-mentioned categories give a broad description of joint structure, this classification does not sufficiently describe the articulations or the movements that occur. In reality, no joint surface is planar or resembles a true geometric form. Instead, joint surfaces are either convex in all directions or concave in all directions (see "Kinesiology")—that is, they resemble either the outer or inner surface of a piece of eggshell.[14] Because the curve of an eggshell varies from point to point, these articular surfaces are called *ovoid*.

Joint Receptors

All synovial joints of the body are provided with an array of corpuscular (mechanoreceptors) and noncorpuscular (nociceptors) receptor endings (**Table 4-5**) embedded in articular, muscular, and cutaneous structures with varying characteristic behaviors and distributions depending on articular tissue.

Anatomy of Specific Joints

Shoulder Complex

The shoulder complex is composed of four articulations:

- The glenohumeral (G-H) joint
- The acromioclavicular (A-C) joint
- The sternoclavicular (S-C) joint
- The scapulothoracic pseudoarticulation

A fifth articulation—the subacromial articulation between the coracoacromial arch (a rigid structure above the humeral head and rotator cuff tendons) and the rotator cuff tendons—is sometimes included.[15]

Complete movement at the shoulder girdle involves a complex interaction between the G-H, A-C, and S-C complex, scapulothoracic (pseudo joint), upper thoracic, costal, and sternomanubrial joints, and the lower cervical spine. The major muscles of the shoulder complex are outlined in **Table 4-6**.

- *Scapular elevators:* Upper trapezius and levator scapulae
- *Scapular depressors:* Latissimus dorsi, pectoralis major, pectoralis minor, and lower trapezius
- *Scapular protractors:* Serratus anterior, pectoralis major, and pectoralis minor
- *Scapular retractors:* Trapezius and rhomboids
- *Scapular rotators:*
  - *Upward:* Upper trapezius, serratus anterior, and lower trapezius
  - *Downward:* Rhomboids, levator scapulae, and pectoralis minor
- *Shoulder flexors:* Anterior deltoid, coracobrachialis, pectoralis major, biceps brachii, and supraspinatus
- *Shoulder extensors:* Latissimus dorsi, subscapularis, posterior deltoid, and teres major
- *Shoulder abductors:* Middle deltoid and supraspinatus
- *Shoulder adductors:* Pectoralis major, latissimus dorsi, and teres major
- *Shoulder external rotators:* Teres minor, infraspinatus, and posterior deltoid
- *Shoulder internal rotators:* Subscapularis, teres major, pectoralis major, latissimus dorsi, and anterior deltoid

TABLE 4-5 — Joint Receptor Types

Type	Location	Function
I: Small Ruffini endings Slow-adapting, low-threshold stretch receptors	Joint capsule and ligaments	Type I receptors are important in signaling actual joint position or changes in joint positions. They contribute to reflex regulation of postural tone, to coordination of muscle activity, and to a perceptional awareness of joint position. An increase in joint capsule tension by active or passive motion, by posture, or by mobilization or manipulation causes these receptors to discharge at a higher frequency.
II: Pacinian corpuscles Rapidly adapting, low-threshold receptors	Adipose tissue, the cruciate ligaments, the anulus fibrosus, ligaments, and the fibrous capsule	Type II receptors sense joint motion and regulate motor-unit activity of the prime movers of the joint. They are entirely inactive in immobile joints and become active for brief periods at the onset of movement and during rapid changes in tension. Type II receptors fire during active or passive motion of a joint, or with the application of traction.
III: Large Ruffini Slowly adapting, high-threshold receptors	Ligaments and the fibrous capsule	Type III receptors detect large amounts of tension. These receptors become active only in the extremes of motion or when strong manual techniques are applied to the joint.
IV: Nociceptors Slowly adapting, high-threshold free nerve endings		Type IV receptors are inactive in normal circumstances but become active with marked mechanical deformation or tension. They are also active in response to direct mechanical or chemical irritation.

Data from Wyke BD: The neurology of joints: A review of general principles. Clin Rheum Dis 7:223–239, 1981; and Wyke BD: Articular neurology and manipulative therapy, in Glasgow EF, Twomey LT, Scull ER, et al (eds): Aspects of Manipulative Therapy (ed 2). New York, Churchill Livingstone, 1985, pp 72–77

TABLE 4-6 — Shoulder Girdle Muscle Function and Innervation

Muscles	Origin	Insertion	Peripheral Nerve	Nerve Root	Motions
Pectoralis major	Anterior surface of the sternal half of the clavicle; anterior surface of the sternum	Intertubercular groove of humerus	Pectoral	Clavicular head: C5 and C6	Adduction, horizontal adduction, and internal rotation
				Sternocostal head: C7, C8, and T1	Clavicular fibers: Forward flexion Sternocostal fibers: Extension
Pectoralis minor	Ribs 3–5	Medial border and superior surface of coracoid process of scapula	Medial pectoral	C8–T1	Stabilizes scapula by drawing it anteriorly and inferiorly against thoracic wall
Latissimus dorsi	Spinous processes of inferior six thoracic vertebrae, thoracolumbar fascia, iliac crest, and inferior three ribs	Floor of intertubercular groove of humerus	Thoracodorsal	C7 (C6, C8)	Adduction, extension, and internal rotation

(continued)

TABLE
4-6

Shoulder Girdle Muscle Function and Innervation (continued)

Muscles	Origin	Insertion	Peripheral Nerve	Nerve Root	Motions
Teres major	Dorsal surface of inferior angle of scapula	Medial lip of intertubercular groove of humerus	Subscapular	C5–C8	Adduction, extension, horizontal abduction, and internal rotation
Teres minor	Superior part of lateral border of scapula	Inferior facet on greater tuberosity of humerus	Axillary	C5 (C6)	Horizontal abduction (also a weak external rotator)
Deltoid	Lateral one-third of clavicle, acromion, and spine of scapula	Deltoid tuberosity of humerus	Axillary	C5 (C6)	Anterior: Forward flexion, horizontal adduction Middle: Abduction Posterior: Extension, horizontal abduction
Supraspinatus	Supraspinatus fossa	Superior facet on greater tuberosity of humerus	Suprascapular	C5 (C6)	Abduction
Subscapularis	Subscapularis fossa	Lesser tuberosity of humerus	Upper and lower subscapular	C5–C8	Adduction and internal rotation
Infraspinatus	Infraspinatus fossa	Middle facet on greater tuberosity of humerus	Suprascapular	C5 (C6)	Abduction, horizontal abduction, and external rotation
Serratus anterior	External surfaces of lateral parts of ribs 1 through 8	Anterior surface of the medial border of scapula	Long thoracic	C5–C7	Protracts and rotates scapula and holds it against thoracic wall
Levator scapula	Posterior tubercles of transverse processes of C1–C4	Superior part of medial border of scapula	Dorsal scapular	C4–5	Elevates scapula and tilts glenoid cavity in inferiorly by rotating scapula downward
Rhomboids	Ligamentum nuchae and spinous processes of C7–T5	Medial border of scapula from level of spine to inferior angle	Dorsal scapular	C4–C5	Retracts scapula and rotates it downward to depress glenoid cavity
Coracobrachialis	Tip of coracoid process of scapula	Middle medial border of humerus	Musculocutaneous	C5–C6	Horizontal flexion and adduction of humerus at shoulder
Biceps brachii	Tip of coracoid and supraglenoid tubercle of scapula	Radial tuberosity and lacertus fibrosis	Musculocutaneous	C5–C6	Flexes arm and supinates forearm
Trapezius	Spinous processes of cervical and thoracic vertebrae	Scapula and acromion	Spinal accessory; branches of ansa cervicalis	CN XI	Elevates, retracts, and upwardly rotates scapula

● **Key Point** *Sprengel deformity* is a failure of the scapula to descend during normal development. It is characterized as a prominent lump in the web of the neck and may be associated with scoliosis, rib abnormalities, and Klippel–Feil syndrome.

● **Key Point** *Snapping scapula* is attributed to friction between the mobile scapula and its attached soft tissues and the relatively stable thoracic wall. Anatomic explanations for snapping scapula include thickened bursa, bone spurs on the scapula or a rib, and osteochondroma.

● **Key Point** *Scaption* refers to the forward elevation of the internally rotated arm in the scapular plane with the thumb pointed toward the floor.

● **Key Point** Scapular dyskinesia (also referred to as abnormal scapulohumeral rhythm, scapular winging, and scapular dysrhythmia) describes abnormal or atypical movement of the scapula during normal active motion tasks. The finding is common in patients with an unstable glenohumeral joint and patients with impingement syndrome. A scapular dyskinesia may occur primary or secondary to shoulder impingement and instability.

Elbow Complex

The elbow is composed of three articulations:

- *Humeroulnar:* The concave ulna articulates with the convex distal humerus (trochlea). This hinged articulation permits motion in a single plane, allowing for flexion and extension of the elbow.
- *Humeroradial (radiocapitellar) joint:* The concave head of the radius articulates with the capitellum, which is the convex lateral articular surface of the distal humerus. This joint permits the radius to rotate, allowing supination and pronation of the forearm (in association with the proximal radioulnar joint).
- *Proximal (superior) radioulnar joint:* A uniaxial pivot joint formed between the periphery of the convex radial head and the fibrous osseous ring formed by the concave radial notch of the ulna.

The muscles of the elbow complex are outlined in **Table 4-7**.

● Key Point An interosseous membrane located between the radius and ulna serves to help distribute forces throughout the forearm and provide muscle attachment.

Wrist and Hand

The wrist joint is composed of the distal radius and ulna, eight carpal bones, and the bases of five metacarpals. The carpal bones lie in two transverse rows. The proximal row contains (radial to ulnar) the scaphoid (navicular), lunate, triquetrum, and pisiform. The distal row holds (radial to ulnar) the trapezium, trapezoid, capitate, and hamate. The midcarpal joint lies between the two rows of carpals. Wrist flexion, extension, and radial deviation are mainly midcarpal joint motions.

The carpal tunnel serves as a conduit for the median nerve and nine flexor tendons (the eighth tendons of the flexor digitorum superficialis and flexor digitorum profundus, and the flexor pollicis longus). Within the tunnel, the median nerve divides into a motor branch and distal sensory branches.

The ulnar artery and ulnar nerve pass through the tunnel of Guyon. The muscles of the forearm, wrist, and hand are outlined in **Table 4-8**.

● Key Point The thumb is the most important digit of the hand, and the sellar (saddle-shaped) carpometacarpal (CMC) joint is the most important joint of the thumb. Motions that can occur at this joint include flexion/extension, adduction/abduction, and opposition (which includes varying amounts of flexion, internal rotation, and palmar adduction).

The *anatomic snuffbox* is represented by a depression on the dorsal surface of the hand at the base of the thumb, just distal to the radius. The tendons of

TABLE 4-7	Muscles of the Elbow and Forearm: Their Actions, Nerve Supply, and Nerve Root Derivation		
Action	**Muscles Acting**	**Peripheral Nerve Supply**	**Nerve Root Deviation**
Elbow flexion	Brachialis	Musculocutaneous	C5–C6, (C7)
	Biceps brachii	Musculocutaneous	C5–C6
	Brachioradialis	Radial	C5–C6, (C7)
	Pronator teres	Median	C6–C7
	Flexor carpi ulnaris	Ulnar	C7–C8
Elbow extension	Triceps	Radial	C7–C8
	Anconeus	Radial	C7–C8, (T1)
Forearm supination	Supinator	Posterior interosseous (radial)	C5–C6
	Biceps brachii	Musculocutaneous	C5–C6
Forearm pronation	Pronator quadratus	Anterior interosseous (median)	C8, T1
	Pronator teres	Median	C6–C7
	Flexor carpi radialis	Median	C6–C7

TABLE 4-8   Muscles of the Wrist and Hand: Their Actions and Nerve Supply

Action	Muscles	Nerve Supply
Wrist extension	Extensor carpi radialis longus	Radial
	Extensor carpi radialis brevis	Posterior interosseous
	Extensor carpi ulnaris	Posterior interosseous
Wrist flexion	Flexor carpi radialis	Median
	Flexor carpi ulnaris	Ulnar
Ulnar deviation of wrist	Flexor carpi ulnaris	Ulnar
	Extensor carpi ulnaris	Posterior interosseous
Radial deviation of wrist	Flexor carpi radialis	Median
	Extensor carpi radialis longus	Radial
	Abductor pollicis longus	Posterior interosseous
	Extensor pollicis brevis	Posterior interosseous
Finger extension	Extensor digitorum communis	Posterior interosseous
	Extensor indicis	Posterior interosseous
	Extensor digiti minimi	Posterior interosseous
Finger flexion	Flexor digitorum profundus	Anteriorinterosseous, lateral two digits
		Ulnar, medial two digits
	Flexor digitorum superficialis	Median
	First and second: median	
	Lumbricals	Third and fourth: ulnar
	Interossei	Ulnar
	Flexor digiti minimi	Ulnar
Abduction of fingers	Dorsal interossei	Ulnar
	Abductor digiti minimi	Ulnar
Adduction of fingers	Palmar interossei	Ulnar
Thumb extension	Extensor pollicis longus	Posterior interosseous
	Extensor pollicis brevis	Posterior interosseous
	Abductor pollicis longus	Posterior interosseous
Thumb flexion	Flexor pollicis brevis	Superficial head: median
		Deep head: ulnar
	Flexor pollicis longus	Anterior interosseous
	Opponens pollicis	Median
Abduction of thumb	Abductor pollicis longus	Posterior interosseous
	Abductor pollicis brevis	Median
Adduction of thumb	Adductor pollicis	Ulnar
Opposition of thumb	Opponens pollicis	Median
Thumb flexion	Flexor pollicis brevis	Superficial head: median
Thumb abduction	Abductor pollicis brevis	Median
Opposition of little finger	Opponens digiti minimi	Ulnar

the abductor pollicis longus (APL) and extensor pollicis brevis (EPB) form the radial border of the snuffbox, while the tendon of the extensor pollicis longus (EPL) forms the ulnar border. Along the floor of the snuffbox are the deep branch of the radial artery and the tendinous insertion of the extensor carpi radialis longus (ECRL). Underneath these structures, the scaphoid and trapezium bones are found.

● **Key Point** Tenderness with palpation in the anatomic snuffbox suggests a scaphoid fracture, but this also can present in minor wrist injuries or other conditions.

● **Key Point** Kienböck disease is an avascular necrosis of the lunate, usually as a result of distant trauma. It has also been associated with relative shortening of the ulnar compared with the radius bone.

Hip

The acetabulum is made up of three bones: the ilium, ischium, and pubis. The acetabular labrum deepens the acetabulum and increases articular congruence. The hip joint is classified as an unmodified ovoid (ball-and-socket) joint. This arrangement permits motion in three planes: sagittal (flexion and extension around a transverse axis), frontal (abduction and adduction around an anterior–posterior axis), and transverse (internal and external rotation around a vertical axis). A number of muscles act across the hip (**Table 4-9**).

- *Hip flexors:* Iliopsoas, sartorius, rectus femoris, and pectineus
- *Hip extensors:* Gluteus maximus and medius, and the hamstrings (semitendinosis, semimembranosus, and biceps femoris)

TABLE 4-9 Muscles Acting Across the Hip Joint

Muscle	Origin	Insertion	Innervation
Adductor brevis	External aspect of the body and inferior ramus of the pubis	By an aponeurosis to the line from the greater trochanter of the linea aspera of the femur	Obturator nerve, L3
Adductor longus	Pubic crest and symphysis	By an aponeurosis to the middle third of the linea aspera of the femur	Obturator nerve, L3
Adductor magnus	Inferior ramus of pubis, ramus of ischium, and the inferolateral aspect of the ischial tuberosity	By an aponeurosis to the linea aspera and adductor tubercle of the femur	Obturator nerve and tibial portion of the sciatic nerve, L2–L4
Biceps femoris (long head)	The sacrotuberous ligament and posterior aspect of the ischial tuberosity	By way of a tendon, on the lateral aspect of the head of the fibula, the lateral condyle of the tibial tuberosity, the lateral collateral ligament, and the deep fascia of the leg	Tibial portion of the sciatic nerve, S1
Gemelli (superior and inferior)	Superior–dorsal surface of the spine of the ischium; inferior–upper part of the tuberosity of the ischium	Superior and inferior–medial surface of the greater trochanter	Sacral plexus, L5–S1
Gluteus maximus	Posterior gluteal line of the ilium, iliac crest, aponeurosis of the erector spinae, dorsal surface of the lower part of the sacrum, side of the coccyx, sacrotuberous ligament, and intermuscular fascia	Iliotibial tract of the fascia lata, gluteal tuberosity of the femur	Inferior gluteal nerve, S1–S2
Gluteus medius	Outer surface of the ilium between the iliac crest and the posterior gluteal line, anterior gluteal line, and fascia	Lateral surface of the greater trochanter	Superior gluteal nerve, L5
Gluteus minimus	Outer surface of the ilium between the anterior and inferior gluteal lines, and the margin of the greater sciatic notch	A ridge laterally situated on the anterior surface of the greater trochanter	Superior gluteal nerve, L5

(continued)

TABLE 4-9   Muscles Acting Across the Hip Joint (continued)

Muscle	Origin	Insertion	Innervation
Gracilis	Body and inferior ramus of the pubis	The anterior–medial aspect of the shaft of the proximal tibia, just proximal to the tendon of the semitendinosus	Obturator nerve, L2
Iliacus	Super two-thirds of the iliac fossa; upper surface of the lateral part of the sacrum	Fibers converge with tendon of the psoas major to lesser trochanter	Femoral nerve, L2
Obturator externus	Rami of the pubis, ramus of the ischium, medial two-thirds of the outer surface of the obturator membrane	Trochanteric fossa of the femur	Obturator nerve, L4
Obturator internus	Internal surface of the anterolateral wall of the pelvis; obturator membrane	Medial surface of the greater trochanter	Sacral plexus, S1
Pectineus	Pecten pubis	Along a line leading from the lesser trochanter to the linea aspera	Femoral or obturator or accessory obturator nerves, L2
Piriformis	Front of the sacrum; gluteal surface of the ilium; capsule of the sacroiliac joint; sacrotuberous ligament	Upper border of the greater trochanter of femur	Sacral plexus, S1
Psoas major	Transverse processes of all the lumbar vertebrae, bodies, and intervertebral discs of the lumbar vertebrae	Lesser trochanter of the femur	Lumbar plexus, L2–L3
Quadratus femoris	Ischial body next to the ischial tuberosity	Quadrate tubercle on femur	Nerve to quadratus femoris
Rectus femoris	By two heads, from the anterior inferior iliac spine, and a reflected head from the groove above the acetabulum	Base of the patella	Femoral nerve, L3–L4
Sartorius	Anterior superior iliac spine and notch below it	Upper part of the medial surface of the tibia in front of the gracilis	Femoral nerve, L2–L3
Semimembranosus	Ischial tuberosity	The posterior–medial aspect of the medial condyle of the tibia	Tibial nerve, L5–S1
Semitendinosus	Ischial tuberosity	Upper part of the medial surface of the tibia behind the attachment of the sartorius and below that of the gracilis	Tibial nerve, L5–S1
Tensor fasciae latae	Outer lip of the iliac crest and the lateral surface of the anterior superior iliac spine	Iliotibial tract	Superior gluteal nerve, L4–L5

- *Hip abductors:* Gluteus medius and minimus, piriformis, and obturator internus
- *Hip adductors:* Adductor magnus, adductor longus, adductor brevis, and gracilis
- *Hip internal rotators:* Tensor fascia latae, gluteus medius, gluteus minimus, pectineus, and adductor longus

- *Hip external rotators:* Gluteus maximus, obturator externus, obturator internus, piriformis, gemelli, and sartorius

The femur is held in the acetabulum by five separate ligaments:

- *Iliofemoral ligament:* Attaches to the anterior inferior iliac spine of the pelvis and the intertrochanteric line of the femur. By limiting the range of hip extension, this ligament, with the assistance of the pubofemoral ligament, allows maintenance of the upright posture and reduces the need for contraction of the hip extensors in balanced stance. The ligament also is thought to limit external rotation, and the superior portion tightens with hip adduction.

- *Pubofemoral ligament:* Originates at the superior ramus of the pubis, also attaching to the intertrochanteric line of the femur. Its fibers tighten in extension and abduction, and they reinforce the joint capsule along the medial surface.
- *Ischiofemoral ligament:* Connects the ischium to the greater trochanter of the femur. This ligament, which tightens with internal rotation of the hip, is more commonly injured than the other hip ligaments. When the hip is flexed, the ligament serves to limit hip adduction.
- *Transverse acetabular ligament:* Consists of the labrum covering the acetabular notch.
- *Femoral head ligament:* Joins the femoral head with the transverse ligament and acetabular notch.

● **Key Point** Given that the hip region is also a common source of symptom referral from other regions, the examination of the hip rarely occurs in isolation. It almost always involves an assessment of the lumbar spine, pelvis, and knee joint complex.

● **Key Point** End-range hip flexion is associated with a posterior rotation of the ilium bone. The end range of hip extension is associated with an anterior rotation of the ilium. Hip abduction/adduction are associated with a lateral tilt of the pelvis.

Knee Joint Complex

The knee joint complex includes three articulating surfaces, which form two distinct joints contained within a single joint capsule: the patellofemoral and tibiofemoral joint.

The tibiofemoral joint is a ginglymoid, or modified hinge joint, that relies upon the static restraints of the joint capsule, ligaments, and menisci, as well as the dynamic restraints of the quadriceps, hamstrings, and gastrocnemius, for joint stability. The patella, the largest sesamoid bone in the body, possesses the thickest articular cartilage. The articular surface, which can have a variable contour, articulates with the trochlear groove of the femur. The motions that occur about the knee consist of flexion

and extension, coupled with other motions such as varus and valgus motions, and external and internal rotation.

● **Key Point** For flexion to be initiated from a position of full extension, the knee joint must first be "unlocked." The service of locksmith is provided by the popliteus muscle, which acts to internally rotate the tibia with respect to the femur, enabling flexion to occur

The muscles that act on the knee are outlined in **Table 4-10**. During flexion of the knee, the femur rolls posteriorly and glides anteriorly, with the opposite occurring with extension of the knee. The quadriceps ("Q") angle can be described as the angle formed by the bisection of two lines, one line drawn from the anterior superior iliac spine (ASIS) to the center of the patella, and the other line drawn from the center of the patella to the tibial tubercle.

● **Key Point** Various normal values for the Q-angle have been reported in the literature. The most common ranges cited are 8° to 14° for males and 15° to 17° for females.[16,17] The discrepancy between males and females is supposedly due to the wider pelvis of the female, although this has yet to be proven.

A number of key ligaments provide stability to the knee joint complex:

- *Anterior cruciate ligament (ACL):* Originates from deep within the notch of the distal femur. Its proximal fibers fan out along the medial wall of the lateral femoral condyle. There are two bundles of the ACL—the anteromedial and the posterolateral, named according to where the bundles insert into the tibial plateau. The ACL attaches in front of the intercondyloid eminence of the tibia, being blended with the anterior horn of the lateral meniscus. These attachments allow it to resist anterior translation of the tibia, in relation to the femur.
- *Posterior cruciate ligament (PCL):* Connects the posterior intercondylar area of the tibia to the medial condyle of the femur. This configuration allows the PCL to resist forces pushing the tibia posteriorly relative to the femur.
- *Medial collateral ligament (MCL):* A broad, flat, membranous band that is attached proximally to the medial condyle of femur immediately below the adductor tubercle, below the medial condyle of the tibia and medial surface of its body. The MCL functions to resists valgus forces.

TABLE
4-10

Muscles of the Knee: Their Actions, Nerve Supply, and Nerve Root Derivation			
Action	**Muscles Acting**	**Nerve Supply**	**Nerve Root Derivation**
Flexion of knee	Biceps femoris	Sciatic	L5, S1–S2
	Semimembranosus	Sciatic	L5, S2–S2
	Semitendinosus	Sciatic	L5, S1–S2
	Gracilis	Obturator	L2–L3
	Sartorius	Femoral	L2–L3
	Popliteus	Tibial	L4–L5, S1
	Gastrocnemius	Tibial	S1–S2
	Tensor fascia latae	Superior gluteal	L4–L5
Extension of knee	Rectus femoris	Femoral	L2–L4
	Vastus medialis	Femoral	L2–L4
	Vastus intermedius	Femoral	L2–L4
	Vastus lateralis	Femoral	L2–L4
	Tensor fascia latae	Superior gluteal	L4–L5
Internal rotation of flexed leg (non–weight bearing)	Popliteus	Tibial	L4–L5
	Semimembranosus	Sciatic	L5, S1–S2
	Semitendinosus	Sciatic	L5, S1–S2
	Sartorius	Femoral	L2–L3
	Gracilis	Obturator	L2–L3
External rotation of flexed leg (non–weight bearing)	Biceps femoris	Sciatic	L5, S1–S2

- *Lateral collateral ligament (LCL):* Stretches obliquely inferiorly and posteriorly from the lateral epicondyle of the femur above, to the head of the fibula. The LCL functions to resists varus forces.

Ankle and Foot Joint Complex

The majority of the support provided to the ankle and foot joints comes by way of the arrangement of the ankle mortise and by the numerous ligaments found here (**Table 4-11**). Further stabilization is afforded by an abundant number of tendons that cross this joint complex (**Table 4-12**). These tendons are also involved in producing foot and ankle movements and are held in place by retinaculae. The intrinsic muscles of the foot are outlined in **Table 4-13**. Motions of the leg foot and ankle consist of single-plane and multi-plane movements. The single-plane motions include:

- *The frontal plane motions of inversion and eversion.* Inversion and eversion are single-plane motions that occur in the frontal plane at the subtalar joint around a sagittal axis.

- *The sagittal plane motions of dorsiflexion and plantarflexion.* These terms indicate movement at the ankle and at the midtarsal joint. Plantar flexion is movement of the foot downward toward the ground, and dorsiflexion is a movement of the foot upward toward the tibia.

- *The horizontal plane motions of adduction and abduction.* These terms describe motions of the forefoot in the horizontal plane about a superior–inferior axis. Abduction moves the forefoot laterally, whereas adduction moves the forefoot medially on the midfoot.

A triplane motion is a movement about an obliquely oriented axis through all three body planes. Triplanar motions occur at the talocrural, subtalar, and midtarsal joints, and at the first and fifth rays. Pronation and supination are considered triplanar motions.

- *Pronation and supination during weight-bearing activities.* During weight-bearing activities, pronation involves a combination of calcaneal eversion, adduction and plantarflexion

TABLE
4-11
Ankle and Foot Joints and Associated Ligaments

Joint	Associated Ligament	Motions Limited
Distal tibiofibular	Anterior tibiofibular	Distal glide of fibula
		Plantar flexion
	Posterior tibiofibular	Distal glide of fibular
		Plantar flexion
Ankle	Deltoid (medial collateral)	
	Superficial	
	Tibionavicular	Plantar flexion, abduction
	Tibiocalcaneal	Eversion, abduction
	Posterior tibiotalar	Dorsiflexion, abduction
	Deep	
	Anterior tibiotalar	Eversion, abduction, plantar flexion
	Lateral or fibular collateral	Plantar flexion
	Anterior talofibular	Inversion
		Anterior displacement of foot
	Calcaneofibular	Inversion
		Dorsiflexion
	Posterior talofibular	Dorsiflexion
		Posterior displacement of foot
	Lateral talocalcaneal	Inversion
		Dorsiflexion
	Anterior capsule	Plantar flexion
	Posterior capsule	Dorsiflexion
Subtalar	Interosseous talocalcaneal	
	Anterior band	Inversion
		Joint separation
	Posterior band	Inversion
		Joint separation
	Lateral talocalcaneal	
	Deltoid	
	Lateral collateral	
	Posterior talocalcaneal	Dorsiflexion
	Medial talocalcaneal	Eversion
	Anterior talocalcaneal	Inversion
	(cervical ligaments)	
Main ligamentous support of longitudinal arches	Long plantar	Eversion
	Short plantar	Eversion
	Plantar calcaneonavicular	Eversion
	Plantar aponeurosis	Eversion
Midtarsal or transverse	Bifurcated	Joint separation
	Medial band	Plantar flexion
	Lateral band	Inversion
	Dorsal talonavicular	Plantar flexion of talus on navicular
	Dorsal calcaneocuboid	Inversion, plantar flexion

TABLE 4-12	Extrinsic Muscle Attachments and Innervation			
Muscle	Proximal	Distal	Innervation	Function
Gastrocnemius	Medial and lateral condyle of femur	Posterior surface of calcaneus through Achilles tendon	Tibial S2 (S1)	Plantarflexion Flexion of the knee
Plantaris	Lateral supracondylar line of femur	Posterior surface of calcaneus through Achilles tendon	Tibial S2 (S1)	Plantarflexion Flexion of the knee
Soleus	Head of fibula, proximal third of shaft, soleal line, and midshaft of posterior tibia	Posterior surface of calcaneus through Achilles tendon	Tibial S2 (S1)	Plantarflexion
Tibialis anterior	Distal to lateral tibial condyle, proximal half of lateral tibial shaft, and interosseous membrane	First cuneiform bone, medial and plantar surfaces, and base of first metatarsal	Deep fibular (peroneal) L4 (L5)	Dorsiflexion Inversion
Tibialis posterior	Posterior surface of tibia, proximal two-thirds posterior of fibula, and interosseous membrane	Tuberosity of navicular bone, tendinous expansion to other tarsals and metatarsals	Tibial L4 and L5	Plantarflexion Inversion
Fibularis (peroneus) longus	Lateral condyle of tibia, head and proximal two-thirds of fibula	Base of first metatarsal and first cuneiform, lateral side	Superficial fibular (peroneal) L5 and S1 (S2)	Eversion Plantarflexion
Fibularis (peroneus) brevis	Distal two-thirds of lateral fibular shaft	Tuberosity of fifth metatarsal	Superficial fibular (peroneal) L5 and S1 (S2)	Plantarflexion Eversion
Fibularis (peroneus) tertius	Lateral slip from extensor digitorum longus	Tuberosity of fifth metatarsal	Deep fibular (peroneal) L5 and S1	Dorsiflexion Eversion
Flexor hallucis longus	Posterior distal two-thirds fibula	Base of distal phalanx of great toe	Tibial S2 (S3)	Flexion of the great toe Plantarflexion Inversion
Flexor digitorum longus	Middle three-fifths of posterior tibia	Base of distal phalanx of lateral four toes	Tibial S2 (S3)	Flexion of toes 2–5 Plantarflexion Inversion
Extensor hallucis longus	Middle half of anterior shaft of fibula	Base of distal phalanx of great toe	Deep fibular (peroneal) L5 and S1	Extension of the great toe Dorsiflexion
Extensor digitorum longus	Lateral condyle of tibia proximal anterior surface of shaft of fibula	One tendon to each lateral four toes, to middle phalanx and extending to distal phalanges	Deep fibular (peroneal) L5 and S1	Extension of toes 2–5 (MTP, PIP, and DIP joints) Dorsiflexion Eversion

TABLE
4-13

Intrinsic Muscles of the Foot

Muscle	Proximal	Distal	Innervation	Function
Extensor digitorum brevis	Distal superior surface of calcaneus	Dorsal surface of second through fourth toes, base of proximal phalanx	Deep fibularis (peroneal) S1 and S2	Extension of the first four toes
Flexor digitorum brevis	Tuberosity of calcaneus	One tendon slip into base of middle phalanx of each of the lateral four toes	Medial and lateral plantar S3 (S2)	Flexion of the MTP and PIP joints of the lesser four toes
Extensor hallucis brevis	Distal superior and lateral surfaces of calcaneus	Dorsal surface of proximal phalanx	Deep fibular (peroneal) S1 and S2	Extension of great toe
Flexor hallucis brevis	Plantar surface of cuboid and third cuneiform bones	Base of proximal phalanx of great toe	Medial plantar S3 (S2)	MTP flexion of the great toe
Quadratus plantae	By two heads to the plantar aspect of the calcaneus	Lateral border of the flexor digitorum longus tendon	Lateral plantar S1 and S2	Helps to stabilize the tendon of the flexor digitorum longus, preventing them from migrating medially when under force
Abductor hallucis	Tuberosity of calcaneus and plantar aponeurosis	Base of proximal phalanx, medial side	Medial plantar L5 and S1 (L4)	Abduction of the great toe
Adductor hallucis	Base of second, third, and fourth metatarsals and deep plantar ligaments	Proximal phalanx of first digit lateral side	Medial and lateral plantar S1 and S2	Flexion and abduction of the MTP joint of the great toe
Lumbricals	Medial and adjacent sides of flexor digitorum longus tendon to each lateral digit	Medial side of proximal phalanx and extensor hood	Medial and lateral plantar L5, S1, and S2 (L4)	Flexion of the MTP joints, simultaneously extending the IP joints
Plantar interossei				
First	Base and medial side of third metatarsal	Base of proximal phalanx and extensor hood of third digit	Medial and lateral plantar S1 and S2	Adduction of toes
Second	Base and medial side of fourth metatarsal	Base of proximal phalanx and extensor hood of fourth digit		
Third	Base and medial side of fifth metatarsal	Base of proximal phalanx and extensor hood of fifth digit		
Dorsal interossei				
First	First and second metatarsal bones	Proximal phalanx and extensor hood of second digit medially	Medial and lateral plantar S1 and S2	Abduction of toes 2–4
Second	Second and third metatarsal bones	Proximal phalanx and extensor hood of second digit laterally		
Third	Third and fourth metatarsal bones	Proximal phalanx and extensor hood of third digit laterally		
Fourth	Fourth and fifth metatarsal bones	Proximal phalanx and extensor hood of fourth digit laterally		
Abductor digiti minimi	Lateral side of fifth metatarsal bone	Proximal phalanx of fifth digit	Lateral plantar S1 and S2	Abduction of the fifth toe
Flexor digiti minimi	Plantar aspect of the base of the fifth metatarsal	Lateral base of the proximal phalanx of the fifth toe	Lateral plantar S1 and S2	MTP flexion of the fifth toe

of the talus, and internal rotation of the tibia, whereas supination involves a combination of calcaneal inversion, abduction and dorsiflexion of the talus, and external rotation of the tibia.

- *Pronation and supination during non-weight-bearing activities.* During non-weight-bearing activities, pronation involves a combination of calcaneal eversion, abduction, and dorsiflexion of the talus, whereas supination involves a combination of calcaneal inversion, adduction, and plantarflexion of the talus.

● **Key Point** During pronation, the forefoot is rotated with the big toe downward and the little toe upward, whereas during supination, the reverse occurs.

Craniovertebral Joints

The *craniovertebral (CV) junction* is a collective term that refers to the region of the cervical spine where the skull and vertebral column articulate. It comprises the bony structures of the foramen magnum, occiput, atlas, axis, and their supporting ligaments. The posterior portion of the foramen magnum houses the brainstem–spinal cord junction.

Occipito–Atlantal (O-A) Joint

The occipito–atlantal (O-A) joint is formed between the occipital condyles and the superior articular facets of the atlas (C1). The paired occipital condyles are ovoid structures with their long axis situated in a posterolateral to anteromedial orientation.

Atlanto-Axial Joint

This relatively complex articulation consists of:

- Two lateral zygapophysial joints between the articular surfaces of the inferior articular processes of the atlas and the superior processes of the axis.
- Two medial joints: one between the anterior surface of the dens of the axis and the anterior surface of the atlas, and the other between the posterior surface of the dens and the anterior hyalinated surface of the transverse ligament.
- The transverse ligament, which stretches between tubercles on the medial aspects of the lateral masses of the atlas and functions to counteract anterior translation of the atlas relative to the axis, thereby maintaining the position of the dens relative to the anterior arch of the atlas. The transverse ligament also limits the amount of flexion between the atlas and axis.[18] These limiting functions are of extreme importance because excessive movement of either type could result in the dens compressing the spinal cord, epipharynx, vertebral artery, or superior cervical ganglion.

- The alar ligaments, which connect the superior part of the dens to fossae on the medial aspect of the occipital condyles, although they can also attach to the lateral masses of the atlas. The function of the ligament is to resist flexion, contralateral side bending, and rotation.[19]
- The tectorial membrane, which is the superior continuation of the posterior longitudinal ligament and connects the body of vertebra C2 to the anterior rim of the foramen magnum. This bridging ligament is an important limiter of upper cervical flexion.

Cervical Spine

The cervical spine is made up of seven vertebrae. C1 articulates with the occiput of the skull above and with C2 below. Vertebrae C3 through C7 allow for varying degrees of flexion, extension, side bending, and rotation as an interdependent group. Eight pairs of cervical spinal nerves exit bilaterally through the intervertebral foramina. Each spinal nerve is named for the vertebra above which it exits; for example, the C6 nerve exits above the C6 vertebra. The muscles of the cervical spine are outlined in **Table 4-14**, **Table 4-15**, and **Table 4-16**.

● **Key Point** With stability being sacrificed for mobility, the cervical spine is rendered more vulnerable to both direct and indirect trauma. The cervical spine can be the source of many pain syndromes, including neck, upper thoracic, and periscapular syndromes, cervical radiculopathy, and shoulder and elbow syndromes.

Temporomandibular Joint

The temporomandibular joint (TMJ) is a synovial compound modified ovoid bicondylar joint formed between the articular eminence of the temporal bone, the intra-articular disc, and the head of the mandible. The TMJ is unique in that, even though the joint is synovial, the articulating surfaces of the bones are covered not by hyaline cartilage, but by fibrocartilage.

● **Key Point** The development of fibrocartilage over the load-bearing surface of the TMJ indicates that the joint is designed to withstand large and repeated stresses, and that this area of the joint surface has a greater capacity to repair itself than would hyaline cartilage.

Located between the articulating surface of the temporal bone and the mandibular condyle is a

TABLE
4-14

Attachments and Innervation of Cervical Muscles

Muscle	Proximal	Distal	Innervation
Upper trapezius	Superior nuchal line Ligamentum nuchae	Lateral third of clavicle and the acromion process	Spinal accessory
Levator scapulae	Transverse processes of upper four cervical vertebrae	Medial border of scapula at level of scapular superior angle	Dorsal scapular C5 (C3 and C4)
Splenius capitis	Inferior ligamentum nuchae, spinous process of C7 and T1–T4 vertebrae	Mastoid process, occipital bone, and lateral third of superior nuchal line	Cervical spinal nerve and ventral primary rami of cervical spinal nerves
Splenius cervicis	Spinous processes of T3–T6 vertebrae	Posterior tubercles of C1–C3	
Scalenus			
Anterior	Anterior tubercles of C3–C6	Superior crest of first rib	Ventral primary rami of cervical spinal nerves
Middle	Posterior tubercles of C2–C7	Superior crest of first rib	
Posterior	Posterior tubercles of C5–C7	Outer surface of second rib	
Longus colli	Anterior tubercles of C3–C5 Anterior surface of C5–C7, T1–T3	Tubercle of the atlas, anterior tubercles of C5 and C6, anterior surface of C2–C4	Ventral primary rami of cervical spinal nerves
Longus capitis	Anterior tubercles of C3–C6	Inferior occipital bone, basilar portion	Ventral primary rami of cervical spine nerves

TABLE
4-15

Prime Movers of the Cervical Spine: Extensors and Flexors

Prime Extensors	Prime Flexors
Trapezius	Sternocleidomastoid—anterior fibers
Sternocleidomastoid—posterior fibers	Accessory muscles
Iliocostalis cervices	Prevertebral muscles
Longissimus cervices	Longus coli
Splenius cervices	Longus capitis
Splenius capitis	Rectus capitis anterior
Interspinales cervices	Scalene group
Spinalis cervices	Scalenus anterior
Spinalis capitis	Infrahyoid group
Semispinalis cervices	Sternohyoid
Semispinalis capitis	Omohyoid
Levator scapulae	Sternothyroid
Suboccipitals	Thyrohyoid

fibrocartilaginous disc (sometimes inappropriately referred to as meniscus). The movements that occur at the TMJ are extremely complex.

Mouth opening (mandibular depression), contralateral deviation, and protrusion all involve an anterior osteokinematic rotation of the mandible and an anterior, inferior, and lateral glide of the mandibular head and disc.

Mouth closing (mandibular elevation), ipsilateral deviation, and retrusion all involve a posterior osteokinematic rotation of the mandible and a posterior, superior, and medial glide of the mandibular head and disc.

Working in combinations, the muscles of the TMJ (Table 4-17) are involved as follows:

- *Mouth opening (mandibular depression):* Bilateral action of the lateral pterygoid and digastric muscles
- *Mouth closing (mandibular elevation):* Bilateral action of the temporalis, masseter, and medial pterygoid muscles
- *Lateral deviation:* Action of the ipsilateral masseter and temporalis, and contralateral medial and lateral pterygoid muscles

TABLE 4-16	Prime Movers of the Cervical Spine: Rotation and Side Bending	

Muscles of Rotation and Side Bending

Ipsilateral Side Bending	*Ipsilateral Rotation*
Longissimus capitis	Splenius capitis
Intertransversarii posteriores	Splenius cervices
	Rotatores breves cervices
Multifidus	Rotatores longi cervices
Rectus capitis lateralis	Rectus capitis posterior major
Intertransversarii anteriores cervices	Obliquus capitis inferior
Scaleni	
Iliocostalis cervicis	
Contralateral Rotation	*Ipsilateral Side Bending and Contralateral Rotation*
Obliquus capitis superior	Sternocleidomastoid
	Scalenus anterior
	Multifidus
	Longus colli

Ipsilateral Side Bending and Ipsilateral Rotation

Longus coli

Scalenus posterior

TABLE 4-17	Muscle Functions of the Temporomandibular Joint	

Motion	Muscle Responsible for Motion
Depression	Lateral pterygoid
	Suprahyoid
	Infrahyoid
Elevation	Temporalis
	Masseter
	Medial pterygoid
Protrusion	Masseter
	Lateral pterygoid
	Medial pterygoid
Retrusion	Temporalis
	Masseter
	Digastric
Lateral deviation (side to side)	Medial pterygoid
	Lateral pterygoid
	Masseter
	Temporalis

- *Protrusion:* Bilateral action of the lateral pterygoid, medial pterygoid, and anterior fibers of the temporalis muscles
- *Retrusion:* Bilateral action of the posterior fibers of the temporalis muscle and the digastric, stylohyoid, geniohyoid, and mylohyoid muscles

Thoracic Spine and Rib Cage

In the thoracic spine, protection and function of the thoracic viscera take precedence over segmental spinal mobility. The rib cage and its articulations provide a significant degree of stability. The increased stability/reduced mobility of the thoracic segments has been reported to produce three primary effects:[20,21]

- It influences the motions available in other regions of the spine and the shoulder girdle.
- It increases the potential for postural impairments in this region.[22]

- It provides an important weight-bearing mechanism for the vertebral column.[23]

The muscles of the thoracic and lumbar spine are outlined in **Table 4-18**.

● **Key Point** The load-bearing capacity of the spine has been found to be up to three times greater with an intact rib cage.[24,25]

Lumbar Spine

Generally, the five similar lumbar vertebral bodies are distinguished from the thoracic bodies by the absence of rib facets. The primary ligamentous support for the lumbar spine is the anterior longitudinal ligament, the posterior longitudinal ligament, the attachments of the annulus fibrosis, the facet joints, and the interosseous ligaments between the spinous processes. Motions at the lumbar spine joints can occur in three cardinal planes: sagittal (flexion and extension), coronal (side bending), and transverse (rotation).

The amount of range available in the lumbar spine decreases with age. Different trunk muscles play differing roles in the provision of dynamic stability to the spine.

Sacroiliac Joint

The sacroiliac joint (SIJ) is a true diarthrodial joint that joins the sacrum to the pelvis. The SIJ contains

TABLE 4-18	Muscle Functions of the Thoracic and Lumbar Spine
Motion	Muscle Responsible for Motion
Flexion	Rectus abdominis
	Internal oblique
	External oblique
Extension	Erector spinae
	Quadratus lumborum
	Multifidus
Rotation and sidebending	Psoas major
	Quadratus lumborum
	External oblique
	Internal oblique
	Multifidus
	Longissimus thoracis
	Iliocostalis thoracis
	Rotatores

numerous ridges and depressions, indicating its function for stability more than motion, although some motion does occur at the joint. Stability at the SIJ is provided not just by the ridges present in the joint but also by the presence of generously sized ligaments. The ligamentous structures offer resistance to shear and loading. There is very little agreement, among disciplines or even within disciplines, about the biomechanics of the pelvic complex.

Kinesiology

When describing joint movements, the *anatomical reference position* is used. The anatomical reference position for the human body is described as the erect standing position with the feet just slightly separated and the arms hanging by the side, the elbows straight and with the palms of the hand facing forward (Figure 4-1).

Directional Terms

Directional terms are used to describe the relationship of body parts or the location of an external object with respect to the body.[26] The following are commonly used directional terms:

- *Superior or cranial:* Closer to the head
- *Inferior or caudal:* Closer to the feet
- *Anterior or ventral:* Toward the front of the body
- *Posterior or dorsal:* Toward the back of the body
- *Medial:* Toward the midline of the body
- *Lateral:* Away from the midline of the body
- *Proximal:* Closer to the trunk
- *Distal:* Away from the trunk
- *Superficial:* Toward the surface of the body
- *Deep:* Away from the surface of the body in the direction of the inside of the body

Movements of the Body Segments

Movements of the body segments occur in three dimensions along imaginary planes and around various axes of the body.

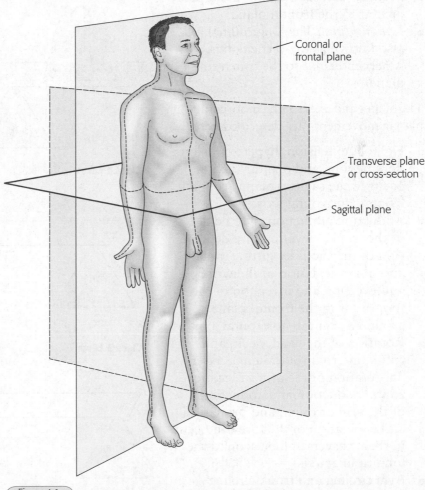

Figure 4-1 Anatomic position and planes of the body.

Planes of the Body

There are three traditional planes of the body, corresponding to the three dimensions of space:[26]

- *Sagittal:* The sagittal plane, also known as the anterior–posterior or median plane, divides the body vertically into left and right sections.
- *Frontal:* The frontal plane, also known as the lateral or coronal plane, divides the body into front and back sections.
- *Transverse:* The transverse plane, also known as the horizontal plane, divides the body equally into top and bottom sections.

Axes of the Body

Three reference axes are used to describe human motion: frontal, sagittal, and longitudinal. The axis around which the movement takes place is always perpendicular to the plane in which it occurs.

- *Frontal:* The frontal axis, also known as the transverse axis, is perpendicular to the sagittal plane.
- *Sagittal:* The sagittal axis is perpendicular to the frontal plane.
- *Longitudinal:* The longitudinal axis, also known as the vertical axis, is perpendicular to the transverse plane.

The planes and axes for the more common planar movements are described here:

- Flexion, extension, hyperextension, dorsiflexion, and plantar flexion occur in the sagittal plane around a frontal–horizontal axis.
- Abduction/adduction, side flexion of the trunk, elevation and depression of the shoulder girdle, radial and ulnar deviation of the wrist, and eversion and inversion of the foot occur in the frontal plane around a sagittal–horizontal axis.
- Rotation of the head, neck, and trunk; internal rotation and external rotation of the arm or leg; horizontal adduction and abduction of the arm or thigh; and pronation and supination of the forearm occur in the transverse plane around the longitudinal axis.
- Arm circling and trunk circling are examples of circumduction.

Circumduction involves an orderly sequence of circular movements that occur in the sagittal, frontal, and intermediate oblique planes, so that segment as a whole incorporates a combination of flexion, extension, abduction, and adduction. Circumduction movements can occur at biaxial and triaxial joints. Examples of these joints include the tibiofemoral, radiohumeral, hip, glenohumeral, and the spinal joints.

Levers

Biomechanical levers can be defined as rotations of a rigid surface about an axis. For simplicity's sake, levers are usually described using a straight bar, which is the lever, and the fulcrum, which is the point on which the bar is resting. The effort force attempts to cause movement of the load. That part of the lever between the fulcrum and the load is the load arm. There are three types of levers (Figure 4-2):

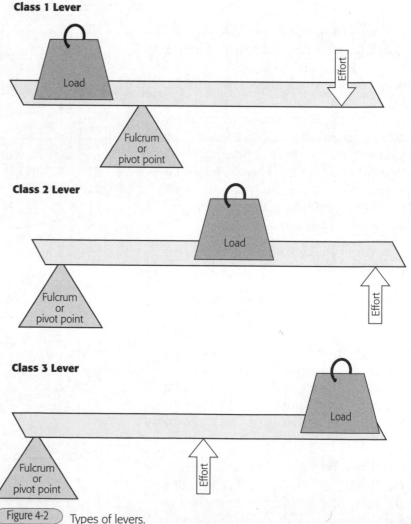

Figure 4-2 Types of levers.

- *First class:* Occurs when two forces are applied on either side of an axis and the fulcrum lies between the effort and the load, like a seesaw. Examples in the human body include the contraction of the triceps at the elbow joint, or tipping of the head forward and backward.
- *Second class:* Occurs when the load (resistance) is applied between the fulcrum and the point at which the effort is exerted. This has the advantage of magnifying the effects of the effort so that it takes less force to move the resistance. Examples of second-class levers in everyday life include the nutcracker and the wheelbarrow—with the wheel acting as the fulcrum. There are numerous examples of second-class levers in the human body. One example is weight-bearing plantarflexion (rising up on the toes). Another is an isolated contraction of the brachioradialis to flex the elbow, which could not occur without the other elbow flexors being paralyzed.
- *Third class:* Occurs when the load is located at the end of the lever and the effort lies between the fulcrum and the load (resistance), like a drawbridge or a crane. The effort is exerted between the load and the fulcrum. The effort expended is greater than the load, but the load is moved a greater distance. Most movable joints in the human body function as third-class levers—for example, flexion at the elbow.

Osteokinematics

Osteokinematics is defined as the study of bone motion. Actual bone movement is a combination of one or more basic movements:

- *Spin:* The motion of the chosen point is only rotation around the mechanical axis of the bone (pure spin). Examples include internal and external rotation of the radius.
- *Swing:* Any motion of the point other than pure spin.
- *Pure swing:* Also known as a cardinal swing. A pure swing involves no spin. The point moves from its initial position to the final position along the shortage path possible, with the path (chord) corresponding to a meridian of latitude or longitude, or a straight line on a flat surface.
- *Impure swing:* Also known as an arcuate swing. An impure swing is a combination of swing and spin. The point moves along a path (arc) that is other than the shortest possible distance.

Degrees of Freedom

The number of independent modes of motion at a joint is called the *degrees of freedom* (DOF). When referring to degrees of freedom, the swings must be cardinal and the axis of swing must be at a 90° angle relative to the other swing axes.

- *1 DOF:* A joint that can swing in one direction or can only spin—for example, the proximal interphalangeal joint.
- *2 DOF:* A joint that can swing in two directions or swing in one direction and spin. Examples include the tibiofemoral joint, the temporomandibular joint, the proximal and distal radioulnar joints, the subtalar joint, and the talocalcaneal joint.
- *3 DOF:* A bone that can spin and also swing in two distinct directions. Examples include ball-and-socket joints, such as the shoulder and hip.

Arthrokinematics

The small motion that is available at joint surfaces is referred to as *accessory* or arthrokinematic motion. Normal arthrokinematic motions must occur for full-range physiological motion to take place. A restriction of arthrokinematic motion results in a decrease in osteokinematic motion. Three types of movement occur at the articulating surfaces (Figure 4-3):

- *Roll:* A roll occurs when the points of contact on each joint surface are constantly changing. This type of movement is analogous to a tire on a car as the car rolls forward. The term *rock* is often used to describe small rolling motions.
- *Slide:* A slide is a pure translation. It occurs if only one point on the moving surface makes contact with varying points on the opposing surface. This type of movement is analogous to a car tire skidding when the brakes are applied suddenly on a wet road. This type of motion is also referred to as translatory or accessory motion. While the roll of a joint always occurs in the same direction as the swing of a bone, the direction of the slide is determined by the shape of the articulating surface. This rule is often referred to as the concave–convex rule: If the joint surface is convex relative to the other surface, the slide occurs in the opposite direction to the osteokinematic motion. If, in contrast, the joint surface is concave, the slide occurs in the same direction as the osteokinematic motion.

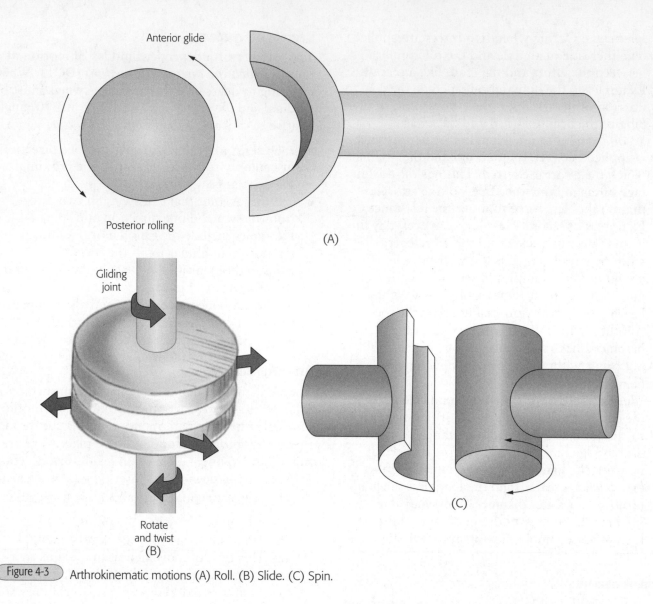

Anterior glide

Posterior rolling

(A)

Gliding joint

Rotate and twist

(B)

(C)

Figure 4-3 Arthrokinematic motions (A) Roll. (B) Slide. (C) Spin.

■ *Spin:* A spin is defined as any movement in which the bone moves but the mechanical axis remains stationary. A spin involves a rotation of one surface on an opposing surface around a longitudinal axis. This type of motion is analogous to the pirouette performed in ballet. Spin motions in the body include internal and external rotation of the glenohumeral joint when the humerus is abducted to 90°, and at the radial head during forearm pronation and supination. Most anatomic joints demonstrate composite motions involving a roll, slide, and spin.

An articulating surface can be either concave (female) or convex (male) in shape (ovoid), or a combination of both shapes (sellar) (**Table 4-19**).

● Key Point The convex–concave rules describe the relationship between arthrokinematics and osteokinematics:

- Convex rule: If the moving joint surface is convex relative to the other surface, the slide occurs in the opposite direction to the movement of the bone shaft of the lever (angular motion) (Figure 4-4).
- Concave rule: If the moving joint surface is concave, the slide occurs in the same direction to the movement of the bone shaft of the lever (angular motion).

This rule is very important to remember for joint mobility testing and for joint mobilizations.

If during mobility testing, there is a limited glide:

- If the limitation occurs when the concave surface is moving, the restriction is likely due to a contracture of the trailing portion of the capsule.
- If the limitation occurs when the convex surface is moving, the restriction is likely due to an inability of the moving surface to move into the contracted portion of the capsule (may be due to adhesions between redundant folds of the capsule).

| TABLE 4-19 | Characteristics of Convex and Concave Surfaces |

Concave (Female) Surfaces	Convex (Male) Surfaces
Concave surfaces can both spin and glide on their convex partners.	Convex surfaces can both spin and glide on their concave partner. In addition, convex surfaces can roll upon the concave surface, and rolling is the primary movement of a convex surface.
Spin and glides of the joint are combined in joints with 1 degree of freedom (DOF).	
Spin and glides can occur independently in a joint with 2 or 3 DOF.	Rolling is always accompanied by gliding, except at the beginning and termination of the movement.
Concave surfaces can roll on the convex surface, except when the joint is in the close-pack position.	Rolling does not occur in the close-pack position.
Rolling is accompanied by gliding, except at the beginning and termination of a movement.	Rolling always takes place in the same direction as the swing of the bone.
Rolling and gliding occur in the same direction, which is also the same direction as the swing of the bone.	Gliding always takes place in the opposite direction of the rolling movement.
Rolling causes the leading edge of the concave surface to approximate the convex surface and the trailing edge to lift up from the convex surface.	Since the convex surface is always larger than the concave surface, the gliding movement in the opposite direction prevents the convex surface from rolling off of the concave surface.
Rolling supplements gliding, the latter of which is the primary movement of the concave surface and makes for economy of articular cartilage.	

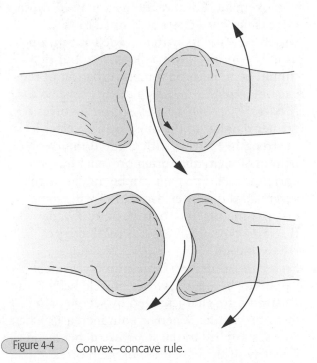

Figure 4-4   Convex–concave rule.

Close-Packed and Open-Packed Positions of the Joint

Joint movements are usually accompanied by a relative compression (approximation) or distraction (separation) of the opposing joint surfaces. These relative compressions or distractions affect the level of *congruity* of the opposing surfaces. The position of maximum congruity of the opposing joint surfaces is termed the *close-packed* position of the joint. The position of least congruity is termed the *open-packed* position.

Close-Packed Position

The close-packed position of a joint is the joint position that results in:

- Maximal tautness of the major ligaments
- Maximal surface congruity
- Least transarticular pressure
- Minimal joint volume
- Maximal stability of the joint

Once the close-packed position is achieved, no further motion in that direction is possible. The close-packed positions for the various joints are given in **Table 4-20**.

Open-Packed Position

In essence, any position of the joint, other than the close-packed position, could be considered an open-packed position. The open-packed position of a joint, also referred to as the *loose-packed* position, is the joint position that results in:

- Slackening of the major ligaments of the joint
- Minimal surface congruity

TABLE 4-20	Close-Packed Positions of the Joints
Joint	**Position**
Zygapophysial (spine)	Extension
Temporomandibular	Teeth clenched
Glenohumeral	Abduction and external rotation
Acromioclavicular	Arm abducted to 90°
Sternoclavicular	Maximum shoulder elevation
Ulnohumeral	Extension
Radiohumeral	Elbow flexed 90°; forearm supinated 5°
Proximal radioulnar	5° of supination
Distal radioulnar	5° of supination
Radiocarpal (wrist)	Extension with radial deviation
Metacarpophalangeal	Full flexion
Carpometacarpal	Full opposition
Interphalangeal	Full extension
Hip	Full extension, internal rotation, and abduction
Tibiofemoral	Full extension and external rotation of tibia
Talocrural (ankle)	Maximum dorsiflexion
Subtalar	Supination
Midtarsal	Supination
Tarsometatarsal	Supination
Metatarsophalangeal	Full extension
Interphalangeal	Full extension

- Minimal joint surface contact
- Maximal joint volume
- Minimal stability of the joint

The open-packed position permits maximal distraction of the joint surfaces. Because the open-packed position causes the brunt of any external force to be borne by the joint capsule or surrounding ligaments, most capsular or ligamentous sprains occur when a joint is in its open-packed position. The open-packed positions of the various joints are described in **Table 4-21**.

● **Key Point** The open-packed position is commonly used during joint mobilization techniques.

Capsular and Noncapsular Patterns of Restriction

Broadly speaking, two patterns of range of motion are used in the interpretation of joint motion:

- A *capsular* pattern of restriction is a limitation of pain and movement in a joint-specific ratio, which is usually present with arthritis, or following prolonged immobilization (**Table 4-22**).
- A *noncapsular* pattern of restriction is a limitation in a joint in any pattern other than a capsular one. It may indicate the presence of either a derangement, a restriction of one part of the joint capsule, or an extra-articular lesion that obstructs joint motion.

Musculoskeletal Injury and Repair

Muscle Injuries

Muscle strains may be classified according to their severity as follows:[27,28]

- *Mild (first-degree) strain:* Involves a tear of a few muscle fibers with minor swelling and local tenderness. Grade I injuries are associated with no or minimal loss of strength and restriction of movement. Local tenderness may be present, increasing when stress is applied to the structure. Patients with a grade I strain can usually continue normal activities, but they should be monitored for exacerbation of the existing injury.
- *Moderate (second-degree) strain:* Involves greater damage to the muscle and a clear loss of strength. Patients with grade II injuries have pain on activity that often prevents further participation. The pain can be moderate to severe, and it is often associated with some loss of function and joint stability. Grade II strains typically require 3 to 28 days of rehabilitation.[29]
- *Severe (third-degree) strain:* Involves a tear extending across the whole muscle belly. Grade III strains are characterized by severe pain or loss of function. Whether pain increases when stress is applied to the structure depends on the integrity of the remaining tissue. For example, there may be no pain in cases of a complete tear. Although grade I and II muscle strains are treated conservatively, surgical intervention is often necessary for grade III injuries.[30] Healing of grade III strains can require up to 3 months of rehabilitation.

TABLE 4-21	Open-Packed (Resting) Positions of the Joints
Joint	Position
Zygapophysial (spine)	Midway between flexion and extension
Temporomandibular	Mouth slightly open (freeway space)
Glenohumeral	55° of abduction, 30° of horizontal adduction
Acromioclavicular	Arm resting by side
Sternoclavicular	Arm resting by side
Ulnohumeral	70° of flexion, 10° of supination
Radiohumeral	Full extension, full supination
Proximal radioulnar	70° of flexion, 35° of supination
Distal radioulnar	10° of supination
Radiocarpal (wrist)	Neutral with slight ulnar deviation
Carpometacarpal	Midway between abduction/adduction and flexion/extension
Metacarpophalangeal	Slight flexion
Interphalangeal	Slight flexion
Hip	30° of flexion, 30° of abduction, slight lateral rotation
Tibiofemoral	25° of flexion
Talocrural (ankle)	10° of plantar flexion, midway between maximum inversion and eversion
Subtalar	Midway between extremes of range of movement
Midtarsal	Midway between extremes of range of movement
Tarsometatarsal	Midway between extremes of range of movement
Metatarsophalangeal	Neutral
Interphalangeal	Slight flexion

Achilles tendon at the heel. Tendinitis is most commonly caused by overuse and can result in pain and loss of function. In specific instances (i.e., calcific tendinitis of the rotator cuff) calcium can be deposited along the course of the tendon. The cause of calcium deposits within the rotator cuff tendon is not entirely understood. Different reasons have been suggested, including blood supply and aging of the tendon, but the evidence to support these conclusions is not conclusive.

- *Tendinosis:* A chronic alteration of the tendon accompanied by tissue degeneration, cell atrophy, and pain that is often associated with tendon thickening.[31]
- *Paratenonitis:* Encompasses peritendinitis, tenosynovitis, and tenovaginitis and is used to describe an inflammatory disorder of tissues surrounding the tendon, such as the tendon sheath. In most cases, these conditions seem to result from a repetitive friction of the tendon and its sheath.[32]

The goal of rehabilitation is to restore the tendon to its optimal length and cellularity, and to enhance its ability to withstand loads.

Tendon Injuries

Tendon injuries are among the most common overuse injuries. Three major types are recognized:

- *Tendinitis:* By definition, tendinitis is an inflammation of the tendon. Common sites of tendinitis include the rotator cuff of the shoulder (e.g., supraspinatus), bicipital tendon, origin of the wrist extensors (e.g., lateral epicondylitis, tennis elbow) and flexors (e.g., medial epicondylitis) at the elbow, the patellar and popliteal tendons and iliotibial band at the knee, the origin of the anterior tibial tendon in the leg (i.e., shin splints), and the

Ligament Injury

The most common mechanism of ligament injury is excessive lengthening of the ligament when the associated joint is moved into an excessive range of motion. Ligament injuries are classified into three grades:

- *Grade I (mild):* Involves stretching of the ligament, but no fiber damage.
- *Grade II (moderate):* Involves stretching of the ligament and tearing of some fibers.
- *Grade III (complete):* Involves almost complete ligament disruption.

The signs and symptoms of the various grades of ligament injury are outlined in **Table 4-23**.

TABLE 4-22 Capsular Patterns of Restriction

Joint	Limitation of Motion (Passive Angular Motion)
Glenohumeral	External rotation > abduction > internal rotation (3:2:1)
Acromioclavicular	No true capsular pattern; possible loss of horizontal adduction, pain (and sometimes slight loss of end range) with each motion
Sternoclavicular	Same as for acromioclavicular joint
Humeroulnar	Flexion > extension (±4:1)
Humeroradial	No true capsular pattern; possible equal limitation of pronation and supination
Superior radioulnar	No true capsular pattern; possible equal limitation of pronation and supination with pain at end ranges
Inferior radioulnar	No true capsular pattern; possible equal limitation of pronation and supination with pain at end ranges
Wrist (carpus)	Flexion = extension
Radiocarpal	Same as for wrist (carpus)
Carpometacarpal	
Mid carpal	
1st carpometacarpal	Retroposition
Carpometacarpal 2–5	Fan > fold
Metacarpophalangeal 2–5	Flexion > extension (±2:1)
Interphalangeal	
Proximal (PIP)	Flexion > extension (±2:1)
Distal (DIP)	
Hip	Internal rotation > flexion > abduction = extension > other motions
Tibiofemoral	Flexion > extension (±5:1)
Superior tibiofibular	No capsular pattern: pain at end range of translatory movements
Talocrural	Plantar flexion > dorsiflexion
Talocalcaneal (subtalar)	Varus > valgus
Midtarsal	
Talonavicular Calcaneocuboid	Inversion (plantar flexion, adduction, supination) > dorsiflexion
1st metatarsophalangeal	Extension > flexion (± 2:1)
Metatarsophalangeal 2–5	Flexion ≥ extension
Interphalangeal 2–5	
Proximal	Flexion ≥ Extension
Distal	Flexion ≥ Extension

Data from Cyriax J: Textbook of Orthopaedic Medicine, Diagnosis of Soft Tissue Lesions (ed 8). London, Bailliere Tindall, 1982

Musculoskeletal Tissue Healing

Acute (Coagulation and Inflammation) Stage

The reaction that occurs immediately after a soft tissue injury involves two processes: coagulation and inflammation. Following an injury to the tissues, capillary blood flow is disrupted, causing hypoxia to the area. This initial period of vasoconstriction, which lasts 5 to 10 minutes, limits the blood loss and causes the inflammatory phase to begin, which in turn prompts a period of vasodilation, and the

TABLE 4-23	Ligament Injuries		
Grade	**Signs and Symptoms**		**Implications**
Grade I (mild)	Minimal loss of structural integrity		Minimal functional loss
	No abnormal motion		Early return to training; some protection may be necessary
	Little or no swelling		
	Localized tenderness		
	Minimal bruising		
Grade II (moderate)	Significant structural weakening		Tendency to recur
	Some abnormal motion		Need protection from risk of further injury
	Solid end feel to stress		May need modified immobilization
	More bruising and swelling		May stretch out further with time
	Often associated hemarthrosis and effusion		
Grade III (complete)	Loss of structural integrity		Needs prolonged protection
	Marked abnormal motion		Surgery may be considered
	Significant bruising		Often permanent functional instability
	Hemarthrosis		

extravasation (the movement of white blood cells from the capillaries to the tissues surrounding them) of blood constituents.[33] Extravasated blood contains platelets, which secrete substances that form a clot to prevent further bleeding and infection, clean dead tissue, and nourish white cells. These substances include macrophages and fibroblasts.[34] Inflammation is mediated by chemotactic substances, which are bodily cells that direct their movements according to certain chemicals in their environment, including anaphylatoxins that attract neutrophils and monocytes.

- *Neutrophils:* Neutrophils are white blood cells of the polymorphonuclear (PMN) leukocyte subgroup that express and release cytokines, which in turn intensify inflammatory reactions by several other cell types. The function of neutrophils is to bind to microorganisms, internalize them, and kill them, thereby controlling the spread of infection.
- *Monocytes:* Monocytes are white blood cells of the mononuclear leukocyte subgroup that migrate into tissues and develop into macrophages, and provide immunological defenses against many infectious organisms. Macrophages serve to orchestrate a "long-term" response (innate and adaptive immunity)

to injured cells subsequent to the acute response.[35]

● Key Point The *innate immune system* comprises the cells and mechanisms that defend the host from infection by other organisms, in a nonspecific manner, but does not confer long-lasting or protective immunity to the host. The *adaptive immune system* is composed of highly specialized, systemic cells and processes that have the ability to recognize and remember specific pathogens (to generate immunity), and to mount stronger attacks each time the pathogen is encountered.

The white blood cells of the inflammatory stage serve to clean the wound debris of foreign substances, increase vascular permeability, and promote fibroblast activity.[35] The extent and severity of the inflammatory response depend on the size and the type of the injury, the tissue involved, and the vascularity of that tissue.[36–40] Four systems work together during this phase:

- *Kinin system:* Causes vasodilation and increased permeability and stimulates pain receptors
- *Clotting system:* Leads to fibrin deposition and clot formation
- *Fibrinolytic system:* Leads to the synthesis of plasmin, which functions to degrade/dissolve the fibrin clot and to trigger activation of the complement system
- *Complement system:* Produces a variety of proteins with activities essential to healing

The complete removal of the wound debris marks the end of the inflammatory process, which usually occurs after 4 to 6 days unless the insult is perpetuated.

Clinical findings during the acute (coagulation and inflammatory) stage include swelling, redness, and increased warmth of the involved area, and impairment or loss of function.

Subacute (Migratory and Proliferative) Stage

The subacute stage of soft tissue healing, characterized by migration and proliferation, usually occurs from the time of the initial injury and overlaps the inflammation phase. Characteristic changes include capillary growth and granulation tissue formation, fibroblast proliferation with collagen synthesis, and increased macrophage and mast cell activity. This stage is responsible for the development of wound tensile strength.

After the wound base is free of necrotic tissue, the body begins to work to close the wound. The connective tissue in healing wounds is composed primarily of collagen, types I and III. Proliferation of collagen results from the actions of the fibroblasts that have been attracted to the area and stimulated to multiply by growth factors. This proliferation produces first fibrinogen and then fibrin, which eventually becomes organized into a honeycomb matrix and walls off the injured site.[41] The wound matrix functions as a glue to hold the wound edges together, giving it some mechanical protection, while also preventing the spread of infection. However, until the provisional extracellular matrix is replaced with a collagenous matrix, the wound matrix has a low tensile strength and is vulnerable to breakdown.

The collagenous matrix facilitates angiogenesis by providing time and protection to new and friable vessels. The process of neovascularization during this phase provides a granular appearance to the wound as a result of the formation of loops of capillaries and migration of macrophages, fibroblasts, and endothelial cells into the wound matrix. Once an abundant collagen matrix has been formed in the wound, the fibroblasts stop producing collagen, and the fibroblast-rich granulation tissue is replaced by a relatively acellular scar, marking the end of this stage. This fibrous tissue repair process can last anywhere from 5 to 15 days or several weeks, depending on the type of tissue and the extent of damage.

Clinically, this stage is characterized by a decrease in pain and swelling and an increase in pain-free active and passive ROM. During passive ROM, the subjective report of pain is synchronous with tissue resistance.

Chronic (Maturation and Remodeling) Stage

The chronic phase involves a conversion of the initial healing tissue to scar tissue. This lengthy phase of contraction, tissue remodeling, and increasing tensile strength in the wound can last for up to one year. From day 21 to day 60 there is a predominance of fibroblasts that are easily remodeled.[42] Fibroblasts are responsible for the synthesis, deposition, and remodeling of the extracellular matrix. Following the deposition of granulation tissue, some fibroblasts are transformed into myofibroblasts, which congregate at the wound margins and start pulling the edges inward, reducing the size of the wound. An increase in collagen types I and III and other aspects of the remodeling process are responsible for wound contraction and visible scar formation. Epithelial cells migrate from the wound edges and continue to migrate until similar cells from the opposite side are met. This contracted tissue, or scar tissue, is functionally inferior to original tissue and is a barrier to diffused oxygen and nutrients.[43] The remodeling time is influenced by factors that affect the density and activity level of the fibroblasts, including the amount of time to mobilize, the stresses placed on the tissue, the location of the lesion, and the quality of the vascular supply.[44] Imbalances in collagen synthesis and degradation during this phase of healing may result in hypertrophic scarring or keloid formation with superficial wounds.

● **Key Point** A keloid is a type of scar that results from an overgrowth of granulation tissue at the site of a healed skin injury. The overgrowth extends beyond the boundaries of an injury, damaging healthy tissues. Keloids are firm, rubbery lesions or shiny, fibrous nodules, and they can vary from pink to flesh-colored or red to dark brown in color. A hypertrophic scar can occur during the healing process when collagen production greatly exceeds collagen lysis. A hypertrophic scar is raised but remains within the borders of the original injury.

If the healing tissues are kept immobile, the fibrous repair is weak and there are no forces influencing the collagen; if left untreated, the scar formed is less than 20% of its original size.[45] Contraction of the scar, due to cross-linking of the collagen fibers and bundles, and the formation of adhesions between the immature collagen and surrounding tissues can cause scar hypomobility. In areas where the skin is loose and mobile, this creates minimal effect.

However, in areas such as the dorsum of the hand where there is no extra skin, wound contracture can have a significant effect on function. Despite the presence of an intact epithelium at 3 to 4 weeks after the injury, the tensile strength of the wound has been measured at approximately 25% of its normal value. Several months later, only 70% to 80% of the strength may be restored.[46] This would appear to demonstrate that the remodeling process may last many months or even years, making it extremely important to continue applying controlled stresses in the form of exercise to the tissue long after healing appears to have occurred.[46]

> ● **Key Point**   Scarring that occurs parallel to the line of force of a structure is less vulnerable to reinjury than a scar that is perpendicular to those lines of force.[47]

During this stage, pain is typically felt at the end of the range when stress is placed on restricted contractures or adhesions or when there is soreness due to the increased stress of resistive exercise.

Articular Cartilage Injury and Disease

Injuries to articular cartilage can be divided into three distinct types:

- *Type 1:* Type 1 injuries (superficial) involve microscopic damage to the chondrocytes and extracellular membrane (ECM).
- *Type 2:* Type 2 injuries (partial thickness) involve microscopic disruption of the articular cartilage surface (chondral fractures or fissuring).[48] This type of injury has traditionally had an extremely poor prognosis because the injury does not penetrate the subchondral bone and therefore does not provoke an inflammatory response.[48]
- *Type 3:* Type 3 injuries (full-thickness) involve disruption of the articular cartilage with penetration into the subchondral bone, which produces a significant inflammatory process.[48] The intrinsic repair capacity of such defects remains limited to the production of fibrocartilage. When symptomatic, small full-thickness injuries may be successfully treated with minimally invasive techniques designed to permit the efflux of marrow elements into the defect, resulting in fibrocartilage formation.[49] However, large defects may respond poorly to such techniques and may therefore require more sophisticated strategies,

including arthroscopic lavage and debridement, microfracture, autologous chondrocyte implantation, or osteochondral grafting.

Fibrocartilage Healing

Fibrocartilage, such as intervertebral discs, the labrum, and the menisci in the knee and temporomandibular joint, differs from hyaline cartilage in that it is composed of type I collagen instead of type II collagen and has a much higher fiber content than other types of cartilage. The nourishment of adult fibrocartilage is largely dependent on diffusion of nutrients through the synovial fluid in synovial joints. In amphiarthrodial joints (e.g., the intervertebral disc), nutrients are diffused across the fluid contained in the adjacent trabecular bone, assisted by the "milking" action produced by intermittent weight bearing.

The perichondrium surrounding fibrocartilage is poorly organized and contains small blood vessels located only near the peripheral rim of the tissue. Therefore, injuries to the fibrocartilage lead to abnormal hydration and an irreversible cascade of tissue alteration.[50] Because fibrocartilage is largely aneural, avascular, and devoid of immune system recognition, it has a very low potential for regeneration. In adult joints, however, some repair of damaged fibrocartilage can occur near the vascularized periphery—for example, the outer third of the meniscus of the knee. Due to these factors, in many cases of fibrocartilage injury, surgical intervention is required.

Bone Healing

A fracture is commonly defined as a break in the continuity of a bone. The most common cause of fractures is trauma, with the incidence and type of fracture sustained varying with age, race, and comorbidities. The striking feature of bone healing, compared with healing in other tissues, is that repair is by the original tissue, not scar tissue. *Regeneration* is perhaps a better descriptor than *repair*. Like other forms of healing, the repair of bone fracture includes the processes of inflammation, repair, and remodeling; the type of healing varies, however, depending on the method of treatment. The process of bone healing involves a combination of intramembranous and endochondral ossification. These two processes participate in the fracture repair sequence by at least four discrete stages of healing: the hematoma formation (inflammation or granulation) phase, the soft callus formation (reparative or revascularization) phase,

Stage 1: Organization

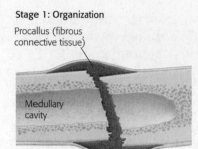

Procallus (fibrous connective tissue)

Medullary cavity

Bleeding and clot formation

Granulation tissue formation
• Fibroblast and blood vessel proliferation

Procallus formation

Day 5

Stage 2: Callus formation

Soft callus (fibrous connective tissue and hyaline cartilage)

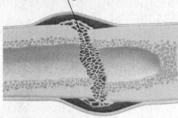

Areas of hyaline cartilage develop within the procallus, converting it to a soft callus

Hard callus (weak, disorganized bone)

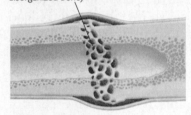

Intramembranous and endochondral ossification convert the soft callus into a hard callus

Day 28

Stage 3: Remodeling

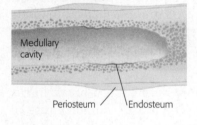

Medullary cavity

Periosteum   Endosteum

Remodeling has removed the callus and replaced the fractured matrix

The only remaining evidence of former injury may be the slight thickening of the endosteum and periosteum

Years later

Figure 4-5 Bone healing.

the hard callus formation (maturing or modeling) phase, and the remodeling phase (**Figure 4-5**).[51]

Hematoma Formation (Inflammatory) Phase

Initially, the tissue volume in which new bone is to be formed is filled with the matrix, generally including a blood clot or hematoma.[48] An effective bone healing response will include an initial inflammatory phase characterized by the release of a variety of products, an increase in regional blood flow, invasion of neutrophils and monocytes, removal of cell debris, and degradation of the local fibrin clot.

Soft Callus Formation (Reparative or Revascularization) Phase

This phase is characterized by the formation of connective tissues, including cartilage, and formation of new capillaries from preexisting vessels (angiogenesis). During the first 7 to 10 days of fracture healing, the periosteum undergoes an intramembranous bone formation response. By the middle of the second week, abundant cartilage overlies the fracture site, and this chondroid tissue initiates biochemical preparations to undergo calcification.

Hard Callus Formation (Modeling) Phase

This phase is characterized by the systematic removal of the initial matrix and tissues that formed in the site, primarily through osteoclastic and chondroclastic resorption, and their replacement with more organized lamellar bone (woven bone) aligned in response to the local loading environment.[48] The calcification of fracture callus cartilage can occur either directly from mesenchymal tissue (intramembranous) or via an intermediate stage of cartilage (endochondral or chondroid routes). Osteoblasts can form woven bone rapidly, but the result is randomly arranged and mechanically weak. Nonetheless, bridging of a fracture by woven bone constitutes *clinical union*. The clinical union is a critical milestone in the healing of a broken long bone as it signals that the woven bone at the fracture site has hardened and become so firmly fixed to the other fragments that they move as a single unit. Splinting is usually reduced at this stage, but the site still requires protection from excessive stresses. Once cartilage is calcified, it becomes a target for the ingrowth of blood vessels.

Remodeling Phase

By replacing the cartilage with bone and converting the cancellous bone into compact bone, the callus is gradually remodeled. During this phase, the woven bone is remodeled into stronger lamellar bone by a combination of osteoclast bone resorption and osteoblast bone formation.

Effects of Immobilization

Continuous immobilization of connective and skeletal muscle tissues in an adaptively shortened state can cause some undesirable consequences.

Cartilage Degeneration

Immobilization of a joint causes atrophic changes in articular cartilage resulting in cartilage softening.[52] As the softened articular cartilage is vulnerable to damage during weight bearing, care must be taken by the PTA during such activities and the use of an assistive device may be warranted.

Decreased Mechanical and Structural Properties of Ligaments

One study[53] showed that after 8 weeks of immobilization, the stiffness of a ligament decreased to 69% of control values, and even after one year of rehabilitation the ligament did not return to its prior level of strength. This results in a compromise in the ability of the ligament to provide stabilization, thereby making the joint more susceptible to injury unless protected using a splinting, bracing, or assistive device when bearing weight.

● **Key Point** Following a period of immobilization, healing connective tissues are more vulnerable to deformation and breakdown than normal tissues subjected to similar amounts of stress.[54]

Decreased Bone Density

The interactions among systemic and local factors to maintain normal bone mass are complex.[55–59] Bone mass is maintained because of a continuous coupling between bone resorption by osteoclasts and bone formation by osteoblasts, and this process is influenced by both systemic and local factors.[60] Mechanical forces acting on bone stimulate osteogenesis (Wolff law), and the absence of such forces inhibits osteogenesis. Marked osteopenia occurs in otherwise healthy patients in states of complete immobilization or weightlessness.[61,62] In children, bone has a high modeling rate and appears to be more sensitive to the absence of mechanical loading than bone in adults.[63] Decreased bone density results in increased vulnerability of the bone to fracture. Therapeutic exercises, particularly closed-chain exercises, have been shown to be beneficial in strengthening bone.

Weakness or Atrophy of Muscle

The longer the duration of immobilization, the greater is the atrophy of muscle and loss of functional strength. Muscle atrophy is an imbalance between protein synthesis and degradation. After modest trauma, there is a decrease in whole-body protein synthesis rather than increased breakdown. With more severe trauma, major surgery, or multiple organ failure, both synthesis and degradation increase, the latter being more enhanced.[64,65] Muscle atrophy can begin within just a few days.[66] The composition of muscle affects its response to immobilization, with atrophy occurring more quickly and more extensively in tonic (slow-twitch) postural muscle fibers than in phasic (fast-twitch) fibers.[67]

Change in Muscle Length

If the muscle is immobilized in a shortened position for several weeks, there is a reduction in the length of the muscle and its fibers and in the number of sarcomeres in series within myofibrils as the result of sarcomere absorption.[68] The absorption rate occurs faster than the muscle's ability to regenerate sarcomeres, resulting in muscle atrophy and weakness and a shift to the left in the length-tension curve of a shortened muscle.[69] This shift decreases the muscle's capacity to produce maximum tension at its normal resting length as it contracts.[70]

● **Key Point** The PTA must remember that the restoration of full strength and range of motion may prove difficult if the connective tissues are allowed to heal without early active motion, or in a shortened position, and that the patient may be prone to repeated strains.[71] Thus, range-of-motion exercises should be started once swelling and tenderness have subsided to the point that the exercises are not unduly painful, and strengthening exercises should be introduced as tolerated.[71]

Musculoskeletal Data Collection

Range of Motion

Range of motion refers to the distance and direction a joint can move. Each specific joint has a normal range of motion that is expressed in degrees (**Table 4-24**). Within the field of physical therapy, goniometry is commonly used to measure the total amount of available motion at a specific joint. Goniometry can be used to measure both active and passive range of motion. The correct selection of which goniometer device to use depends on the joint angle to be measured. The length of arms varies among instruments and can range from 3 to 18 inches. Extendable goniometers allow varying ranges from 9½ inches to 26 inches. The longer-armed goniometers or the bubble inclinometer is recommended when the landmarks are further apart, such as when measuring trunk, hip, knee, elbow, and shoulder movements. In the smaller joints such as the wrist/hand and foot/ankle, a traditional goniometer with a shorter arm is used.

Procedure

The patient is positioned in the recommended testing position. While stabilizing the proximal joint

TABLE 4-24 Active Ranges of the Major Joints

Joint	Action	Degrees of Motion
Cervical	Flexion	0–45
	Extension	0–45
	Sidebending (R/L)	0–45 to each side
	Rotation (R/L)	0–60 to each side
Thoracolumbar	Flexion	0–80 (tape measure = 4 inches)
	Extension	0–20 to 30
	Sidebending (R/L)	0–35 to each side
	Rotation (R/L)	0–45 to each side
Shoulder	Flexion	0–180
	Extension	0–40
	Abduction	0–180
	Internal rotation	0–80
	External rotation	0–90
Elbow	Flexion	0–150
Forearm	Pronation	0–80
	Supination	0–80
Wrist	Flexion	0–60
	Extension	0–60
	Radial deviation	0–20
	Ulnar deviation	0–30
Thumb	Carpometacarpal abduction	0–70
	Carpometacarpal opposition	Tip of thumb to base of 5th digit
	Carpometacarpal flexion	0–15
	Carpometacarpal extension	0–20
	MCP flexion	0–50
	IP flexion	0–80
Digits (2–5)	MCP flexion	0–90
	MCP hyperextension	0–45
	PIP flexion	0–100
	DIP flexion	0–90
	DIP hyperextension	0–10
Hip	Flexion	0–100
	Extension	0–30
	Abduction	0–40
	Adduction	0–20
	Internal rotation	0–40
	External rotation	0–50
Knee	Flexion	0–150
Ankle	Plantarflexion	0–40
	Dorsiflexion	0–20
	Inversion	0–35
	Eversion	0–15
Subtalar	Inversion	0–5
	Eversion	0–5

component, the clinician gently moves the distal joint component through the available range of motion until the end feel is determined. An estimate is made of the available range of motion and the distal joint component is returned to the starting position. The clinician palpates the relevant bony landmarks and aligns the goniometer. The starting measurement is recorded. The goniometer is then removed and the patient moves the joint through the available range of motion. Once the joint has been moved through the available range of motion, the goniometer is replaced and realigned, and a measurement is read and recorded (**Table 4-25** and **Table 4-26**).

● Key Point Active range of motion testing gives the clinician information about:

- The quantity of available physiological motion
- The presence of muscle substitutions
- The willingness of the patient to move
- The integrity of the contractile and inert tissues
- The quality of motion
- Symptom reproduction
- The pattern of motion restriction (capsular/noncapsular)

The term *painful arc* is used to describe an occurrence of temporary pain during active or passive motion that disappears before the end of the movement. The presence of a painful arc indicates that some structure is being compressed or impinged.

TABLE 4-25 Goniometric Techniques for the Upper Extremity

Joint	Motion	Axis	Stationary Arm	Movable Arm	Range of Motion
Shoulder	Flexion	Acromion process	Midaxillary line of the thorax	Lateral midline of the humerus using the lateral epicondyle of the humerus for reference	180°
	Extension	Acromion process	Midaxillary line of the thorax	Lateral midline of the humerus using the lateral epicondyle of the humerus for reference	60°
	Abduction	Anterior aspect of the acromion process	Parallel to the midline of the anterior aspect of the sternum	Medial midline of the humerus	180°
	Horizontal Adduction	Anterior aspect of the acromion process	Parallel to the midline of the anterior aspect of the sternum	Medial midline of the humerus	135°
	Internal rotation	Olecranon process	Parallel or perpendicular to the floor	Ulna using the olecranon process and ulnar styloid for reference	70°
	External rotation	Olecranon process	Parallel or perpendicular to the floor	Ulna using the olecranon process and ulnar styloid for reference	90°
Elbow	Flexion	Lateral epicondyle of the humerus	Lateral midline of the humerus using the center of the acromion process for reference	Lateral midline of the radius using the radial head and radial styloid process for reference	150°
Forearm	Pronation	Lateral to the ulnar styloid process	Parallel to the anterior midline of the humerus	Dorsal aspect of the forearm, just proximal to the styloid process of the radius and ulna	80°
	Supination	Medial to the ulnar styloid process	Parallel to the anterior midline of the humerus	Ventral aspect of the forearm, just proximal to the styloid process of the radius and ulna	80°

(continued)

TABLE 4-25

Goniometric Techniques for the Upper Extremity (continued)

Joint	Motion	Axis	Stationary Arm	Movable Arm	Range of Motion
Wrist	Flexion	Lateral aspect of the wrists over the triquetrum	Lateral midline of the ulna using the olecranon and ulnar styloid process for reference	Lateral midline of the fifth metacarpal	80°
	Extension	Lateral aspect of the wrists over the triquetrum	Lateral midline of the ulna using the olecranon and ulnar styloid process for reference	Lateral midline of the fifth metacarpal	70°
	Radial deviation	Over the middle of the dorsal aspect of the wrist over the capitate	Dorsal midline of the forearm using the lateral epicondyle of the humerus for reference	Dorsal midline of the third metacarpal	20°
	Ulnar deviation	Over the middle of the dorsal aspect of the wrist over the capitate	Dorsal midline of the forearm using the lateral epicondyle of the humerus for reference	Dorsal midline of the third metacarpal	30°
Thumb	Carpometa-carpal flexion	Over the palmar aspect of the first carpometacarpal joint	Ventral midline of the radius using the ventral surface of the radial head and radial styloid process for reference	Ventral midline of the first metacarpal	
	Carpometa-carpal extension	Over the palmar aspect of the first carpometacarpal joint	Ventral midline of the radius using the ventral surface of the radial head and radial styloid process for reference	Ventral midline of the first metacarpal	
	Carpometa-carpal abduction	Over the lateral aspect of the radial styloid process	Lateral midline of the second metacarpal using the center of the second metacarpal or phalangeal joint for reference	Lateral midline of the first metacarpal using the center of the first metacarpal or phalangeal joint for reference	
	Carpometa-carpal adduction	Over the lateral aspect of the radial styloid process	Lateral midline of the second metacarpal using the center of the second metacarpal or phalangeal joint for reference	Lateral midline of the first metacarpal using the center of the first metacarpal or phalangeal joint for reference	
Fingers	Metacarpo-phalangeal flexion	Over the dorsal aspect of the metacarpophalangeal joint	Over the dorsal midline of the metacarpal	Over the dorsal midline of the proximal phalanx	
	Metacarpo-phalangeal extension	Over the dorsal aspect of the metacarpophalan-geal joint	Over the dorsal midline of the metacarpal	Over the dorsal midline of the proximal phalanx	
	Metacarpo-phalangeal abduction	Over the dorsal aspect of the metacarpophalan-geal joint	Over the dorsal midline of the metacarpal	Over the dorsal midline of the proximal phalanx	
	Metacarpo-phalangeal adduction	Over the dorsal aspect of the metacarpophalan-geal joint	Over the dorsal midline of the metacarpal	Over the dorsal midline of the proximal phalanx	

| TABLE 4-25 | Goniometric Techniques for the Upper Extremity (continued) |

Joint	Motion	Axis	Stationary Arm	Movable Arm	Range of Motion
	Proximal inter-phalangeal flexion	Over the dorsal aspect of the proximal interphalan-geal joint	Over the dorsal midline of the proximal phalanx	Over the dorsal midline of the middle phalanx	
	Proximal inter-phalangeal extension	Over the dorsal aspect of the proximal interphalan-geal joint	Over the dorsal midline of the proximal phalanx	Over the dorsal midline of the middle phalanx	
	Distal inter-phalangeal flexion	Over the dorsal aspect of the proximal interphalan-geal joint	Over the dorsal midline of the middle phalanx	Over the dorsal midline of the distal phalanx	
	Distal inter-phalangeal extension	Over the dorsal aspect of the proximal interphalan-geal joint	Over the dorsal midline of the middle phalanx	Over the dorsal midline of the distal phalanx	

| TABLE 4-26 | Goniometric Techniques for the Lower Extremity |

Joint	Motion	Axis	Stationary Arm	Movable Arm	Range of Motion
Hip	Flexion	Over the lateral aspect of the hip joint using the greater trochanter of the femur reference	Lateral midline of the pelvis	Lateral midline of the femur using the lateral epicondyle for reference	120°
	Extension	Over the lateral aspect of the hip joint using the greater trochanter of the femur reference	Lateral midline of the pelvis	Lateral midline of the femur using the lateral epicondyle for reference	30°
	Abduction	Over the ASIS of the extremity being measured	Aligned with imaginary horizontal line extending from one ASIS to the other ASIS	Anterior midline of the femur using the midline of the patella for reference	45°
	Adduction	Over the ASIS of the extremity being measured	Aligned with imaginary horizontal line extending from one ASIS to the other ASIS	Anterior midline of the femur using the midline of the patella for reference	30°
	Internal rotation	Anterior aspect of the patella	Perpendicular to the floor or parallel to the supporting surface	Anterior midline of the lower leg using the crest of the tibia and a point midway between the two malleoli for reference	45°
	External rotation	Anterior aspect of the patella	Perpendicular to the floor or parallel to the supporting surface	Anterior midline of the lower leg using the crest of the tibia and a point midway between the two malleoli for reference	45°

(continued)

| TABLE 4-26 | Goniometric Techniques for the Lower Extremity (continued) |

Joint	Motion	Axis	Stationary Arm	Movable Arm	Range of Motion
Knee	Flexion	Lateral epicondyle of the femur	Lateral midline of the femur using the greater trochanter for reference	Lateral midline of the fibula using the lateral malleolus and fibular head for reference	135°
Ankle	Dorsiflexion	Lateral aspect of the lateral malleolus	Lateral midline of the fibular using the head of the fibula for reference	Parallel to the lateral aspect of the fifth metatarsal	20°
	Plantar flexion	Lateral aspect of the lateral malleolus	Lateral midline of the fibular using the head of the fibula for reference	Parallel to the lateral aspect of the fifth metatarsal	50°
Subtalar	Inversion	Posterior aspect of the ankle midway between the malleoli	Posterior midline of the lower leg	Posterior midline of the calcaneus	35°
	Eversion	Posterior aspect of the ankle midway between the malleoli	Posterior midline of the lower leg	Posterior midline of the calcaneus	15°

End Feels

Cyriax[72] introduced the concept of the end feel, which can be defined as the quality of resistance at the end range. The end feel can indicate to the clinician the cause of the motion restriction (**Table 4-27** and **Table 4-28**). For example, a hard, capsular end feel indicates a pericapsular hypomobility, while a jammed or pathomechanical end feel indicates a pathomechanical hypomobility. A normal end feel would indicate normal range, whereas an abnormal end feel would suggest abnormal range, either hypomobile or hypermobile. An association between an increase in pain and abnormal–pathological end feels compared with normal end feels has been demonstrated.[73]

Leg Length Assessment

There are two leg length assessments:

- *True leg-length discrepancy:* The patient lies supine with hips and knees extended. Using a tape measure, the clinician assesses the distance from the ASIS to the distal most part of the medial malleolus and compares bilaterally. Differences greater than 1 centimeter may be indicative of femoral or tibial length discrepancies, or coxa vara/coxa valgus.

- *Apparent leg-length discrepancy:* The patient lies supine with hips and knees extended. Using a tape measure, the clinician measures the length from the umbilicus to the most distal part of the medial malleolus and compares bilaterally. Distances greater than 1 centimeter may be indicative of abnormal pelvic positioning.

Manual Muscle Testing

An important component of an examination is the assessment of muscle strength. The assessment of strength provides the clinician with information about the ability of the musculotendinous units to act across a bone-joint lever-arm system to actively generate motion or to passively resist movement against gravity and variable resistance.[74] Manual muscle testing (MMT) is traditionally used by the clinician to assess the strength of a muscle or muscle group, although a number of other methods can be used to measure strength, including dynamometry, isokinetics, and cable tensiometry.

TABLE
4-27

Normal End Feels

Type	Cause	Characteristics and Examples
Bony	Produced by bone-to-bone approximation.	Abrupt and unyielding, with the impression that further forcing will break something. *Examples*: Normal: Elbow extension. Abnormal: Cervical rotation (may indicate osteophyte).
Muscular	1. Insufficiency: Produced by the muscle–tendon unit; may occur with adaptive shortening. 2. Slow guarding: Resistance that is felt; slowly releases with sustained force.	Stretch with elastic recoil and exhibits constant-length phenomenon. Similar to capsular (see below). Further forcing feels as if it will snap something. *Examples*: Normal: Wrist flexion with finger flexion, the straight leg raise, and ankle dorsiflexion with the knee extended. Abnormal: Decreased dorsiflexion of the ankle with the knee flexed.
Soft tissue approximation	Produced by the contact of two muscle bulks on either side of a flexing joint where the joint range exceeds other restraints.	A very forgiving endfeel that gives the impression that further normal motion is possible if enough force could be applied. *Examples*: Normal: Knee flexion, elbow flexion in extremely muscular subjects. Abnormal: Elbow flexion with the obese subject.
Capsular	Produced by capsule or ligaments.	Various degrees of stretch without elasticity. Stretch ability is dependent on thickness of the tissue. Strong capsular or extracapsular ligaments produce a hard capsular endfeel, while a thin capsule produces a softer one. The impression given to the clinician is that if further force is applied, something will tear. *Examples*: Normal: Wrist flexion (soft), elbow flexion in supination (medium) and knee extension (hard). Abnormal: Inappropriate stretch ability for a specific joint. If too hard, may indicate a hypomobility due to arthrosis; if too soft, a hypermobility.

Data from Dutton M: Mcgraw-Hill's National Physical Therapy Examination (ed1). New York Mcgraw-Hill, 2009

TABLE
4-28

Abnormal End Feels

Type	Causes	Characteristics and Examples
Springy	Produced by the articular surface rebounding from an intra-articular meniscus or disc. The impression is that if forced further, something will collapse.	A rebound sensation as if pushing off from a Sorbo rubber pad. *Examples:* Normal: Axial compression of the cervical spine. Abnormal: Knee flexion or extension with a displaced meniscus.
Boggy	Produced by viscous fluid (blood) within a joint.	A "squishy" sensation as the joint is moved toward its end range. Further forcing feels as if it will burst the joint. *Examples:* Normal: None. Abnormal: Hemarthrosis at the knee.

(continued)

| TABLE 4-28 | Abnormal End Feels (continued) |

Type	Causes	Characteristics and Examples
Fast guarding (spasm)	Produced by reflex and reactive muscle contraction in response to irritation of the nociceptor predominantly in articular structures and muscle. Forcing it further feels as if nothing will give.	An abrupt and "twangy" end to movement that is unyielding while the structure is being threatened but disappears when the threat is removed (kicks back). With joint inflammation, it occurs early in the range, especially toward the close-pack position, to prevent further stress. With an irritable joint hypermobility, it occurs at the end of what should be normal range as it prevents excessive motion from further stimulating the nociceptor. Spasm in grade II muscle tears becomes apparent as the muscle is passively lengthened and is accompanied by a painful weakness of that muscle. Note: Muscle guarding is not a true end feel as it involves a co-contraction. *Examples*: Normal: None. Abnormal: Significant traumatic arthritis, recent traumatic hypermobility, grade II muscle tears.
Empty	Produced solely by pain. Frequently caused by serious and severe pathological changes that do not affect the joint or muscle and so do not produce spasm. Demonstration of this endfeel is, with the exception of acute subdeltoid bursitis, de facto evidence of serious pathology. Further forcing simply increases the pain to unacceptable levels.	The limitation of motion has no tissue resistance component, and the resistance is from the patient being unable to tolerate further motion due to severe pain. It is not the same feeling as voluntary guarding, but rather it feels as if the patient is both resisting and trying to allow the movement simultaneously. *Examples*: Normal: None. Abnormal: Acute subdeltoid bursitis, sign of the buttock.
Facilitation	Not truly an endfeel, as facilitated hypertonicity does not restrict motion. It can, however, be perceived near the end range.	A light resistance as from a constant light muscle contraction throughout the latter half of the range that does not prevent the end of range being reached. The resistance is unaffected by the rate of movement. *Examples*: Normal: None. Abnormal: Spinal facilitation at any level.

Data from Dutton M: McGraw-Hill's National Physical Therapy Examination (ed1). New York McGraw-Hill, 2009

● Key Point Dynamometry is a method of strength testing using sophisticated strength measuring devices (e.g., hand-grip, hand-held, fixed, and isokinetic dynamometry). A handheld dynamometer (HHD) is a precision measurement instrument (demonstrates intrarater reliability of >0.94) designed to obtain more discrete, objective measures of strength during MMT than can be achieved via traditional MMT.

- When subject strength is clearly beyond a tester's capability to control, use of an HHD is not indicated.
- Aside from limitations regarding mechanical advantage and strength when using an HHD, there also is the issue of patient comfort as a potential limitation. Even though the HHD is padded, it does not and cannot conform to a given body part like a tester's hand can, and a common subject complaint is tenderness over the dynamometer placement site.

● Key Point MMT is an ordinal level of measurement,[75] and it has been found to have both interrater and intrarater reliability, especially when the scale is expanded to include plus or minus a half or a full grade.[76–78]

The various test positions and procedures for MMT as per Kendall[79] are outlined in **Table 4-29,** and examples of common grading scales used with MMT are given in **Table 4-30.** Choosing a particular grading system is based on the skill level of the clinician while ensuring consistency for each patient, so that

Patient Positioning and Procedures for MMT

Patient Positioning	Muscle Tested	Test
Supine	Pectoralis major	Upper fibers: starting with the elbow extended, and the shoulder in 90° of flexion and slight internal rotation, the humerus is horizontally adducted toward the sternal end of the clavicle
		Lower fibers: starting with the elbow extended, and the shoulder in flexion and slight internal rotation, adduction of the arm obliquely toward the opposite iliac crest
	Pectoralis minor	Forward thrust of the shoulder with the arm at the side but with no downward pressure by the patient's hand
	Serratus anterior	Abduction of the scapula projecting the upper extremity upward from the table with the arm extended
	Flexor hallucis brevis	Flexion of the metatarsophalangeal joint of the great toe
	Flexor digitorum brevis	Flexion of the proximal interphalangeal joints of the second, third, fourth, and fifth digits
	Flexor hallucis longus	Flexion of the interphalangeal joint of the great toe
	Flexor digitorum longus	Flexion of the distal interphalangeal joints of the second, third, fourth, and fifth digits
	Extensor digitorum longus and brevis	Extension of all joints of the second, third, fourth, and fifth digits
	Fibularis tertius	Dorsiflexion of the ankle joint, with eversion of the foot
	Extensor hallucis longus and brevis	Extension of the metatarsophalangeal and interphalangeal joints of the great toe
	Tibialis anterior	Dorsiflexion of the ankle joint and inversion of the foot, without extension of the great toe
	Tibialis posterior	Inversion of the foot with plantarflexion of the ankle joint
	Fibularis longus and brevis	Eversion of the foot with plantarflexion of the ankle joint
Prone	Triceps brachii and anconeus	Extension of the elbow joint (to slightly less than full extension)
	Latissimus dorsi	Adduction of the arm, with extension, in the internally rotated position
	Teres major	Extension and adduction of the humerus in the internally rotated position, with the back of the hand resting on the posterior iliac crest
	Infraspinatus and teres minor	External rotation of the humerus with the shoulder abducted to 90° and the elbow held at right angle
	Rhomboid and levator scapulae	Adduction and elevation of the scapula with internal rotation of the inferior angle
	Middle trapezius	Supporting the weight of the arm (thumb pointing upward), the clinician places the scapula in a position of adduction, with some external rotation of the inferior angle, and without elevation of the shoulder girdle
	Lower trapezius	Depression, external rotation of the inferior angle, and adduction of the scapula with the arm placed diagonally overhead and the shoulder externally rotated
	Soleus	Plantarflexion of the ankle joint without inversion or eversion of the foot with the knee flexed to 90°
Sitting	Adductor pollicis	Adduction of the thumb toward the palm
	Abductor pollicis brevis	Abduction of the thumb anteriorly away from the palm

(continued)

TABLE 4-29 Patient Positioning and Procedures for MMT (continued)

Patient Positioning	Muscle Tested	Test
	Opponens pollicis	Flexion, abduction, and slight internal rotation of the metacarpal bone so that the thumbnail shows in palmar view
	Flexor pollicis longus	Flexion of the interphalangeal joint of the thumb
	Flexor pollicis brevis	Flexion of the metacarpophalangeal joint of the thumb without flexion of the interphalangeal joint
	Extensor pollicis longus	Extension of the interphalangeal joint of the thumb
	Extensor pollicis brevis	Extension of the metacarpophalangeal joint of the thumb
	Abductor pollicis longus	Abduction and slight extension of the first metacarpal bone
	Abductor digiti minimi	Abduction of the little finger
	Opponens digiti minimi	Opposition of the fifth metacarpal toward the first
	Flexor digiti minimi	Flexion of the metacarpophalangeal joint with interphalangeal joints extended
	Lumbricales and interossei	Extension of interphalangeal joints with simultaneous flexion of metacarpophalangeal joint
	Palmaris longus	Tensing of the palmar fascia by strongly cupping the palm of the hand, and flexion of the wrist
	Extensor digitorum	Extension of the metacarpophalangeal joints of the second through fifth digits, with interphalangeal joints relaxed
	Flexor digitorum superficialis	Flexion of the proximal interphalangeal joint with the distal interphalangeal joint extended, of the second, third, fourth, and fifth digits
	Flexor digitorum profundus	Flexion of the distal interphalangeal joint of the second, third, fourth, and fifth digits
	Flexor carpi radialis	Flexion of the wrist toward the radial side
	Flexor carpi ulnaris	Flexion of the wrist toward the ulnar side
	Extensor carpi radialis longus	Extension of the wrist toward the radial side (with the elbow flexed about 30°)
	Extensor carpi radialis brevis	Extension of the wrist toward the radial side (with the elbow fully flexed)
	Extensor carpi ulnaris	Extension of the wrist toward the ulnar side
	Pronator teres	Pronation of the forearm with the elbow partially flexed
	Pronator quadratus	Pronation of the forearm with the elbow fully flexed
	Supinator and biceps	Supination of the forearm with the elbow at right angle or slightly below
	Brachioradialis	Flexion of the elbow with forearm neutral between pronation and supination
	Coracobrachialis	Shoulder flexion in external rotation with the elbow completely flexed and the forearm supinated
	Biceps brachii	Elbow flexion slightly less than or at right angle, with forearm in supination
	Brachialis	Elbow flexion slightly less than or at right angle, with forearm in pronation
	Supraspinatus and middle deltoid	Shoulder abduction without rotation
	Anterior deltoid	Shoulder abduction and slight flexion, with the humerus in slight external rotation

TABLE
4-29

Patient Positioning and Procedures for MMT (continued)

Patient Positioning	Muscle Tested	Test
	Posterior deltoid	Shoulder abduction in slight extension, with the humerus in slight internal rotation
	Upper trapezius	Elevation of the acromial end of the clavicle and scapula; extension and rotation of the head and neck toward the elevated shoulder with the face rotated in the opposite direction
Standing	Supraspinatus	Initiation of abduction of the humerus
	Gastrocnemius	Standing on one leg, the patient rises on toes, pushing the bodyweight directly upward

TABLE 4-30

Comparison of MMT Grades[a]

Medical Research Council[b]	Daniels and Worthingham[c]	Kendall and McCreary[d]	Explanation
5	Normal (N)	100%	Holds test position against maximal resistance
4+	Good + (G+)		Holds test position against moderate to strong pressure
4	Good (G)	80%	Holds test position against moderate resistance
4–	Good – (G–)		Holds test position against slight to moderate pressure
3+	Fair + (F+)		Holds test position against slight resistance
3	Fair (F)	50%	Holds test position against gravity
3–	Fair– (F–)		Gradual release from test position
2+	Poor + (P+)		Moves through partial ROM against gravity OR Moves through complete ROM gravity eliminated and holds against pressure
2	Poor (P)	20%	Able to move through full ROM gravity eliminated
2–	Poor– (P–)		Moves through partial ROM gravity eliminated
1	Trace (T)	5%	No visible movement; palpable or observable tendon prominence/ flicker contraction

(continued)

TABLE 4-30

Comparison of MMT Grades[a] (continued)

Medical Research Council[b]	Daniels and Worthingham[c]	Kendall and McCreary[d]	Explanation
0	0	0%	No palpable or observable muscle contraction
The grades of 0, 1, and 2 are tested in the gravity-minimized position (contraction is perpendicular to the gravitational force). All other grades are tested in the antigravity position.	The more functional of the three grading systems because it tests a motion that utilizes all of the agonists and synergists involved in the motion.[a]	Designed to test a specific muscle rather than the motion, and requires both selective recruitment of a muscle by the patient and a sound knowledge of anatomy and kinesiology on the part of the clinician to determine the correct alignment of the muscle fibers.[a]	

Data from (a) Palmer ML, Epler M: Principles of examination techniques, in Palmer ML, Epler M (eds): Clinical Assessment Procedures in Physical Therapy. Philadelphia, J. B. Lippincott, 1990, pp 8–36; (b) Frese E, Brown M, Norton B: Clinical reliability of manual muscle testing: Middle trapezius and gluteus medius muscles. Phys Ther 67:1072–1076, 1987; (c) Daniels K, Worthingham C: Muscle Testing Techniques of Manual Examination (ed 5). Philadelphia, W. B. Saunders, 1986; and (d) Kendall FP, McCreary EK, Provance PG: Muscles: Testing and Function. Baltimore, Williams & Wilkins, 1993

coworkers who may be reexamining the patient are using the same testing methods.

> **● Key Point** Note the following definitions:
> - *Make test:* An evaluation procedure where the patient is asked to apply a force against the clinician or dynamometer.
> - *Break test:* An evaluation procedure in which the patient is asked to hold a contraction against pressure that is applied in the opposite direction to the contraction.

To be a valid test, strength testing must elicit a maximum contraction of the muscle being tested. Five strategies ensure this:

1. Placing the joint which the muscle to be tested crosses in, or close to, its open-packed position.
2. Placing the muscle to be tested in a shortened position. This puts the muscle in an ineffective physiological position and has the effect of increasing motor neuron activity.
3. Having the patient perform an eccentric muscle contraction by using the command "Don't let me move you." As the tension at each cross-bridge and the number of active cross-bridges is greater during an eccentric contraction, the maximum eccentric muscle tension developed is greater with an eccentric contraction than a concentric one.
4. Breaking the contraction. It is important to break the patient's muscle contraction in order to ensure that the patient is making a maximal effort and that the full power of the muscle is being tested.
5. Holding the contraction for at least 5 seconds. Weakness due to nerve palsy has a distinct fatigability. If a muscle appears to be weaker than normal, further investigation is required.

The test is repeated three times. Muscle weakness resulting from disuse will be consistently weak and should not get weaker with several repeated contractions.

Another muscle that shares the same innervation (spinal nerve or peripheral nerve) is tested. Knowledge of both spinal nerve and peripheral nerve innervation will aid the clinician in determining which muscle to select.

Substitutions by other muscle groups during testing indicate the presence of weakness. They do not, however, tell the clinician the cause of the weakness. Whenever possible, the same muscle is tested on the opposite side, using the same testing procedure, in order to make a comparison.

In addition to examining the integrity of the contractile and inert structures, strength testing may be used to examine the integrity of the myotomes.

A *myotome* is defined as a muscle or group of muscles served by a single nerve root. *Key muscle* is a better, more accurate term, as the muscles tested are the most representative of the supply from a particular segment.

- *Shoulder shrug:* Tests the upper trapezius muscle for CN XI (spinal accessory nerve) and spinal roots C2, C3 (posterior surface of the neck), and C4 (A-C joint).
- *Shoulder abduction:* Tests the deltoid muscle for axillary nerve and spinal roots C5 (lateral aspect of the arm) and C6 (lateral aspect of forearm; hand and thumb; index finger).
- *Elbow flexion of supinated arm:* Tests the biceps brachii muscle for the musculocutaneous nerve and spinal roots C5 and C6.
- *Elbow flexion of neutral arm:* Tests the brachioradialis muscle for the full radial nerve and spinal roots C5 and C6.
- *Elbow extension test:* Tests the triceps brachii muscle for the full radial nerve and spinal roots C6, C7 (middle finger), and C8 (little and ring finger; medial aspect of the hand and wrist).
- *Radial wrist extension:* Tests the extensor carpi ulnaris (ECU) muscle for the radial nerve and spinal roots C6, C7, and C8.
- *Wrist flexion:* Tests the flexor carpi ulnaris (FCU) muscle for all the nerves and spinal
- root C8 and T1 (medial forearm).
- *Thumb extension:* Tests the extensor pollicis longus (EPL) muscle for radial nerve and spinal roots C6, C7, and C8.
- *Fifth digit abduction:* Tests the abductor digiti minimi muscle for ulnar nerve and spinal roots C8 and T1.
- *Hip flexion:* Tests iliopsoas muscles for lumbar plexus and spinal roots L1 (proximal medial thigh), L2 (proximal anterior thigh), and L3 (distal anterior and medial thigh and knee).
- *Knee extension:* Tests quadriceps femoris muscles for femoral nerve and spinal roots L2, L3, and L4 (anterior and medial lower extremity).
- *Ankle dorsiflexion:* Tests anterior tibialis muscle for deep fibularis nerve and spinal roots L4 and L5 (anterior and lateral lower extremity; medial dorsal foot; plantar aspect of big toe).
- *Big toe extension:* Tests extensor hallucis longus (EHL) muscle for deep fibularis nerve and spinal roots L5 and S1 (lateral dorsal foot; most of plantar foot).
- *Knee flexion:* Tests hamstring muscles for sciatic nerve and spinal roots L5, S1, and S2 (posterior thigh; proximal lower extremity).
- *Ankle plantar flexion:* Tests gastrocnemius muscle for tibial nerve and spinal roots S1 and S2.

> ● **Key Point** The *Guide to Physical Therapist Practice*[80] lists both MMT and dynamometry as appropriate measures of muscle strength.

Deep Tendon Reflexes

A reflex is a subconscious, programmed unit of behavior in which a certain type of stimulus from a receptor automatically leads to the response of an effector. Reflexes can be controlled by spinal or supraspinal (brain stem) pathways. The stretch reflex (myotatic or deep tendon) is an example of the spinal reflex. A number of processes involved in locomotor function are oriented around these reflexes and are referred to as postural reflexes.

> ● **Key Point** The assessment of reflexes is extremely important in the diagnosis and localization of neurologic lesions.[81]

Any muscle that possesses a tendon is capable of producing a deep tendon reflex. Five of these are regularly tested: the biceps (C5), brachioradialis (C6), and triceps (C7) in the upper extremity, and the quadriceps (L4) and Achilles (S1) in the lower extremities.

Deep tendon reflexes are graded by the PT as follows:

0   Absent (areflexia)
1+ Decreased (hyporeflexia)
2+ Normal
3+ Hyperactive (brisk)
4+ Hyperactive with clonus (hyperreflexive)

Upper and Lower Quarter Screens

Designed by Cyriax,[72] the screening examination is based on sound anatomic and pathologic principles. The Cyriax screening examination is traditionally performed after the history and is often incorporated as part of the systems review. The scanning examination is used when there is no history to explain the signs and symptoms, or when the signs and symptoms are unexplainable. The clinician must choose which scanning examination to use based on the presenting signs and symptoms. The upper quarter scanning examination

(**Table 4-31**) is appropriate for upper thoracic, upper extremity, and cervical problems, whereas the lower quarter scanning examination (**Table 4-32**) is typically used for thoracic, lower extremity, and lumbosacral problems. The preferred sequence of the scanning examination is outlined in **Table 4-33**.

Posture Analysis

A simple plumbline or a wall grid is used.

- *Side view:* The plumbline passes through the mastoid process of the temporal bone, bisecting the cervical bodies, the auditory meatus, the tip of the acromion process, and the midthoracic region; is anterior to the second sacral vertebra and the greater trochanter of the hip; is slightly anterior and lateral to the femoral condyle; and is slightly anterior to the lateral malleolus of the ankle.[82]

- *Anterior view:* The shoulders are equal in height or the dominant side is slightly lower, and there is an even space between the feet. The plumbline bisects the head, nose, and frontal bone and should be evenly spaced between the acromion processes. Moving inferiorly, it bisects the jugular notch, sternum, and umbilicus.

TABLE 4-31   Upper Quarter-Quadrant Scanning Motor Examination

Muscle Action	Muscle Tested	Root Level	Peripheral Nerve
Shoulder abduction	Deltoid	Primarily C5	Axillary
Elbow flexion	Biceps brachii	Primarily C6	Musculocutaneous
Elbow extension	Triceps brachii	Primarily C7	Radial
Wrist extension	Extensor carpi radialis longus, brevis, and extensor carpi ulnaris	Primarily C6	Radial
Wrist flexion	Flexor carpi radialis and flexor carpi ulnaris	Primarily C7	Median nerve for radialis and ulnar nerve for ulnaris
Finger flexion	Flexor digitorum superficialis, flexor digitorum profundus, and lumbricales	Primarily C8	Median nerve for superficialis, both median and ulnar nerves for profundus and lumbricales
Finger abduction	Dorsal interossei	Primarily T1	Ulnar

TABLE 4-32   Lower Quarter-Quadrant Scanning Motor Examination

Muscle Action	Muscle Tested	Root Level	Peripheral Nerve
Hip flexion	Iliopsoas	L1–L2	Femoral to iliacus and lumbar plexus to psoas
Knee extension	Quadriceps	L2–L4	Femoral
Hamstrings	Biceps femoris, semimembranosus, and semitendinosus	L4–S3	Sciatic
Dorsiflexion with inversion	Tibialis anterior	Primarily L4	Deep peroneal
Great toe extension	Extensor hallucis longus	Primarily L5	Deep peroneal
Ankle eversion	Peroneus longus and brevis	Primarily S1	Superficial peroneal nerve
Ankle plantarflexion	Gastrocnemius and soleus	Primarily S1	Tibial
Hip extension	Gluteus maximus	L5–S2	Inferior gluteal nerve

TABLE 4-33	Typical Sequence of Upper or Lower Quarter Scanning Examinations

1. Initial observation: Involves everything from initial entry of patient, including gait, demeanor, standing, and sitting postures, obvious deformities and postural defects, scars, radiation burns, creases, and birthmarks

2. Patient history

3. Scanning examination

4. Active range of motion

5. Passive overpressure

6. Resistive tests

7. Deep tendon reflexes

8. Sensation testing

9. Special tests

Negative Scan

If, at end of scan, the clinician has determined that the patient's condition is appropriate for physical therapy but has not determined a diagnosis to treat the patient, the clinician will need to perform further testing.

Positive Scan (Results in a Diagnosis)

1. Specific interventions (traction, manual techniques, and specific exercises) can be given if diagnosis is one that will benefit from physical therapy.

2. Patient is returned to physician for more tests if signs and symptoms are cause for concern.

The iliac crest, fibular heads, and lateral malleoli should be at equal heights bilaterally.

- *Posterior view:* The shoulder should be of equal height or the dominant side is slightly lower; there is even space between the feet. The plumbline bisects the occipital protuberance and the spinous processes. The spaces between the acromion processes and scapulae are even, and there is no winging of the scapulae.

Pelvic and Lumbar Region

The more common faulty postures of the pelvic and lumbar region are described in the following sections.[83]

Lordotic Posture

Lordotic posture is characterized by an increase in the lumbosacral angle, an increase in lumbar lordosis, and an increase in the anterior pelvic tilt and hip flexion.[84] This posture is commonly seen in pregnancy, obesity, and individuals with weakened abdominal muscles. Potential muscle impairments include:

- Decreased mobility in the hip flexor muscles (iliopsoas, tensor fascia latae, rectus femoris) and lumbar extensor muscles (erector spinae).
- Impaired muscle performance due to stretched and weakened abdominal muscles (rectus abdominis, internal and external obliques, and transversus abdominis).

This posture places stress on the anterior longitudinal ligament and the zygapophyseal (facet) joints, and it narrows the posterior disc space and the intervertebral foramen, all of which are potential sources of symptoms.

Slouched Posture

This posture, also referred to as swayback,[79] is characterized by a shifting of the entire pelvic segment anteriorly, resulting in relative hip extension and a shifting of the thoracic segment posteriorly, which in turn results in a relative flexion of the thorax on the upper lumbar spine. There is an increased lordosis in the lower lumbar region, increased kyphosis in the thoracic region, and usually a forward (protracted) head. This posture is commonly seen throughout most age groups and is typically the result of fatigue or muscle weakness. Potential muscle impairments include:

- Decreased mobility in the upper abdominal muscles (upper segments of the rectus abdominis and obliques), internal intercostal, hip extensor, and lower lumbar extensor muscles and related fascia.

- Impaired muscle performance due to stretched and weakened lower abdominal muscles (lower segments of the rectus abdominis and obliques), extensor muscles of the lower thoracic region, and hip flexor muscles.

This posture places stress on the iliofemoral ligaments, the anterior longitudinal ligament of the lower lumbar spine, and the posterior longitudinal ligament of the upper lumbar on thoracic spine. In addition, there is narrowing of the intervertebral foramen in the lower lumbar spine and approximation of the zygapophyseal (facet) joints in the lower lumbar spine.

Flat Low Back Posture

This posture is characterized by a decreased lumbosacral angle, decreased lumbar lordosis, extension, and posterior tilting of the pelvis. It is commonly seen in individuals who spend long periods slouching or flexing in the sitting or standing positions. The potential muscle impairments include:

- Decreased mobility in the trunk flexor (rectus abdominis, intercostals) and hip extensor muscles.
- Impaired muscle performance due to stretched and weak lumbar extensor and possibly hip flexor muscles.

This posture can apply stress on the posterior longitudinal ligament, the posterior disc space, and the normal physiological lumbar curve, which reduces the shock-absorbing effects of the lumbar region and predisposes the patient to injury.

Cervical and Thoracic Region

The more common faulty postures of the cervical and thoracic region include round back with forward head, and flat upper back and neck.[83]

Round Back with Forward Head

This posture is characterized by increased kyphotic thoracic curve, protracted scapulae (round shoulders), and forward head. The causes for this posture are similar to those found with the flat low back posture. The potential muscle impairments include:

- Decreased mobility in the muscles of the anterior thorax (intercostal muscles), of the upper extremity originating on the thorax (pectoralis major and minor, latissimus dorsi, serratus anterior), of the cervical spine and head that attach to the scapular and upper thorax (levator scapulae, sternocleidomastoid, scalene, upper trapezius), and of the suboccipital region (rectus capitis posterior major and minor, obliquus capitis inferior and superior).

- Impaired muscle performance due to stretched and weak lower cervical and upper thoracic erector spinae and scapular retractor muscles (rhomboids, middle trapezius), anterior throat muscles (suprahyoid and infrahyoid), and capital flexors (rectus capitis anterior and lateralis, superior oblique longus colli, longus capitis).

This posture can place excessive stress on any or all of the following structures:

- Anterior longitudinal ligament in the upper cervical spine and posterior longitudinal ligament in the lower cervical and thoracic spine
- Irritation of the zygapophyseal (facet) joints in the upper cervical spine
- Impingement on the neurovascular bundle from anterior scalene or pectoralis minor muscle tightness (thoracic outlet syndrome)
- Impingement of the cervical plexus from levator scapulae muscle tightness
- Temporomandibular joint dysfunction
- Lower cervical disc lesions

Flat Upper Back and Neck

This posture is characterized by a decrease in the thoracic curve, depressed scapulae, depressed clavicles, and decreased cervical lordosis with increased flexion of the occiput on the atlas. Although not common, this posture occurs primarily with exaggeration of the military posture. The potential muscle impairments include:

- Decreased mobility in the anterior neck muscles, thoracic erector spinae, and scapular retractors, with potentially restricted scapular movement, which can interfere with shoulder elevation.
- Impaired muscle performance in the scapular protractor and intercostal muscles of the anterior thorax.

This posture can place stress on the neurovascular bundle in the thoracic outlet between the clavicle and ribs, and it can decrease the shock-absorbing function of the kyphotic curvature, thereby predisposing the neck to injury. The most common postural findings and faults are listed in **Table 4-34**.

Palpation

Palpation, using varying levels of tactile pressure, requires a detailed knowledge of anatomy and a systematic approach. The following should be noted during palpation:

- Myofascial mobility
- Skin temperature
- Areas of localized tenderness
- Skin and soft tissue density and extensibility

TABLE
4-34

Good and Faulty Posture Summary

	Good Posture	Faulty Posture
Head	Head is held erect in a position of good balance.	Chin is up too high. Head is protruding forward. Head is tilted orrotated to one side.
Shoulder and arms	Shoulders are level, and neither one is more forward or backward than the other when seen from the side. Arms hang relaxed at the sides with palms of the hands facing toward the body. Elbows are slightly bent, so forearms hang slightly forward. Scapulae lie flat against the rib cage. Scapulae are neither too close together nor too wide apart (in adults; a separation of approximately 10 centimeters [4 inches] is average).	Arms are held stiffly in any position forward, backward, or out from the body. Arms are turned so that palms of hands face backward. One shoulder is higher than the other. Both shoulders are hiked up. One or both shoulders is drooping forward or sloping. Shoulders are rotated either clockwise or counterclockwise. Scapulae are pulled back too hard. Scapulae are too far apart. Scapulae are too prominent, standing out from the rib cage ("winged scapulae").
Chest	Chest should be slightly up and slightly forward (while the back remains in good alignment) and in a position about halfway between that of a full inspiration and a forced expiration.	Chest is in a depressed, or "hollow-chest," position. Chest is lifted and held up too high, caused by arching the back. Ribs are more prominent on one side than on the other. Lower ribs are flaring out or protruding.
Abdomen	In young children up to about the age of 10, the abdomen normally protrudes somewhat. In older children and adults, it should be flat.	The entire abdomen protrudes. The lower part of the abdomen protrudes while the upper part is pulled in.
Spine and pelvis (side view)	The front of the pelvis and the thighs are in a straight line. The buttocks are not prominent in back but instead slope slightly downward. The spine has four natural curves. In the neck and lower back, the curve is forward, and in the upper back and lowest part of the spine (sacral region), it is backward. The sacral curve is a fixed curve, whereas the other three are flexible.	The low back arches forward too much (lordosis). The pelvis tilts forward toomuch. The front of the thigh forms anangle with the pelvis when this tilt is present. The normal forward curve in the low back has straightened out. The pelvis tips backward, and there is a slightly backward slant to the line of the pelvis in relation to the front of the hips (flat back). There is an increased backward curve in the upper back (kyphosis or round upper back). The neck has an increased forward curve, almost always accompanied by round upper back and seen as a forward head. There is a lateral curve of the spine (scoliosis), toward one side (C-curve) or toward both sides (S-curve).
Hips, pelvis, and spine (back view)	Ideally, the body weight is borne evenly by both feet, and the hips are level. One side is not more prominent than the other as seen from front or back, nor is one hip more forward or backward than the other as seen from the side. The spine does not curve to the left or the right side.	One hip is higher than the other (lateral pelvic tilt). Sometimes it is not really much higher but appears so because a sideways sway of the body has made it more prominent. The hips are rotated so that one is farther forward than the other (clockwise or counterclockwise rotation).

(continued)

TABLE 4-34 Good and Faulty Posture Summary (continued)

	Good Posture	Faulty Posture
Knees and legs	Legs are straight up and down. Patellae face straight ahead when feet are in good position. Looking at the knees from the side, the knees are straight (i.e., neither bent forward nor "locked" backward).	Knees touch when feet are apart (genu valgum). Knees are apart when feet touch (genu varum). Knee curves slightly backward (hyperextended knee) (genu recurvatum). Knee bends slightly forward—that is, it is not as straight as it should be (flexed knee). Patellae face slightly toward each other (medially rotated femurs). Patellae face slightly outward (laterally rotated femurs).
Foot	In standing, the longitudinal arch has the shape of a half dome. Barefoot, the feet toe-out slightly.	There is a low longitudinal arch or flatfoot. There is a low metatarsal arch, usually indicated bycalluses under the ball of the foot. Weight is borne on the inner side of the foot(pronation;"Ankle rolls in"). Weight is borne on the outer border of the foot (supination;"Ankle rolls out"). Toeing-out occurs while walking or while standing inshoes with heels ("outflared" or "slue-footed"). Toeing-in occurs while walking or standing ("pigeon-toed").
Toes	Toes should be straight—that is, neither curled downward nor bent upward. They should extend forward in line with the foot and not be squeezed together or overlap.	Toes bend up at the first joint and down at middle and end joints so that the weight rests on the tips of the toes (hammer toes).This fault is often associated with wearing shoes that are too short. The big toe slants inward toward the midline of the foot (hallus valgus). This fault is often associated with wearing shoes that are too narrow and pointed at the toes.

Data from Magee DJ: Assessment of posture, in Magee DJ (ed): Orthopedic Physical Assessment. Philadelphia, W.B. Saunders, 2002, pp 873–903; and Kendall FP, McCreary EK, Provance PG: Muscles: Testing and Function. Baltimore, Williams & Wilkins, 1993

- Peripheral pulses as indicated
- Areas of edema

Girth Measurement

Girth measurements of an extremity can be measured using two methods:

- *Tape measure:* The circumferential girth of an extremity can be measured using a tape measure and established limb landmarks proximal and distal to the edema location. These measurements are then compared bilaterally using consistent locations and landmarks. At the ankle a figure-eight measurement is taken around the posterior heel and lateral longitudinal arch.
- *Volumetric displacement:* A volumeter is filled with water, and the patient's lower leg or arm is placed slowly into the volumeter to a consistent landmark on the extremity. As the extremity is lowered into the volumeter, water overflows into a runoff spout and into a collection bowl. Once the water has settled, the amount of water displaced is measured and compared bilaterally.

Joint Mobility

The passive articular mobility tests involve the clinician assessing the arthrokinematic, or accessory, motions of a joint. A variety of measurement scales have been proposed for judging the amount of accessory joint motion present between two joint surfaces, most of which are based on a comparison with a comparable contralateral joint, using manually applied forces in a logical and precise manner.[85] Using these techniques, joint accessory motion can be determined as being hypomobile, normal, or hypermobile:[86–88]

- *Normal:* The joint surfaces possess normal movement.

- *Hypomobile:* The joint surfaces possess limited or less than normal movement.
- *Hypermobile:* The joint surfaces possess excessive or beyond normal movement.

The accessory motions can be graded as follows:

0 Ankylosed
1 Considerable hypomobility
2 Slight hypomobility
3 Normal
4 Slight hypermobility
5 Considerable hypermobility
6 Pathologically unstable

Within these grades:

- Grades 0 and 6 require surgery.
- Grades 1 and 2 require joint mobilizations (discussed in **Table 4-35**, **Table 4-36**, and **Table 4-37**). Whether joint mobilizations may be performed by the PTA is determined by state regulations.
- Grade 4 requires postural corrections and stabilization exercises.
- Grade 5 requires postural corrections and the use of some form of stabilization device (corset or collar).

Special Tests

The evidence-based tests are described in **Tables 4-38** through **4-45**.

TABLE 4-35	Indications and Contraindications for Joint Mobilizations
Indications	**Contraindications**
Mild musculoskeletal pain.	**Absolute**
A nonirritable musculoskeletal condition, demonstrated by pain that is provoked by motion but that disappears very quickly.	Bacterial infection
	Malignancy
	Systemic localized infection
Intermittent musculoskeletal pain.	Sutures over the treatment site
Pain reported by the patient that is relieved by rest.	Recent fracture
	Cellulitis
Pain reported by the patient that is relieved or provoked by particular otions or positions.	Febrile state
	Hematoma
Pain that is altered by changes related to sitting or standing posture.	Acute circulatory condition
	An open wound at the treatment site
To stretch supporting tissue in order to restore normal joint accessory motion, reduce pain, and reduce muscle guarding.	Osteomyelitis
	Advanced diabetes
	Hypersensitivity of the skin
	Inappropriate endfeel (spasm, empty, and bony)
	Constant, severe pain, including pain that disturbs sleep, indicating that the condition is likely to be in the acute stage of healing
	Extensive radiation of pain
	Pain unrelieved by rest
	Severe irritability (pain that is easily provoked and that does not go away within a few hours)
	Relative
	Joint effusion or inflammation
	Rheumatoid arthritis
	Presence of neurologic signs
	Osteoporosis
	Hypermobility
	Pregnancy, if a technique is to be applied to the spine
	Dizziness
	Steroid or anticoagulant therapy

TABLE 4-36

Correct Application of Joint Mobilization

Knowledge of the relative shapes of the joint surfaces (concave or convex).[a–d] If the joint surface is convex relative to the other surface, the joint glide occurs in the direction opposite to the osteokinematic movement (angular motion). If, in contrast, the joint surface is concave, the joint glide occurs in the same direction as osteokinematic movement.

Duration, type, and irritability of symptoms.[a,b] This information can provide the clinician with some general guidelines in determining the intensity of the application of a selected technique.

Patient and clinician position. Correct positioning of the patient is essential both to help the patient relax and to ensure safe body mechanics from the clinician. When patients feel relaxed, their muscle activity is decreased, reducing the amount of resistance encountered during the technique.

Position of joint to be treated. The position of the joint to be treated must be appropriate for the stage of healing and the skill of the clinician. It is recommended that the resting position of the joint be used when the patient has an acute condition or the clinician is inexperienced. The resting position in this case refers to the position that the injured joint adopts, rather than the classic resting (open-packed) position for a normal joint. Other positions for starting the mobilization may be used by a skilled clinician in patients with nonacute conditions.

Hand placement. Wherever possible, contact with the patient should be maximized. The hand should conform to the area being treated, so that the forces are spread over a larger area. A gentle and confident touch inspires confidence from the patient. Accurate hand placement is essential for efficient stabilization and for the accurate transmission of force.

Specificity. Specificity refers to the exactness of the procedure, and is based on its intent. Whenever possible, the forces imparted by a technique should occur at the point where they are needed.

Direction of force. The direction of the force can be either *direct*, which is toward the motion barrier or restriction,[e] or *indirect*, which is away from the motion barrier or restriction.[f,g] Although the rationale for a direct technique is easy to understand, the rationale for using an indirect technique is more confusing. A good analogy is the stuck drawer that cannot be opened. Often the movement that eventually frees the drawer is an inward motion, followed by a pull.[h]

Amount of force. The amount of force used depends on the intent of the manual procedure and a number of other factors, including but not limited to

- Age, sex, and general health status of the patient
- Barrier to motion and endfeel (stage of healing)
- Type and severity of the movement disorder

Reinforcement of any gains made. It has been demonstrated that movement gained by a specific manual technique performed in isolation will be lost within 48 hours, if the motions gained are not reinforced.[i] Thus, motion gained by a manual technique must be reinforced by both the mechanical and the neurophysiologic benefits of active movement.[j] These active movements must be as local and precise as possible to the involved segment or myofascial structure.

Data from (a) Maitland G: Peripheral Manipulation (ed 3). London, Butterworth, 1991; (b) Maitland G: Vertebral Manipulation. Sydney, Butterworth, 1986; (c) Kaltenborn FM: Manual Mobilization of the Extremity Joints: Basic Examination and Treatment Techniques (ed 4). Oslo, Norway, Olaf Norlis Bokhandel, Universitetsgaten, 1989; (d) Nitz AJ: Physical therapy management of the shoulder. Phys Ther 66:1912–1919, 1986; (e) Kappler RE: Direction action techniques. J Am Osteopath Assn 81:239–243, 1981; (f) Mitchell FL, Moran PS, Pruzzo NA: An Evaluation and Treatment Manual of Osteopathic Muscle Energy Procedures. Manchester, MO, Mitchell, Moran and Pruzzo Associates, 1979; (g) Greenman PE: Principles of Manual Medicine (ed 2). Baltimore, Williams & Wilkins, 1996; (h) Nyberg R: Manipulation: Definition, types, application, in Basmajian JV, Nyberg R (eds): Rational Manual Therapies. Baltimore, Maryland, Williams & Wilkins, 1993, pp 21–47; (i) Nansel D, Peneff A, Cremata E, et al: Time course considerations for the effects of unilateral cervical adjustments with respect to the amelioration of cervical lateral flexion passive end-range asymmetry. J Manip Physiol Ther 13:297–304, 1990; and (j) Jull GA: Physiotherapy management of neck pain of mechanical origin, in Giles LGF, Singer KP (eds): Clinical Anatomy and Management of Cervical Spine Pain. The Clinical Anatomy of Back Pain. London, England, Butterworth-Heinemann, 1998, pp 168–191

TABLE 4-37 Joint Mobilization Techniques

Technique	Grades	Purpose
Kaltenborn	Grade I: piccolo (loosen)	Utilized for pain relief
	Grade II: slack (take up the slack)	Utilized to maintain integrity of joint play
	Grade III: stretch	Utilized in conjunction with mobilization glides according to the convex–concave rules to treat joint hypomobility in the remodeling stage of healing
Maitland	Grade I (low amplitude)	Rhythmic oscillation performed at the beginning of joint motion used as introductory technique to reduce pain
	Grade II (high amplitude)	Rhythmic oscillation performed in the middle of joint motion to reduce pain and muscle guarding
	Grade III (high amplitude)	Rhythmic oscillation performed at the end of joint motion to increase tissue mobility
	Grade IV (low amplitude)	Rhythmic oscillation performed at the end of joint motion to increase tissue mobility
	Grade V (manipulation)	Not within the scope of practice

TABLE 4-38 Evidence-Based Special Tests of the Cervical Spine and TMJ

Name of Test	Brief Description	Positive Findings	Evidence-Based
Temporomandibular joint screen[a]	Patient is asked to open and close the mouth, and to laterally deviate the jaw as clinician observes the quality and quantity of motion, and notes any reproduction of symptoms.	Positive for TMJ if patient reports tenderness in the masticatory muscles, the preauricular area, or the TMJ area.	Sensitivity: 0.87 Specificity: 0.67
Lateral palpation of TMJ[b]	Clinician palpates the lateral and posterior aspects of the TMJ with the index finger.	Positive for TMJ dysfunction if pain is elicited.	Sensitivity: 0.88 Specificity: 0.36
Auscultation of TMJ using a stethoscope[c]	Clinician auscultates for the presence of sounds during mouth opening/closing.	Presence of a click sound is considered positive for TMJ dysfunction.	Sensitivity: 0.69 Specificity: 0.51
Auscultation of TMJ using a stethoscope	Clinician auscultates for the presence of crepitus (grating or grinding) during mouth opening/closing.	Positive for TMJ dysfunction if crepitus is present.	Sensitivity: 0.70 Specificity: 0.43
Joint mobility testing of TMJ—condylar translation[d]	Clinician palpates condylar movement while patient maximally opens mouth.	Positive for anterior disc displacement if limited motion is detected.	Sensitivity: 0.32 Specificity: 0.83
Spurling(1)[e]	Patient bends to the side and extends the neck, and clinician applies compression.	Positive if pain or tingling starts in the shoulder and radiates distally to the elbow.	Sensitivity: 0.30 Specificity: 0.93
Spurling (2)[f]	Patient is seated, the neck is bent toward the ipsilateral side, and clinician applies 7 kilograms of overpressure.	Positive if symptoms are reproduced.	Sensitivity: 0.50 Specificity: 0.88
Neck compression test[g]	Patient is seated. Clinician sidebends and slightly rotates patient's head. A compression force of 7 kilograms is exerted.	Positive if test aggravates radicular pain, numbness, or paresthesias.	Sensitivity: 0.28 (right), 0.33 (left) Specificity: 0.92 (right), 1.0 (left)
Axial manual traction[h]	With patient supine, clinician provides actual distraction force between 10 and 15 kilograms.	Positive if symptoms are reduced or disappear.	Sensitivity: 0.26 Specificity: 1.0

(continued)

TABLE 4-38

Evidence-Based Special Tests of the Cervical Spine and TMJ (continued)

Name of Test	Brief Description	Positive Findings	Evidence-Based
Shoulder abduction test[g]	Patient lifts the hand above the head.	Positive if symptoms are reduced or disappear.	Sensitivity: 0.31 (right), 0.42 (left) Specificity: 1.05 (right), 1.0 (left)
Sharp-Purser Test[i]	Patient sits with neck in a semiflexed position. Clinician places palm of one hand on patient's forehead and index finger of the other hand on the spinous process of the axis.	When posterior pressure is applied to the forehead, a sliding motion of the head posteriorly in relation to the axis indicates a positive test for atlantoaxial instability.	Sensitivity: 0.69 Specificity: 0.96
Compression of brachial[j] plexus	Clinician applies firm compression and squeezing of the brachial plexus with the thumb.	Positive only when the pain radiates to the shoulder or upper extremity.	Sensitivity: 0.69 Specificity: 0.83
Pain provocation using active flexion and extension[k]	Patient performs active flexion and extension to the extremes of the range.	Positive for neck dysfunction if subject reports pain with procedure.	Sensitivity: 0.27 Specificity: 0.90

Data from (a) Cleland J: Temporomandibular Joint, Orthopedic Clinical Examination: An Evidence-Based Approach for Physical Therapists. Carlstadt, NJ, Icon Learning Systems, 2005, pp 39–89; (b) Stegenga B, de Bont LG, van der Kuijl B, et al: Classification of temporomandibular joint osteoarthrosis and internal derangement. 1. Diagnostic significance of clinical and radiographic symptoms and signs. Cranio 10:96–106; discussion 116–117, 1992; (c) Manfredini D, Tognini F, Zampa V, et al: Predictive value of clinical findings for temporomandibular joint effusion. Oral Surg Oral Med Oral Pathol Oral Radiol Endod 96:521–526, 2003; (d) Orsini MG, Kuboki T, Terada S, et al: Clinical predictability of temporomandibular joint disc displacement. J Dent Res 78:650-660, 1999; (e) Tong HC, Haig AJ, Yamakawa K: The Spurling test and cervical radiculopathy. Spine 27:156–159, 2002; (f) Wainner RS, Gill H: Diagnosis and nonoperative management of cervical radiculopathy. J Orthop Sports Phys Ther 30:728–744, 2000; (g) Viikari-Juntura E, Porras M, Laasonen EM: Validity of clinical tests in the diagnosis of root compression in cervical disc disease. Spine 14:253–257, 1989; (h) Viikari-Juntura E, Takala E, Riihimaki H, et al: Predictive validity of symptoms and signs in the neck and shoulders. J Clin Epidemiol 53:800–808, 2000; (i) Uitvlugt G, Indenbaum S: Clinical assessment of atlantoaxial instability using the Sharp-Purser test. Arthritis Rheum 31:918–922, 1988; (j) Uchihara T, Furukawa T, Tsukagoshi H: Compression of brachial plexus as a diagnostic test of a cervical cord lesion. Spine 19:2170–2173, 1994; and (k) Sandmark H, Nisell R: Validity of five common manual neck pain provoking tests. Scand J Rehabil Med. 27:131–136, 1995

TABLE 4-39

Evidence-Based Special Tests of the Lumbar Spine and SIJ

Name of Test	Brief Description	Positive Findings	Evidence-Based
Two-stage treadmill test[a]	Patient ambulates on a level and inclined (15°) treadmill 10 minutes. A 10-minute rest period sitting upright in a chair follows each test.	Positive for lumbar spinal stenosis if symptoms are reproduced based on time to onset of symptoms, and prolonged recovery after level walking.	Sensitivity: 0.68–0.82, respectively Specificity: 0.83–0.68 respectively
Segmental hypomobility testing[b]	Assessment of AROM, AbAROM, PAIVM, and PPIVM.	Presence of hypomobility with any of the tests.	*AROM* Sensitivity: 0.75 Specificity: 0.60 *AbAROM* Sensitivity: 0.43 Specificity: 0.88 *PAIVM* Sensitivity: 0.75 Specificity: 0.35 *PPIVM* Sensitivity: 0.42 Specificity: 0.89

Name of Test	Brief Description	Positive Findings	Evidence-Based
Straight leg raise for detecting disc herniation[c]	Patient lies supine with the knee fully extended and the ankle in neutral dorsiflexion. Clinician passively flexes the hip while maintaining the knee extension to the point where pain or paresthesia is experienced in the back or lower limb. Various sensitizing maneuvers (dorsiflexion of the ankle and flexion of the cervical spine) are then added.	Positive if the sensitizing maneuvers exacerbate the symptoms.	Sensitivity: 0.91 Specificity: 0.26
Crossed straight leg raise for detecting disc herniation[c]	Clinician performs a straight leg raise on the uninvolved lower extremity.	Positive if symptoms in the involved extremity are reproduced.	Sensitivity: 0.29 Specificity: 0.88
Patrick test (SIJ pain provocation test)[d]	Patient's hip is flexed, abducted, and externally rotated by placement of the lateral malleolus on the knee of the contralateral leg. The pelvis is stabilized, and overpressure is applied to the medial aspect of the knee.	Positive if buttock and groin pain is reproduced.	Sensitivity: 0.77 Specificity: 1.0
Posterior gapping of the SIJ[e]	Patient lies on side. Clinician applies firm downward pressure to the contralateral ilium.	Positive for ankylosing spondylitis if pain over the sacrum or into the buttocks is provoked.	Sensitivity: 0.70 Specificity: 0.90
Anterior gapping of the SIJ[f]	Patient lies supine. Clinician applies crossover pressure to both anterior superior iliac spines.	Positive if familiar symptoms are produced or increased.	Sensitivity: 0.23 Specificity: 0.81
Gaenslen test (SIJ dysfunction)[e]	Patient lies supine with both legs extended. The leg being tested is passively brought into full knee flexion, while the opposite hip remains in extension. Overpressure is then applied to the flexed extremity.	Positive if pain is reproduced.	Sensitivity: 0.21 Specificity: 0.72
Long sitting test[g]	Patient lies supine. Clinician palpates inferior border of medial malleoli and makes a determination of symmetry. Patient assumes the long sitting position, and clinician again records symmetry of the malleoli.	Positive for iliosacral dysfunction if asymmetric malleoli lengths reverse from supine to long sit.	Sensitivity: 0.17 Specificity: 0.38
Thigh thrust[h]	Patient lies supine with hip flexed 90° and slightly adducted. Clinician cups the sacrum with one hand and uses the other to apply a posteriorly directed force to the femur.	Positive for SIJ dysfunction if familiar symptoms are reproduced or increased.	Sensitivity: 0.88 Specificity: 0.69
Compression test[f]	Patient lies on side, involved side up, with the hips flexed approximately 45° and the knees flexed approximately 90°. Clinician applies a force vertically downward on the anterior superior iliac crest.	Positive for SIJ dysfunction if there is reproduction of or an increase in familiar symptoms.	Sensitivity: 0.22 Specificity: 0.83
Sacral thrust test[h]	Patient lies prone. Clinician applies a force vertically downward to the center of the sacrum.	Positive for SIJ dysfunction if there is reproduction or an increase in familiar symptoms.	Sensitivity: 0.63 Specificity: 0.75

(continued)

TABLE 4-39 Evidence-Based Special Tests of the Lumbar Spine and SIJ (continued)

Name of Test	Brief Description	Positive Findings	Evidence-Based
Mennell test[f]	Patient lies on side, involved side down, with the involved side hip and knee flexed toward the abdomen. Clinician puts one hand over the ipsilateral buttock and iliac crest and with the other hand grasps the semi-flexed ipsilateral knee and lightly forces the leg into extension.	Positive for SIJ dysfunction if there is reproduction of or increase in familiar symptoms.	Sensitivity: Right: 0.66 Left: 0.45 Specificity: Right: 0.80 Left: 0.86
Gillet test[i]	Patient stands with feet spread 12 inches apart. Clinician palpates the S2 spinous process with one hand and the PSIS with the other. Patient then flexes the hip and knee on the side being tested.	Positive for SIJ dysfunction if the PSIS fails to move in a posteroinferior direction relative to S2.	Sensitivity: 0.08 Specificity: 0.93
Standing flexion test[i]	Patient stands. Clinician palpates the inferior slope of the PSIS. Patient is asked to bend forward completely.	Positive for sacroiliac hypomobility if one PSIS moves more cranially than the contralateral side.	Sensitivity: 0.17 Specificity: 0.79
Sitting flexion test[i]	Patient is in seated position. Clinician palpates the inferior aspect of each PSIS. Patient is asked to bend forward as far as possible.	Positive for sacroiliac joint dysfunction if inequality of PSIS movement is found.	Sensitivity: 0.09 Specificity: 0.93

Abbreviations: AbAROM, abnormality of segmental range of motion; AROM, active range of motion; PAIVM, passive accessory intervertebral motion; PPIVM, passive physiologic intervertebral motion; PSIS, posterior superior iliac spine; SIJ, sacroiliac joint

Data from (a) Fritz JM, Erhard RE, Delitto A, et al: Preliminary results of the use of a two-stage treadmill test as a clinical diagnostic tool in the differential diagnosis of lumbar spinal stenosis. J Spinal Disord 10:410–416, 1997; (b) Abbot J, Mercer S: Lumbar segmental hypomobility: Criterion-related validity of clinical examination items (a pilot study). NZJ Physiother 31:3–9, 2003; (c) Deville WL, van der Windt DA, Dzaferagic A, et al: The test of Lasegue: systematic review of the accuracy in diagnosing herniated discs. Spine25:1140-1147, 2000; (d) Broadhurst NA, Bond MJ: Pain provocation tests for the assessment of sacroiliac joint dysfunction. J Spinal Disord 11:341–345, 1998; (e) Russel AS, Maksymowych W, LeClercq S: Clinical examination of the sacroiliac joints: A prospective study. Arthritis Rheum 24:1575–1577, 1981; (f) Ozgocmen S, Bozgeyik Z, Kalcik M, et al: The value of sacroiliac pain provocation tests in early active sacroiliitis. Clin Rheumatol 27:1275–1282, 2008; (g) Bemis T, Daniel M: Validation of the long sitting test on subjects with Iliosacral dysfunction. J Orthop Sports Phys Ther 8:336–345, 1987; (h) Laslett M, Aprill CN, McDonald B, et al: Diagnosis of sacroiliac joint pain: Validity of individual provocation tests and composites of tests. Man Ther 10:207–218, 2005; and (i) Levangie PK: Four clinical tests of sacroiliac joint dysfunction: The association of test results with innominate torsion among patients with and without low back pain. Phys Ther 79:1043–1057, 1999

TABLE 4-40 Evidence-Based Special Tests for the Shoulder Complex

Name of Test	Brief Description	Positive Finding	Evidence-Based Sensitivity	Specificity
Hornblower sign[a]	Patient is seated. Clinician places patient arm in 90° of scaption and asks patient to externally rotate against resistant.	Positive for infraspinatus or teres minor tear if the patient is unable to externally rotate the shoulder.	1.0	0.93
Empty can test for supraspinatus tendon tears[b]	Patient's arm is positioned in the scaption plane—internal rotation and approximately 90° of shoulder flexion. Clinicial applies manual resistance in a direction toward the floor.	Positive for supraspinatus tear if pain, weakness, or both is reproduced.	Pain 0.63 Weak 0.77 Both 0.89	0.55 0.68 0.50

TABLE 4-40

Evidence-Based Special Tests for the Shoulder Complex (continued)

Name of Test	Brief Description	Positive Finding	Evidence-Based Sensitivity	Specificity
Full can test for supraspinatus tendon tears[b]	Patient's arm is positioned in the scaption plane—external rotation and approximately 90° of shoulder flexion. Clinician applies manual resistance in a direction toward the floor.	Positive for supraspinatus tear if pain, weakness, or both is reproduced.	Pain 0.66 Weak 0.77 Both 0.86	0.64 0.74 0.57
Dropping sign for infraspinatus degeneration[a]	Patient is seated. Clinician places patient shoulder in 0° of abduction and 45° of external rotation with elbow flexed to 90°. Patient is asked to hold position when clinician releases forearm.	Positive for infraspinatus degeneration if patient is unable to hold position and arm returns to 0° of external rotation.	1.00	1.00
Palm up test (Speed test) for biceps tendon tear[c]	Patient elevates humerus to 60° with elbow extended and forearm supinated. Patient holds this position while the clinician applies resistance against elevation.	Positive if pain is elicited.	0.63	0.35
Combined tests[d]	Clinician tests for supraspinatus and external rotator weakness, and impingement sign.	Positive for subacromial impingement if weakness found in the supraspinatus and external rotators, and there is a positive impingement sign.	Not applicable	0.00
Transdeltoid palpation (rent test)[e]	Patient seated with arm by side. Clinician palpates anterior margin of acromion through the deltoid. Clinician then passively extends patient's arm and internally and externally rotates to palpate the rotator cuff tendons.	Positive for rotator cuff tear if clinician palpates eminence or rent.	0.957	0.968
Lift-off test for subscapularis tendon	Patient is seated with the arm internally rotated so that the posterior surface of the hand rests on the lower back. Patient is asked to actively lift the hand away from the back.	Positive for subscapularis weakness/ subacromial impingement if the patient unable to lift the hand away from the back.	0.89[f] 0.89[g]	1.00[f] 0.36[g]
Supraspinatus test[g]	Patient is standing, shoulders abducted to 90° in scapular plane and internal rotation of the humerus. Clinician applies isometric resistance.	Positive if weakness or pain is detected.	1.00	0.53
Combined tests[h]	Clinician performs supraspinatus and infraspinatus manual muscle test, and palpation.	Positive for rotator cuff involvement if weakness detected and pain is elicited with palpation.	0.91	0.75
Neer impingement sign for rotator cuff tear	Patient is seated. Clinician stabilizes scapula with one hand and forces patient's arm into maximal elevation with the other hand.	Positive for rotator cuff tear if pain is produced.	0.84[i] 0.33[g] 0.39[j] 0.93[k] 0.00[l] 0.89[m] 0.89[c]	0.51[i] 0.61[g] 1.0[j] ---- ---- ---- 0.31[c]
Neer impingement sign for subacromial bursitis	Same as for the previous test.	Positive for subacromial bursitis if pain is produced.	0.75[i]	0.48[i]

(continued)

Name of Test	Brief Description	Positive Finding	Evidence-Based	
			Sensitivity	Specificity
Hawkins impingement sign for rotator cuff tear	Patient's arm is passively flexed to 90° and forcefully moved into internal rotation.	Positive for rotator cuff tear if pain is produced.	0.88[i] 0.44[g]	0.43[i] 0.53[g]
Hawkins–Kennedy test for subacromial impingement	Patient's arm is passively flexed to 90° and forcefully moved into internal rotation.	Positive for subacromial impingement if pain is reproduced.	0.80[i] 0.78[l] 0.62[g] 0.87[m] 0.92[c]	0.76[i] 1.00[l] 0.69[g] — 0.25[c]
Hawkins impingement sign for subacromial bursitis	Pain produced by forced internal rotation of the humerus in 90 degrees of abduction.[i]		0.92	0.44
Horizontal adduction	Clinician flexes shoulder to 90° and then adducts it horizontally across the body.	Positive for an A-C lesion if pain is reproduced at the A-C joint.	0.82[c]	0.28[c]
Speed test (for subacromial impingement)	Patient elevates humerus to 60° with elbow extended and forearm supinated. The patient holds this position while the clinician applies resistance against elevation.	Positive if pain is elicited.	0.69[c]	0.56[c]
Speed test for biceps or superior labrum anterior and posterior (SLAP)	Same as for the previous test.	Positive if pain is elicited.	0.90[o]	0.14[o]
Yergason test	Patient's elbow is flexed to 90° with forearm in pronation. Patient is then instructed to actively supinate forearm against resistant.	Positive for subacromial impingement if pain is elicited.	0.37[c]	0.86[c]
Painful arc	Patient is instructed to perform straight-plane abduction of the arm throughout full range of motion.	Positive if pain occurs between 60° and 100° of abduction.	0.33[c]	0.81[c]
Internal rotation resisted strength test	Patient stands. Clinician positions the patient's arm in 90° of abduction and 80° of external rotation. Clinician applies resistance against external rotation, then internal rotation in the same position.	Positive for intra-articular disease if the patient exhibits greater weakness in internal rotation when compared with external rotation, and for impingement syndrome if there is greater weakness with external rotation.	0.88[o]	0.96[o]
Bicipital groove tenderness[p]	Clinician gently presses the biceps groove with the shoulder adducted 10°.	Positive for labral tear if pain is reproduced.	0.27	0.66
Biceps palpation[q]	Point tenderness of the biceps tendon in the biceps groove 3–6 centimeters below anterior acromion.	Positive for labral tear if pain is reproduced.	0.53	0.54

TABLE 4-40

Evidence-Based Special Tests for the Shoulder Complex (continued)

Name of Test	Brief Description	Positive Finding	Evidence-Based Sensitivity	Specificity
Crank test[r]	Patient lies supine. Clinician elevates the humerus 160° in the scapular plane and then applies an axial load to the humerus while the shoulder is internally and externally rotated.	Positive for a labral tear if pain is elicited.	0.61	0.55
O'Brien test[p]	Patient stands and flexes the arm to 90° with the elbow in full extension. Patient then adducts the arm 10° and internally rotates the humerus. Clinician applies a downward force to the arm as patient resists. Patient then fully supinates the arm and the procedure is repeated.	Positive if pain is elicited with the first maneuver and reduced with the second maneuver.	0.63	0.53
Compression rotation test[p]	Patient lies supine with the arm abducted to 90° and the elbow flexed to 90°. Clinician applies an axial force to the humerus. The humerus is circumducted and rotated.	Positive for a labral tear if pain or clicking is elicited.	0.61	0.54
Anterior apprehension test[p]	Patient lies supine. Clinician passively abducts and externally rotates the humerus.	Positive for shoulder instability if patient complains of pain or instability.	0.62	0.42
Gilcreest test: Palm up test for biceps long-head	Patient elevates arm with elbow extended and forearm supinated against resistance applied by clinician.	Positive if patient feels pain at anterior aspect of arm along course of biceps brachii.	0.63[m]	0.35[m]
Yocum test	Patient is seated or standing and is asked to place hand on involved shoulder on contralateral shoulder and raise the elbow.	Positive for subacromial impingement if pain is elicited.	0.78[m]	—
Shoulder relocation test (no force on humerus at start position)	Patient lies supine with glenohumeral joint at edge of table. Clinician places shoulder in 90° of abduction and 90° of elbow flexion and then externally rotates the shoulder.	Positive if there is either pain or apprehension.	0.30 for pain[s] 0.57 for apprehension[s]	0.58 for pain[s] 1.0 for apprehension[s]
Shoulder relocation test (anterior-directed force on humerus at start position)	Patient lies supine with glenohumeral joint at edge of table. Clinician places shoulder in 90° of abduction and 90° of elbow flexion and then externally rotates the shoulder and applies an anterior directed force on the humerus.	Positive if there is either pain or apprehension.	0.54 for pain[s] 0.68 for apprehension[s]	0.44 for pain[s] 1.0 for apprehension[s]
Anterior release test for anterior instability	Patient is supine with arm in 90° of abduction and external rotation while clinician applies a posterior force over the humeral head. Clinician quickly releases the posterior force.	Positive if there is either pain or apprehension.	0.92[t]	0.89[t]

(continued)

TABLE 4-40 — Evidence-Based Special Tests for the Shoulder Complex (continued)

Name of Test	Brief Description	Positive Finding	Evidence-Based Sensitivity	Evidence-Based Specificity
Load and shift[u]	Patient lies supine. Clinician grasps patient elbow with one hand and the proximal humerus with the other hand. The arm is placed in 90° of abduction in the scapular plane. Clinician attempts to shift the humeral head in anterior, posterior, and inferior directions.	Amount of laxity is graded from 0 to 3, with 0 indicating little or no movement and 3 indicating that the humeral head can be dislocated off the glenoid and remains so when the pressure is released.	Anterior: 0.5 Posterior: 0.14 Inferior: 0.08	Anterior: 1.00 Posterior: 1.00 Inferior: 1.00

Data from (a) Walch G, Boulahia A, Calderone S, et al: The "dropping" and "hornblower's" signs in evaluation of rotator-cuff tears. J BoneJoint Surg Br80:624–628, 1998; (b) Itoi E, Tadato K, Sano A, et al: Which is more useful, the "full can test" or the "empty can test" in detecting the torn supraspinatus tendon? Am J Sports Med 27:65–68, 1999; (c) Calis M, Akgun K, Birtane M, et al: Diagnostic values of clinical diagnostic tests in subacromial impingement syndrome. Ann Rheumatic Dis 59:44–47, 2000; (d) Murrell GA, Walton JR: Diagnosis of rotator cuff tears. Lancet. 357:769–770, 2001; (e) Wolf EM, Agrawal V: Transdeltoid palpation (the rent test) in the diagnosis of rotator cuff tears. J Shoulder Elbow Surg. 10:470–473, 2001; (f) Gerber C, Krushell RJ: Isolated rupture of the tendon of the subscapularis muscle: clinical features in 16 cases. J Bone Joint Surg 73B:389–394, 1991; (g) Ure BM, Tiling T, Kirschner R, et al: The value of clinical shoulder examination in comparison with arthroscopy: A prospective study. Unfallchirurg 96:382–386, 1993; (h) Lyons AR, Tomlinson JE: Clinical diagnosis of tears of the rotator cuff. J Bone Joint Surg Br 74:414–415, 1992; (i) MacDonald PB, Clark P, Sutherland K: An analysis of the diagnostic accuracy of the Hawkins and Neer subacromial impingement signs. J Shoulder Elbow Surg 9:299–301, 2000; (j) Bak K, Faunl P: Clinical findings in competitive swimmers with shoulder pain. Am J Sports Med 25:254–60, 1997; (k) Post M, Cohen J: Impingement syndrome: a review of late stage II and early stage III lesions. Clin Orth Rel Res 207:127–132, 1986; (l) Rupp S, Berninger K, Hopf T: Shoulder problems in high level swimmers: Impingement, anterior instability, muscular imbalance. Int J Sports Med 16:557–562, 1995; (m) Leroux JL, Thomas E, Bonnel F, et al: Diagnostic value of clinical tests for shoulder impingement. Rev Rheum 62:423–428, 1995; (n) Bennett WF: Specificity of the Speed's test: arthroscopic technique for evaluating the biceps tendon at the level of the bicipital groove. Arthroscopy 14:789–796, 1998; (o) Zaslav KR: Internal rotation resistance strength test: A new diagnostic test to differentiate intra-articular pathology from outlet (Neer) impingement syndrome in the shoulder. J Shoulder Elbow Surg 10:23–27, 2001; (p) Oh JH, Kim JY, Kim WS, et al: The evaluation of various physical examinations for the diagnosis of type II superior labrum anterior and posterior lesion. Am J Sports Med 36:353–359, 2008; (q) Gill HS, El Rassi G, Bahk MS, et al: Physical examination for partial tears of the biceps tendon. Am J Sports Med 35:1334-40, 2007; (r) Walsworth MK, Doukas WC, Murphy KP, et al: Reliability and diagnostic accuracy of history and physical examination for diagnosing glenoid labral tears. Am J Sports Med 36:162–168, 2008; (s) Speer KP, Hannafin JA, Altchek DW, et al: An evaluation of the shoulder relocation test. Am J Sports Med 22:177–183, 1994; (t) Gross ML, Distefano MC: Anterior release test: A new test for occult shoulder instability. Clin Orth Rel Res 339:105–108, 1997; and (u) Tzannes A, Murrell GA: Clinical examination of the unstable shoulder. Sports Med 32:447–457, 2002

TABLE 4-41 — Evidence-Based Special Tests for the Elbow Complex

Name of Test	Brief Description	Positive Findings	Evidence-Based
Elbow extension test[a]	Patient sits with arms supinated, then flexes shoulders to 90° and extends both elbows.	Positive for bony or joint injury if the involved elbow has less extension than the contralateral side.	Sensitivity: 0.96 Specificity: 0.48
Pressure provocative test[b]	Patient's elbow is positioned in 20° of flexion and forearm supination. Clinician applies pressure to the ulnar nerve just proximal to the cubital tunnel for 60 seconds.	Positive for cubital tunnel syndrome if the patient reports symptoms in the distribution of the ulnar nerve.	Sensitivity: 0.89 Specificity: 0.98
Moving valgus stress test[c]	Patient's shoulder is abducted to 90° with maximal external rotation. Clinician maximally flexes the elbow and applies a valgus stress, and then quickly extends the elbow to 30°.	Positive if patient experiences maximal medial elbow pain between 120° and 70° of elbow flexion.	Sensitivity: 1.0 Specificity: 0.75

Data from (a) Appelboam A, Reuben AD, Benger JR, et al: Elbow extension test to rule out elbow fracture: Multicentre, prospective validation and observational study of diagnostic accuracy in adults and children. BMJ 337:a2428, 2008; (b) Novak CB, Lee GW, Mackinnon SE, et al: Provocative testing for cubital tunnel syndrome. J Hand Surg Am 19:817–820, 1994; and (c) O'Driscoll SW, Lawton RL, Smith AM: The "moving valgus stress test" for medial collateral ligament tears of the elbow. Am J Sports Med 33:231–239, 2005

TABLE 4-42 — Evidence-Based Tests for the Wrist and Hand

Name of Test	Brief Description	Positive Findings	Evidence-Based
Scaphoid fracture test[a]	Clinician exerts passive overpressure into ulnar deviation of wrist while forearm is pronated.	Positive if patient reports pain in the anatomical snuffbox.	Sensitivity: 1.0 Specificity: 0.34
Pain with longitudinal compression of thumb[b]	Clinician holds patient's thumb and applies a long axis compression through the metacarpal bone into the scaphoid.	Positive for a scaphoid fracture if patient reports pain in the anatomical snuffbox.	Sensitivity: 0.98 Specificity: 0.98
Tinel sign[c]	Clinician taps the median nerve at the wrist 4 to 6 times.	Positive for carpal tunnel syndrome if patient reports pain or paresthesias in the distribution of the median nerve.	Sensitivity: 0.68 Specificity: 0.90
Phalen test[c]	Patient holds the wrist in complete flexion with the elbow extended and the forearm pronated for 60 seconds.	Positive if symptoms are reproduced.	Sensitivity: 0.68 Specificity: 0.91
Carpal compression test[d]	Patient is seated with the elbow flexed to 30°, the forearm supinated, and the wrist in neutral. Clinician places both thumbs over the transverse carpal ligament and applies 6 pounds of pressure for 30 seconds maximum.	Positive for carpal tunnel syndrome if the patient experiences exacerbation of symptoms in the median nerve distribution.	Sensitivity: 0.64 Specificity: 0.30
Scaphoid shift test	Patient's elbow is stabilized on the table with forearm in slight pronation. With one hand, clinician grasps the radial side of patient's wrist with the thumb on the palmar prominence of the scaphoid. With the other hand, clinician grasps patient's hand at the metacarpal level to stabilize the wrist. Clinician maintains pressure on the scaphoid tubercle and moves patient's wrist into ulnar deviation with slight extension, then radial deviation with slight flexion. Clinician releases pressure on the scaphoid while the wrist is in radial deviation and flexion.	Positive for instability of the scaphoid if the scaphoid shifts, or patient's symptoms are reproduced when the scaphoid is released.	Sensitivity: 0.69 Specificity: 0.66
Ballottement test	Clinician stabilizes patient's lunate bond between the thumb and index finger of one hand, while the other hand moves the piso-triquetral complex in a palmar and dorsal direction.	Positive for instability of the lunotriquetral joint if patient's symptoms are reproduced or excessive laxity of the joint is revealed.	Sensitivity: 0.64 Specificity: 0.44

Data from (a) Powell JM, Lloyd GJ, Rintoul RF: New clinical test for fracture of the scaphoid. Can J Surg 31:237–238, 1988; (b) Waeckerle JF: A prospective study identifying the sensitivity of radiographic findings and the efficacy of clinical findings in carpal navicular fractures. Ann Emerg Med 16:733–737, 1987; (c) Ahn DS: Hand elevation: A new test for carpal tunnel syndrome. Ann Plast Surg 46:120–124, 2001; and (d) Wainner RS, Fritz JM, Irrgang JJ, et al: Development of a clinical prediction rule for the diagnosis of carpal tunnel syndrome. Arch Phys Med Rehabil. 86:609–618, 2005

TABLE 4-43 — Evidence-Based Special Tests of the Hip Joint Complex

Name of Test	Brief Description	Positive Findings	Evidence-Based
Internal rotation–flexion–axial compression maneuver[a]	Patient lies supine. Clinician flexes and internally rotates the hip, then applies an axial compression force through the femur.	Provocation of pain is considered positive for acetabular labrum tear.	Sensitivity: 0.75 Specificity: 0.43
Thomas test (acetabular labrum tear)[a]	Patient lies supine. Clinician extends involved extremity from the flexed position.	Provocation of pain is considered positive for acetabular labrum tear.	Sensitivity: 0.25 Specificity: not provided

(continued)

TABLE 4-43

Evidence-Based Special Tests of the Hip Joint Complex (continued)

Name of Test	Brief Description	Positive Findings	Evidence-Based
Flexion–adduction test[b]	Patient lies supine with hip flexed to 90° and in neutral rotation. The hip is then allowed to adduct.	Provocation of pain is considered positive for hip disease.	Demonstrated that the test possessed diagnostic utility (sensitivity) for detecting the involved extremity but should not be used in isolation
Positive Trendelenburg test[c]	Patient stands and lifts one foot off the ground at a time.	Positive if the patient is unable to elevate his/her pelvis on the non-stance side and hold the position for at least 30 seconds.	Sensitivity: 0.23 Specificity: 0.94
Patrick test[d]	With patient supine, clinician flexes, abducts, and externally rotates the involved hip so that the lateral ankle is placed just proximal to the contralateral knee. While stabilizing the anterior superior iliac spine, the involved leg is lowered toward the tables to end range.	Positive for hip dysfunction if it reproduces the patient symptoms.	Sensitivity: 0.60 Specificity: 0.18
Scour test[e]	With patient supine, clinician passively flexes the symptomatic hip to 90°, moves the knee toward the opposite shoulder, and applies an axial load to the femur.	Positive if it causes lateral hip pain or groin pain.	Sensitivity: 0.62 Specificity: 0.75
Patellar pubic percussion test[f]	With patient supine, clinician percusses (taps) one patella at a time while auscultating the pubic symphysis with a stethoscope.	Positive if there is a diminution of the percussion note on the involved side.	Sensitivity: 0.94 Specificity: 0.96

Data from (a) Narvani AA, Tsiridis E, Kendall S, et al: A preliminary report on prevalence of acetabular labrum tears in sports patients with groin pain. Knee Surg Sports Traumatol Arthroscopy 11:403–408, 2003; (b) Woods D, Macnicol M: The flexion-adduction test: An early sign of hip disease. J Pediatr Orthop B 10:180–185, 2001; (c) Woodley SJ, Nicholson HD, Livingstone V, et al: Lateral hip pain: Findings from magnetic resonance imaging and clinical examination. J Orthop Sports Phys Ther 38:313–328, 2008; (d) Martin RL, Irrgang JJ, Sekiya JK: The diagnostic accuracy of a clinical examination in determining intra-articular hip pain for potential hip arthroscopy candidates. Arthroscopy 24:1013–1018, 2008; (e) Sutlive TG, Lopez HP, Schnitker DE, et al: Development of a clinical prediction rule for diagnosing hip osteoarthritis in individuals with unilateral hip pain. J Orthop Sports Phys Ther 38: 542–550, 2008; and (f) Adams SL, Yarnold PR: Clinical use of the patellar-pubic percussion sign in hip trauma. Am J Emerg Med 15:173–175, 1997

TABLE 4-44

Evidence-Based Special Tests of the Knee Joint Complex

Name of Test	Brief Description	Positive Findings	Evidence-Based
Lachman	Patient lies supine. Knee joint is flexed between 10° and 20°, and femur is stabilized with one hand.	Lack of end feel for tibial translation or subluxation is positive.	Sensitivity: 0.82[a] 0.65[b] 0.78[c] Specificity: 0.97[a] 0.42[b] 1.0[c]

TABLE 4-44

Evidence-Based Special Tests of the Knee Joint Complex (continued)

Name of Test	Brief Description	Positive Findings	Evidence-Based
Anterior drawer	Patient lies supine. Knee is flexed between 60° and 90° with the foot on the examination table. Clinician draws the tibia anteriorly.	Increased anterior tibial displacement compared with opposite side.	Sensitivity: 0.41[a] 0.78[c] Specificity: 0.95[a] 1.0[c]
Pivot shift test[a]	Patient lies supine. Knee is placed in 10° to 20° of flexion, and the tibia is rotated internally while clinician applies a valgus force.	Positive if lateral tibial plateau subluxes anteriorly.	Sensitivity: 0.82 Specificity: 0.98
Posterior sag sign[d]	Patient lies supine withnnee and hip flexed to 90°.	Increase posterior tibial displacement is positive for PCL injury.	Sensitivity: 0.79 Specificity: 1.0
Varus test[e]	Patient lies supine. Clinician places patient's knee in 20° of flexion and applies a varus stress to the knee.	Positive if pain or laxity is present.	Sensitivity: 0.25 Specificity: not provided
Valgus stress test[e]	Patient lies supine. Clinician places patient's knee in 20° of flexion and applies a valgus stress to the knee.	Positive if pain or laxity is present.	Sensitivity: 0.86 Specificity: not provided
McMurray test[f]	Patient lies supine. Clinician brings the leg from extension into 90° of flexion while the foot is held first in internal rotation, then in external rotation.	Positive for meniscal tear if there is a palpable clunk.	Sensitivity: 0.16 Specificity: 0.98
Apley grind test[g]	Patient lies prone with knee flexed to 90°. Clinician places downward pressure on foot, compressing the knee while internally and externally rotating the tibia.	Positive for meniscal tear if tibial rotation reproduces the patient's pain.	Sensitivity: 0.97 Specificity: 0.87
Ballottement test[h]	Patient is positioned in supine. Clinician quickly pushes patient's patella posteriorly with two or three fingers.	Positive for knee swelling if the patella bounces off the trochlear with a distinct impact.	Sensitivity: 0.83 Specificity: 0.49
Thessaly test	Patient stands on the symptomatic leg while holding clinician's hands. Patient then rotates the body and leg internally and externally with the knee flexed to 20°.	Positive for meniscal tear when the patient feels pain and/or a click in the joint line.	Sensitivity: 0.90[i] Specificity: 0.98[i] Sensitivity: 0.79[j] Specificity: 0.40[j]

Data from (a) Katz JW, Fingeroth RJ: The diagnostic accuracy of ruptures of the anterior cruciate ligament comparing the Lachman test, the anterior drawer sign, and the pivot shift test in acute and chronic knee injuries. Am J Sports Med 14:88–91, 1986; (b) Cooperman JM, Riddle DL, Rothstein JM: Reliability and validity of judgments of the integrity of the anterior cruciate ligament of the knee using the Lachman's test. Phys Ther 70:225–233, 1990; (c) Lee JK, Yao L, Phelps CT, et al: Anterior cruciate ligament tears: MR imaging compared with arthroscopy and clinical tests. Radiology 166:861–864, 1988; (d) Rubinstein RA Jr, Shelbourne KD, McCarroll JR, et al: The accuracy of the clinical examination in the setting of posterior cruciate ligament injuries. Am J Sports Med 22:550–557, 1994; (e) Harilainen A: Evaluation of knee instability in acute ligamentous injuries. Ann Chir Gynaecol 76:269–273, 1987; (f) Evans PJ, Bell GD, Frank C: Prospective evaluation of the McMurray test. Am J Sports Med 21:604–608, 1993; (g) Fowler PJ, Lubliner JA: The predictive value of five clinical signs in the evaluation of meniscal pathology. Arthroscopy 5:184–186, 1989; (h) Kastelein M, Luijsterburg PA, Wagemakers HP, et al: Diagnostic value of history taking and physical examination to assess effusion of the knee in traumatic knee patients in general practice. Arch Phys Med Rehabil 90:82–86, 2009; (i) Harrison BK, Abell BE, Gibson TW: The Thessaly test for detection of meniscal tears: validation of a new physical examination technique for primary care medicine. Clin J Sport Med 19:9–12, 2009; and (j) Mirzatolooei F, Yekta Z, Bayazidchi M, et al: Validation of the Thessaly test for detecting meniscal tears in anterior cruciate deficient knees. Knee 17:221–223, 2010

<table>
<tr><td colspan="2">

TABLE 4-45   Evidence-Based Special Tests for the Foot and Ankle

</td></tr>
</table>

Name of Test	Brief Description	Positive Findings	Evidence-Based
Anterior drawer[a]	Patient lies supine. Clinician maintains the ankle in 10° to 15° of plantarflexion while drawing the heel gently forward.	Positive for anterior talofibular ligament tear if talus rotates out of the ankle mortise anteriorly.	Sensitivity: 0.71 (<48 hours after injury), 0.96 (5 days after injury) Specificity: 0.33 (<48 hours after injury), 0.84 (5 days after injury)
Impingement sign[b]	Patient sits. Clinician grasps calcaneus with one hand and uses other hand to grasp forefoot and bring it into plantarflexion. Clinician uses thumb to place pressure over anterolateral ankle. Foot is then brought from plantarflexion to dorsiflexion while thumb pressure is maintained.	Positive for anterolateral ankle impingement if pain provoked with pressure from clinician's thumb is greater in dorsiflexion than in plantarflexion.	Sensitivity: 0.95 Specificity: 0.88
Gap test[c]	Patient lies prone. Clinician palpates the course of the Achilles tendon.	Positive for Achilles tendon tear if gap in Achilles tendon is noted.	Sensitivity: 0.73 Specificity: not provided
Windlass test[d]	Patient stands on a step stool with toes over the stool's edge. Clinician extends the MTP joint of the great toe while allowing the IP joint to flex.	Positive for plantar fasciitis if pain is reproduced at the end range of MTP extension.	Sensitivity: 0.32 Specificity: 1.0
Paper grip test[e]	The patient is in sitting position with the hips, knees, and ankles at 90° and toes placed on a piece of cardboard. The clinician stabilizes the feet while attempting to slide cardboard away from the toes.	Positive for toe plantarflexion weakness if participant cannot maintain cardboard under the toes.	Sensitivity: 0.80 Specificity: 0.79

Data from (a) van Dijk CN, Mol BW, Lim LS, et al: Diagnosis of ligament rupture of the ankle joint. Physical examination, arthrography, stress radiography and sonography compared in 160 patients after inversion trauma. Acta Orthop Scand 67:566–570, 1996; (b) Molloy S, Solan MC, Bendall SP: Synovial impingement in the ankle: A new physical sign. J Bone Joint Surg Br 85:330–333, 2003; (c) Maffulli N: The clinical diagnosis of subcutaneous tear of the Achilles tendon: A prospective study in 174 patients. Am J Sports Med 26:266–270, 1998; (d) De Garceau D, Dean D, Requejo SM, et al: The association between diagnosis of plantar fasciitis and Windlass test results. Foot Ankle Int 24:251–255, 2003; and (e) Menz HB, Zammit GV, Munteanu SE, et al: Plantarflexion strength of the toes: Age and gender differences and evaluation of a clinical screening test. Foot Ankle Int 27:1103–1108, 2006

Musculoskeletal Pathologies

Fractures

A number of fracture types exist (**Table 4-46**). Fractures may be classified according to direction, mechanism, whether the skin is broken or not, and location.

● **Key Point**   Growth plate fractures can occur in the skeletally immature patient and are associated with a number of complications.

The standard form of treatment for a fracture is some form of immobilization for a period of time. Following the immobilization period, the therapeutic goals are to restore ROM and strength to the involved region.

● **Key Point**   Osteoporosis accounts for the largest number of fractures among the elderly.

Bursitis

Bursitis is defined as inflammation of a bursa and occurs when the synovial fluid becomes infected by

| TABLE 4-46 | Types of Fractures |

Types of Fracture	Description
Avulsion	An avulsion fracture is an injury to the bone where a tendon or ligament pulls off a piece of the bone.
Closed	When there is a closed fracture there is no broken skin. The bones that broke do not penetrate the skin (but may be seen under the skin) and there is no contusion from external trauma.
Comminuted	A comminuted fracture has more than two fragments of bone that have broken off. It is a highly unstable type of bone fracture with many bone fragments.
Complete	A fracture in which the bone has been completely fractured through its own width.
Complex	This type of fractured bone severely damages the soft tissue that surrounds the bone.
Compound (open)	When this occurs, the bone breaks and fragments of the bone will penetrate through the internal soft tissue of the body and break through the skin from the inside. There is a high rise of infection if external pathogenic factors enter into the interior of the body.
Compression	This type of bone fracture occurs when the bone is compressed beyond its limits of tolerance. These fractures generally occur in the vertebral bodies as a result of a flexion injury or without trauma in patients with osteoporosis. Compression fractures of the calcaneus also are common when patients fall from a height and land on their feet.
Epiphyseal	A fracture of the epiphysis and physisgrowth plate. These injuries are classified using the Salter–Harris Classification.
Greenstick	The pathology of this type of fracture includes an incomplete fracture in which only one side of the bone has been broken. The bone is usually "bent" and broken only on the outside of the bend. It is mostly seen in children and is considered a stable fracture due to the fact that the whole bone has not been broken. As long as the bone is kept rigid, healing is usually quick.
Hairline	This bone fracture has minimal trauma to the bone and surrounding soft tissues. It is an incomplete fracture with no significant bone displacement and is considered a stable fracture. In this type of fracture the crack extends only into the outer layer of the bone, not completely through the entire bone. It is also known as a fissure fracture.
Impaction	Occurs when one fragment is driven into another. This type of fracture is common in tibial plateau fractures in adults.
Oblique	A fracture that goes at an angle to the axis to the bone.
Pathologic	A pathologic fracture occurs when a bone breaks in an area that is weakened by another disease process. Causes of weakened bone include tumors, infection, and certain inherited bone disorders.
Spiral	In this pattern a bone has been broken due to a twisting-type motion. It is highly unstable and may be diagnosed as an oblique fracture unless a proper x-ray has been taken. The spiral fracture will look like a corkscrew type that runs parallel to the axis of the broken bone.
Stress	These fractures may extend through all or only part of the way through the bone. These types of fractures are common in soldiers or runners and are far more common in women. They often occur in the spine and lower extremities (most often in the fibula, tibia, or metatarsals). Stress fractures occur in a variety of age groups, ranging from young children to elderly persons. Stress fractures do not necessarily occur in association with a history of increased activity. Therefore, it is important to remember that the absence of a history of trauma or increased activity does not eliminate the possibility of stress or insufficiency fracture as a cause of musculoskeletal pain.

bacteria or irritated because of too much friction. When inflamed, the synovial cells increase in thickness and may show villous hyperplasia. Symptoms of bursitis include inflammation, localized tenderness, warmth, edema, erythema of the skin (if superficial), and loss of function. Common forms of bursitis include:

- Subacromial (subdeltoid) bursitis
- Olecranon bursitis

- Iliopsoas bursitis
- Trochanteric bursitis
- Ischial bursitis
- Prepatellar bursitis
- Infrapatellar bursitis
- Anserine bursitis

For the treatment of bursitis, the following is recommended:

- Apply the principles of PRICEMEM (Protection, Rest, Ice, Compression, Elevation, Manual therapy, Early motion, and Medications) to aid healing.
- Remove any extrinsic factors (damaging stimuli). This often involves absence from abuse rather than absolute rest.
- Identify any faulty mechanics/technique and educate patient on correct warm-up.
- Apply ultrasound and cross-section massage to the bursa as tolerated.

Degenerative Joint Disease

Historically, osteoarthritis (OA) has been divided into primary and secondary forms:

- *Primary:* An idiopathic phenomenon, occurring in previously intact joints, with no apparent initiating factor. It is related to the aging process, occurring in older individuals and most commonly affecting the hands, particularly the distal interphalangeal joints (Heberden nodes), proximal interphalangeal joints, and first carpometacarpal joints.
- *Secondary:* A degenerative disease of the synovial joints that results from some predisposing condition, usually trauma, that has adversely altered the articular cartilage and/or subchondral bone of the affected joints.

Therapeutic goals include:

- Pain management and control of inflammation (physical agents and modalities)
- Joint protection and function (orthotics, splints, assistive devices, and task modifications)
- Increase flexibility and strength (ROM, stretching, and progressive resisted exercises)
- Patient education with regards to joint protection

Rheumatoid Arthritis

Rheumatoid arthritis (RA) is a disease that affects the entire body and the whole person. The cycle of stretching, healing, and scarring that occurs as a result of the inflammatory process seen in rheumatoid arthritis causes significant damage to the soft tissues and periarticular structures. The more commonly involved joints include the proximal interphalangeal (PIP; pannus formation and ulnar drift), metacarpalphalangeal (MCP), wrist, elbow, knee, ankle, and metatarsusphalangeal (MTP) joints. In the hand, many common deformities can be seen, such as ulnar deviation of the MCP joints, radial deviation of the carpometacarpal block, boutonnière deformity, and swan neck deformities of the digits. Therapeutic goals are based on the stage of the disease:

Acute

- Pain management and control of inflammation (physical agents and thermal/cryo modalities)
- Maintenance of ROM and prevention of deformities (body mechanics, orthotic devices, and splints for ADLs)
- Patient education for regular rest periods, joint protection, energy conservation, and recognition of disease progression

Chronic

- Gait training with assistive devices and task modifications
- Increase flexibility, strength, and functional endurance using ROM exercises, stretching exercises, and gentle functional/strengthening exercises, including swimming or stationary cycling

Systemic Lupus Erythematosus

Systemic lupus erythematosus (SLE), sometimes referred to as lupus, is a chronic inflammatory autoimmune disorder that can affect any organ or system of the body. According to the American Rheumatism Association, a person is considered to have SLE if four of the following criteria are present:

- Abnormal titer of antinuclear antibodies
- Butterfly rash
- Discoid rash
- Hemolytic anemia, leukopenia, leukopenia, or thrombocytopenia
- Nonerosive arthritis of two or more peripheral joints characterized by tenderness, swelling, or effusion
- Photosensitivity
- Pleuritis or pericarditis
- Arthralgias and arthritis

- Cardiopulmonary signs—pleuritis, pericarditis, dyspnea
- Central nervous system involvement—headaches, depression, seizures, peripheral neuropathy (Raynaud phenomenon)
- Kidney dysfunction or failure

> **● Key Point** The seronegative arthropathies include ankylosing spondylitis, Reiter syndrome (the classic triad of arthritis, conjunctivitis, and urethritis), psoriatic arthritis, and arthritis associated with inflammatory bowel disease.

Therapeutic goals include:

- Careful observation for signs of renal failure such as weight gain, edema, or hypertension
- Pain management (physical agents and modalities)
- Increase strength (aquatic therapy)
- Decrease chronic fatigue (energy conservation and activity pacing techniques)
- Joint protection (gait training with assistive devices)
- Patient education for postural awareness
- If Raynaud phenomenon is present, patient education on how to warm and protect the hands and feet

Ankylosing Spondylitis

Ankylosing spondylitis (AS, also known as Bekhterev or Marie–Strümpell disease) is a chronic, progressive rheumatoid disorder of unknown etiology. A human leukocyte antigen (HLA) haplotype association (HLA-B27) has been found with ankylosing spondylitis and remains one of the strongest known associations of disease with HLA-B27, but other diseases are also associated with the antigen.[89] Thoracic involvement in AS occurs almost universally. The patient is usually between 15 and 40 years of age.[90] Although males are affected more frequently than females, mild courses of AS are more common in the latter.[89] The disease includes ossification of the:

- Anterior longitudinal ligament
- Costovertebral joints
- Zygapophyseal joints
- Intervertebral disc
- Sacroiliac joint

This ossification eventually results in spinal deformities, including flattening of the lumbar lordosis, kyphosis of the thoracic spine, and hyperextension of the cervical spine. These changes, in turn, result in flexion contractures of the hips and knees, with significant morbidity and disability.[89] Late in the disease process, the joints away from the spine may be involved, in addition to a number of organs (eyes, heart, lungs, and kidneys). Calin and colleagues[91] describe five screening questions for AS:

1. Is there morning stiffness?
2. Is there improvement in discomfort with exercise?
3. Was the onset of back pain before age 40 years?
4. Did the problem begin slowly?
5. Has the pain persisted for at least 3 months?

Using at least four positive answers to define a "positive" result, the sensitivity of these questions was 0.95, and specificity was 0.85.[91]

Therapeutic goals include:

- Customized exercise programs. A strict regimen of daily exercises, which include positioning and spinal extension exercises, deep breathing exercises, and exercises for the peripheral joints, must be followed.[92] Several times a day, patients should lie prone for 5 minutes, and they should be encouraged to sleep on a hard mattress (without pillows) and avoid the side-lying position. Swimming is the best routine sport.
- Maintenance of proper posture.
- Task modifications and ergonomic modifications.

Psoriatic Arthritis

Psoriatic arthritis is an inflammatory arthritis associated with psoriasis, which affects men and women with equal frequency.[93] Psoriatic arthritis can manifest in one of a number of patterns, including distal joint disease (affecting the distal interphalangeal joints of the hands and feet), asymmetric oligoarthritis (arthritis affecting one to four joints), polyarthritis (arthritis of five or more joints), and arthritis mutilans (an extremely severe form of chronic rheumatoid arthritis characterized by resorption of bones and the consequent collapse of soft tissue).[93] Therapeutic goals include:

- Joint protection and maintenance of joint mobility (splints and orthotics)
- Gait training using assistive devices
- Stretching exercises
- Patient education for joint protection

Gout

Gout is a chronic genetic disease caused by the accumulation of uric acid crystals in synovial joints. Gout is typically observed at the knee and great toe of the foot. Therapeutic goals include:

- Pain management (transcutaneous electrical nerve stimulation, or TENS) and stress reduction (relaxation exercises)
- Joint protection and maintenance of joint mobility
- Patient education about the disease
- Stretching and strengthening exercises

Fibromyalgia

Primary fibromyalgia (FM) is characterized by widespread and generalized body aches of at least 3 months' duration, which can cause pain or paresthesias, or both, in a nonradicular pattern.[94-96] FM is not a disease but rather a syndrome with a common set of characteristic symptoms, including constitutional symptoms of fatigue, nonrestorative sleep, and the presence of a defined number of tender points.[97] Therapeutic goals include:

- Pain management and promotion of relaxation (TENS, massage, whirlpool, biofeedback, and relaxation exercises)
- Increase flexibility
- Aerobic exercise program (walking, biking, swimming, and water aerobics)

Achilles Tendinitis

Achilles tendinitis is the most common overuse syndrome of the lower leg.[98] A number of factors appear to contribute to the development of Achilles tendinitis:

- *Biomechanical factors:* The rapid and repeated transitions from pronation to supination cause the Achilles tendon to undergo a "whipping" or "bow-string" action.[98] Moreover, if the foot remains in a pronated position after knee extension has begun, the lateral tibial rotation at the knee and the medial tibial rotation at the foot results in a "wringing" or twisting action of the tendon.[99]
- *Training variables:* A lack of a stretching program, a faster training pace, and hill training have all been found to correlate with increased incidence.[98]
- *Fatigue:* Overtraining has been found to correlate to calf muscle fatigue and microtears

of the tendon.[99,100] Muscular insufficiency has been cited as a significant factor in the inability to eccentrically restrain dorsiflexion during the beginning of the support phase of running.[98,101-103]

- *Shoe type:* High-heeled shoes shorten the Achilles tendon.

The therapeutic goals are:

- Control pain and inflammation (PRICEMEM)
- Increase flexibility through Achilles stretching and correction of any lower chain asymmetries, particularly low back, pelvic, and hip flexor asymmetries
- Lower kinetic chain strengthening
- Patient education about correct shoe wear
- Orthotics (made from a mold of the foot held in subtalar neutral and non–weight-bearing can be of significant benefit)

> **● Key Point** The recommended amount of rest with Achilles tendinitis varies depending on the severity of the symptoms:[104]
>
> - Type I: Characterized by pain that is only experienced after activity. Type I patients should reduce their exercise by 25%.
> - Type II: Characterized by pain that occurs both during and after activity, but does not affect performance. Type II patients should reduce activity levels by 50%.
> - Type III: Characterized by pain during and after activity that does affect performance. Type III patients should temporarily discontinue heavy activity.

Rupture of the Achilles Tendon

The etiology of a spontaneous Achilles tendon rupture remains incompletely understood, although a number of theories have been proposed, including microtrauma,[105] decreased perfusion,[106] and systemic or locally injected steroids.[107] However, the fact that the peak incidence of Achilles tendon rupture occurs in the middle age group rather than in the older population tends to lend credence to a mechanical etiology.[108] Three activities have been implicated in rupturing an Achilles tendon:[109]

- Pushing off with weight bearing on the forefoot while extending the knee.
- Sudden dorsiflexion with full weight bearing, as might occur with a slip or fall.
- Violent dorsiflexion, such as that occurs when jumping or falling from a height and landing on a plantar flexed foot.

The diagnosis of an Achilles tendon rupture is based almost solely on history and physical findings.

The classic history is reports of sudden pain in the calf area, often associated with an audible snap, followed by difficulty in stepping off on the foot.[108] Physical examination reveals swelling of the calf as well as a palpable defect in the tendon (sometimes called a hatchet strike), as well as ecchymosis around the malleoli.[110] Perhaps the most reliable sign of a complete rupture is a positive result on the Thompson squeeze test (passive plantarflexion with squeezing of the involved calf muscle).[111,112]

The conservative intervention of Achilles tendon rupture consists of short- or long-leg cast immobilization in the gravity equinus position (10° to 20° of plantar flexion). However, this approach appears to result in a high incidence of re-rupture (10% to 30%)[113–116] and a decrease in maximal function.[117–119] This may be because it is impossible to restore the correct length of the Achilles tendon with nonoperative treatment.[108] If a patient requires surgical intervention, then a cast or a brace is required for 6 to 8 weeks. The physical therapy intervention is the same for surgical and nonsurgical cases once the cast is removed and includes assistive device training, range of motion, stretching, icing, endurance training, gait training, strengthening, plyometrics, and skills-specific training.

Acromioclavicular Joint Injuries

Injuries to the A-C joint can be categorized as either acute traumatic or chronic injuries.[120] The chronic disorder may be atraumatic or posttraumatic, with the former being attributed to generalized osteoarthritis, inflammatory arthritis, or mechanical problems of the meniscus of this joint.[121] The majority of traumatic injuries occur from a fall onto the shoulder with the arm adducted at the side with the ground reaction force producing displacement of the scapula in relation to the distal clavicle.[120] Injuries to the A-C joint were originally classified by Tossy and colleagues[122] and Allman[123] as incomplete (grades I and II) and complete (grade III). This classification has been expanded to include six types of injuries based on the direction and amount of displacement (**Table 4-47**).[124–127] The therapeutic goals for grades I through III (the grades with the best physical therapy outcomes) are outlined in **Table 4-48**.

Adhesive Capsulitis

Adhesive capsulitis, often termed *frozen shoulder*, is associated with female gender, age older than 40 years, post-trauma, diabetes, prolonged immobilization, certain orthopedic diagnoses (supraspinatus tendinitis, partial rotator cuff tear, and

bicipital tendinitis), thyroid disease, post-stroke or post-myocardial infarction, certain psychiatric conditions, and the presence of certain autoimmune diseases.[128] Two types have been described:[129]

- *Primary:* Idiopathic with no known etiology in origin and insidious onset.
- *Secondary:* Either traumatic in origin, or related to a disease process, neurological, or cardiac condition.

Adhesive capsulitis results from progressive inflammation and stiffness of the shoulder capsule and the connective tissues surrounding the glenohumeral joint develop adhesions, greatly restricting motion and causing chronic pain.

Adhesive capsulitis is characterized by restricted active and passive range of motion of the glenohumeral joint. The movement that is most severely inhibited is external rotation of the shoulder. In the acute phase, pain radiates below the elbow and awakens the patient at night. In the chronic phase, pain is usually localized around the lateral brachial region. Adhesive capsulitis can be diagnosed if limits to the active range of motion are the same or almost the same as the limits to the passive range of motion. An arthrogram or magnetic resonance imaging (MRI) scan may confirm the diagnosis, though in practice this is rarely required.

The therapeutic goals include:

- Control of pain and inflammation (PRICEMEM)
- Restoration of the range of motion through the application of controlled tensile stresses to produce elongation of the restricting tissues
- Appropriate progression of range of motion and then strengthening exercises

> ● **Key Point** Nicholson[130] found that mobilization significantly improved range of motion into abduction but offered no significant advantage of exercise alone in other motions.
>
> • The patient with capsular restriction and low irritability may require aggressive soft tissue and joint mobilization.
>
> • The patient with high irritability may require pain-easing manual therapy techniques.
>
> • Treatment for the patient with limited ROM due to nonstructural changes is aimed at addressing the cause of the pain

Ankle Sprains

Ankle sprains are the most common injuries in sports and recreational activities, and if left untreated, they can lead to chronic instability and impairment.

TABLE 4-47	Classification of A-C Injuries and Clinical Finding
Type I	Isolated sprain of acromioclavicular ligaments with intact coracoclavicular ligaments, and deltoid and trapezoid muscles.
	Clinical findings include: Tenderness and mild pain at A-C joint, high (160° to 180°), painful arc, and pain with resisted horizontal adduction.
Type II	A-C ligament is disrupted and there is a sprain of the coracoclavicular ligament.
	Clinical findings include: A wider A-C joint gap with possible slight vertical separation when compared with the normal shoulder. In addition, the coracoclavicular interspace may be slightly increased, but the deltoid and trapezoid muscles remain intact. There is moderate to severe local pain, and tenderness in coracoclavicular space. PROM is painful in all end ranges but especially with horizontal adduction. Resisted abduction and abduction are also often painful.
Type III	A-C joint is dislocated and the shoulder complex displaced inferiorly. The A-C ligament is disrupted and the coracoclavicular interspace is 25% to 100% greater than normal shoulder due to coracoclavicular ligament disruption. In addition, the deltoid and trapezoid muscles are usually detached from the distal end of the clavicle.
	Clinical findings include: The arm is held in an adducted position by the patient and there is an obvious gap visible between acromion and clavicle. AROM is always painful, but PROM is painless if done carefully.
Type IV	A-C ligament is disrupted and the A-C joint is dislocated with the clavicle anatomically displaced posteriorly into or through the trapezius muscle. The deltoid and trapezoid muscles are detached from the distal end of the clavicle. In addition, the coracoclavicular ligaments are completely disrupted, but, although the coracoclavicular interspace may be displaced, it may appear normal.
	Clinical findings include: A posteriorly displaced clavicle.
	Surgery indicated.
Type V	A-C and coracoclavicular ligaments disrupted. The A-C joint is dislocated and there is gross disparity between the clavicle and the scapula (300% to 500% greater than normal). In addition, the deltoid and trapezoid muscles are detached from the distal end of the clavicle.
	Clinical findings include: Tenderness over the entire lateral half of the clavicle.
	Surgery indicated.
Type VI	A-C ligaments disrupted, and the coracoclavicular ligaments are completely disrupted. The A-C joint is dislocated and the clavicle anatomically displaced inferiorly to the clavicle or the coracoid process. Inaddition, the deltoid and trapezoid muscles are detached from the distal end of the clavicle. Often accompanied with clavicle or upper rib fracture and/or brachial plexus injury.
	Clinical findings include: The coracoclavicular interspace is reversed with the clavicle being inferior to the acromion or the coracoid process. The superior aspect of shoulder is flatter than opposite side.
	Surgery indicated.

Abbreviations: AROM, active range of motion; PROM, passive range of motion.

TABLE 4-48	Physical Therapy Intervention for A-C Joint Injuries

Injury Type	Intervention
Type I	Does not require immobilization.
	Ice is recommended for pain.
	If return to sport involves contact or impact forces, a doughnut pad placed over the shoulder helps to protect the joint.
Type II	Patients are typically prescribed a sling as desired.
	ROM exercises are initiated as tolerated, often beginning with PROM to minimize muscle activation of the trapezius and deltoid. However, because the deltoid and trapezius fibers reinforce the A-C joint capsule, specific strengthening exercises for these muscles are part of the long-term rehabilitation program.
	Return to function usually occurs within 2 to 3 weeks after injury.
Type III	The most appropriate intervention is somewhat controversial and can be either surgical or conservative.
	The most commonly used device for reduction is the Kenny–Howard harness.

Sprains of the lateral ligamentous complex represent 85% of ankle ligament sprains.[131,132]

The therapeutic goals in the acute stage center around aggressive attempts to:

■ Minimize effusion so as to speed healing (cryotherapy, compression, and elevation).

■ Promote early protected motion and early supported/protected weight bearing as tolerated. Protected weight bearing with an orthosis is permitted, with weight bearing to tolerance as soon as possible following injury.

■ Enable protected return to activity. As the healing progresses and the patient is able to bear more weight on his or her ankle, there is a corresponding increase in the use of weight-bearing (closed-chain) exercises.

■ Prevent reinjury.

The therapeutic goals in the subacute stages of the rehabilitation process include:

■ Dynamic balance and proprioceptive exercises. An external support/brace may still be required during this phase.

■ Increase range of motion. Long-sitting gastrocnemius stretching with a strap can be introduced in this phase (6 reps of 20 seconds each) to promote ankle dorsiflexion past the neutral position, enabling a closer to normal walking pattern.

■ Increase strength. Open-chain (non-weight-bearing) progressive resistive exercises with rubber tubing resistance are performed (2 sets of 30 reps each) for isolated plantarflexion, dorsiflexion, inversion, and eversion. Stationary cycling can also be performed (at a comfortable intensity for up to 30 minutes) to provide cardiovascular endurance training and controlled ankle range of motion.[137]

The therapeutic goals in the advanced healing stage (2 to 4 weeks post injury) are:

■ Restoration of normal active range of motion (AROM)

■ Normal gait without an assistive device

■ Pain-free performance of full weight-bearing functional activities

■ Enhancement of proprioception for return to normal activities and sport as appropriate

Anterior Cruciate Ligament Tear

Anterior cruciate ligament (ACL) injury factors have been divided into intrinsic and extrinsic factors.[138] Intrinsic factors include a narrow intercondylar notch, a weak ACL, generalized overall joint laxity, and lower extremity malalignment. Extrinsic factors include abnormal quadriceps and hamstring interactions, altered neuromuscular control, shoe-to-surface interface, the playing surface, and the athlete's playing style.

Gender has also been implicated. ACL injury rates are two to eight times higher in women than in men participating in the same sports.[138,139]

The typical clinical presentation is one of significant pain, effusion, and edema that significantly limits range of motion. In addition, the patient may be unable to bear weight on the involved extremity. Ligament laxity testing (anterior drawer and Lachman) is typically positive if the ligament is ruptured (grade III). The therapeutic goals depend on the severity of the injury. A nonsurgical approach is recommended for:

- Patients with either partial (grades I and II) ACL tears (negative pivot shifts) or "isolated" ACL tears who lead a less active lifestyle and participate in linear, nondeceleration activities.
- The middle-aged and older athlete. Physical therapy often is the treatment of choice, unless the patient plans to participate in sports activities that expose the knees to vigorous twisting forces.

The nonsurgical approach includes:

- ROM exercises, which are initiated as early as possible, and performed carefully, so as not to further aggravate soft tissue injury or prolong pain and effusion.
- Progressive strengthening of the quadriceps, gastrocnemius–soleus, and hamstrings muscles to prevent, or minimize, atrophy and maintain or improve strength.

> ● **Key Point**   Posterior cruciate ligament (PCL) tears are far less common than ACL tears. Because of the PCL's inherent strength, damage to the PCL usually occurs only with significant trauma such as a motor vehicle accident (dashboard injury)[142] or when landing in a hyperflexed knee position from a jump.[143] Clinical findings for a PCL tear include pain in the posterior aspect of the knee joint that may be aggravated with kneeling. Instability may or may not be present, depending on the severity of the tear.

Bicipital Tendinitis

Tendinitis of the long head of the biceps occurs more often as a secondary condition related to an impingement syndrome.[144,145] Because the tendon passes beneath the anterior edge of the acromion, impingement can cause biceps tendinopathy as well as rotator cuff problems. In addition, the biceps tendon sheath is a direct extension of the G-H joint, and inflammatory conditions such as rheumatoid arthritis can involve the biceps tendon. The pain associated with inflammation of the long head of the biceps is typically felt along the anterior lateral aspect of the shoulder with radiation into the biceps muscle, and tenderness is noted directly over the bicipital groove. The typical clinical presentation includes:

- Full active and passive ROM, although pain is often reported at the end range of flexion and abduction
- Normal accessory glides at the G-H joint (negating the need to use joint mobilizations)[144,145]
- Pain upon palpation of the bicipital groove while the arm is in 10° of internal rotation
- Pain with resisted elbow flexion or resisted forward flexion of the shoulder
- Pain on passive stretch of the biceps tendon
- Positive Speed test

The conservative intervention for biceps tendinitis secondary to chronic impingement is similar to that described for rotator cuff tendinitis. These include electrotherapeutic modalities, physical agents, nonsteroidal anti-inflammatory drugs (NSAIDs), transverse friction massage (TFM), and gentle stretching of the contractile tissues. Care must be taken with the TFM not to exacerbate the acutely or chronically inflamed tissue. Once the pain and inflammation is under control, the patient is progressed through range-of-motion exercises within the pain-free ranges. Intensive strengthening is initiated when full pain-free active range of motion has been restored.

Carpal Tunnel Syndrome

Carpal tunnel syndrome (CTS) results from entrapment of the median nerve in the relatively unyielding space of the carpal tunnel, which may result in numbness, pain, or paresthesia of the fingers and may severely hinder a patient's ability to perform precision maneuvers of the thumb, index, and middle fingers.

> ● **Key Point**   Although CTS occurs in all age groups, it more commonly occurs between the fourth and sixth decades.

The clinical features of this syndrome include intermittent pain and paresthesias in the median nerve distribution of the hand, which can become persistent as the condition progresses.[146–149] Muscle weakness and paralysis can occasionally occur. The symptoms are typically worse at night, exacerbated by strenuous wrist movements, and can be associated with morning stiffness. The pain may radiate proximally into the forearm and arm. The therapeutic goals for mild cases typically include:

- Symptom management (ice massage, electrical stimulation, ultrasound, phonophoresis, and iontophoresis).
- Joint protection through the use of splints, activity, and ergonomic modification. Night splints appear to help reduce the nocturnal symptoms and allow the wrist to rest fully.
- Increase range of motion using isolated tendon excursion exercises.
- Patient education to avoid sustained pinching or gripping, repetitive wrist motions, and sustained positions of full wrist flexion.

De Quervain Tenosynovitis

De Quervain disease is a progressive stenosing tenosynovitis that affects the tendon sheaths of the first dorsal compartment of the wrist (abductor pollicis longus and extensor pollicis brevis), resulting in a thickening of the extensor retinaculum, a narrowing of the fibro-osseous canal, and an eventual entrapment and compression of the tendons, especially during radial deviation.[150] Overuse, repetitive tasks that involve overexertion of the thumb or radial and ulnar deviation of the wrist, and arthritis are the most common predisposing factors, as they cause the greatest stresses on the structures of the first dorsal compartment.[151,152] Such activities include golfing, fly-fishing, typing, sewing, knitting, and cutting. The therapeutic goals include:

- Pain management and control of inflammation (physical agents and modalities).
- Maintenance of ROM and prevention of deformities (continuous immobilization through splinting with a thumb spica for 3 weeks).
- Strengthening following the removal of the splint. ROM exercises are prescribed, with a gradual progression to strengthening.

Epicondylitis

Lateral Epicondylitis (Tennis Elbow)

Lateral epicondylitis represents a pathological condition of the tendons of the muscles that control wrist extension and radial deviation, resulting in pain on the lateral side of the elbow. This pain is aggravated with movements of the wrist, by palpation of the lateral side of the elbow, or by contraction of the exensor muscles of the wrist. Individuals who perform repetitive wrist extension against resistance are particularly at risk—for example, participants of tennis, baseball, javelin, golf, squash, racquetball, swimming, and weightlifting. The exact etiology of tennis elbow is uncertain, but the strongest risk factor for lateral epicondylitis is age. The peak incidence is between 30 and 60 years of age. No difference in incidence between men and women or association between tennis elbow and the dominant hand has been demonstrated.

> ● **Key Point** While the terms *epicondylitis* and *tendinitis* are commonly used to describe tennis elbow, they are misnomers. Histopathological studies have demonstrated that tennis elbow is not an inflammatory condition; rather, it is a degenerative condition, a tendinosis.[153,154]

The typical presentation of tennis elbow includes:

- Pain along the lateral aspect of the elbow, especially over the lateral epicondyle, but sometimes radiating into the dorsum of the hand.
- Pain with gripping and movements of the wrist, especially wrist extension and lifting movements.
- Pain with activities involving the wrist extensors (e.g., pouring a pitcher or gallon of milk, lifting with the palm down).
- Localized point tenderness over the lateral epicondyle.

Medical management focuses on alleviating pain and inflammation. Physical therapy goals include:

- Pain management (PRICEMEM) and joint protection (counterforce brace). Once the acute phase as passed, the focus is to restore the range of motion.
- Patient education (to avoid repetitive motions; improve technique; address racket size, grip size, and string tension).
- Activity modification.
- An exercise regimen to correct imbalances of flexibility and strength of the elbow wrist and hand. These exercises typically consist of progressive resistance concentric and eccentric exercises for the wrist extensors, with the elbow flexed to 90° and also with the elbow straight.

Medial Epicondylitis (Golfer's Elbow)

Medial epicondylitis is only one-third as common as lateral epicondylitis and primarily involves a tendinopathy of the common flexor origin, specifically the flexor carpi radialis, and the humeral head of the pronator teres.[155] To a lesser extent the palmaris longus, flexor carpi ulnaris, and flexor digitorum superficialis may also be involved.[156] The mechanism for medial epicondylitis is similar to that of lateral epicondylitis—repetitive overuse. The therapeutic goals for medial epicondylitis mimic those for lateral epicondylitis except that the strengthening program involves concentric and eccentric exercises for the flexor pronator muscles.

Finger Injuries

Boutonnière Deformity

The boutonnière or "buttonhole" deformity occurs when the common extensor tendon that inserts on the base of the middle phalanx is damaged. The realignment of the extensor mechanism, coupled with the loss of certain muscle influence, produces a deformity of extension of the MCP and DIP joints, and flexion of the PIP joint—the classic boutonnière deformity. If traumatic in origin, this condition can be difficult to diagnose, due to the degree of swelling, but if more than a 30° extension lag is present at the PIP joint, a boutonnière lesion should be suspected.

The presence of a mobile correctable deformity requires little more than immobilizing the PIP in full extension for 6 to 8 weeks, and the DIP and MCP joints held free. Gentle AROM exercises can begin for flexion and extension of the PIP joint at 4 to 8 weeks, with the splint being reapplied between exercises. General strengthening usually begins at 10 to 12 weeks. For a return to competition, an additional 2 months is required.

Swan-Neck (Recurvatum) Deformity

The swan-neck deformity is characterized by a flexion deformity at the DIP and hyperextension of the PIP joint. This rearrangement leads to an increased extensor force across the PIP joint with a resulting hyperextension of the PIP joint. The resultant loss of function includes an inability to bring the tips of the fingers into grasp. Clinical findings include a hyperextended PIP joint with a flexed DIP joint of the same digit.

The intervention for swan-neck deformity depends on the etiological status of the PIP joint and its related anatomical structures. The intervention for a swan-neck deformity with no loss of PIP joint flexion is usually conservative, with a silver ring splint used for the correction of the PIP hyperextension.

Mallet Finger

Mallet finger deformity is a traumatic disruption of the terminal tendon resulting in a loss of active extension of the DIP joint. This is one of the most common hand injuries sustained by the athletic population, especially common in the baseball catcher and football receiver. The physical examination reveals a flexion deformity of the distal interphalangeal (DIP) joint, which can be extended passively but not actively. This lack of active extension at the DIP joint is due to the zero tension being provided by the extensor digitorum communis (EDC), in addition to the resulting increased tone in the flexor digitorum profundus (FDP).

Conservative intervention involves 6 weeks of immobilization. Mallet deformities with an associated large fracture fragment are typically treated with 6 weeks of immobilization following open reduction and internal fixation, usually with K-wires.[157] Closed reduction is used for other types, followed by 6 weeks of continuous dorsal splinting of the DIP in 0° of extension to 15° of hyperextension.[157] The PIP joint should be free to move. Gentle progressive resistive exercises (PREs) using putty or a hand exerciser are initiated at week 8. Usually the splint is discontinued at 9 weeks if the DIP extension remains at 0° to 5° and there is no extensor lag. Unrestricted use usually occurs after 12 weeks.

Rupture of the Terminal Phalangeal Flexor (Jersey Finger)

The rupture of the FDP tendon from its insertion on the distal phalanx (Jersey finger) is often misdiagnosed as a sprained or "jammed" finger, as there is no characteristic deformity associated with it.[157] The injury is typically caused by forceful passive extension while the flexor digitorum profundus muscle is contracting. A common example is in football when the flexed finger is caught in a jersey while the athlete is attempting to make a tackle, hence the term "jersey finger."

The intervention can involve doing nothing if function is not seriously affected, or surgical reattachment of the tendon, which requires a 12-week course of rehabilitation.

Groin Pain

The hip adductor muscles, including the gracilis, pectineus, and adductor longus, brevis, and magnus are the most frequent cause of groin region pain, with the adductor longus being the most commonly injured.[158,159] Adductor strains have been known to cause long-standing problems. There are a number of causative factors for an adductor strain, including a muscular imbalance of the combined action of the muscles stabilizing the hip joint, resulting from fatigue or an abduction overload, especially as the adductor muscles act as important stabilizers of the hip joint. Adductor strains are associated with jumping, running, kicking, and twisting activities, particularly when external rotation of the affected leg is an added component of the activity.

The signs and symptoms are easily recognizable:[160]

- Twinging or stabbing pain in the groin area with quick starts and stops
- Edema or echemosis several days post injury
- Pain with manual resistance to hip adduction when tested in different degrees of hip flexion: 0° (gracilis), 45° (adductor longus and brevis), 90° (if combined with adduction—pectineus)
- Possibly a palpable defect in severe ruptures
- Muscle guarding

The differential diagnosis includes abdominal muscle strains, inguinal hernia, osteitis pubis, and referred pain from the hip joint or lumbar spine.

The intervention involves the principles of PRICEMEM in the acute stage. This is followed by heat applications, hip adductor isometrics, and gentle stretching during the subacute phase, progressing to a graded resistive program and a gradual return to full activity. As part of the rehabilitation program, any imbalance between the adductors and the abdominals needs to be addressed. In addition, the clinician should examine the patient's technique in his or her required activity as poor technique can overload and fatigue the adductors.

Hallux Valgus

Hallux valgus is the term used to describe a deformity of the first MTP joint in which the proximal phalanx is deviated laterally with respect to the first metatarsal. Hallux valgus has been observed to occur almost exclusively in populations that wear shoes, although some predisposing anatomic factors make some feet more vulnerable than others to the effects of extrinsic factors.[161–166] Women have been observed to have hallux valgus in a ratio of 9:1 compared with men.[167] With increasing lateral deviation of the hallux, the MTP joint becomes incongruent, the sesamoids subluxate laterally, the hallux pronates, the medial aspect of the first metatarsal head becomes more prominent, and weight bearing shifts from the first metatarsal head to the second metatarsal, and possibly the third.

The intervention includes recommendations for wider shoes and orthotics. Achilles stretching should be used in cases of Achilles contracture. A simple toe spacer can be used between the first and second toes. In cases of pes planus associated with hallux valgus, a medial longitudinal arch support with Morton extension under the first MTP joint may also alleviate symptoms. If pain persists, however, structural realignment of the first metatarsal varus is usually necessary, as the bunion deformity becomes more severe and decompensated.

Lumbar Herniated Nucleus Pulposus

The water-retaining ability of the nucleus pulposus progressively declines with age resulting in a decrease in the mechanical stiffness of the disc, allowing the annulus to bulge with a corresponding loss of disc and foramina height. The etiology of pain for a particular individual cannot be determined because of the multiplicity of potential sources. However, the degenerating disc is known to have neurovascular elements associated with the periphery, including pain fibers. Disc deterioration and loss of disc height may shift the balance of weight bearing to the facet joint. Nuclear material, which is displaced into the spinal canal, is associated with a significant inflammatory response—macrophages respond to this displaced foreign material and seek to clear the spinal canal. Compression of a motor nerve results in weakness, and compression of a sensory nerve results in numbness. Radicular pain results from inflammation of the nerve, explaining the lack of correlation between the actual size of a disc herniation or even the consequent degree of neural compression with the correlating clinical symptoms. Furthermore, degeneration may result in radial tears and leakage from the nuclear material, which is toxic to the nerves. The resultant inflammatory response causes neural irritation with radiating pain without numbness, weakness, or loss of reflex, as neural compression is absent.

A pain drawing can be very helpful in assessing the pattern of pain regarding a dermatomal distribution or in assessing the organicity of the complaints. The physical assessment is essentially a neurological assessment of weakness, dermatomal numbness, reflex change, or, most importantly in the lumbar spine, sciatic or femoral nerve root tension. The provocation of radiating pain down the leg is the most sensitive test for a lumbar disc herniation. For a higher lumbar lesion, reverse straight-leg raising or hip extension stretching the femoral nerve is analogous to a straight-leg raising sign.

The intervention focus should address the reduction of inflammation. Therefore, a period of rest is appropriate, and warm, moist heat or modalities and gentle exercises based on patient tolerance. Exercises mobilize muscles and joints to facilitate the removal of edema and promote recovery. A TENS unit may be helpful in some patients with chronic conditions. Patients should be encouraged to maintain flexibility by initiating lifelong exercise regimens, including aerobic conditioning, particularly swimming, which allows gravity relief.

Iliotibial Band Friction Syndrome

As its name suggests, iliotibial band friction syndrome (ITBFS) is a repetitive stress injury, common in runners and cyclists, that results from friction of the iliotibial band as it slides over the prominent lateral femoral epicondyle at approximately 30° of knee flexion. The friction has been found to occur at the posterior edge of the band, which is felt to be tighter against the lateral femoral condyle than the anterior fibers. The friction causes a gradual development of a reddish-brown bursal thickening at the lateral femoral epicondyle.

Subjectively, the patient reports pain with the repetitive motions of the knee. There is rarely a history of trauma. Although walking on level surfaces does not generally reproduce symptoms, especially if a stiff-legged gait is used, climbing or descending stairs often aggravates the pain. Patients do not complain of pain during squatting or stop-and-go activities. The lateral knee pain is described as diffuse and hard to localize. Objectively, there is localized tenderness to palpation at the lateral femoral condyle and/or Gerdy tubercle on the anterior–lateral portion of the proximal tibia. The resisted tests are likely to be negative for pain. The special tests for the iliotibial band (ITB)—Ober test, prone lying test, and retinacular test—should be positive for pain, crepitus, or both, especially at 30° of weight-bearing knee flexion. In addition to the finding of a tight iliotibial band, a cavus foot (calcaneal varus) structure, leg length difference (with the syndrome developing on the shorter side), fatigue, internal tibial torsion (increased lateral retinaculum tension), an anatomically prominent lateral femoral epicondyle, and genu varum have all been associated with ITB friction problems, although they have yet to be substantiated.

The intervention for ITBFS consists of activity modification to reduce the irritating stress (in the athlete this may include decreasing mileage, changing the bike seat position, changing the training surfaces, or using new running shoes), heat or ice applications, strengthening of the hip abductors, and stretching of the iliotibial band.

Surgical intervention, consisting of a resection of the posterior half of the ITB at the level that passes over the lateral femoral condyle, is reserved for the more recalcitrant cases.

Medial Collateral Ligament Sprain

A medial collateral ligament (MCL) sprain is typically caused by a valgus stress to a slightly flexed knee, often when landing or bending or on high impact to the outside of the knee. The typical clinical presentation depends on the severity of the injury but can include:

- An inability to fully extend and flex the knee
- Pain and tenderness along the medial aspect of the knee
- An antalgic gait
- A positive valgus stress test

Medical management typically focuses on controlling pain and inflammation, which can include pharmacological intervention, a prescription for a knee immobilizer or a hinge brace, and crutches.

● **Key Point** A grade 1 MCL sprain can take between 2 and 10 weeks to fully heal. Recovery times for grades 2 and 3 are difficult to predict; depending on the amount of damage done, recovery can take weeks to several months.

The physical therapy intervention focuses on:

- Progressively increasing range of motion and strength while avoiding valgus stress through the knee
- Functional training, including gait and stair climbing
- Therapeutic modalities, including electrical stimulation
- Transverse frictional massage

Meniscal Injuries

Meniscal injuries are a common sports-related problem and the most frequent injury to the knee joint.

Such injuries are especially prevalent among competitive athletes, particularly those who play soccer, football, and basketball.

Meniscal tears can be classified into two types:

- *Traumatic tears:* Most commonly found in young, athletically active individuals. These injuries are not necessarily associated with contact injuries, but they are frequently associated with ACL tears and less commonly with PCL tears. Vertical longitudinal tears are the most common; transverse or radial tears are also common.
- *Degenerative tears:* Tend to occur in patients older than 40 years. No history of a traumatic event is present. These tears have minimal or no healing capacity, and horizontal cleavage tears, flap tears, and complex tears are most common.

The most common report is one of joint-line pain. The patient may also report joint clicking or locking, and the knee giving way. Injuries to the healthy meniscus are usually produced by a combination of compressive forces coupled with rotation of the flexed knee as it starts to move into extension. The final type and location of the tear are determined by the direction and magnitude of the force acting on the knee and the position of the knee when injured.

Treatment options depend on knowledge of the exact type, location, and extent of the meniscal tear. Severe damage, loss, or removal of the menisci frequently leads to joint instability and later accelerated degenerative joint disease (DJD), resulting in further disability and joint replacement.

Osteoarthritis

Osteoarthritis (OA), also known as degenerative joint disease or degenerative arthritis, is a process involving degradation of joints, including the subchondral bone and articular cartilage (see Chapter 12).

Patella Tendinitis

Patellar tendinitis (jumper's knee) and quadriceps tendinitis are overuse conditions that are frequently associated with eccentric overloading during deceleration activities (e.g., repeated jumping and landing, downhill running). The high stresses placed upon these areas during closed kinetic chain functioning place them at high risk for overuse injuries. Overuse is simply a mismatch between stress on a given structure and the ability of that structure to dissipate the forces, resulting in inflammatory changes.

The diagnosis of tendinitis is based on a detailed history and careful palpation of the tendons in both flexion and extension. Pain upon palpation near the patellar insertion is present in both patellar and quadriceps tendinitis. These are usually self-limiting conditions that respond to rest, stretching, eccentric strengthening, bracing, and other conservative techniques. When treating overuse injuries, it is essential that the clinician limits both the chronic inflammation and degeneration by working on both sides of the problem—tissue strength should be maximized through proper training, and adequate healing time must be allowed before returning to full participation.

A number of protocols have been advocated for the conservative intervention of patella tendinitis:

- *Grade I lesions:* Characterized by no undue functional impairment and pain only after the activity, these injuries are addressed with adequate warm-up before training and ice massage after.
- *Grade II–III strains:* These injuries are treated through activity modification, localized heating of the area, a detailed flexibility assessment, and an evaluation of athletic techniques. In addition, a concentric–eccentric program for the anterior tibialis muscle group is prescribed that progresses into a purely eccentric program as the pain decreases.[168]

Surgical intervention is usually required only if significant tendinosis develops. It is successful in the majority of patients.

Patellofemoral Dysfunction

Anterior knee pain or patellofemoral pain syndrome (PFS) is a commonly recognized symptom complex characterized by pain in the vicinity of the patella, which is worsened by sitting and climbing stairs, or inclined walking and squatting, and is a common reason for referral to physical therapy. The pain is characteristically located behind the kneecap (i.e., retropatellar) and most often manifests during activities that require knee flexion and forceful contraction of the quadriceps (e.g., during squats, ascending/descending stairs).

The pain may worsen in intensity, duration, and rapidity of onset if the aggravating activity is performed repeatedly. Sitting with the knee flexed for a protracted period of time may exacerbate the pain, such as while watching a movie (hence it is sometimes called "moviegoer's knee"). Symptoms often occur during the activity, or they may occur later, after the activity has been completed. Symptoms sometimes manifest as late as the next day.

The usual physical findings are localized around the knee:

- Tenderness often is present along the facets of the patella. The facets are most accessible to palpation while the knee is fully extended and the quadriceps muscle is relaxed.
- Crepitus may be present, but, if present in isolation, crepitus does not allow for definitive diagnosis.
- An alteration in the Q-angle is often present.
- Gait analysis may demonstrate excessive foot pronation, excessive knee valgus, or an antalgic gait pattern.
- Repetitive squatting may reproduce knee pain.
- Genu recurvatum and hamstring weakness are present.

Ice packs are frequently used to decrease pain and inflammation associated with this condition. Other modalities that may be useful and commonly are incorporated into physical therapy include electrical stimulation and biofeedback. The basic exercise principles for management of PFS are:

- Restoration of muscle balance within the quadriceps group. Quadriceps strengthening is traditionally performed while the knee is flexed 0° to 30°. Controversy remains as to the extent that the individual muscle groups composing the quadriceps can selectively be strengthened. Stretching of the quadriceps should be of long duration (20 to 30 seconds) and with low force.
- Improving flexibility. Exercises are performed to stretch the iliotibial band, hip, hamstring, and gastrocnemius. Manual stretching of the lateral retinaculum may be used as a conservative approach, partially mimicking the effect of lateral retinacular release.
- Improving range of motion.
- Restricting the offending physical activity.
- Engaging in home exercise programs that include both stretching and strengthening exercises.
- Using patellar taping techniques (McConnell method) to reduce the friction on the patella. If successful, the clinician can teach the patient self-taping techniques to use at home.
- Using proper footwear. The clinician can evaluate the patient's biomechanics and recommend proper shoes and/or orthotics.

- Using soft knee braces. Bracing involves control of the tracking position of the patella and restriction of full knee flexion.

Plantar Fasciitis

Plantar fasciitis is an inflammatory process of the plantar fascia and is reported to be the most common cause of inferior heel pain. The role of the heel spur in plantar fasciitis is controversial. Common findings include a history of pain and tenderness on the plantar medial aspect of the heel, especially during initial weight bearing in the morning. Interference with daily activities is common. Plantar fasciitis is usually unilateral, although both feet can be affected. The heel pain often decreases during the day but worsens with increased activity (such as jogging, climbing stairs, or going up on the toes) or after a period of sitting. Upon assessment, there will be localized pain on palpation along the medial edge of the fascia or at its origin on the anterior edge of the calcaneus, although firm finger pressure is often necessary to localize the point of maximum tenderness. The main area of tenderness is typically just over and distal to the medial calcaneal tubercle, and usually there is one small, exquisitely painful area. Tenderness in the center of the posterior part of the heel may be due to bruising or atrophy of the heel pad or to subcalcaneal bursitis. Slight swelling in the area is common.

A number of interventions have been suggested over the years for the intervention of plantar fasciitis. These include:

- Night splinting
- Orthotics
- Taping
- Heel cups
- Stretching (gastrocnemius and plantar fascia) and strengthening of the leg muscles and foot intrinsics
- Deep frictional massage
- Dexamethasone iontophoresis
- Shoe modifications
- Casting

Rotator Cuff Tendinitis

Rotator cuff tendinitis (RCT), also referred to as shoulder impingement syndrome (SIS), is a progressive overuse disorder caused by trauma (repetitive mechanical impingement of the distal attachment of the rotator cuff on the anterior acromion or cora-coacromial ligament), attrition, and the anatomical structure of the subacromial space. The supraspinatus is the tendon most often affected.

> **● Key Point** Subacromial impingement syndrome (SIS) is a recurrent and troublesome condition closely related to rotator cuff disease. It is characterized by one or more of the following:
>
> • Anterior (external) impingement.
> • Primary impingement: Mechanical impingement of the rotator cuff beneath the coracromial arch typically resulting from subacromial overcrowding.
> • Secondary impingement: Results from glenohumeral instability and/or tensile overload of the rotator cuff resulting in poor control of the humeral head during overhead activities.[169–171]
> • Posterior (internal) impingement: Abnormal contact between the rotator cuff undersurface and the posterosuperior glenoid rim.

Therapeutic goals include:

- Pain management and joint protection (ice massage, electrical stimulation, ultrasound, phonophoresis, and iontophoresis).
- Patient education to avoid shoulder flexion or abduction between 60° and 120° (painful arc) during activities of daily living and exercise.
- Gradual progression of pain-free range of motion, and strengthening exercises for the scapular stabilizers initially, and then the rotator cuff muscles.[172–175] Strengthening exercises are initiated by the patient in order to prevent the possibility of impingement. It is important for the entire rotator cuff to be strong prior to initiating overhead activities.
- Posterior capsule stretching exercises.

Scaphoid Fracture

The scaphoid is the most commonly fractured carpal bone due to its location.[176–179] Due to the scaphoid's scant blood supply, there is a high incidence of delayed healing or nonunion with scaphoid fractures.

> **● Key Point** Accurate early diagnosis of scaphoid fracture is critical as the morbidity associated with a missed or delayed diagnosis is significant and can result in long-term pain, loss of mobility, and decreased function.[180]

> **● Key Point** Although a fracture can occur in any part of the scaphoid, the common areas are at the waist and at the proximal pole.

Classically, the injury results from a fall on an outstretched hand (FOOSH) with the wrist pronated. Patients typically complain of dorsal wrist pain and have tenderness over the anatomic snuffbox. Conservative management of a scaphoid fracture is controversial, with no agreement on the optimum position for immobilization. Current management is immobilization in a long-arm or short-arm thumb spica cast, with the wrist position and length of immobilization dependent on the location of the fracture. Following the removal of the splint, AROM exercises are initiated, with passive range of motion (PROM) to the same motions and progression to strengthening exercises beginning after 2 weeks. A wrist and thumb immobilization splint can be fabricated to wear between exercises and at night for comfort and protection.

> **● Key Point** Scapholunate advanced collapse (SLAC) wrist is a late complication of scaphoid fracture, scapholunate dissociation, Keinböck disease, and fracture of the distal radius.[181] The SLAC wrist is thought to result from a loss of the stabilizing effect of the scaphoid, with the development of an arthrosis at the radioscaphoid articulation.

Spinal Stenosis (Degenerative)

Degenerative spinal stenosis (DSS) is defined as narrowing of the spinal canal, nerve root canal (lateral recess), or intervertebral foramina of the lumbar spine. It is predominantly a disorder of the elderly and is the most common diagnosis associated with lumbar spine surgery in patients older than 65 years.[182] Lumbar spinal stenosis may be classified as central or lateral.[183]

Central Stenosis

Central stenosis is characterized by a narrowing of the spinal canal around the thecal sac containing the cauda equina. The causes of this type of stenosis include facet joint arthrosis and hypertrophy, thickening and bulging of the ligamentum flavum, bulging of the intervertebral disc (IVD), and spondylolisthesis.

Lateral Stenosis

Lateral stenosis is characterized by encroachment of the spinal nerve in the lateral recess of the spinal canal or in the intervertebral foramen.[184] The causes of this type include facet joint hypertrophy, loss of IVD height, IVD bulging, and spondylolisthesis.[185] A compression of the nerve within the canal results in a limitation of the arterial supply or claudication due to the compression of the venous return. The compression of the foraminal contents in the canal may occur more with certain movements or changes in posture:[184]

- The length of the canal is shorter in lumbar lordosis than kyphosis.
- Extension and, to a lesser degree, side bending of the lumbar spine toward the involved side produce a narrowing of the canal.
- Flexion of the lumbar spine reverses the process, returning both the venous capacity and blood flow to the nerve.

Both the history and the examination findings for DSS are very specific. Patients with lumbar spinal stenosis who are symptomatic often relate a long history of low back pain. Unilateral or bilateral leg pain is usually a predominant symptom. Approximately 65% of patients with lumbar spinal stenosis present with neurogenic claudication (also referred to as pseudoclaudication).[186] Subjectively, the patient reports an increase in symptoms with lumbar extension activities such as walking, prolonged standing, and to a lesser degree side bending. On observation the patient presents with a flattened lumbar lordosis. The assessment usually reveals evidence of reduced flexibility or shortening of the hip flexors (iliopsoas and rectus femoris). The hip extensor muscles (gluteus maximus and hamstrings) are usually lengthened. This lengthening places them at a mechanical disadvantage, which leads to early recruitment of the lumbar extensor muscles and may lead to excessive lumbar extension.[187]

Therapeutic exercise is one of numerous treatments that have been proposed for the conservative treatment of patients with lumbar spinal stenosis. The therapeutic exercise progression includes postural education, hip flexor, rectus femoris and lumbar paraspinal stretching, lumbar (core) stabilization exercises targeting the abdominals and gluteals, aerobic conditioning, and positioning through a posterior pelvic tilt.[188–190]

Spondylolysis/Spondylolisthesis

Spondylylosis is a defect of the pars interarticularis of the spine, which lies between the superior and inferior articular facets of the vertebral arch. The actual defect in the pars covers a broad range of etiologies, from stress fracture to a traumatic bony fracture with separation. Spondylolisthesis is a diagnostic term that identifies anterior slippage and inability to resist shear forces of a vertebral segment in relation to the vertebral segment immediately below it. Spondylolisthesis usually occurs in the lumbar spine. Newman[191] described five groups represented by this deformity based on etiology:

1. *Congenital:* Congenital spondylolisthesis results from dysplasia of the fifth lumbar and sacral arches and zygapophyseal joints.
2. *Isthmic:* Isthmic spondylolisthesis is caused by a defect in the pars interarticularis, which can be an acute fracture, a stress fracture, or an elongation of the pars.
3. *Degenerative:* Degenerative spondylolisthesis occurs due to disc and zygapophyseal joint degeneration. It usually affects older people and occurs most commonly at L4–L5. The slip occurs because of arthritis in the zygapophyseal joint with loss of the ligamentous support. The zygapophyseal joints sustain approximately 33% of the static compression load on the lumbar motion segment and dynamically as much as 33% of the axial load dependent on spine position.[192]
4. *Traumatic:* Traumatic spondylolisthesis occurs with a fracture or acute dislocation of the zygapophyseal joint. It is fairly rare.
5. *Pathologic:* Pathologic spondylolisthesis may result from a systemic disease causing a weakening of the pars, pedicle, or zygapophyseal joint, or from a local condition such as a tumor.

Spondylolisthesis aquisita, a sixth etiologic category, was added to represent the slip caused by the surgical disruption of ligaments, bone, and disc.

Clinically, patients with spondylolisthesis will complain of low back pain that is mechanical in nature. This pain is worsened with activity and alleviated with rest. A patient may also complain of leg pain, which either can be of a radicular type pattern or more commonly will be one of neurogenic claudication. If neurogenic claudication is present, the patient may complain of bilateral thigh and leg tiredness, aches, and fatigue.[193] The questions regarding bicycle use versus walking can be helpful in differentiation of neurogenic versus vascular claudication. Vascular claudication occurs because not enough blood is flowing to a muscle. While enough blood flows to the muscle to meet the needs of the muscle at rest, when the muscle is involved with exercise the working muscle needs more blood and the narrowed artery may not let enough through.

> **● Key Point** Patients with neurogenic claudication should have minimization of symptoms while riding the bicycle. These patients are far more comfortable leaning forward or sitting, which flexes the spine, than walking.[194] The forward flexion increases the anterior–posterior (AP) diameter of the canal, which allows more volume of the neural elements and improves the microcirculation. Patients with vascular claudication will have pain when walking and when riding the bicycle.

The therapeutic exercise progression for this population includes postural education, hip flexor, rectus femoris and lumbar paraspinal stretching, lumbar (core) stabilization exercises targeting the abdominals and gluteals, aerobic conditioning, and positioning through a posterior pelvic tilt.[188-190]

Temporomandibular Joint Disorders

Temporomandibular joint internal derangement is one of the most common forms of TMD and is associated with characteristic clinical findings such as pain, joint sounds, and irregular or deviating jaw function.[195,196] The term *internal derangement* when related to TMD denotes an abnormal positional relationship of the articular disc to the mandibular condyle and the articular eminence.[197] This abnormal positional relationship may result in mechanical interference and restriction of the normal range of mandibular activity.[198-200] Magnetic resonance imaging is currently the most accurate imaging modality for identification of disc positions of the TMJ and may be regarded as the gold standard for disc position identification purposes.[201] The conservative intervention for this condition depends on the causative factors. Typically, the focus is on:[202]

- Pain management techniques.
- Postural education.
- Elimination of any occlusal disharmony.
- Joint mobilizations performed by the PT based on state regulations.
- Psychological stress reduction. Biofeedback can help the patient recognize periods of stress.
- Habit training to develop a path of mandibular movement that avoids any interference.
- Reduction or elimination of parafunctional habits (cheek biting, nail biting, pencil chewing, teeth clenching, or bruxism).
- A reduction in the force of chewing, while encouraging chewing on the affected side to decrease the interarticular pressure.
- Methods to prevent the disc–condyle complex from returning to the closed position. This can be accomplished by applying a permanent stabilization splint for a few months. The splint should be fabricated without any repositioning component and should be balanced for both day and night wear. When symptoms have been reduced, the patient should be weaned off the splint during the day and, eventually, at night.

Thoracic Outlet Syndrome

The thoracic outlet is the anatomical space bordered by the first thoracic rib, the clavicle, and the superior border of the scapula through which the great vessels and nerves of the upper extremity pass. The outlet passage is further defined by the interscalene interval, a triangle with its apex directed superiorly. This triangle is bordered anteriorly by the anterior scalene muscle, posteriorly by the middle scalene muscle, and inferiorly by the first rib. Thoracic outlet syndrome (TOS) is a clinical syndrome characterized by symptoms attributable to compression of the neural or vascular anatomic structures that pass through the thoracic outlet. The lowest trunk of the brachial plexus, which is made up of rami from the C8 and T1 nerve roots, is the most commonly compressed neural structure in thoracic outlet syndrome. These nerve roots provide sensation to the fourth and fifth fingers of the hand and motor innervation to the hand intrinsic muscles.

The chief complaint is usually one of diffuse arm and shoulder pain, especially when the arm is elevated beyond 90°. Potential symptoms include pain localized in the neck, face, head, upper extremity, chest, shoulder, or axilla, and upper extremity paresthesias, numbness, weakness, heaviness, fatiguability, swelling, discoloration, ulceration, or Raynaud phenomenon.[203] Neural compression symptoms occur more commonly than vascular symptoms.[204]

Conservative intervention should be directed toward the cause, and it typically focuses on the correction of postural abnormalities of the neck and shoulder girdle by strengthening the weak muscles (i.e., scapular adductors and upward rotators, shoulder external rotators, deep anterior cervical flexor muscles, and thoracic extensors), stretching the adaptively shortened muscles (i.e., scalene, levator scapulae, pectoralis minor, pectoralis major, anterior portion of the intercostals, short suboccipital muscles), and mobilizing the hypomobile joints of the shoulder complex, clavicle, and the first rib.

Wrist Fractures

Colles Fracture

Colles fracture is defined as a complete fracture of the distal radius with dorsal displacement of the distal fragment.[205] The typical mechanism of injury is a FOOSH. The fracture displacement and angulation are evident on the lateral film—the Colles fracture has the characteristic dorsiflexion or "silver fork" deformity. Radiographs of the anterior–posterior view show the usual comminuted fracture. Management of this fracture requires an accurate reduction of the fracture and maintenance of the normal length of the radius. The method of reduction, as well as the position of immobilization, is quite variable. In most cases, closed reduction and a cast are effective. In other cases, open reduction and external fixation are necessary.[206] Loss of full rotation of the forearm is common in this type of fracture.

Smith Fracture

A Smith fracture, sometimes called a reverse Colles fracture, is a complete fracture of the distal radius with palmar displacement of the distal fragment.[207] The usual mechanism for this type of fracture is a fall on the back of a flexed hand.

Customary management for a Smith fracture is with closed reduction and long-arm casting in supination for 3 weeks, followed by 2 to 3 weeks in a short-arm cast.[207] Types II and III are frequently unstable, however, and thus require an open reduction and internal fixation (ORIF).

Barton Fracture

A Barton fracture involves a dorsal or volar articular fracture of the distal radius resulting in a subluxation of the wrist.[207] The mechanism of injury for this type of fracture usually includes some form of direct and violent injury to the wrist, or from a sudden pronation of the distal forearm on a fixed wrist. The fracture is reduced and an above-elbow cast is then applied for 4 weeks, followed by a forearm cast for a further 3 weeks with the wrist in ulnar deviation. Other techniques describe using an ORIF, with 16 weeks being the average healing time.

Buckle Fracture

A buckle fracture is an incomplete, undisplaced fracture of the distal radius commonly seen in children. Immobilization for 3 to 4 weeks in a short-arm cast or palmar splint is adequate.[176]

> ● **Key Point** The possibility of abuse should be considered in the child with a fracture. Consultation with an orthopedist is advisable for fractures in the pediatric population.

The fracture is treated with a cast, ORIF, or external fixation. The fracture site is immobilized for 6 weeks if casted, 8 weeks with an external fixator, or 2 weeks if an ORIF with plate and screws is performed. If the fracture is nondisplaced, rehabilitation may last 2 to 6 weeks, whereas displaced fractures typically require 8 to 12 weeks.

The physical therapy intervention for wrist fractures can begin while the fracture is immobilized. It involves AROM of the shoulder in all planes, elbow flexion and extension, and finger flexion and extension. The finger exercises must include isolated MCP flexion, composite flexion (full fist), and intrinsic minus fisting (MCP extension with interphalangeal [IP] flexion). If a fixator or pins are present, pin site care should be performed according to physician preference. Following the period of immobilization, an immobilization capsular pattern will initially be present. Commonly, extension and supination are limited and need to be mobilized. AROM exercises of wrist flexion, extension, and ulnar and radial deviation are initiated. Wrist extension exercises are performed with the fingers flexed, especially at the MCP joints. PROM is performed according to physician preference, either immediately or after 1 to 2 weeks.

The AROM exercises of the wrist and forearm are progressed to strengthening exercises, using light weights and tubing. Putty can be used to increase grip strength if necessary.

Plyometrics and neuromuscular reeducation exercises are next, followed by return to function or sports activities.

Orthopedic Surgical Repairs

Spinal Surgery

Lumbar Discectomy

Lumbar discectomy involves removing a small window of bone in the spine, moving the nerve to one side and removing either some or all of the herniated disc. Percutaneous discectomy uses x-ray and a video screen to guide small instruments toward the disc. Postoperative recovery is relatively fast, with relief from nerve root compression often immediate.

Laminectomy

Laminectomy is the most commonly performed surgery on the lower spine. It involves removing part of all of the lamina to remove pressure on one or more nerve roots. Because the procedure requires an incision of two more inches, a hospital stay is required.

Vertebroplasty

This procedure, usually performed on an outpatient basis, is used to repair fractured vertebrae. A small incision is made in the skin over the affected area, and a light cement mixture is injected into the vertebra. The cement hardens to stabilize the bones of the spine.

Kyphoplasty

Kyphoplasty is similar to vertebroplasty. It involves making a small incision in the back and injecting a cementlike material to repair a fractured vertebra(e). However, in kyphoplasty, prior to injecting the cement, the surgeon inserts a balloon device to help restore the height and shape of the spine.

Foraminotomy

This procedure, used to enlarge the foramen, involves removing any bone or tissue that is obstructing the foramen and compressing the nerve root. This procedure is often combined with other procedures, such as a laminectomy.

Total Joint Replacement

Total Shoulder Arthroplasty

Total shoulder arthroplasty (TSA) is a surgical option for elderly patients with cuff-deficient arthritic shoulders.[208] Other patients who may require a TSA include those with bone tumors, rheumatoid arthritis, Paget disease, avascular necrosis of the humeral head, fracture dislocations, and recurrent dislocations.[209,210]

The main indication for surgical intervention is unremitting pain, rather than decreased motion, and a failure of conservative measures. Additional considerations include patient age, activity level, job requirements, and general health.[208]

> ● **Key Point** A course of shoulder stretching before a prosthetic arthroplasty may improve postsurgical function.[211] The key muscles to address include the rotator cuff, deltoid, trapezius, rhomboids, serratus anterior, latissimus dorsi, teres major, and pectoralis major and minor.[212]

The patient is usually placed in a sling or an elastic shoulder immobilizer following the operation that positions the humerus in adduction, internal rotation, and slight forward flexion. The shoulder immobilizer is worn between exercise sessions and at night. Sometimes, a continuous passive motion machine is prescribed by the physician. An abduction splint may be issued if a rotator cuff repair is performed and is worn for 6 to 8 weeks, according to the surgeon's instructions.

> ● **Key Point** The amount of external rotation and active internal rotation that the patient can perform in the first 4 to 6 weeks is limited to motion parameters that are achieved at the time of surgery. Typically, the only motions not allowed in the early weeks are active internal rotation and active and passive external rotation beyond 35° to 40°.

The goal of the postoperative rehabilitation process is to decrease pain and improve functional status while providing greater joint stability to the patient. The final outcome following shoulder arthroplasty will depend on many factors, including the quality of the soft tissue (especially the status of the rotator cuff), the quality of the bone, the type of implant and fixation used, the patient's expectations, and the quality of the rehabilitation program.[212]

> ● **Key Point** Only the surgeon knows the extent of soft tissue damage and repair, and the guidelines communicated to the PTA must be strongly adhered to.

Total Hip Arthroplasty

Total hip arthroplasty (THA) is performed in cases of severe joint damage resulting from osteoarthritis, aseptic necrosis, congenital abnormalities, rheumatoid arthritis, and Paget disease.[213] Arthroplasty of the hip may be categorized as a total hip arthroplasty or a hemiarthroplasty (see next section). In a total hip arthroplasty, the articular surfaces of both the acetabulum and femur are replaced. This involves either replacement of the femoral head and neck (conventional total hip arthroplasty) or replacement of the surface of the femoral head (resurfacing total hip arthroplasty); both procedures also replace the acetabulum. The most common indications for a THA are:[214]

- Pain
- Functional limitations
- Loss of mobility

> ● **Key Point** Although most THAs are performed in patients between 60 and 80 years of age, hip replacement is occasionally performed in younger patients, including patients in their teens and early 20s.[215,216]

A number of surgical approaches exist, each with its own advantages and diadvantages:

- *Anterolateral approach:* There are numerous variations of the anterolateral approach. All variations approach the hip through the interval between the tensor fascia lata and the gluteus medius muscle. Some portion of the hip abductor is released from the greater trochanter, and the hip is dislocated anteriorly.[216]

- *Direct lateral approach:* The direct lateral approach leaves the posterior portion of the gluteus medius attached to the greater trochanter. Because the posterior soft tissues and capsule are left intact, this approach is preferred in the more noncompliant patients to prevent postsurgical dislocation.[216]
- *Posterolateral approach:* The posterolateral approach, the most commonly used approach, gains access to the hip joint by splitting the gluteus maximus muscle. The short external rotators are then released, and the hip abductors are retracted anteriorly. The femur is then dislocated posteriorly.

● **Key Point** During the surgical approach to the hip joint, a trochanteric osteotomy may be necessary, especially in revision surgery. This procedure involves detaching the hip abductor mechanism. After this mechanism is repaired, the patient should avoid abduction exercises.

More recently, the *minimally invasive anterior approach* has become more popular. Despite being classed as an open approach, this procedure is approached through one or two small incisions. The rationale for minimally invasive procedures is that compared with traditional procedures, the use of small incisions potentially lessens soft tissue trauma during surgery and therefore should improve and accelerate a patient's postoperative recovery.[217] Other benefits are reduced blood loss, reduce postoperative pain, shorter length of hospital stay and lower cost of hospitalization, more rapid recovery of functional mobility, and a better cosmetic appearance of the surgical scar.[217]

The hip joint may be replaced with a variety of materials, including metal, polyethylene, and ceramic. There are also various methods of arthroplasty fixation, such as polymethylmethacrylate (PMMA) cement and screw fixation, although cementless press fit and porous ingrowth arthroplasties may also be used. The most common materials used for a total hip replacement articulation are a metal femoral head (cobalt–chromium), which articulates with an acetabular cup (polyethylene with metal backing). The PTA must be aware of several potential complications associated with THA. These include but are not limited to the following:

- Deep vein thrombosis (DVT)
- Heterotopic ossification
- Femoral fractures
- Dislocation
- Neurovascular injury

● **Key Point** Standard precautions given to patients who underwent a lateral or posterolateral approach to prevent posterior hip dislocation include the following:

• Do not cross your legs (avoid hip adduction). Typically an abduction wedge or pillow is prescribed.

• Put a pillow between your legs if you lie on your side.

• Do not turn your leg inward (avoid hip internal rotation).

• Do not bend forward at the hip.

• Sit only on elevated chairs or toilet seats and do not bend over from the hips to reach objects or tie your shoes (avoid hip flexion greater than 90°).

In addition, an assistive device or reacher is necessary to safely perform activities of daily living (ADL). Combinations of hip flexion, internal rotation, and adduction must be avoided for up to 4 months after surgery.

Following the surgery, thromboembolic disease (TED) hose are placed on the patient. For patients who have undergone either a posterolateral approach or a transtrochanteric approach, a triangular foam cushion is strapped between the legs to keep the hip in an abducted position. Patients at a high risk of dislocation, such as those who have undergone a postrevision arthroplasty or those with cognitive impairments, may need to wear a hip abduction orthosis that maintains the hip in abduction for 6 to 12 weeks. These orthoses may make ambulation difficult if the abduction is more than 5° to 10°.

● **Key Point** Patients with cemented joint replacements can weight bear as tolerated (WBAT) unless the operative procedure involved a soft-tissue repair or internal fixation of bone. Patients with cementless, or ingrowth, joint replacements are put on partial weight bearing (PWB) or toe-touch weight bearing (TTWB) for 6 weeks to allow maximum bony ingrowth to take place.

Total Knee Arthroplasty

Although pain and loss of function are the primary reasons for a total knee arthroplasty (TKA), the procedure can also be used to correct knee instability and lower extremity alignment and for the treatment of isolated but severe patellofemoral disease.[218,219]

The fate of the PCL in primary TKA is controversial. Retaining the PCL has the potential to restore more normal knee kinematics and better stair-climbing ability. If the PCL is sacrificed, a posterior stabilizer is used. However, the long-term results of PCL-retaining and posterior-stabilized TKAs are similar.[220,221]

Many early designs of TKA replaced only the tibiofemoral joint and did not address the patellofemoral articulation. The posterior stabilizer was developed to increase the arc of motion of these earlier models and thereby improve the functional results of TKA. Whether to resurface the patella remains among the most controversial topics in TKA.

Complications associated with TKA include the following:[223]

- Thromboembolic disease
- Fat embolism
- Poor wound healing
- Infection
- Periprosthetic fractures
- Neurologic problems; peroneal nerve palsy is the most common neurologic complication of TKA
- Vascular problems; injuries to the superficial femoral, popliteal, and genicular vessels have all been reported following TKA
- Arthrofibrosis
- Disruption of the extensor mechanism

REVIEW **Questions**

1. Define the terms *shoulder dislocation* and *shoulder separation*.
2. What is the triangular fibrocartilage complex?
3. When manual testing the sartorius muscle, in which three planes of motion at the hip should your resistance be in?
4. Which three muscles attach to the first cuneiform bone?
   a. The anterior tibialis, the posterior tibialis, and the fibularis (peroneus) longus
   b. The extensor digitorum, the flexor hallucis, and the fibularis (peroneus) longus
   c. The anterior tibialis, the peroneus brevis, and the fibularis (peroneus) longus
   d. The flexor hallucis longus, the posterior tibialis, and the fibularis (peroneus) brevis
5. Which is the only joint that directly attaches the upper extremity to the thorax?
6. The tendons of which muscles attach to the greater tuberosity of the humerus?
7. Which muscle covers the obturator foramina and the lesser sciatic foramina?
8. Which joint is damaged in a shoulder separation?
9. In which position is the hip in its most stable position?
10. What is the close-packed position of the ankle?
11. Which three tendons form the pes anserine?
12. Which muscle unlocks the fully extended knee?

13. What is a Colles fracture?
14. What is a Pott fracture?
15. What is a common complication of a proximal humerus fracture?
16. What is the close-packed position of the humeroulnar joint?
17. What is the resting position of the humeroulnar joint?
18. What is the resting position of the proximal radioulnar joint?
19. Which carpal bone is the most commonly fractured?
20. A fracture to the scaphoid can cause what complication?
21. Which artery is compressed in an anterior compartment syndrome?
22. Which is the most commonly injured ankle ligament with a mechanism of plantar flexion and inversion?
23. In the knee, which of the two menisci is more prone to injury?
24. What is the primary function of the posterior cruciate ligament?
25. Which muscles act as the secondary restraint for the anterior cruciate ligament?
26. Which gender and age range tend to suffer more from patellofemoral dysfunction?
27. Strengthening of which muscle is used to help with patellofemoral dysfunction?
28. List two special tests the supervising PT may use to help diagnose a tear of the posterior cruciate ligament.
29. What is the close-packed position of the hip?
30. Which special test might the supervising PT use to test for iliotibial band tightness?
31. What is the name of the ligament that maintains the dens against the Atlas?
32. Which muscle functions to open the mouth?
33. Which four joints make up the shoulder complex?
34. Name the two major ligaments of the acromioclavicular joint.
35. In addition to flexing the shoulder and flexing the elbow, what other functions does the bicep perform?
36. What motions do the lumbricals perform?
37. At which cervical joint does most of the rotation occur?
38. How many degrees of freedom are available at the hip joint?
39. In which direction does the pelvis tilt in order to increase the lumbar lordosis?
40. Which muscles are capable of producing external rotation at the glenohumeral joint?
41. Which two muscles originate from the anterior superior iliac spine?
42. The most limited motion of the lumbar spine is:
    a. Flexion
    b. Lateral bending
    c. Rotation
    d. Extension
    e. The lumbar spine is not limited in any direction of movement.
43. The subtalar joint of the foot is an articulation between which two bones?
44. The flexor digitorum profundus muscle is primarily a flexor of which joints?
45. The "spring" ligament, which provides some elasticity to the arch of the foot, is also known by which name?
46. In a patient with excessive lumbar lordosis, which muscles will not need stretching?
    a. Hip flexors
    b. Hamstrings
    c. Back extensors
    d. Pectoralis major
47. Which structure serves as the apex of the medial longitudinal arch of the foot?
    a. The base of the first metatarsal
    b. The head of the first metatarsal
    c. The midshaft of the first metatarsal
    d. The navicular tuberosity
48. While palpating a patient's wrist and hand, you elicit tenderness on a line between the radial tubercle and the base of the third metacarpal. Which bones are probably affected?
    a. Scaphoid and capitate
    b. Capitate and hamate
    c. Trapezium and scaphoid
    d. Trapezium and trapezoid
49. Which of the following structures of the knee joint is primarily responsible for preventing anterior movement of the tibia on the femur?
    a. Medial collateral ligaments
    b. Posterior cruciate ligament
    c. Anterior cruciate ligament
    d. Quadriceps tendon
50. A coxa valga deformity is:
    a. An increase in the angle of inclination between the neck of the femur and the shaft.
    b. A lengthening of the extremity on the involved side.
    c. A deformity of the knee.
    d. None of the above.

51. An osteotomy is:
    a. Fusion of a joint
    b. A bag that collects fluid from the colon
    c. Operative sectioning of a bone
    d. A form of debridement

52. In differentiating osteoarthritis from rheumatoid arthritis, the latter:
    a. More often involves weight-bearing joints
    b. Involves the distal interphalangeal joints
    c. Is a systemic disease
    d. Is often associated with increasing age

53. A supracondylar fracture of the humerus would most likely cause a peripheral nerve injury involving:
    a. The median nerve
    b. The radial nerve
    c. The ulnar nerve
    d. The musculocutaneous nerve

54. Atrophy of the muscles of the thenar eminence would indicate injury to which nerve?
    a. Musculocutaneous
    b. Median
    c. Radial
    d. Ulnar

55. You are assessing a patient who demonstrates an inability to fully flexed the index finger and middle finger, thumb opposition is lost, and the sensory deficit includes the lateral half of the ring finger, the middle and index finger, and the thumb. Which nerve do you suspect is involved?
    a. Ulnar nerve
    b. Radial nerve
    c. Median nerve
    d. None of the above

56. You are assessing a patient with a history of knee trauma. There is marked swelling of the knee joint, the tibia can be displaced forward on the femur, and there is pain and marked instability of the knee joint. Which of the following structures is likely to be involved?
    a. Medial collateral ligament
    b. Lateral collateral ligament
    c. Anterior cruciate ligament
    d. Posterior cruciate ligament

57. Which of the following muscles has the most important function as a downward rotator of the scapula?
    a. Levator scapulae
    b. Upper trapezius
    c. Pectoralis major
    d. Rhomboid major

58. While examining a patient's shoulder the PT decides to test for the presence of a tear in the supraspinatus muscle. Which test could the PT use?
    a. Apley scratch test
    b. Tinel sign
    c. Drop-arm test
    d. Yergason test

59. Which of the following muscles does not attach to the humerus?
    a. Teres major
    b. Pectoralis major
    c. Pectoralis minor
    d. Supraspinatus

60. You are assessing a patient with a hip flexion contracture. Which special test used by the PT to confirm this would likely be found in the patient's chart?
    a. Yergason
    b. Thomas
    c. Ober
    d. Lachman

61. Which of the following muscles are most important for crutch walking?
    a. Anterior deltoid and biceps
    b. Middle deltoid and triceps
    c. Posterior deltoid and subscapularis
    d. Latissimus dorsi and lower trapezius

62. Which of the following muscles are important stabilizers of the scapula?
    a. Levator scapulae
    b. Latissimus dorsi
    c. Serratus anterior
    d. Deltoid

63. Which of the following muscles is not supplied by the median nerve?
    a. Flexor carpi radialis
    b. Flexor digitorum superficialis
    c. Flexor pollicus longus
    d. Abductor pollicus longus

64. All of the following muscles have an action at the wrist except:
    a. Flexor carpi radialis
    b. Extensor carpi ulnaris
    c. Flexor carpi ulnaris
    d. Extensor digitorum communis

65. A positive Ober test indicates:
    a. Contracted biceps
    b. Contracted gastrocnemius
    c. Contracted iliotibial band
    d. Contracted iliopsoas

66. To test for a medial collateral ligament tear at the knee, the clinician must apply:
    a. Valgus stress
    b. Varus stress
    c. Posterior stress
    d. Anterior stress

67. A 17-year-old high school basketball player who you are treating for a left ankle sprain resprains his left ankle. He complains of moderate pain (6/10), and there is moderate swelling that seems to be worsening, causing him to ambulate with an antalgic gait. In this case, the *best* intervention would be:
    a. Cold/intermittent compression combination followed by elevation
    b. Cold whirlpool, followed by elastic compression and elevation
    c. Contrast baths and elastic compression
    d. None of the above

68. During your assessment you notice that the patient cannot fully extend his knee while positioned in supine with the foot dorsiflexed and the hip flexed first to 60° and then 90°. The tightness is most likely caused by the:
    a. Hamstrings
    b. Hip flexors
    c. Gastrocnemius
    d. None of the above

69. You are examining a patient for TMJ dysfunction. The patient states that she has had a number of episodes of her jaw locking in an open position. The most likely structure involved is:
    a. The masseter
    b. The disc
    c. The lateral pterygoid
    d. The infrahyoid

70. You are examining a female dancer with a diagnosis of unilateral spondylolysis at L4. The patient reports generalized low back pain when she stands for longer than 30 minutes and an inability to sleep on her stomach. Objective findings from the PT's examination include excessive lumbar lordosis, a positive Ober test of the right hip. Which POC would the PT likely recommend?
    a. Stretching the iliopsoas and iliotibial (IT) band; strengthening the abdominals
    b. Stretching the gluteus medius and maximus; strengthening the abdominals
    c. Advising the patient not to stand for long periods and not to sleep on her stomach
    d. None of the above

References

1. Barnes J: Myofascial Release: A Comprehensive Evaluatory and Treatment Approach. Paoli, PA, MFR Seminars, 1990
2. Smolders JJ: Myofascial pain and dysfunction syndromes, in Hammer WI (ed): Functional Soft Tissue Examination and Treatment by Manual Methods: The Extremities. Gaithersburg, MD, Aspen, 1991, pp 215–234
3. Teitz CC, Garrett WE, Jr, Miniaci A, et al: Tendon problems in athletic individuals. J Bone Joint Surg 79:A:138–152, 1997
4. Garrett WE Jr: Muscle strain injuries: clinical and basic aspects. Med Sci Sports Exerc 22:436–443, 1990
5. Garrett WE: Muscle strain injuries. Am J Sports Med 24:S2–S8, 1996
6. Safran MR, Seaber AV, Garrett WE: Warm-up and muscular injury prevention: An update. Sports Med 8:239–249, 1989
7. Huijbregts PA: Muscle injury, regeneration, and repair. J Man Manip Ther 9:9–16, 2001
8. Safran MR, Benedetti RS, Bartolozzi AR, III., et al: Lateral ankle sprains: A comprehensive review: Part 1: Etiology, pathoanatomy, histopathogenesis, and diagnosis. Med Sci Sports Exercise 31:S429–S437, 1999
9. Smith RL, Brunolli J: Shoulder kinesthesia after anterior glenohumeral dislocation. Phys Ther 69:106–112, 1989
10. McGaw WT: The effect of tension on collagen remodelling by fibroblasts: A stereological ultrastructural study. Connect Tissue Res 14:229, 1986
11. Cohen NP, Foster RJ, Mow VC: Composition and dynamics of articular cartilage: structure, function, and maintaining healthy state. J Orthop Sports Phys Ther 28:203–215, 1998
12. Junqueira LC, Carneciro J: Bone, in Junqueira LC, Carneciro J (eds): Basic Histology (ed 10). New York, McGraw-Hill, 2003, pp 141–159
13. Van de Graaff KM, Fox SI: Histology, in Van de Graaff KM, Fox SI (eds): Concepts of Human Anatomy and Physiology. New York, WCB/McGraw-Hill, 1999, pp 130–158
14. Williams GR, Chmielewski T, Rudolph KS, et al: Dynamic knee stability: Current theory and implications for clinicians and scientists. J Orthop Sports Phys Ther 31:546–566, 2001
15. Wiater JM: Functional anatomy of the shoulder, in Placzek JD, Boyce DA (eds): Orthopaedic Physical Therapy Secrets. Philadelphia, Hanley & Belfus, 2001, pp 243–248
16. Woodland LH, Francis RS: Parameters and comparisons of the quadriceps angle of college aged men and women in the supine and standing positions. Am J Sports Med 20:208–211, 1992
17. Olerud C, Berg P: The variation of the quadriceps angle with different positions of the foot. Clin Orthop 191:162–165, 1984
18. White AA, Johnson RM, Panjabi MM, et al: Biomechanical analysis of clinical stability in the cervical spine. Clin Orthop 109:85–96, 1975
19. Panjabi M, Dvorak J, Crisco J, et al: Flexion, extension, and lateral bending of the upper cervical spine in response to alar ligament transections. J Spinal Disord 4:157–167, 1991

20. Refshauge KM, Bolst L, Goodsell M: The relationship between cervicothoracic posture and the presence of pain. J Manual Manip Ther 3:21–24, 1995

21. Edmondston SJ, Singer KP: Thoracic spine: anatomical and biomechanical considerations for manual therapy. Manual Ther 2:132–143, 1997

22. Raine S, Twomey LT: Attributes and qualities of human posture and their relationship to dysfunction or musculoskeletal pain. Crit Rev Phys Rehabil Med 6:409–437, 1994

23. Singer KP, Malmivaara A: Pathoanatomical characteristics of the thoracolumbar junctional region, in Giles LGF, Singer KP (eds): Clinical Anatomy and Management of the Thoracic Spine. Oxford, Butterworth-Heinemann, 2000, pp 100–113

24. Andriacchi T, Schultz A, Belytschko T, et al: A model for studies of mechanical interactions between the human spine and rib cage. J Biomech 7:497–505, 1974

25. Shea KG, Schlegel JD, Bachus KN, et al: The contribution of the rib cage to thoracic spine stability, International Society for the Study of the Lumbar Spine. Vermont, 1996, p 150

26. Hall SJ: Kinematic Concepts for Analyzing Human Motion, in Hall SJ (ed): Basic Biomechanics. New York, McGraw-Hill, 1999, pp 28–89

27. Jarvinen TA, Kaariainen M, Jarvinen M, et al: Muscle strain injuries. Curr Opin Rheumatol 12:155–61, 2000

28. Reid DC: Sports Injury Assessment and Rehabilitation. New York, Churchill Livingstone, 1992

29. Watrous BG, Ho G Jr: Elbow pain. Prim Care 15:725–735, 1988

30. Glick JM: Muscle strains: Prevention and treatment. Phys Sports Med 8:73–77, 1980

31. Peers KH, Lysens RJ: Patellar tendinopathy in athletes: Current diagnostic and therapeutic recommendations. Sports Med 35:71–87, 2005

32. Backman C, Boquist L, Friden J, et al: Chronic Achilles paratenonitis with tendinosis: an experimental model in the rabbit. J Orthop Res 8:541–547, 1990

33. Singer AJ, Clark RAF: Cutaneous wound healing. N Engl J Med 341:738–746, 1999

34. Heldin C-H, Westermark B: Role of platelet-derived growth factor in vivo, in Clark RAF (ed): The Molecular and Cellular Biology of Wound Repair (ed 2). New York, Plenum Press, 1996, pp 249–273

35. Sen CK, Khanna S, Gordillo G, et al: Oxygen, oxidants, and antioxidants in wound healing: An emerging paradigm. Ann N Y Acad Sci 957:239–249, 2002

36. Kellett J: Acute soft tissue injuries: A review of the literature. Med Sci Sports Exerc 18:5, 1986

37. Amadio PC: Tendon and ligament, in Cohen IK, Diegelman RF, Lindblad WJ (eds): Wound Healing: Biomechanical and Clinical Aspects. Philadelphia, W. B. Saunders, 1992, pp 384–395

38. Hunt TK: Wound healing and wound infection: Theory and surgical practice. New York, Appleton-Century-Crofts, 1980

39. Peacock EE: Wound Repair (ed 3). Philadelphia, W. B. Saunders, 1984

40. Ross R: The fibroblast and wound repair. Biol Rev 43:51–96, 1968

41. Arem A, Madden J: Effects of stress on healing wounds: Intermittent non-cyclical tension. J Surg Res 42:528–543, 1971

42. Tillman LJ, Cummings GS: Biologic mechanisms of connective tissue mutability, in Currier DP, Nelson M (eds): Dynamics of human biologic tissue. Philadelphia, F. A. Davis, 1992

43. Chvapil M, Koopman CF: Scar formation: physiology and pathological states. Otolaryngol Clin North Am 17:265–272, 1984

44. Kisner C, Colby LA: Soft tissue injury, repair, and management, in Kisner C, Colby LA (eds): Therapeutic Exercise: Foundations and Techniques (ed 5). Philadelphia, F. A. Davis, 2002, pp 295–308

45. Levenson SM, Geever EF, Crowley LV, et al: The healing of rat skin wounds. Ann Surg 161:293–308, 1965

46. Orgill D, Demling RH: Current concepts and approaches to wound healing. Crit Care Med 16:899, 1988

47. Farfan HF: The scientific basis of manipulative procedures. Clin Rheum Dis 6:159–177, 1980

48. Vereeke West R, Fu F: Soft tissue physiology and repair, Orthopaedic Knowledge Update 8: Home Study Syllabus. Rosemont, IL, American Academy of Orthopaedic Surgeons, 2005, pp 15–27

49. Lewis PB, McCarty LP 3rd, Kang RW, et al: Basic science and treatment options for articular cartilage injuries. J Orthop Sports Phys Ther 36:717–727, 2006

50. Alford W, Cole BJ: The indications and technique for meniscal transplant. Orthop Clin North Am 36:469–484, 2005

51. Marsh DR, Li G: The biology of fracture healing: optimising outcome. Br Med Bull 55:856–869, 1999

52. Jurvelin J, Kiviranta I, Tammi M, et al: Softening of canine articular cartilage after immobilization of the knee joint. Clin Orthop 207:246–252, 1986

53. Noyes FR, Torvik PJ, Hyde WB, et al: Biomechanics of ligament failure: II. An analysis of immobilization, exercise, and reconditioning effects in primates. J Bone Joint Surg 56A:1406–1418, 1974

54. Deyo RA: Measuring functional outcomes in therapeutic trials for chronic disease. Controlled Clin Trials 5:223, 1984

55. Akeson WH, Amiel D, Woo SL-Y: Immobility effects on synovial joints: The pathomechanics of joint contracture. Biorheology 17:95–110, 1980

56. Akeson WH, Amiel D, Abel MF, et al: Effects of immobilization on joints. Clin Orthop 219:28–37, 1987

57. Akeson WH, Woo SL, Amiel D, et al: The connective tissue response to immobility: Biochemical changes in periarticular connective tissue of the immobilized rabbit knee. Clin Orthop 93:356–362, 1973

58. Bailey DA, Faulkner RA, McKay HA: Growth, physical activity, and bone mineral acquisition, in Hollosky JO (ed): Exercise and sport sciences reviews. Baltimore, MD, Williams and Wilkins, 1996, pp 233–266

59. Lane JM, Riley EH, Wirganowicz PZ: Osteoporosis: Diagnosis and treatment. J Bone Joint Surg 78A:618–632, 1996

60. Harris WH, Heaney RP: Skeletal renewal and metabolic bone disease. N Engl J Med 280:193–202, 253–259, 303–311, 1969

61. Donaldson CL, Hulley SB, Vogel JM, et al: Effect of prolonged bed rest on bone mineral. Metabolism 19:1071–1084, 1970

62. Mazess RB, Whedon GD: Immobilization and bone. Calcif Tiss Int 35:265–267, 1983

63. Rosen JF, Wolin DA, Finberg L: Immobilization hypercalcemia after single limb fractures in children and adolescents. Am J Dis Child 132:560–564, 1978

64. Birkhahn RH, Long CL, Fitkin D, et al: Effects of major skeletal trauma on whole body protein turnover in man measured by L-(1,14C)-leucine. Surgery 88:294–300, 1980

65. Arnold J, Campbell IT, Samuels TA, et al: Increased whole body protein breakdown predominates over increased whole body protein synthesis in multiple organ failure. Clin Sci 84:655–61, 1993

66. Kannus P, Jozsa L, Kvist M, et al: The effect of immobilization on myotendinous junction: an ultrastructural, histochemical and immunohistochemical study. Acta Physiol Scand 144:387–394, 1992

67. Lieber RL, Bodine-Fowler SC: Skeletal muscle mechanics: Implications for rehabilitation. Phys Ther 73:844–56, 1993

68. Jokl P, Konstadt S: The effect of limb immobilization on muscle function and protein composition. Clin Orthop Relat Res 222–229, 1983

69. Kisner C, Colby LA: Stretching for impaired mobility, in Kisner C, Colby LA (eds): Therapeutic Exercise: Foundations and Techniques (ed 5th). Philadelphia, F. A. Davis, 2002, pp 65–108

70. Gossman MR, Sahrmann SA, Rose SJ: Review of length-associated changes in muscle. Phys Ther 62:1799–1808, 1982

71. Booher JM, Thibodeau GA: The body's response to trauma and environmental stress, in Booher JM, Thibodeau GA (eds): Athletic Injury Assessment (ed 4). New York, McGraw-Hill, 2000, pp 55–76

72. Cyriax J: Textbook of Orthopaedic Medicine, Diagnosis of Soft Tissue Lesions (ed 8). London, Bailliere Tindall, 1982

73. Petersen CM, Hayes KW: Construct validity of Cyriax's selective tension examination: association of end-feels with pain ath the knee and shoulder. J Orthop Sports Phys Ther 30:512–527, 2000

74. American Medical Association: Guides to the Evaluation of Permanent Impairment (ed 5). Chicago, American Medical Association, 2001

75. Sapega AA: Muscle performance evaluation in orthopedic practice. J Bone Joint Surg 72A:1562–1574, 1990

76. Iddings DM, Smith LK, Spencer WA: Muscle testing: part 2. Reliability in clinical use. Phys Ther Rev 41:249–256, 1961

77. Silver M, McElroy A, Morrow L, et al: Further standardization of manual muscle test for clinical study: applied in chronic renal disease. Phys Ther 50:1456–1465, 1970

78. Marx RG, Bombardier C, Wright JG: What we know about the reliability and validity of physical examination tests used to examine the upper extremity. J Hand Surg 24A:185–193, 1999

79. Kendall FP, McCreary EK, Provance PG: Muscles: Testing and Function. Baltimore, Williams & Wilkins, 1993

80. Guide to Physical Therapist Practice (ed 2): Phys Ther 81:S13–S95, 2001

81. Waxman SG: Correlative Neuroanatomy (ed 24). New York, McGraw-Hill, 1996

82. Jackson-Manfield P, Neumann DA: Structure and function of the vertebral column, in Jackson-Manfield P, Neumann DA (eds): Essentials of Kinesiology for the Physical Therapist Assistant. St. Louis, MO, Mosby Elsevier, 2009, pp 177–225

83. Kisner C, Colby LA: The spine and posture: structure, function, postural impairments, and management guidelines, in Kisner C, Colby LA (eds): Therapeutic Exercise: Foundations and Techniques (ed 5th). Philadelphia, F. A. Davis, 2002, pp 383–406

84. Cailliet R: Low Back Pain Syndrome (ed 4). Philadelphia, F. A. Davis, 1991, pp 263–268

85. Riddle DL: Measurement of accessory motion: Critical issues and related concepts. Phys Ther 72:865–874, 1992

86. Maitland G: Peripheral Manipulation (ed 3). London, Butterworth, 1991

87. Maitland G: Vertebral manipulation. Sydney, Butterworth, 1986

88. Kaltenborn FM: Manual Mobilization of the Extremity Joints: Basic Examination and Treatment Techniques (ed 4). Oslo, Norway, Olaf Norlis Bokhandel, Universitetsgaten, 1989

89. Haslock I: Ankylosing spondylitis. Baillieres Clin Rheumatol 7:99, 1993

90. Gladman DD, Brubacher B, Buskila D, et al: Differences in the expression of spondyloarthropathy: A comparison between ankylosing spondylitis and psoriatic arthritis: genetic and gender effects. Clin Invest Med 16:1–7, 1993

91. Calin A, Porta J, Fries JF, et al: Clinical history as a screening test for ankylosing spondylitis. JAMA 237:2613–2614, 1977

92. Kraag G, Stokes B, Groh J, et al: The effects of comprehensive home physiotherapy and supervision on patients with ankylosing spondylitis: An 8-month follow-up. J Rheumatol 21:261–263, 1994

93. Gladman DD: Clinical aspects of the spondyloarthropathies. Am J Med Sci 316:234–238, 1998

94. Freundlich B, Leventhal L: The fibromyalgia syndrome, in Schumacher HR, Klippel JH, Koopman WJ (eds): Primer on the Rheumatic Diseases. Atlanta, Arthritis Foundation, 1993, pp 227–230

95. Stockman R: The courses, pathology and treatment of chronic rheumatism. Edinb Med J 15:107–116, 1904

96. Grodin AJ, Cantu RI: Soft tissue mobilization, in Basmajian JV, Nyberg R (eds): Rational Manual Therapies. Baltimore, Maryland, Williams & Wilkins, 1993, pp 199–221

97. Schneider MJ: Tender points/fibromyalgia vs. trigger points/myofascial pain syndrome: A need for clarity in terminology and differential diagnosis. J Man Physiol Ther 18:398–406, 1995

98. McCrory JL, Martin DF, Lowery RB, et al: Etiologic factors associated with Achilles tendinitis in runners. Med Sci Sports Exerc 31:1374–1381, 1999

99. Clement DB, Taunton JE, Smart GW: Achilles tendinitis and peritendinitis: Etiology and treatment. Am J Sports Med 12:179–183, 1984

100. James SL, Bates BT, Osternig LR: Injuries to runners. Am J Sports Med 6:40–49, 1978

101. Clement DB, Taunton JE, Smart GW, et al: A survey of overuse running injuries. Physician Sportsmed. 9:47–58, 1981

102. Renstrom P, Johnson RJ: Overuse injuries in sports: A review. Sports Med 2:316–333, 1985

103. Hess GP, Cappiello WL, Poole RM, et al: Prevention and treatment of overuse tendon injuries. Sports Med 8:371–384, 1989

104. Nichols AW: Achilles tendinitis in running athletes. J Am Bd Fam Pract 2:196–203, 1989

105. Fox JM, Blazina ME, Jobe FW, et al: Degeneration and rupture of the Achilles tendon. Clin Orthop 107:221–224, 1975

106. Langergren C, Lindholm A: Vascular distribution in the Achilles tendon. Acta Chir Scand 116:491–495, 1958

107. Maffulli N, Dymond NP, Regine R: Surgical repair of ruptured Achilles tendon in sportsmen and sedentary patients: A longitudinal ultrasound assessment. Int J Sports Med 11:78–84, 1990

108. Popovic N, Lemaire R: Diagnosis and treatment of acute ruptures of the Achilles tendon: Current concepts review. Acta Orthop Belg 65:458–471, 1999

109. Arner O, Lindholm A, Orell SR: Histologic changes in subcutaneous rupture of the Achilles tendon. Acta Chir Scand 116:484, 1958/1959

110. Wills CA, Washburn S, Caiozzo V, et al: Achilles tendon rupture: A review of the literature comparing surgical versus nonsurgical treatment. Clin Orthop 207:156–163, 1986

111. Thompson TC, Doherty JH: Spontaneous rupture of tendon of Achilles: A new clinical diagnostic test. J Trauma 2:126, 1962

112. Fierro NL, Sallis RE: Achilles tendon rupture: Is casting enough. Postgrad Med 98:145–151, 1995

113. Cetti A, Christensen SE, Ejsted R, et al: Operative versus non-operative treatment of Achilles tendon rupture. Am J Sports Med 21:791–799, 1993

114. Jacobs D, Martens M, Van Audekercke R, et al: Comparison of conservative and operative treatment of Achilles tendon rupture. Am J Sports Med 6:107–111, 1978

115. Lea RB, Smith L: Non-surgical treatment of tendo Achilles rupture. J Bone and Joint Surg 54A:1398–1407, 1972

116. Leppilahti J, Orava S: Total Achilles tendon rupture. Sports Med 25:79–100, 1998

117. Soma CA, Mandelbaum BR: Repair of acute Achilles tendon ruptures. Orthop Clin North Am 26:241–246, 1995

118. Nistor L: Surgical and non-surgical treatment of Achilles tendon rupture. J Bone and Joint Surg 63A:394–399, 1981

119. Inglis AE, Scott WN, Sculco TP, et al: Surgical repair of ruptures of the tendo Achillis. J Bone Joint Surg 58A:990–993, 1976

120. Turnbull JR: Acromioclavicular joint disorders. Med Sci Sports Exerc 30:S26–S32, 1998

121. Daigneault J, Cooney LM Jr: Shoulder pain in older people. J Am Geriatr Soc 46:1144–51, 1998

122. Tossy JD, Mead MC, Simond HM: Acromioclavicular separations: Useful and practical classification for treatment. Clin Orthop 28:111–119, 1963

123. Allman, F.L. Jr: Fractures and ligamentous injuries of the clavicle and its articulation. J Bone Joint Surg 49A:774–784, 1967

124. Rockwood CA Jr: Injuries to the acromioclavicular joint, in Rockwood CA Jr, Green DP (eds): Fractures in Adults (ed 2). Philadelphia, J. B. Lippincott, 1984, pp 860–910

125. Rockwood CA Jr, Young DC: Disorders of the acromioclavicular joint, in Rockwood CA Jr, Matsen FA, III.

(eds): The Shoulder. Philadelphia, W. B. Saunders, 1990, pp 413–468

126. Williams GR, Nguyen VD, Rockwood CA Jr: Classification and radiographic analysis of acromioclavicular dislocations. Appl Radiol 29–34, 1989

127. Wirth MA, Rockwood CA Jr: Chronic Conditions of the acromioclavicular and sternoclavicular joints, in Chapman MW (ed): Operative Orthopaedics (ed 2). Philadelphia, J. B. Lippincott, 1993, pp 1673–1683

128. Brue S, Valentin A, Forssblad M, et al: Idiopathic adhesive capsulitis of the shoulder: A review. Knee Surg Sports Traumatol Arthrosc, 2007

129. Nash P, Hazelman BD: Frozen Shoulder. Baillieres Clin Rheumatol 3, 1989

130. Nicholson GG: The effects of passive joint mobilization on pain and hypomobility associated with adhesive capsulitis of the shoulder. J Orthop Sports Phys Ther 6:238–246, 1985

131. Garrick JG: The frequency of injury, mechanism of injury, and epidemiology of ankle sprains. Am J Sports Med 5:241–242, 1977

132. O'Donoghue DH: Treatment of ankle injuries. Northwest Med 57:1277–1286, 1958

133. Thorndike A: Athletic Injuries: Prevention, Diagnosis and Treatment. Philadelphia, Lea and Febiger, 1962

134. Inman VT: Sprains of the ankle, in Chapman MW (ed): AAOS Instructional Course Lectures, 1975, pp 294–308

135. O'Donoghue DH: Treatment of Injuries to Athletes. Philadelphia, W. B. Saunders, 1976, pp 698–746

136. Iversen LD, Clawson DK: Manual of Acute Orthopaedics. Boston, Little, Brown, and Company, 1982

137. Roy S, Irvin R: Sports Medicine: Prevention, Evaluation, Management, and Rehabilitation. Englewood Cliffs, NJ, Prentice-Hall, 1983

138. Arendt E, Dick R: Knee injury patterns among men and women in collegiate basketball and soccer: NCAA data and review of literature. Am J Sports Med 23:694–701, 1995

139. Bjordal JM, Arnly F, Hannestad B, et al: Epidemiology of anterior cruciate ligament injuries in soccer. Am J Sports Med 25:341–345, 1997

140. Arnoczky SP: Anatomy of the anterior cruciate ligament, in Urist MR (ed): Clinical Orthopedics and Related Research. Philadelphia, J. B. Lippincott, 1983, pp 19–20; 26–30

141. Cabaud HE: Biomechanics of the anterior cruciate ligament, in Urist MR (ed): Clinical Orthopedics and Related Research. Philadelphia, J. B. Lippincott, 1983, pp 26–30

142. Trickey EL: Injuries to the PCL: Diagnosis and treatment of early injuries and reconstruction of late instability. Clin Orthop 147:76–81, 1980

143. Insall JN, Hood RW: Bone block transfer of the medial head of the gastrocnemius for posterior cruciate insufficiency. J Bone and Joint Surg 65A:691–699, 1982

144. Neviaser RJ: Painful conditions affecting the shoulder. Clin Orthop 173:63–69, 1983

145. Neviaser TJ: The role of the biceps tendon in the impingement syndrome. Orthop Clin North Am 18:383–386, 1987

146. D'Arcy CA, McGee S: Does this patient have carpal tunnel syndrome? JAMA 283:3110–3117, 2000

147. Barnes CG, Curry HLE: Carpal tunnel syndrome in rheumatoid arthritis: A clinical and electrodiagnostic survey. Ann Rheum Dis 26:226–233, 1970

148. Feuerstein M, Burrell LM, Miller VI, et al: Clinical management of carpal tunnel syndrome: A 12 year review of outcomes. Am J Ind Med 35:232–245, 1999

149. Szabo RM: Carpal tunnel syndrome-general, in Gelberman RH (ed): Operative Nerve Repair and Reconstruction. Philadelphia, J. B. Lippincott, 1991, pp 882–883

150. Lapidus PW, Fenton R: Stenosing tenovaginitis at the wrist and fingers: Report of 423 cases in 269 patients. Arch Surg 64:475–487, 1952

151. Muckart RD: Stenosing tendovaginitis of abductor pollicis brevis at the radial styloid (de Quervain's disease). Clin Orthop 33:201–208, 1964

152. Finkelstein H: Stenosing tenovaginitis at the radial styloid process. J Bone and Joint Surg 12A:509, 1930

153. Nirschl RP: Elbow tendinosis: Tennis elbow. Clin Sports Med 11:851–870, 1992

154. Nirschl RP: Tennis elbow tendinosis: Pathoanatomy, nonsurgical and surgical management, in Gordon SL, Blair SJ, Fine LJ (eds): Repetitive Motion Disorders of the Upper Extremity. Rosemont, IL, American Academy of Orthopaedic Surgeons, 1995, pp 467–479

155. Jobe FW, Ciccotti MG: Lateral and medial epicondylitis of the elbow. J Am Acad Orthop Surgeons 2:1–8, 1994

156. Nirschl RP: Prevention and treatment of elbow and shoulder injuries in the tennis player. Clin Sports Med 7:289–308, 1988

157. Burton RI, Eaton RG: Common hand injuries in the athlete. Orthop Clin North Am 4:809–838, 1973

158. Hasselman CT, Best TM, Garrett WE: When groin pain signals an adductor strain. Physician Sports Med 23:53–60, 1995

159. Lovell G: The diagnosis of chronic groin pain in athletes: a review of 189 cases. Aust J Sci Med Sport 27:76–79, 1995

160. Casperson PC, Kauerman D: Groin and hamstring injuries. Athletic Training 17:43, 1982

161. Geissele AE, Stanton RP: Surgical treatment of adolescent hallux valgus. J Pediatr Orthop 10:642–648, 1990

162. McDonald MD, Stevens. DB: Modified Mitchell bunionectomy for management of adolescent hallux valgus. Clin Orthop 332:163–169, 1996

163. Cole S: Foot inspection of the school child. J Am Podiatry Assoc 49:446–454, 1959

164. Coughlin MJ: Juvenile bunions, in Mann RA, Coughlin MJ (eds): Surgery of the Foot and Ankle (ed 6). St. Louis, Mosby-Year Book, 1993, pp 297–339

165. Craigmile DA: Incidence, origin, and prevention of certain foot defects. Br Med J 2:749–52, 1953

166. Scranton PE Jr, Zuckerman JD: Bunion surgery in adolescents: Results of surgical treatment. J Pediatr Orthop 4:39–43, 1984

167. Frey C: Foot health and shoewear for women. Clin Orthop Related Re 372:32–44, 2000

168. Black JE, Alten SR: How I manage infrapatellar tendinitis. Physician Sports Med 12:86–90, 1984

169. Jobe FW, Kvitne RS, Giangarra CE: Shoulder pain in the overhand and throwing athlete: The relationship of anterior instability and rotator cuff impingement. Orthop Rev 18:963–975, 1989

170. Jobe CM et al: Anterior shoulder instability, impingement and rotator cuff tear, in Jobe FW (ed): Operative Techniques in Upper Extremity Sports Injuries. St. Louis, Mosby-Year Book, 1996

171. Jobe FW, Pink M: Classification and treatment of shoulder dysfunction in the overhead athlete. J Orthop Sports Phys Ther 18:427–431, 1993

172. Gordon EJ: Diagnosis and treatment of common shoulder disorders. Med Trial Tech Q 28:25–73, 1981

173. Nixon JE, DiStefano V: Ruptures of the rotator cuff. Orthop Clin North Am 6:423–445, 1975

174. Ellman H: Diagnosis and treatment of incomplete rotator cuff tears. Clin Orthop 254:64–74, 1990

175. Goldberg BA, Nowinski RJ, Matsen FA III: Outcome of Nonoperative Management of Full-Thickness Rotator Cuff Tears. Clin Orthop Related Res 1:99–107, 2001

176. Onieal M-E: Essentials of musculoskeletal care. Rosemont, IL, American Academy of Orthopaedic Surgeons, 1997

177. Onieal M-E: The hand: Examination and diagnosis, American Society for Surgery of the Hand (ed 3). New York, Churchill Livingstone, 1990

178. Onieal M-E: Common wrist and ankle injuries. ADVANCE for Nurse Practitioners 4:31–36, 1996

179. Gates SJ, Mooar PA: Orthopaedics and sports medicine for nurses: Common problems in management. Baltimore, Williams & Wilkins, 1999

180. Wackerle JF: A prospective study identifying the sensitivity of radiographic findings and the efficacy of clinical findings in carpal navicular fractures. Ann Emerg Med 16:733–737, 1987

181. Watson HK, Kao SD: Degenerative disorders of the carpus, in Lichtman DM, Alexander AH (eds): The wrist and its disorders (ed 2). Philadelphia, WB Saunders, 1997, pp 583–91

182. Turner JA, Ersek M, Herron L, et al: Surgery for lumbar spinal stenosis: Attempted meta-analysis of the literature. Spine 17:1–8, 1992

183. Arnoldi CC, Brodsky AE, Cauchoix J: Lumbar spinal stenosis and nerve root encroachment syndromes: Definition and classification. Clin Orthop 115:4–5, 1976

184. Verbiest H: A radicular syndrome from developmental narrowing of the lumbar vertebral canal. J Bone Joint Surg 26B:230, 1954

185. Huijbregts PA: Lumbopelvic Region: Aging, Disease, Examination, Diagnosis, and Treatment, in Wadsworth C (ed): Current Concepts of Orthopaedic Physical Therapy—Home Study Course. La Crosse, WI, Orthopaedic Section, APTA, 2001

186. Katz JN, Dalgas M, Stucki G, et al: Degenerative lumbar spinal stenosis: Diagnostic value of the history and physical examination. Arthritis Rheum 38:1236–1241, 1995

187. Weinstein SM, Herring SA: Rehabilitation of the patient with low back pain, in DeLisa JA, Gans BM (eds): Rehabilitation Medicine: Principles and Practice (ed 2). Philadelphia, J. B. Lippincott, 1993, pp 996–1017

188. Fast A: Low back disorders: Conservative management. Arch Phys Med Rehabil 69:880–891, 1988

189. Fritz JM, Erhard RE, Vignovic M: A nonsurgical treatment approach to patients with lumbar spinal stenosis. Phys Ther 77:962–973, 1997

190. Bodack MP, Monteiro M: Therapeutic exercise in the treatment of patients with lumbar spinal stenosis. Clin Orthop Related Res 384:144–152, 2001

191. Newman PH: The etiology of spondylolisthesis. J Bone Joint Surg 45B:39–59, 1963

192. Yang K, King A: Mechanism of facet load transmission as a hypothesis for low back pain. Spine 9:557–565, 1984

193. Laus M, Tigani D, Alfonso C, et al: Degenerative spondylolisthesis: Lumbar stenosis and instability. Chir Organi Mov 77:39–49, 1992

194. Postacchinia F, Perugia D: Degenerative lumbar spondylolisthesis. Part I: Etiology, pathogenesis, pathomorphology, and clinical features. Ital J Orthop Traumatol 17:165–173, 1991

195. Isacsson G, Linde C, Isberg A: Subjective symptoms in patients with temporomandibular disk displacement versus patients with myogenic craniomandibular disorders. J Prosthet Dent 61:70–77, 1989

196. Paesani D, Westesson P-L, Hatala M, et al: Prevalence of temporomandibular joint internal derangement in patients with craniomandibular disorders. Am J Orthod Dentofacial Orthop 101:41–47, 1992

197. Dolwick MF: Clinical diagnosis of temporomandibular joint internal derangement and myofascial pain and dysfunction. Oral Maxillofac Surg Clin North Am 1:1–6, 1989

198. Juniper RP: Temporomandibular joint dysfunction: A theory based upon electromyographic studies of the lateral pterygoid muscle. Br J Oral Maxillofac Surg 22:1–8, 1984

199. Porter MR: The attachment of the lateral pterygoid muscle to the meniscus. J Prosthet Dent 24:555–62, 1970

200. Wongwatana S, Kronman JH, Clark RE, et al: Anatomic basis for disk displacement in temporomandibular joint (TMJ) dysfunction. Am J Orthod Dentofacial Orthop 105:257–264, 1994

201. Tasaki MM, Westesson PL: Temporomandibular joint: Diagnostic accuracy with sagittal and coronal MR imaging. Radiology 186:723–729, 1993

202. Bell WE: Orofacial Pains: Classification, Diagnosis, Management (ed 3). Chicago, New Year Medical Publishers, 1985

203. Thompson JF, Jannsen F: Thoracic outlet syndromes. Br J Surg 83:435–436, 1996

204. Roos DB: The place for scalenectomy and first-rib resection in thoracic outlet syndrome. Surgery 92:1077–1085, 1982

205. Onieal M-E: Common wrist and elbow injuries in primary care. Lippincott's Primary Care Practice. Musculoskeletal Conditions 3:441–450, 1999

206. McLatchie GR: Essentials of Sports Medicine (ed 2). Edinburgh, Churchill Livingstone, 1993

207. Wilson RL, Carter MS: Management of hand fractures, in Hunter J, Schneider LH, Mackin EJ, et al (eds): Rehabilitation of the hand. St. Louis, C. V. Mosby, 1990, p 284

208. Zeman CA, Arcand MA, Cantrell JS, et al: The rotator cuff-deficient arthritic shoulder: Diagnosis and surgical management. J Am Acad Orthop Surgeons 6:337–348, 1998

209. Sisk TD, Wright PE: Arthroplasty of the shoulder and elbow, in Crenshaw AH (ed): Campbell's Operative Orthopaedics (ed 8). St. Louis, Mosby, 1992

210. Bergmann G: Biomechanics and pathomechanics of the shoulder joint with reference to prosthetic joint replacement, in Koelbel R, et al (eds): Shoulder Replacement. Berlin, Spring-Verlag, 1987, p 33

211. Williams GR Jr, Rockwood CA Jr: Massive rotator cuff defects and glenohumeral arthritis, in Friedman RJ (ed): Arthroplasty of the Shoulder. New York, Thieme Medical Publishers, 1994, pp 204–214

212. Brown DD, Friedman RJ: Postoperative rehabilitation following total shoulder arthroplasty. Orthop Clin North Am 29:535–547, 1998

213. Harris WH: Traumatic arthritis of the hip after dislocation and acetabular fractures. Treatment by mold arthroplasty: An end-result study using a new method of result evaluation. J Bone Joint Surg 51:737–755, 1969

214. Mulliken BD, Rorabeck CH, Bourne RB, et al: A modified direct lateral approach in total hip arthroplasty: A comprehensive review. J Arthroplasty 13:737–747, 1998

215. Mallory TH, Lombardi AV, Fada RA, et al: Dislocation after total hip arthroplasty using the anterolateral abductor split approach. Clin Orthop 358:166–172, 1999

216. Dee R, DiMaio F, Pae R: Inflammatory and degenerative disorders of the hip joint, in Dee R, Hurst LC, Gruber MA, et al (eds): Principles of Orthopaedic Practice (ed 2). New York, McGraw-Hill, 1997, pp 839–893

217. Baerga-Varela L, Malanga GA: Rehabilitation and minimally invasive surgery, in Hozack WJ, Krismer M, Nogler M, et al (eds): Minimally invasive total joint arthroplasty. Heidelberg, Springer-Verlag, 2004, pp 2–5

218. Greenfield B, Tovin BJ, Bennett JG: Knee, in Wadsworth C (ed): Current Concepts of Orthopedic Physical Therapy. La Crosse, WI, Orthopaedic Section, APTA, 2001

219. Kolettis GT, Stern SH: Patellar resurfacing for patellofemoral arthritis. Orthop Clin North Am 23:665–673, 1992

220. Aglietti P, Buzzi R, De Felice R, et al: The Insall-Burstein total knee replacement in osteoarthritis: A 10-year minimum follow-up. J Arthroplasty 14:560–565, 1999

221. Banks SA, Markovich GD, Hodge WA: In vivo kinematics of cruciate-retaining and substituting knee arthroplasties. J Arthroplasty 12:297–304, 1997

222. Auberger SS, Mangine RE: Innovative Approaches to Surgery and Rehabilitation, Physical Therapy of the Knee. New York, Churchill Livingstone, 1988, pp 233–262

223. Ecker ML, Lotke PA: Postoperative care of the total knee patient. Orthop Clin North Am 20:55–62, 1989

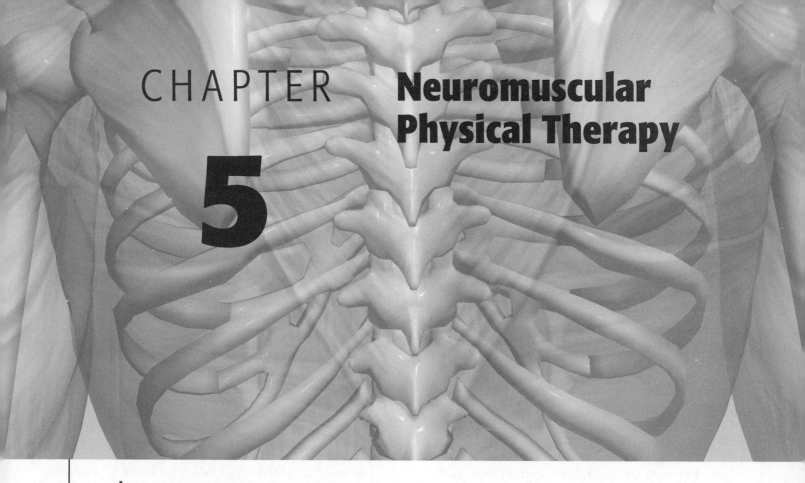

Neuromuscular Physical Therapy

5

Basic Anatomy and Physiology

The *nerve cell*, or *neuron*, is the functional unit of the nervous system. The other cellular constituent is the *neuroglial cell*, or *glia*, which functions to provide structural and metabolic support for the neurons. **Table 5-1** provides a list of these supporting cells and their functions.[1] Although neurons come in a variety of sizes and shapes, each nerve has four functional parts:

- *Dendrite:* Serves a receptive function, receiving information from other nerve cells or the environment
- *Axon:* Conducts information to other nerve cells
- *Cell body:* Contains the nucleus of the cell and has important integrative functions
- *Axon terminal:* The transmission site for action potentials, the messengers of the nerve cell

● **Key Point** The communication of information from one nerve cell to another occurs at junctions called *synapses*, where a chemical is released in the form of a neurotransmitter.

Nervous System Organization

The nervous system can be divided into two anatomical divisions, each with its own subdivisions. The *central nervous system* (CNS) comprises the brain and the spinal cord, and the *peripheral nervous system* is made up of cranial and spinal nerves. The peripheral nervous system is further subdivided into somatic and autonomic divisions.

- The *somatic system* is made up of all of the fibers going from the CNS to skeletal muscle cells. It innervates the skin, muscles, and joints.

TABLE 5-1	Supporting Cells and Their Functions
Cell Type	**Functions**
Schwann cells	Surround axons of all peripheral nerve fibers, forming a neurolemmal sheath; wrap around many peripheral fibers to form myelin sheaths
Satellite cells (ganglionic gliocytes)	Support ganglia within the peripheral nervous system (PNS)
Oligodendrocytes	Form myelin sheaths around axons, producing white matter of the central nervous system (CNS)
Astrocytes	Vascular processes cover that capillaries within the brain and contribute to the blood-brain barrier
Microglia	Phagocytize pathogens and cellular debris within the CNS
Ependymal cells	Form the epithelial lining of brain cavities (ventricles) and the central canal of the spinal cord

Data from Van de Graaff KM, Fox SI: Central nervous system, in Van de Graaff KM, Fox SI (eds): Concepts of Human Anatomy and Physiology. New York, WCB/McGraw-Hill, 1999, pp 407–446

- Fibers of the *autonomic system* innervate the glands and smooth muscle of the viscera.[1] Fibers within this system are further subdivided into two components: parasympathetic and sympathetic.

Myelin is a lipid-rich membrane that coats, protects, and insulates nerves. Most of the axons of the PNS and CNS are covered by myelin, which is divided into segments about 1 millimeter long by small gaps where the myelin is absent, called *nodes of Ranvier*. As the brain sends messages through the nerves of the spinal cord, the impulses jump from node to node through a process called *salutatory conduction*. Because myelin has a high electrical resistance and low capacitance, it functions to increase the nerve conduction velocity of neural transmissions.

● **Key Point** Myelin contains proteins that can be targeted by the immune system. The destruction of the myelin in the CNS is what triggers many of the symptoms of diseases like multiple sclerosis (MS).

Central Nervous System

As mentioned above, the central nervous system has two subdivisions: the brain and the spinal cord. Nerves within the CNS are referred to as *upper motor neurons* (UMN). The CNS is enclosed by a system of membranes called *meninges*. The meninges consist of three layers: the dura mater, the arachnoid mater, and the pia mater. The primary function of the meninges and of the cerebrospinal fluid is to protect the central nervous system. Cerebrospinal fluid (CSF) flows through the meningeal spaces and within the four ventricles of the brain. The CSF provides a type of blood-brain barrier through selective secretion between the capillaries of the choroid plexus and the CSF that flows next to the neural tissue.

Brain

The brain, contained within the skull (*cranium*), begins its embryonic development as the cephalic end of the neural tube, before rapidly growing and differentiating into three distinct swellings: the prosencephalon, the mesencephalon, and the rhombencephalon (**Table 5-2**).[2]

The brainstem attaches to the spinal cord and includes the mesencephalon (midbrain), pons, and medulla oblongata, the latter of which contains nuclei for autonomic functions of the body and their connecting tracts. The brainstem gives rise to 10 of the 12 pairs of cranial nerves. The brain is completely dependent upon a continuous supply of arterial blood to provide it with glucose and oxygen.

TABLE
5-2

Derivation and Functions of the Major Brain Structures

Region		Structure	Description/Function
Prosencephalon (Forebrain)	Telencephalon	Cerebrum	Lies in front or on top of the brainstem and is the largest and most developed of the major divisions of the brain.
			Consists of six paired lobes within two hemispheres, which are folded into many gyri (crests) and sulci (grooves), thus allowing the cortex to expand in surface area without taking up much greater volume.
			Controls most sensory processing; conscious and volitional movements; language and communication; learning and memory.
		Limbic system	A set of brain structures including the hippocampus, amygdala, anterior thalamic nuclei, and limbic cortex, which support a variety of functions, including emotion, behavior, long-term memory, and olfaction.
		Basal ganglia	Associated with a variety of functions, including motor control, motor learning, and action selection.
	Diencephalon	Thalamus	Functions include the relaying of sensation, spatial sense, and motor signals to the cerebral cortex, along with the regulation of consciousness, sleep, and alertness.
		Hypothalamus	Regulates food and water intake, body temperature, and heart rate. One of the most important functions of the hypothalamus is to link the nervous system to the endocrine system via the pituitary gland.
		Pituitary gland	Considered to be the "master gland," it regulates homeostasis and various endocrine functions.
Mesencephalon (Midbrain)	Mesencephalon	Superior colliculi	Visual reflexes (hand–eye coordination).
		Inferior colliculi	Auditory reflexes.
		Cerebral peduncles	Important fibers running through the cerebral peduncles include the corticospinal tract and the corticobulbar tract, among others. This area contains many nerve tracts conveying motor information to and from the brain to the rest of the body.
Rhombencephalon (Hindbrain)	Metencephalon	Cerebellum	Balance/equilibrium and coordination of skeletal muscle contractions (force, direction, extent, and sequencing of movement).
		Pons	Relay center; contains nuclei (pontine nuclei).
	Myelencephalon	Medulla oblongata	Relay center; contains many nuclei; visceral autonomic center (e.g., respiration, heart rate, vasoconstriction).

Data from Van de Graaff KM, Fox SI: Central nervous system, in Van de Graaff KM, Fox SI (eds): Concepts of Human Anatomy and Physiology. New York, WCB/McGraw-Hill, 1999, pp 407–446

● **Key Point** The *blood–brain barrier* is a capillary barrier comprising a complex group of both anatomical structures and physiological transport systems that precisely regulate the chemical composition of the extracellular fluid (ECF) of the brain and closely monitor both the kinds of substances that enter the ECF and the rate at which they enter.

Spinal Cord

The spinal cord is the portion of the CNS that extends through the vertebral canal of the vertebral column and is continuous with the medulla and brainstem at its upper end through the foramen magnum of the skull. The conus medullaris serves as the lower end of the cord. In adults, the conus ends at the L1 or L2 level of the vertebral column.

> **● Key Point** The *cauda equina* (CE) is formed by nerve roots caudal to the level of spinal cord termination. The CE nerve roots are particularly susceptible to compressive and tensile stresses, since they have a poorly developed epineurium. Due to increased permeability of the microvascular system that serves these nerves, there is a tendency toward edema formation of the nerve roots, which may result in compounding an initial and sometimes seemingly slight injury.

> **● Key Point** The spinal cord participates directly with the control of body movements, the processing and transmission of sensory information from the trunk and limbs, and the regulation of visceral functions.[1] The spinal cord also provides a conduit for the two-way transmission of messages between the brain and the body.

Two prominent enlargements of the spinal cord can be seen in a posterior view: the cervical enlargement located between C3 and T2, and the lumbar enlargement between T9 and T12.

> **● Key Point** The spinal cord has an external segmental organization. Each of the 31 pairs of spinal nerves that arise from the spinal cord has a ventral root and a dorsal root, with each root made up of one to eight rootlets. Each root consists of bundles of nerve fibers.[3]

Peripheral Nervous System

Peripheral nerves are referred to as *lower motor neurons* (LMN). The *peripheral nervous system* (PNS) consists of 43 pairs of nerves: 12 pairs connect with the brain and are called cranial nerves, and 31 pairs connect with the spinal cord as the spinal nerves. The PNS can be divided into two major divisions:

- *Afferent division:* The neurons of this division (sometimes referred to as primary afferents or first-order neurons) convey information from receptors in the periphery to the CNS. The cell bodies of afferent neurons are located outside of the brain or spinal cord in structures called ganglia.
- *Efferent division:* This division is further divided into the autonomic nervous system and the somatic nervous system.

Peripheral nerve fibers are classified as one of the following types:

- *A fibers:* Large, myelinated, fast conducting
- *Alpha:* Responsible for proprioception, somatic motor

- *Beta:* Responsible for touch, pressure
- *B fibers:* Small, myelinated, conduct less rapidly; preganglionic autonomic
- *C fibers:* Smallest, unmyelinated, slowest conducting
- *Delta:* Responsible for pain, temperature, touch
- *Dorsal root:* Pain, reflex responses
- *Gamma:* Responsible for motor to the muscle spindles
- *Sympathetic:* Postganglionic sympathetics

Autonomic Nervous System

The autonomic system (ANS) is the division of the PNS that functions primarily at a subconscious level. The ANS has two divisions: sympathetic and parasympathetic, each of which is differentiated by its site of origin as well as the transmitters it releases.[4] In general, these two systems have antagonist effects on their end organs.

Somatic Nervous System

The somatic nervous system is associated with voluntary control of body movements. The various nerves of the somatic nervous system are described in the following section.

Nerves of the Somatic Nervous System

The somatic nervous system, which consists of efferent nerves responsible for stimulating muscle contraction, including all the neurons connected with skeletal muscles, skin, and sense organs, is associated with the voluntary control of body movements via skeletal muscles, and with sensory reception of external stimuli (e.g., touch, hearing, sight).

Cranial Nerves

The 12 pairs of cranial nerves (CN) are typically referred to by the roman numerals I through XII. The cranial nerve roots enter and exit the brainstem to provide sensory and motor innervation to the head and muscles of the face. CN I and II (olfactory and optic, respectively) are not true nerves but are fiber tracts of the brain. The anatomy, function, and examination of the cranial nerve system are described in the "Cranial Nerve Examination" section.

Spinal Nerves

A total of 31 symmetrically arranged pairs of spinal nerves exit from all levels of the vertebral column, except for those of C1 and C2,[5] each derived from the spinal cord. The spinal nerves are divided topographically into eight cervical pairs (C1–8), 12 thoracic pairs (T1–12), 5 lumbar pairs (L1–5), 5 sacral pairs (S1–5), and a coccygeal pair. The dorsal and ventral roots of the spinal nerves are located within the vertebral canal.

> ● **Key Point** The portion of the spinal nerve that is not within the vertebral canal, and which usually occupies the intervertebral foramen, is referred to as a peripheral nerve.

As the nerve roots begin to exit the vertebral canal, they must penetrate the dura mater, before passing through dural sleeves within the intervertebral foramen. The dural sleeves are continuous with the epineurium of the nerves.

Essentially, there are three types of spinal nerves:[3]

- *Primary dorsal:* Usually consists of a medial sensory branch and a lateral motor branch. The dorsal roots of the spinal nerves are represented by restricted peripheral sensory regions called *dermatomes.* The peripheral sensory nerves are represented by more distinct and circumscribed areas.
- *Primary ventral:* Forms the cervical, brachial, and lumbosacral plexuses.
- *Communicating ramus:* Serves as a connection between the spinal nerves and the sympathetic trunk.

> ● **Key Point** Only the thoracic and upper lumbar nerves contain a white ramus communicans, but the gray ramus is present in all spinal nerves.

> ● **Key Point** Because in the majority of patients there is no C1 dorsal root, there is no C1 dermatome. When present, the C1 dermatome covers a small area in the central part of the neck close to the occiput.[3]

Peripheral Nerves

Peripheral nerves are enclosed in three layers of tissue of differing character. From the inside outward, these are the endoneurium, perineurium, and epineurium.[6] Peripheral nerve fibers can be categorized according to function: sensory, motor, or mixed.

Cervical Nerves and the Brachial Plexus

The eight pairs of cervical nerves are derived from cord segments between the level of the foramen magnum and the middle of the seventh cervical vertebra.[7]

- *Posterior primary divisions:* The C1 (suboccipital) nerve is the only branch of the first posterior primary divisions. It is a motor nerve, serving the muscles of the suboccipital triangle, with very few sensory fibers.[7]
- *Anterior primary divisions:* The anterior primary divisions of the first four cervical nerves (C1–4) form the cervical plexus, which is depicted in (Figure 5-1).

> ● **Key Point** The *phrenic nerve* is the largest branch of the cervical plexus and plays a vital role in respiration.

The brachial plexus is formed by the anterior rami of the lower four cervical and first thoracic nerve roots (C5-T1). It proceeds through the neck, the axilla, and into the arm where it is divided into *trunks, divisions, cords,* and *branches.* The brachial plexus is depicted in (Figure 5-2).

From the Trunks

A nerve extends to the subclavius muscle (C5–6) from the upper trunk, or fifth root. The subclavius muscle acts mainly on the stability of the sternoclavicular joint, with more or less intensity according to the degree of the clavicular interaction with the movements of the peripheral parts of the superior limb. It seems to act as a substitute for the ligaments of the sternoclavicular joint.[8]

The suprascapular nerve originates from the upper trunk of the brachial plexus formed by the roots of C5 and C6. It supplies the supraspinatus and infraspinatus muscles, and it also provides articular branches to the glenohumeral and acromioclavicular joints. In addition, it provides sensory and sympathetic fibers to two-thirds of the shoulder capsule and to the glenohumeral and acromioclavicular joints.

From the Cords

The medial and lateral pectoral nerves extend from the medial and lateral cords, respectively. They supply the pectoralis major and pectoralis minor muscles. The pectoralis major muscle has dual innervation.[9]

The three subscapular nerves from the posterior cord are:

- The upper subscapular nerve (C5–6), which supplies the subscapularis muscle.

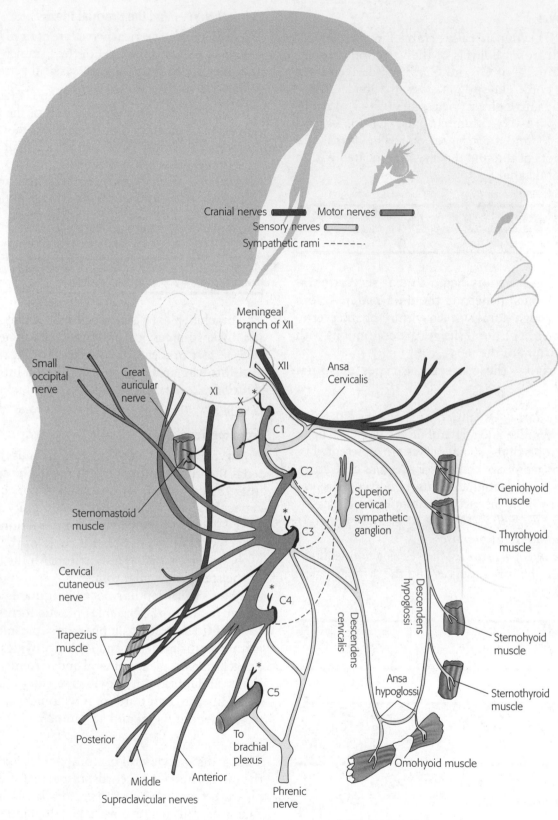

Cranial nerves

Motor nerves

Sensory nerves

Sympathetic rami

Meningeal
branch of XII

XII

Ansa
Cervicalis

Small
occipital
nerve

Great
auricular
nerve

XI

X

*

C1

Sternomastoid
muscle

C2

Superior
cervical
sympathetic
ganglion

Geniohyoid
muscle

Thyrohyoid
muscle

Cervical
cutaneous
nerve

*

C3

Descendens
hypoglossi

Descendens
cervicalis

Trapezius
muscle

*

C4

Sternohyoid
muscle

*

C5

Ansa
hypoglossi

Sternothyroid
muscle

Posterior

To
brachial
plexus

Omohyoid muscle

Middle

Anterior

Phrenic
nerve

Supraclavicular nerves

Figure 5-1   The cervical plexus.

*To adjacent vertebral musclature

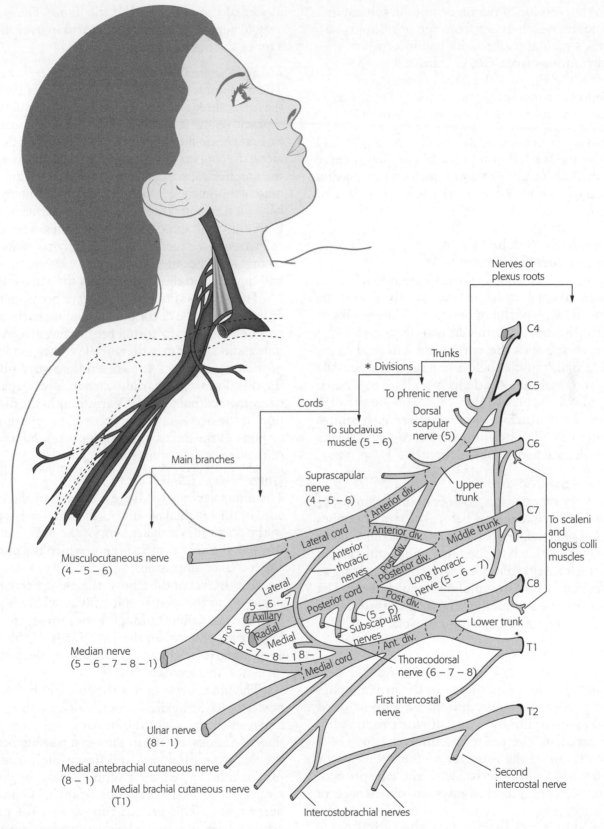

Figure 5-2   The brachial plexus.

*Splitting of the plexus into anterior and posterior divisions is one of the most significant features in the redistribution of nerve fibers, because it is here that fibers supplying the flexor and extensor groups of muscles of the upper extremity are separated. Similar splitting is noted in the lumber and sacral plexuses for the supply of muscles of the lower extremity.

- The thoracodorsal nerve, or middle subscapular nerve, which arises from the posterior cord of the brachial plexus with its motor fiber contributions from C6, C7, and C8.
  This nerve supplies the latissimus dorsi.
- The lower subscapular nerve (C5–6) to the teres major and part of the subscapularis muscle.

Sensory branches of the medial cord (C8–T1) comprise the medial antebrachial cutaneous nerve to the medial surface of the forearm and the medial brachial cutaneous nerve to the medial surface of the arm.

Branches of the Brachial Plexus

Musculocutaneous Nerve (C5–6)
The musculocutaneous nerve is the terminal branch of the lateral cord, which in turn is derived from the anterior division of the upper and middle trunks of the fifth through seventh cervical nerve roots.[10,11] The nerve supplies the coracobranchials, biceps, and brachialis muscles before emerging between the biceps and the brachioradialis muscles 2 to 5 centimeters above the elbow.[11–13] The nerve, now called the *lateral antebrachial cutaneous nerve*, separates into anterior and posterior divisions to innervate the anterior-lateral aspect of the forearm.[11]

Axillary Nerve (C5–6)
The axillary nerve is the last nerve of the posterior cord of the brachial plexus before the latter becomes the radial nerve. The posterior trunk of the axillary nerve gives a branch to the teres minor muscle and the posterior deltoid muscle before terminating as the superior lateral brachial cutaneous nerve. The anterior trunk continues, giving branches to supply the middle and anterior deltoid muscle.

Radial Nerve (C6–8, T1)
The radial nerve is the largest branch of the brachial plexus. The radial nerve in the arm supplies the triceps, the anconeus, and the upper portion of the extensor-supinator group of forearm muscles. In the forearm, the posterior interosseous nerve innervates all of the muscles of the six extensor compartments of the wrist, with the exception of the extensor carpi radialis brevis and extensor carpi radialis longus.

The skin areas supplied by the radial nerve include the posterior brachial cutaneous nerve, to the dorsal aspect of the arm; the posterior antebrachial cutaneous nerve, to the dorsal surface of the forearm; and the superficial radial nerve, to the dorsal aspect of the radial half of the hand. The isolated area of supply is a small patch of skin over the dorsum of the first interosseous space.

Median Nerve (C5–T1)
The trunk of the median nerve derives its fibers from the lower three (sometimes four) cervical and the first thoracic segments of the spinal cord. Although it has no branches in the upper arm, the nerve trunk descends along the course of the brachial artery and passes onto the anterior aspect of the forearm, where it gives off muscular branches, including the anterior interosseous nerve. It then enters the hand, where it terminates with both muscular and cutaneous branches. The sensory branches of the median nerve supply the skin of the palmar aspect of the thumb and the lateral two and a half fingers, and the distal ends of the same fingers.

The anterior interosseous nerve provides motor innervation to the flexor pollicis longus; to the medial part of the flexor digitorum profundus, involving the index and sometimes the middle finger; and to the pronator quadratus. It also sends sensory fibers to the distal radioulnar, radiocarpal, intercarpal, and carpometacarpal joints.[14] Variations in the distribution of the nerve have been noted; it may supply all or none of the flexor digitorum profundus and part of the flexor digitorum superficialis.[15]

Ulnar Nerve (C8, T1)
The ulnar nerve is the largest branch of the medial cord of the brachial plexus. As the ulnar nerve passes to the posterior compartment of the arm, it courses through the arcade of Struthers, which is a potential site for its compression.

At the level of the elbow, the ulnar nerve passes posterior to the medial epicondyle, where it passes through the cubital tunnel. From there, the ulnar nerve passes between the two heads of the flexor carpi ulnaris origin and traverses the deep flexor–pronator aponeurosis.[16,17]

The ulnar nerve enters the forearm by coursing posterior to the medial humeral condyle and passing between the heads of the flexor carpi ulnaris.[18] It then continues distally to the wrist passing between the flexor carpi ulnaris and flexor digitorum profundus muscles, which it supplies. Proximal to the wrist, the palmar cutaneous branch of the ulnar nerve arises. This branch runs across the palmar aspect of the forearm and wrist outside of the tunnel of Guyon to supply the proximal part of the ulnar side of the palm. A few centimeters more distally to the tunnel, a dorsal cutaneous branch arises and supplies the ulnar side of the dorsum of the hand, the dorsal aspect of the fifth finger, and the ulnar half of the forefinger. The ulnar nerve supplies the flexor carpi ulnaris, the ulnar head of the flexor digitorum profundus, and all of the small muscles deep and medial to the long flexor tendon of the thumb, except the first two lumbricales. Its sensory distribution includes the skin of the little finger and the medial half of the hand and the ring finger.

Thoracic Nerves

Dorsal Rami

The thoracic dorsal rami travel posteriorly, close to the vertebral zygapophysial joints, before dividing into medial and lateral branches.

Medial Branches

The medial branches supply the short, medially placed back muscles (the iliocostalis thoracis, spinalis thoracis, semispinalis thoracis, thoracic multifidi, rotatores thoracis, and intertransversarii muscles) and the skin of the back as far as the midscapular line.[19] The medial branches of the upper six thoracic dorsal rami pierce the rhomboids and trapezius, reaching the skin in close proximity to the vertebral spines, which they occasionally supply.

Lateral Branches

The lateral branches supply smaller branches to the sacrospinalis muscles. The lateral branches increase in size the more inferior they are. They penetrate, or pass, the longissimus thoracis to the space between it and the iliocostalis cervicis, supplying both of these muscles, as well as the levatores costarum.[19] The 12th thoracic lateral branch sends a filament medially along the iliac crest, which then passes down to the anterior gluteal skin.

Ventral Rami

There are 12 pairs of thoracic ventral rami, and all but the 12th are between the ribs, serving as intercostal nerves. The 12th ventral ramus, the subcostal nerve, is located below the last rib. The intercostal nerve has a lateral branch, providing sensory distribution to the skin of the lateral aspect of the trunk, and an anterior branch, supplying the intercostal muscles, parietal pleura, and the skin over the anterior aspect of the thorax and abdomen. All of the intercostal nerves mainly supply the thoracic and abdominal walls, with the upper two also supplying the upper limb. The thoracic ventral rami of T3 to T6 supply only the thoracic wall, whereas the lower five rami supply both the thoracic and abdominal walls. The subcostal nerve supplies both the abdominal wall and the gluteal skin.

Lumbar Plexus

The lumbar plexus is formed from the ventral nerve roots of the second, third, and fourth lumbar nerves (in approximately 50% of cases, the plexus also receives a contribution from the last thoracic nerve) as they lie between the quadratus lumborum muscle and the psoas muscle (Figure 5-3). It then travels anteriorly into the body of the psoas muscle to form the lateral femoral cutaneous, femoral, and obturator nerves. L1, L2, and L4 divide into upper and lower branches. The upper branch of L1 forms the

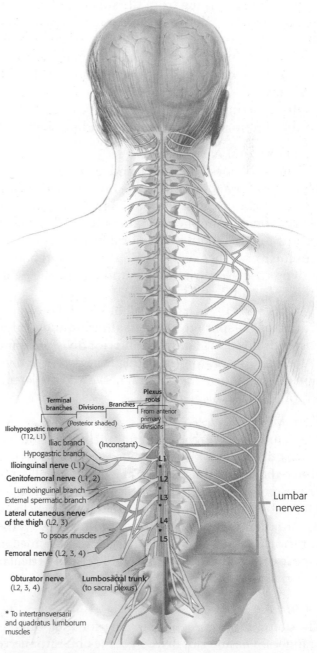

Figure 5-3   The lumbar plexus.

Nerves of the Somatic Nervous System   **171**

iliohypogastric and ilioinguinal nerves. The lower branch of L1 joins the upper branch of L2 to form the genitofemoral nerve. The lower branch of L4 joins L5 to form the lumbosacral trunk.

Iliohypogastric Nerve (T12, L1)
This nerve divides into lateral and anterior cutaneous branches. The lateral (iliac) branch supplies the skin of the upper lateral part of the thigh, while the anterior (hypogastric) branch descends anteriorly to supply the skin over the symphysis.

Ilioinguinal Nerve (L1)
This nerve pierces the internal oblique, which it supplies, before emerging from the superficial inguinal ring to supply the skin of the upper medial part of the thigh and the root of the penis and scrotum or mons pubis and labium majores. An entrapment of this nerve results in pain in the groin region, usually with radiation down to the proximal inner surface of the thigh, sometimes aggravated by increasing tension on the abdominal wall through standing erect.

Genitofemoral Nerve (L1, 2)
This nerve divides into genital and femoral branches. The genital branch supplies the cremasteric muscle and the skin of the scrotum or labia, whereas the femoral branch supplies the skin of the middle upper part of the thigh and the femoral artery. Collateral muscular branches supply the quadratus lumborum and intertransversarii from L1 and L4 and the psoas muscle from L2 and L3.

The lower branch of L2, all of L3, and the upper branch of L4 split into a small anterior and a large posterior division. The three anterior divisions unite to form the obturator nerve; the three posterior divisions unite to form the femoral nerve and the lateral femoral cutaneous nerve.

Femoral Nerve (L2–4)
The femoral nerve, the largest branch of the lumbar plexus, arises from the lateral border of the psoas just above the inguinal ligament. The nerve supplies the sartorius, pectineus, and quadriceps femoris muscles. The sensory distribution of the femoral nerve includes the anterior and medial surfaces of the thigh via the anterior femoral cutaneous nerve, and the medial aspect of the knee, the proximal leg, and articular branches to the knee via the saphenous nerve.

Obturator Nerve (L2–4)
The obturator nerve splits into anterior and posterior branches. The anterior division of the obturator nerve gives an articular branch to the hip joint near its origin.

The anterior division divides into numerous branches, including the cutaneous branches to the subsartorial plexus and directly to a small area of skin on the middle internal part of the thigh, vascular branches to the femoral artery, and communicating branches to the femoral cutaneous and accessory obturator nerves.

The posterior division of the obturator nerve pierces the anterior part of the obturator externus, which it supplies, and descends deep to the adductor brevis. It also supplies the adductors magnus and brevis (if it has not received supply from the anterior division) and gives an articular branch to the knee joint.

Lateral (Femoral) Cutaneous Nerve of the Thigh
The lateral (femoral) cutaneous nerve of the thigh is purely sensory and is derived primarily from the second and third lumbar nerve roots, with occasional contributions from the first lumbar nerve root.[20,21] Sympathetic afferent and efferent fibers also are contained within the nerve.[22] The site at which the lateral (femoral) cutaneous nerve of the thigh exits the pelvis varies.[23]

Sacral Plexus
The lumbosacral trunk (L4, L5) descends into the pelvis, where it enters the formation of the sacral plexus (Figure 5-4). The sacral plexus is formed by the ventral rami of the L4 and L5 and the S1 through S4 nerves. The L4 and L5 nerves join to become the

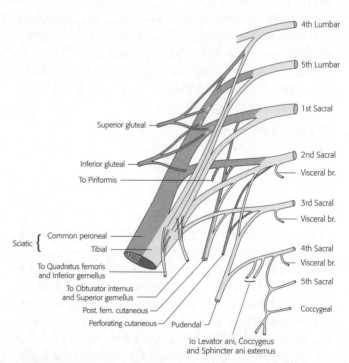

Figure 5-4   The sacral plexus.

Source: Gray H: Anatomy of the Human Body (ed 20). Philadelphia, Lea and Febiger, 1918.

lumbosacral trunk. The S1 through S4 nerves converge to form the broad triangular band of the sacral plexus.

The collateral branches of the posterior division include the following:

- *Superior gluteal nerve:* The roots of the superior gluteal nerve (L4, L5, S1) arise within the pelvis from the sacral plexus. The superior gluteal nerve innervates the gluteus medius and gluteus minimus.[24]
- *Inferior gluteal nerve:* The inferior gluteal nerve (L5, S1, S2) innervates the gluteus maximus muscle. Nerves to the piriformis consist of short, smaller branches from S1 and S2.
- *Superior cluneal nerve:* The medial branch of the superior cluneal nerve passes superficially over the iliac crest, where it is covered by two layers of dense fibrous fascia.
- *Posterior gemoral cutaneous nerve:* The posterior femoral cutaneous nerve constitutes a collateral branch, with roots from both anterior and posterior divisions of S1 and S2, and the anterior divisions of S2 and S3. Perineal branches pass to the skin of the upper medial aspect of the thigh and the skin of the scrotum or labium majores.

Collateral branches from the anterior division extend to the quadratus femoris and gemellus inferior muscles (from L4, L5, and S1) and to the obturator internus and gemellus superior muscles (from L5, S1, and S2). These branches include the sciatic nerve, the tibial nerve, the sural nerve, and the terminal branches of the tibial nerve, which are described in the following section.

Sciatic Nerve

The sciatic nerve is the largest nerve in the body. It arises from the L4, L5, and S1 through S3 nerve roots as a continuation of the lumbosacral plexus. The nerve is composed of the independent tibial (medial) and common fibular (peroneal) (lateral) divisions, which are usually united as a single nerve down to the lower portion of the thigh. The tibial division is the larger of the two divisions. The common fibular (peroneal) nerve is formed by the upper four posterior divisions (L4, L5, S1 S2) of the sacral plexus, and the tibial nerve is formed from all five anterior divisions (L4, L5, S1–3).

Innervation for the short head of the biceps comes from the common fibular (peroneal) division, the only muscle innervated by this division above the knee.

Rami from the tibial trunk pass to the semitendinosus and semimembranosus muscles, the long head of the biceps, and the adductor magnus muscle.

Tibial Nerve

The portion of the tibial trunk below the popliteal space is called the *posterior tibial nerve;* the portion within the space is called the *internal popliteal nerve.* The tibial nerve supplies the gastrocnemius, plantaris, soleus, popliteus, tibialis posterior, flexor digitorum longus, and flexor halluces longus muscles.

Sural Nerve

The sural nerve is a sensory branch of the tibial nerve. It is formed by the lateral sural cutaneous nerve from the common fibular (peroneal) nerve and the medial calcaneal nerve from the tibial nerve. The sural nerve supplies the skin on the posterior-lateral aspect of the lower one-third of the leg and the lateral side of the foot.

Terminal Branches of the Tibial Nerve

In the distal leg, the tibial nerve lies laterally to the posterior tibial vessels, and it supplies articular branches to the ankle joint and to the posterior-medial aspect of the ankle. From this point, its terminal branches include:

- *Medial plantar nerve:* Comparable to the median nerve in the hand, this nerve supplies the flexor digitorum brevis, abductor halluces, flexor halluces brevis, and first lumbrical muscles. It also supplies sensory branches to the medial side of the sole, the plantar surfaces of the medial three and a half toes, and the ungual phalanges of the same toes.
- *Lateral plantar nerve:* Comparable to the ulnar nerve in the hand, this nerve supplies the small muscles of the foot, except those innervated by the medial plantar nerve. It also supplies sensory branches to the lateral portions of the sole, the plantar surface of the lateral one and a half toes, and the distal phalanges of these toes. The interdigital nerves are most commonly entrapped between the second and third web spaces, the third and fourth web spaces, and the intermetatarsal ligaments as a result of a forced hyperextension of the toes, eventually resulting in an interdigital neuroma.
- *Medial calcaneal nerve:* As it passes beneath the flexor retinaculum, the tibial nerve gives off medial calcanean branches to the skin of the heel. An irritation of this nerve may result in heel pain.

- *Common fibular (peroneal) nerve:* The common fibular (peroneal) nerve gives off sensory branches in the popliteal space. These sensory branches include the superior and inferior articular branches to the knee joint and the lateral sural cutaneous nerve.

At the apex of the popliteal fossa, the common fibular (peroneal) nerve begins its independent descent along the posterior border of the biceps femoris, then crosses the dorsum of the knee joint to the upper external portion of the leg near the head of the fibula. The nerve curves around the lateral aspect of the fibula toward the anterior aspect of the bone before passing deep to the two heads of the fibularis (peroneus) longus muscle, where it divides into three terminal nerves:

- *Recurrent articular:* The recurrent articular nerve accompanies the anterior tibial recurrent artery, supplying the tibiofibular and knee joints, as well as a twig to the tibialis anterior muscle.
- *Superficial fibular:* The superficial fibular (peroneal) nerve arises deep within the fibularis (peroneus) longus, supplying the peroneus longus and brevis muscles and providing sensory distribution to the lower front of the leg, the dorsum of the foot, part of the big toe, and adjacent sides of the second to fifth toes up to the second phalanges. When this nerve is entrapped, it causes pain over the lateral distal aspect of the leg and ankle, and thus it is often confused with a disc herniation involving the L5 nerve root.
- *Deep fibular:* The deep fibular (peroneal) nerve supplies the tibialis anterior, extensor digitorum longus, extensor halluces longus, and fibularis tertius muscles. The deep fibular nerve divides into a medial and lateral branch approximately 1.5 centimeters above the ankle joint. These terminal branches extend to the skin of the adjacent sides of the medial two toes (medial branch), to the extensor digitorum brevis muscle (lateral branch), and to the adjacent joints. When the deep fibular nerve is entrapped, there is a complaint of pain in the great toe, which can be confused with a post-traumatic, sympathetic dystrophy.

● **Key Point** Compared with the tibial division, the common fibular (peroneal) division is relatively tethered at the sciatic notch and the neck of the fibula and may, therefore, be less able to tolerate or distribute tension, such as occurs in acute stretching or with changes in limb position or length.

Pudendal and Coccygeal Plexuses

The pudendal and coccygeal plexuses are the most caudal portions of the lumbosacral plexus and supply nerves to the perineal structures. The pudendal plexus supplies the coccygeus, levator ani, and sphincter ani externus muscles. The pudendal nerve is a mixed nerve, and a lesion that affects it or its ascending pathways can result in voiding and erectile dysfunctions.[25]

● **Key Point** A lesion in the afferent pathways of the pudendal nerve is often suspected clinically by suggestive patient histories, including organic neurologic disease or neurologic trauma. Lesions are also suspected when a neurologic physical examination to assess the function of signal segments S2, S3, and S4 is abnormal.

The pudendal nerve divides into:

- The inferior hemorrhoidal nerves to the external anal sphincter and adjacent skin
- The perineal nerve
- The dorsal nerve of the penis

The nerves of the coccygeal plexus are the small sensory anococcygeal nerves derived from the last three segments (S4, S5, C). They pierce the sacrotuberous ligament and supply the skin in the region of the coccyx.

Reflexes

A *reflex* is a subconscious programmed unit of behavior in which a certain type of stimulus from a receptor automatically leads to the response of an effector. Reflexes can be controlled by spinal or supraspinal (brainstem) pathways. Reflexes are classified on the basis of the relevant pathways and central connections as follows:

- *Segmental reflexes:* The stimulus and the response have a fixed spatial relationship.
- *Monosynaptic reflex:* The stretch (myotatic) reflex. The term *deep tendon reflex* is a misnomer—there are no deep tendons used and no reflexes that are conversely superficial. However, as most texts use this term, it will be used throughout.
- *Polysynaptic and oligosynaptic (superficial) reflexes:* The plantar response (sign of Babinski) and the blink reflex.

Monosynaptic Reflex

The *stretch* or *myotatic reflex* is one of the simplest known examples of a reflex, consisting of just two neurons and one synapse. The tap of the reflex hammer on the tendon produces a brief stretch of the tendon (afferent Ia reflex arc involving the muscle spindle; **Table 5-3**), which in turn, causes a contraction of the tendon and muscle belly—the inverse stretch reflex (afferent Ib reflex arc involving the Golgi tendon organ).

Superficial Reflexes

A *superficial reflex* is typically elicited by cutaneous sensory (nociceptive) stimuli that results in a withdrawal (protective) response. The most widely studied superficial reflex is the flexor reflex, which results in a typical withdrawal response with simultaneous facilitation of flexor muscles and inhibition of the extensor muscles on the side of the stimulus, and facilitation of extensors and inhibition of flexors in the contralateral limb, resulting in the *crossed extensor reflex*.

● **Key Point** The presence of an abnormal superficial reflex is suggestive of CNS (upper motor neuron) impairment and requires an appropriate referral.

Examples of superficial reflexes include the abdominal reflex, the cremasteric and the bulbocavernosus reflexes, and the ones outlined in **Table 5-4**.

● **Key Point** Patients with upper motor neuron syndrome demonstrate poor volitional control of movements and limitations in functional skills.[26] The limbs are typically held in fixed, abnormal postures. Antigravity muscles are primarily affected.[26]

Pathologic Reflexes

There are two basic pathologic reflexes: the Babinski and its variants (Chaddock, Oppenheim, and Gordon) and the Hoffman and its variants (ankle and wrist clonus). Some reflexes occur only in specific periods of development and are not evident later in development as they become integrated by the CNS. Pathologic reflexes occur when an injury or a disease process results in a loss of the normal suppression of primitive reflexes that are normally integrated by the cerebrum on the segmental level of the brain stem or spinal cord.[2,14] Thus, the presence of pathologic reflexes is suggestive of CNS

TABLE 5-3	Muscle Spindle and Golgi Tendon Organ
Muscle Spindle	**Golgi Tendon Organs**
Essentially, the purpose of the muscle spindle is to compare the length of the spindle with the length of the muscle that surrounds the spindle. Within each muscle spindle there are 2–12 long, slender, and specialized skeletal muscle fibers called *intrafusal fibers.* The central portion of the intrafusal fiber is devoid of actin or myosin and, thus, is incapable of contracting. As a result, these fibers are capable of putting tension on the spindle only. The intrafusal fibers are of two types: nuclear bag fibers and nuclear chain fibers. • Nuclear bag fibers primarily serve as sensitivity meters for the changing lens of the muscle.[a,b] • Nuclear chain fibers each contain a single row or chain of nuclei and are attached at their ends to the bag fibers. While muscles are innervated by alpha motor neurons, muscle spindles have their own motor supply—namely, gamma motor neurons. The muscle spindle can be stimulated in two different ways: • By stretching the whole muscle, which stretches the mid portion of the spindle thereby exciting the receptor. • By contracting only the end portion of the intrafusal fibers, thereby exciting the receptor (even if muscle length does not change).	Golgi tendon organs (GTOs) are relatively simple sensory receptors that that are arranged in series with the extrafusal muscle fibers and, therefore, become activated by stretch. In the normal person, the Golgi tendon organ contributes to control of muscle activity over the whole range of movement, not just at its extremes.[c] They appear to serve a protective function, while supplying tension information for complicated tension-maintaining reflexes or supplying inhibition at the appropriate moment to switch from flexion to extension movements in walking or running. They may also play a role in increasing muscle force during fatigue. Thus, during fatigue the muscle produces less force, which reduces Golgi tendon organ activity, thereby decreasing inhibition. Activity in the group Ib afferent fibers, associated with Golgi tendon organs, inhibit a process called *autogenic inhibition* (reflex inhibition of a motor unit in response to excessive tension in the muscle fibers it supplies). It was originally thought that this inhibition served only to protect the muscle from being injured when contracting against too heavy a load. Now it is thought that it occurs at the point where autogenic inhibition is great enough to overcome the stretch reflex excitation.

Data from (a) Grigg P: Peripheral neural mechanisms in proprioception. J Sport Rehabil 3:1–17, 1994; (b) Swash M, Fox K: Muscle spindle innervation in man. J Anat 112:61–80, 1972; and (c) de Jarnette B: Sacro-occipital technique. Nebraska City, Major Bertrand de Jarnette, DC, 1972

TABLE 5-4 Superficial (Cutaneous) Reflexes

Reflex	Stimulus	Normal Response	Pertinent Segment
Upper abdominal	Lateral to medial scratching of the skin toward the umbilicus in each of the two upper quadrants	Umbilicus moves up and toward area being stroked	T7–9
Lower abdominal	Lateral to medial scratching of the skin toward the umbilicus in each of the two lower quadrants	Umbilicus moves down and toward area being stroked	T11–12
Cremasteric	Stroking the skin on the proximal and medial thigh	Scrotum/testicle elevates	T12, L1
Plantar	Stroking lateral sole of foot from calcaneus to base of fifth metatarsal and medially across the metatarsal heads	Plantarflexion of toes	S1–2
Gluteal	A stroke over the skin of the buttocks	Skin tenses in gluteal area	L4–5, S1–3
Anal	Scratching the perianal skin	Contraction of anal sphincter muscles	S2–4

(upper motor neuron) impairment and requires an appropriate referral.

Babinski

The Babinski exists as a primitive reflex (the plantar reflex) in infants up to the age of approximately 6 months when it elicits a downward response. The term *Babinski's sign* refers to an upward response that is pathological in origin. To perform the test, the clinician applies noxious stimuli to sole of the patient's foot by running a pointed object along the plantar aspect.[27] A positive test, demonstrated by extension of the big toe and a splaying (abduction) of the other toes, is indicative of an injury to the corticospinal tract.[28]

● **Key Point** As a general rule, influence of the primitive reflexes is not readily observed in the healthy, normally developing child after 6 months of age (exceptions include the symmetric tonic neck reflex and the plantar grasp reflex).

Patterned Behavioral Reflexes

A number of reflex responses to tactile stimuli occur in association with dementia and disorders of the frontal lobes.

- *Grasp reflex of the hand:* An instinctive or orienting grasp reflex is evoked with the application of a light tactile stimulus applied to the lateral margin of the ulna or radial side of the hand.
- *Grasp reflex of the foot:* This reflex is elicited by firm pressure on the metatarsal head, which evokes a slow, sustained flexion of all the toes that may outlast the stimulus by many seconds.
- *Suck reflex:* The stimulus consists of a light stroking of the lip with a tongue blade or finger; the response is a pursing of the lips and an opening of the mouth. There may also be an orienting of the lips or following of the stimulus if it is moved away or toward one side.

Supraspinal Reflexes

The *supraspinal reflexes* produce movement patterns that can be modulated by descending pathways and the cortex. A number of processes involved in locomotor function are oriented around these reflexes, and they are referred to as *postural reflexes*. The postural reflexes constantly react and compensate for changes during body motions and require input from the somatosensory, vestibular, and visual systems.

● **Key Point** Postural reflexes help maintain postural equilibrium and stability during head, trunk, and extremity motions, as well as those that react in situations that have the potential to cause serious injury.

The head and neck are areas of intense reflex activity. Head movements, which occur almost constantly, must be regulated in order to maintain normal eye-head-neck-trunk relationships, and to allow for visual fixation during head movements. There are three main reflex mechanisms:

- *Vestibuloocular reflex (VOR):* The VOR is stimulated by movement of the head in space and has a strong influence on eye movement and positioning.
- *Vestibulospinal reflex (VSR):* The VSR functions to stabilize the body and control movement.
- *Cervico-ocular reflex (COR):* Mechanoreceptors in the cervical muscles are the primary source of afferent input in the elicitation of the COR.

The COR and VOR work together to maintain the visual fixation of the eyes during head and neck movements.

Protective Reflexes

Protective reflexes are a function of the midbrain/cortical regions. They include righting reactions and equilibrium reactions.

Righting reactions can be broken into five different reflexes that serve to keep the head in a normal position, right the body to a normal position, and adjust the body parts in relation to the head and vice versa. These reactions are:

- Labyrinthine righting reflexes acting on the head
- Body-righting reflexes acting on the head
- Neck-righting reflexes
- Body-righting reflexes acting on the body
- Optical righting reflexes

Equilibrium reactions are developed during childhood for the purpose of maintaining or regaining control over the body's center of gravity to prevent falls. There are several categories of equilibrium reactions:

- Protective reaction of the arms (protective extension) and legs
- Tilting reactions
- Postural fixating reactions

Proprioception

Proprioception is a specialized variation of the sensory modality of touch, which plays an important role in coordinating muscle activity. It involves the integration of sensory input concerning static joint position (joint position sensibility), joint movement (kinesthetic sensibility), velocity of movement, and force of muscular contraction, from the skin, muscles, and joints.[29,30] Proprioception can be both conscious, as occurs in the accurate placement of a limb, and unconscious, as occurs in the modulation of muscle function.[30,31]

Other reflex actions include preparatory postural adjustments[33] and reaction movements. Preparatory postural adjustments are preprogrammed neural mechanisms. Reaction movements occur too fast for the feedback loops of the CNS; they are automatic and occur subconsciously.

Proprioceptive deficits can be found with fatigue, aging,[34] arthrosis,[35] and joint instability.[31,32,36–41]

Balance

Balance is the process by which the body's center of mass is controlled with respect to the base of support, whether that base of support is stationary or moving.[41] Normal balance requires input from:

- *The somatosensory system*: Input from mechanoreceptors located in skin, joints, muscles, and ligaments provides proprioceptive information.

- *The visual system:* Involves CN II, III, IV, and VI and assists in balance control by providing input about the position of the head and/or the body in space. Through the vestibulo-ocular input, signals from the muscle spindles in the extra-ocular muscles, the position of the eyeball is controlled so that a visual image is maintained on the fovea.
- *The vestibular system:* Provides feedback about the position and movement of the head with relation to gravity.

Proprioception can be conscious or unconscious, whereas balance is typically conscious. According to Berg, balance can be defined as the ability to:[45]

- Maintain a position
- Move voluntarily
- React to a perturbation

> **● Key Point** Outcome measurement tools for functional balance include:
> - Dynamic Gait Index[46,47]
> - Get Up and Go Test[48,49]
> - Functional Reach Test[50-52]
> - Berg Balance Scale[53-57]
> - Performance-oriented mobility assessment (POMA)[58,59]

Kinesthesia

Kinesthesia refers to the sense of position and movement. While the articular receptors quite clearly play an active role, two other sensors, the muscle spindle and the Golgi tendon organ (GTO), also are important. Information about movement and position sense travels up the spinocerebellar tract.

Neuromuscular Examination

Levels of Consciousness

The levels of consciousness can be documented in descending order:

- *Alert:* The patient's quality of mind is characterized by attentiveness to normal levels of stimulation, self-awareness, subjectivity, sapience, and sentience.
- *Clouding of consciousness:* The patient appears quiet and confused and has difficulty in focusing or maintaining attention on the question or task.

- *Delirium:* The patient appears disoriented, confused, agitated, and loud.
- *Obtunded:* The patient's state of consciousness is characterized by a state of sleep, reduced alertness to arousal, and delayed responses to stimuli.
- *Stupor (semicoma):* The patient responds only to strong, generally noxious stimuli and returns to the unconscious state when stimulation is stopped. When aroused, the patient is unable to interact with the clinician.
- *Vegetative state (unresponsive vigilance):* The patient lacks the capacity for self-aware mental activity due to overwhelming damage or dysfunction of the cerebral hemispheres with sufficient sparing of the diencephalon and brainstem to preserve autonomic and motor reflexes. The patient lacks cognitive responsiveness but has normal sleep/wake cycles and vegetative functions (respiration, heart rate, blood pressure, digestion).
- *Coma:* The patient is unarousable and unresponsive, and any response to repeated stimuli is only primitive avoidance reflexes; in profound coma, all brainstem and myotatic reflexes may be absent.

The most commonly used standardized examination of comatose patients is the Glasgow Coma Scale (GCS) (**Table 5-5**). The scale is intended for grading coma severity and establishing prognosis following head injury. Scoring range is from 3 to 15:

Score	Prognosis
8 or less	Severe brain injury
9–12	Moderate brain injury
13–15	Minor brain injury

Upper and Lower Quarter Scanning Examination

The scanning examination is used when there is no history to explain the presence of signs and symptoms that warrant concern. The clinician must choose which scanning examination to use, based on the presenting signs and symptoms. The upper quarter scanning examination is appropriate for upper thoracic, upper extremity, and cervical problems, whereas the lower quarter scanning examination is typically used for thoracic, lower extremity, and lumbosacral problems.

Upper Quarter Scanning Examination

The upper quarter scanning examination encompasses the following:

- Postural assessment. The assessment of posture is described in Chapter 4.

	Test	Patient Response	Score
TABLE 5-5 Glasgow Coma Scale (GCS)			
Eyeopening	Spontaneous	Opens eyes	4
	Response to speech	Opens eyes	3
	Response to pain	Opens eyes	2
	Response to pain	Doesn't open eyes	1
Best verbal response	Speech	Conversation carried out correctly	5
		Confused, disoriented	4
		Inappropriate words	3
		Unintelligible sounds only	2
		Mute	1
Best motor response	Commands	Follow simple commands	6
	Response to pain	Pulls/pushes examiner's hand away	5
	Response to pain	Pulls part of body away	4
	Response to pain	Flexes body in response to pain	3
	Response to pain	Decerebrates	2
	Response to pain	No motor response	1

- Range of motion assessment. The patient performs AROM of the cervical spine and upper extremities. The clinician applies passive overpressure at the end of the available AROM if the patient does not exhibit signs and symptoms.
- Resistive testing. To screen the various innervation levels, the following resisted tests are completed: cervical rotation (C1), shoulder elevation (C2–4), shoulder abduction (C5), elbow flexion (C5–6), wrist extension (C6), elbow extension (C7), wrist flexion (C7), thumb extension (C8), and finger adduction (T1).
- Reflex testing of the biceps (C5), brachioradialis (C6), and triceps (C7).
- Dermatomes testing of the posterior head (C2), posterolateral neck (C3), acromioclavicular joint (C4), lateral arm (C5), lateral forearm and thumb (C6), palmar distal phalanxmiddle finger (C7), little finger and ulnar border of the hand (C8), and medial forearm (T1).

Lower Quarter Scanning Examination

The lower quarter scanning examination encompasses the following:

- Postural assessment. The assessment of posture is described in Chapter 4.

- Range of motion assessment. The patient performs AROM of the lumbosacral spine and lower extremities. The clinician applies passive overpressure at the end of the available AROM if the patient does not exhibit signs and symptoms.
- Resistive testing. To screen the various innervation levels, the following resisted tests are completed: heel walking (L4–5), toe walking (S1), straight leg raise (L4–S1), hip flexion (L1–2), knee extension (L3–4), ankle dorsiflexion (L4–5), great toe extension (L5), and ankle plantarflexion (S1).
- Reflex testing of the patellar (L4) and Achilles tendon (S1).
- Dermatomes testing of the anterior thigh (L2), middle third of the anterior thigh (L3), patella and medial malleolus (L4), fibular head and dorsum of foot (L5), lateral and plantar aspect of foot (S1), medial aspect of the posterior thigh (S2), and perianal area (S3–5).

Cranial Nerve Examination

With practice, the entire cranial nerve examination[60] can be performed in approximately 5 minutes (**Table 5-6**).[61] The following poem is helpful to remember the order and tests for the cranial nerve examination:[62]

TABLE 5-6	Cranial Nerves and Their Function
Cranial Nerve	**Function and Testing**
I: Olfactory	The olfactory nerve is responsible for the sense of smell. The sense of smell is tested by having the patient identify familiar odors (coffee, lavender, vanilla) with each nostril.
II: Optic	The optic nerve is responsible for vision. The optic nerve is tested by examining visual acuity and confrontation.
III: Oculomotor	The somatic portion of the oculomotor nerve supplies the levator palpabrae superioris muscle; the superior, medial, and inferior rectus muscles; and the inferior oblique muscles, which are responsible for some eye movements. The visceral efferent portion of this nerve is responsible for papillary constriction. The nerve is tested using eye movements and assessing pupil dilation. Cranial nerves III, IV, and VI are typically tested together.
IV: Trochlear	The trochlear nerve supplies the superior oblique muscle of the eye. This nerve is tested using eye movements.
V: Trigeminal	The trigeminal nerve supplies sensory information to the soft and hard palate, maxillary sinuses, upper teeth and upper lip, and the mucous membrane of the pharynx, and it supplies motor information to the muscles of mastication, both pterygoids, the anterior belly of the digastric muscle, the tensor tympani, the tensor veli palatini, and the mylohyoid. The sensory branches of the trigeminal nerve are tested, with a pinprick, close to the midline of the face. The clinician tests the motor components by asking the patient to clench the teeth while the clinician palpates the temporal and masseter muscles.
VI: Abducens	The abducens nerve innervates the lateral rectus muscle of the eye. This nerve is tested through assessment of eye movements.
VII: Facial	The facial nerve is composed of a sensory (intermediate) root, which conveys taste, and a motor root, the facial nerve proper, which supplies the muscles of facial expression, the platysma muscle, and the stapedius muscle of the inner ear. The clinician inspects the face at rest and in conversation with the patient, noting any asymmetry. The patient is asked to smile. If there is asymmetry, the clinician asks the patient to frown or wrinkle the forehead.
VIII: Vestibulocochlear (Auditory)	The cochlear portion is concerned with the sense of hearing. The vestibular portion is part of the system of equilibrium, the vestibular system. The vestibular nerve can be tested in a number of ways depending on the objective. If hearing loss is present, then the clinician should test for lateralization and then compare air and bone conduction.
	Lateralization: The clinician places a tuning fork over the vertex, middle of the forehead, or front teeth. The patient is asked whether the vibration is heard more in one ear (Weber test). Normal individuals cannot lateralize the vibration to either ear. In conduction deafness (e.g., that caused by middle ear disease), the vibration is heard more in the affected ear. In sensorineural deafness, the vibration is heard more in the normal ear.
	Air and bone conduction: Air conduction is assessed by placing the tuning fork in front of the external auditory meatus, whereas bone conduction is assessed by placing the tuning fork on the mastoid process (Rinne test). In a normal individual, the tuning fork is heard louder and longer by air than by bone conduction. In conduction deafness, bone conduction hearing is better. In sensorineural deafness, both air and bone conduction are reduced, although air conduction is the better of the two.
IX: Glossopharyngeal	The glossopharyngeal nerve serves a number of functions. The gag reflex is used to test this nerve, but it is reserved only for the severely affected patients.
X: Vagus	The vagus nerve contains somatic motor, visceral efferent, visceral sensory, and somatic sensory fibers. The functions of the vagus nerve are numerous. The patient is asked to open the mouth and say "aah." The clinician watches the movements of the soft palate and pharynx.
XI: (Spinal) Accessory	The cranial root is often viewed as an aberrant portion of the vagus nerve. The spinal portion of the nerve supplies the sternocleidomastoid and the trapezius muscles. The patient is asked to shrug both shoulders upward against the clinician's hand, and the strength of contraction is noted.
XII: Hypoglossal	The hypoglossal nerve is the motor nerve of the tongue, innervating the ipsilateral side of the tongue, as well as helping to innervate the infrahyoid muscles. The patient is asked to stick out the tongue. The clinician looks for asymmetry, atrophy, or deviation from the midline.

Smell and see
And look around,
Pupils large and smaller.
Smile, hear!
Then say ah . . .
And see if you can swallow.
If you're left in any doubt,
Shrug and stick your tongue right out.

Reflex Testing

The assessment of reflexes is extremely important in the diagnosis and localization of neurological lesions.[3] Reflex testing utilizes the muscle spindle to determine the state of both the afferent and efferent peripheral nervous systems, and the ability of the CNS to inhibit the reflex. The tendon is struck directly and smartly with the reflex hammer. When applying a slight tap to the tendon, a brisk reflex is a normal finding, provided that it is not masking a hyperreflexia due to an incorrect testing technique. Stretch reflexes (**Table 5-7**) may be graded in a variety of ways, including the following:

0   Absent (areflexia)
1+ Decreased (hyporeflexia)
2+ Normal
3+ Hyperactive (brisk)
4+ Hyperactive with clonus (hyperreflexive)

● Key Point   Hyporeflexia, if not generalized to the whole body, indicates a lower motor neuron (LMN) or sensory paresis, which may be segmental (root), multisegmental (cauda equina), or nonsegmental (peripheral nerve).

● Key Point   *Spasticity* is defined as velocity-dependent (resistance increases with velocity) hypertonia and hyperactive tendon reflexes (increased deep tendon reflexes, DTRs) resulting from hyperexcitability of the stretch reflex. Spasticity is a common sequela of an anatomic or physiologic anomaly of the CNS, specifically an injury to the corticospinal system (suprasegmental/upper motor neuron lesions).[63–65] If left untreated, spasticity can lead to the development of secondary impairment such as contracture, postural asymmetries, and deformity.[26]

The superficial (cutaneous) and pathological reflexes (**Table 5-8**) also can be tested.

Diagnostic Procedures

The clinician should review the results of any diagnostic tests that have been performed, if available.

Cerebral Angiography

Cerebral angiography[66–68] is an x-ray procedure used to visualize the vascular system of the brain. Radiopaque contrast material is injected into the carotid, subclavian, brachial, or femoral artery x-rays are taken at specific intervals. Cerebral angiography is useful in determining areas of increased and

---

TABLE 5-7   Common Deep Tendon Reflexes

Reflex	Site of Stimulus	Normal Response	Pertinent Central Nervous System Segment
Jaw	Mandible	Mouth closes	Cranial nerve V
Biceps	Biceps tendon	Biceps contraction	C5–6
Brachioradialis	Brachioradialis tendon or just distal to the musculotendinous junction	Flexion of elbow and/or pronation of forearm	C5–6
Triceps	Distal triceps tendon above the olecranon process	Elbow extension	C7–8
Patella	Patellar tendon	Leg extension	L3–4
Medial hamstrings	Semimembranosus tendon	Knee flexion	L5, S1
Lateral hamstrings	Biceps femoris tendon	Knee flexion	S1–2
Tibialis posterior	Tibialis posterior tendon behind medial malleolus	Plantar flexion of foot with inversion	L4–5
Achilles	Achilles tendon	Plantar flexion of foot	S1–2

TABLE 5-8 — Pathological Reflexes

Reflex	Elicitation	Positive Response	Pathology
Babinski	Stroking of lateral aspect of side of foot	Extension of big toe and fanning of four small toes Normal reaction in newborns	Pyramidal tract lesion Organic hemiplegia
Chaddock	Stroking of lateral side of foot beneath lateral malleolus	Same response as above	Pyramidal tract lesion
Oppenheim	Stroking of anteromedial tibial surface	Same response as above	Pyramidal tract lesion
Gordon	Squeezing of calf muscles firmly	Same response as above	Pyramidal tract lesion
Brudzinski	Passive flexion of one lower limb	Similar movement occurs in opposite limb	Meningitis
Hoffmann	"Flicking" of terminal phalanx of index, middle, or ring finger	Reflex flexion of distal phalanx of thumb and of distal phalanx of index or middle finger whichever one was not "flicked"	Increased irritability of sensory nerves in tetany Pyramidal tract lesion
Lhermitte	Neck flexion	An electric shock–like sensation that radiates down the spinal column into the upper or lower limbs	Abnormalities (demyelination) in the posterior part of the cervical spinal cord

decreased vascularity. It also provides information about the dynamics of cerebral circulation. It does have disadvantages, however: it is invasive, and it may cause meningeal irritation, hemorrhage, vasospasm, and anaphylactic reaction to the dye.

Computed Tomography

Computed tomography (CT)[69–76] uses x-rays emitted from a source and confined to a plane oriented perpendicular to the long axis of the body to provide a detailed cross-section of tissue structure. The narrowly collimated beam of x-rays that rotates in a continuous 360° motion around the patient is transmitted through tissues of varying densities and is converted to an electrical signal. The computer-generated image uses multiple readings of the patient in cross-sectional slices to produce a three-dimensional picture. Contrast enhancement can be used to provide more detail.

CT is best at showing calcific structures, including the skull and calcific abnormalities in the brain, and blood, including subarachnoid blood and epidural, subdural, and cerebral hematomas. It is also very good at showing the ventricles and cerebral spinal fluid spaces. CT imaging of the spine is excellent for showing the team the lesions of no value or for showing the spinal cord or the nerve roots. Its major advantages over magnetic resonance imaging

(described later) include speed, greater availability, and less expense.

Electroencephalography

Electroencephalography (EEG)[77–79] is a process of measuring and recording temporal changes in brainwave activity via electrodes attached to various areas of the patient's head. The test can be used to diagnose seizure, alterations in mental status, and brainstem disorders, and to localize intracranial lesions of the brain.

Electromyogram

The electromyogram (EMG)[26,80–83] is designed to record intrinsic electric activity in a skeletal muscle. Surface electrodes are applied, or a needle electrode (needle EMG) is inserted, into the muscles. Electrical activity is detected within an oscilloscope and transmitted to a loudspeaker. Normal muscle is electrically silent away from the endplate region. With electrode movement, normal insertional activity consists of a brief electrical discharge.

An EMG study can be useful in diagnosing lower motor neuron or primary muscle disease (mononeuropathy, plexopathy, radiculopathy, polyneuropathy, or defective neuromuscular transmission at the neuromuscular junction). The following findings can occur with EMG testing:

- The burst of action potentials when the EMG needle is inserted is increased in denervated muscle.
- Alterations in the size, duration, and shape of the motor unit potentials occur with re-innervation of previously denervated muscles.
- The number of motor unit potentials is decreased in a lower motor neuron injury.

Evoked Potential

Evoked potentials (EPs)[84–89] are responses produced from different levels of the nervous system with a relatively fixed latency following a stimulus. Responses may be recorded from the nerves, the cortical tracts and nuclei, or cortical segments of a stimulated pathway. In clinical practice the most commonly used potentials are visual, auditory, and somatosensory, with each producing a characteristic brainwave pattern.

The evoked potential studies are useful in detecting lesions in multiple sclerosis (prolonged latency without loss in amplitude), evaluating visual or auditory function in patients who cannot cooperate with more formal testing of vision or hearing, and providing useful prognostic information in comatose patients.

Lumbar Puncture

The most common purpose of lumbar puncture (LP) is to obtain cerebrospinal fluid. The CSF is obtained by using a hollow needle and stylet that is inserted into the subarachnoid space of the lumbar portion of the spinal canal at the level of the third and fourth lumbar vertebrae. The CSF sample is used to provide a specific diagnosis, as for some types of meningitis, leptomeningeal carcinoma, and subarachnoid hemorrhage. Two other purposes for a lumbar puncture include:

- To give intrathecal (contrast agent for myelography) injections[90–92]
- To obtain a CSF pressure measurement;[93–95] for example, when there is a suspected idiopathic intracranial hypertension or chronic hydrocephalus
- The complications of lumbar puncture may include severe headaches, infections, and epidural hematomas

Contraindications for lumbar puncture include the presence of a large intracranial mass/lesion or obstructive hydrocephalus.

Magnetic Resonance Imaging

Magnetic resonance imaging (MRI)[96–103] uses a large magnet with a strong magnetic field and relies on the interaction of the spin and associated protons (and, to a lesser extent, neutrons) with its magnetic field (nuclear magnetic resonance). MRI can be used for brain imaging for nearly any clinical indication, but because it costs more than CT, it is usually reserved for situations in which it has advantages over CT. It is clearly superior for evaluating patients with:

- Epilepsy
- Cerebral vasculitis
- Vascular malformations
- Suspected multiple sclerosis and other white matter diseases
- Small, deep infarcts
- Lesions of any type in the brainstem and cerebellum

> **● Key Point** Every tissue in the human body has its own T1 and T2 value. T1-weighted images are useful for showing overall brain anatomy and for a valuation of CSF spaces; they are most useful for demonstrating hydrocephalus, atrophy, cysts, and malformations. T2-weighted images are sensitive to subtle changes in tissue characteristics. As with CT, MRI enhancement of images, which is useful for demonstrating vascular structures such as aneurysms and vascular malformations, can be utilized.

This procedure is noninvasive and painless for the patient, although some patients experience claustrophobia that interferes with completion.

Magnetic Resonance Angiography

Magnetic resonance angiography (MRA)[104–107] provides excellent visualization of large vessels and effectively shows thrombosis, embolism, stenosis, and dissection of large vessels in the head or neck. It is also good for showing aneurysms and arteriovenous and venous malformations.

Myelography

Used to identify a variety of spinal lesions, myelography is a radiographic process by which the spinal cord and spinal subarachnoid space are viewed and photographed after a contrast medium is introduced.[108–112]

Nerve Conduction Velocity

Nerve conduction velocity (NCV) is a test that measures the speed with which an electrical impulse can be transmitted through excitable tissue. The speed of action potential conduction can be measured along any accessible nerve. Conduction velocities of the fastest-conducting fibers are determined by stimulating the nerve at two sites, measuring the latency from each stimulus to onset of response, and dividing the distance between the two sites by the difference in latency between the two responses. Conduction velocity is expressed as meters per second. Decreased conduction velocities are seen in peripheral neuropathies characterized by demyelination—for example, Guillain–Barre.[113] Slowed conduction velocities are seen with focal compression of a peripheral nerve.[114–119]

Positron Emission Tomography

Positron emission tomography (PET)[120–122] is a neuroimaging technique in which radioisotopes are injected and emissions are measured by a gamma ray detector system. This test provides information on the cerebral blood flow and brain metabolism; however, it is not as detailed as CT or MRI.

Ventriculography

Ventriculography[123,124] is an x-ray examination of the head after any injection of air or another contrast medium into the cerebral ventricles; for example, an x-ray examination of the ventricle of the heart after an injection of a radiopaque contrast medium.

Electronystagmography

Electronystagmography (ENG) involves a battery of tests that assess central and peripheral vestibular function and organization. Central vestibular function is reflected in oculomotor tests for nystagmus, reflexes (optokinetic nystagmus), and integrated motion (saccade, pursuit). Peripheral VIII cranial nerve and labyrinthine function are evaluated in response to various stimuli (e.g., positional/positioning, caloric, rotational chair testing).

Nystagmus can be observed, recorded, and quantified. Electro-oculography (EOG) indirectly measures eye movement by detecting changes in the electrical charges produced by the corneal–retinal potential using skin electrodes. Eye movements can also be quantified directly using infrared oculography (IRO). IRO techniques allow direct observation of eye movements and eliminate many artifactual elements present on EOG.

Neurologic Dysfunction

At the most fundamental level, all neurologic dysfunctions can be classified as an upper motor neuron lesion, a lower motor neuron lesion, or a combination of both.

● **Key Point** An upper motor neuron (UMN) lesion is a lesion of the neural pathway above the anterior horn cell or motor nuclei of the cranial nerves. An UMN lesion is characterized by spastic paralysis or paresis, little or no muscle atrophy, hyperreflexive stretch reflexes in a nonsegmental distribution, and the presence of pathological signs and reflexes. It is important that the PTA be aware of the signs and symptoms associated with UMN lesions, as they can constitute a medical emergency.

● **Key Point** A lower motor neuron lesion affects nerve fibers traveling from the anterior horn of the spinal cord to the relevant muscle(s). The characteristics of an LMN include muscle atrophy and hypotonus, a diminished or absent stretch reflex of the areas served by a spinal nerve root, or a peripheral nerve and an absence of pathological signs or reflexes.

Infectious Diseases

Meningitis

Meningitis is an inflammation of the leptomeninges and underlying subarachnoid cerebrospinal fluid (CSF).[125–133] A number of factors influence the development of meningitis, including virulence of the strain, host defenses, and invader–host interactions. Swift identification by the PTA can be life saving. Classic symptoms (not evident in infants or seen often in the elderly) include the following: headache, nuchal rigidity (discomfort on neck flexion), fever and chills, photophobia, vomiting, seizures, focal neurologic symptoms, and altered sensorium (confusion may be the sole presenting complaint, especially in elderly patients).

● **Key Point** Positive signs of meningeal irritation:
- *Kernig sign:* Passive knee extension in supine patient elicits neck pain and hamstring resistance.
- *Brudzinski sign:* Passive neck or single hip flexion is accompanied by involuntary flexion of both hips.

Encephalitis

Encephalitis is an inflammation of the brain parenchyma. The etiology of encephalitis is usually infectious, but it may be noninfectious (acute disseminated encephalitis). The clinical presentation and course can be markedly variable. The classic presentation is encephalopathy with diffuse or focal neurologic symptoms, including the following:

- Behavioral and personality changes, decreased level of consciousness

- Stiff neck, photophobia, and lethargy
- Generalized or localized seizures
- Acute confusion or amnestic states
- Flaccid paralysis

Neural Injuries and Noninfectious Diseases

Cerebrovascular Accident

For description of the cerebrovascular accident (CVA) and its etiology and manifestations, refer to Chapter 11.

Transient Ischemic Attack

A transient ischemic attack (TIA)[134–140] is an acute episode of temporary and focal loss of cerebral function of a vascular (occlusive) origin. As a TIA may last only several minutes, historical questions should be addressed not just to the patient but also to family members and other witnesses. Of concern is the careful detection of changes in behavior, speech, gait, memory, movement, and vision. Contacting the patient's primary physician is important.

Cerebral Aneurysm

An aneurysm[141–147] is an abnormal local dilatation in the wall of a blood vessel, usually an artery, due to a defect, disease, or injury. Causes of aneurysms include:

- Developmental or inherited conditions.
- Hemodynamically induced degenerative vascular injury. The occurrence, growth, thrombosis, and even rupture of intracranial saccular aneurysms can be explained by abnormal hemodynamic shear stresses on the walls of large cerebral arteries, particularly at bifurcation points.
- Trauma, infection, tumor, drug abuse (cocaine), and high-flow states associated with arteriovenous malformations (AVMs) or fistulae.
- Congenital abnormalities of the intracranial vasculature.
- Vasculopathies such as fibromuscular dysplasia (FMD), connective tissue disorders, and spontaneous arterial dissection are associated with an increased incidence of intracranial aneurysm.

Aneurysms commonly arise at the bifurcations of major arteries. Most aneurysms do not cause symptoms until they rupture; when they rupture, they are associated with significant morbidity and mortality.

Traumatic Brain Injury

Traumatic brain injury (TBI)[148–160] is a nondegenerative, noncongenital insult to the brain from an external mechanical force, possibly leading to permanent or temporary impairments of cognitive, physical, and psychosocial functions with an associated diminished or altered state of consciousness. TBI is the major cause of death related to injury among Americans younger than 45 years. The risk of TBI peaks when individuals are aged 15–30 years, with the risk being highest for individuals aged 15–24 years. In individuals aged 75 years and older, falls are the most common cause of TBI. Motor vehicle accidents (MVAs) are the leading cause of TBI in the general population.

TBI can manifest clinically from concussion to coma and death. Injuries are divided into a number of categories:

- *Focal injuries:* Tend to be caused by contact forces.
- *Diffuse injuries:* Are more likely to be caused by noncontact, acceleration–deceleration, or rotational forces. Diffuse axonal injury (DAI), caused by forces associated with acceleration–deceleration and rotational injuries— for example, high-impact MVAs, contact sports, and shaken-baby syndrome.
- *Hypoxic–ischemic injuries:* Result from a lack of oxygenated blood flow to the brain tissue.
- *Increased intracranial pressure (ICP):* Can lead to cerebral hypoxia, cerebral ischemia, cerebral edema, hydrocephalus, and brain herniation.

The physical mechanisms of brain injury are classified using the following categories:

- *Impact loading* (i.e., collision of the head with a solid object at a tangible speed): Causes brain injury through a combination of contact forces and inertial forces.
  - *Inertial forces:* Inertial force ensues when the head is set in motion with or without any contact force, leading to acceleration of the head.
  - *Contact forces:* Coup contusions occur at the area of direct impact to the skull and occur because of the creation of negative pressure when the skull, distorted at the site of impact, returns to its normal shape.

Contrecoup contusions are similar to coup contusions but are located opposite the site of direct impact. Cavitation in the brain, from negative pressure due to translational acceleration impacts from inertial loading, may cause contrecoup contusions as the skull and dura matter start to accelerate before the brain on initial impact.

- *Impulsive loading:* Impulsive loading is uncommon and occurs when the head is set in motion, and then the moving head is stopped abruptly without it being directly struck.
- *Static or quasistatic loading:* This type of loading is rare and occurs if a slowly moving object traps the head against a rigid structure, slowly compressing the skull and producing numerous comminuted fractures.

The three basic types of tissue deformation involved in TBI are the following:

- *Compressive:* Tissue compression
- *Tensile:* Tissue stretching
- *Shear:* Tissue distortion produced when tissue slides over other tissue

Complications associated with TBI include:

- *Epidural hematoma:* Occurs from impact loading to the skull with associated laceration of the dural arteries or veins, often by fractured bones and sometimes by veins in the skull's marrow. More often, a tear in the middle meningeal artery causes this type of hematoma. When hematoma occurs from laceration of an artery, blood collection can cause rapid neurologic deterioration.
- *Subdural hematoma:* Tends to occur in patients with injuries to the cortical veins or pial artery in severe TBI.
- *Intracerebral hemorrhage:* Occurs within the cerebral parenchyma secondary to lacerations or contusion of the brain with injury to larger deeper cerebral vessels with extensive cortical contusion.
- *Intraventricular hemorrhage:* Tends to occur in the presence of very severe TBI and is, therefore, associated with an unfavorable prognosis.
- *Subarachnoid hemorrhage:* May occur in cases of TBI in a manner other than secondary to ruptured aneurysms caused by lacerations of the superficial microvessels in the subarachnoid space.

- *Increased intracranial pressure (ICP):*
  - *Cerebral edema:* May be caused by effects of neurochemical transmitters and by increased ICP.
  - *Hydrocephalus:* The communicating type of hydrocephalus is more common in TBI than the noncommunicating type.
  - *Brain herniation:* Supratentorial herniation is attributable to direct mechanical compression by an accumulating mass or to increased intracranial pressure.

Impairments associated with TBI include:

- Cognitive
- Behavioral
- Communication
- Visual–perceptual
- Swallowing
- Indirect (soft tissue contractures, skin breakdown, deep vein thrombosis, heterotropic ossification, decreased bone density, muscle atrophy, decreased endurance, infection, and pneumonia)

A number of clinical rating scales are used to evaluate change in the patient over time. Two of the more commonly used scales are the Glasgow Coma Scale (GCS), which defines severity of TBI within 48 hours of injury (Table 5-5), and the Ranchos Los Amigos Cognitive Functioning Scale (**Table 5-9**), which can be used to determine the severity of deficit in cognitive functioning.

The physical therapy role involves an interdisciplinary approach. The interdisciplinary team includes the patient and family, physician, speech language pathologist, occupational therapist, rehabilitation nurse, case manager, medical social worker, and neuropsychologist. The goals of the physical therapy intervention include:[161]

- Preventing indirect impairments. Proper positioning both in bed and in a wheelchair is essential to prevent skin breakdown and contractures, improve pulmonary hygiene and circulation, and help modify muscle tone.[162,163] The patient should be turned every two hours when in bed.
- Improving arousal through sensory stimulation. Multisensory stimulation involves the presentation of sensory stimulation in a highly structured and consistent manner.[161] The following sensory systems are systematically stimulated:

TABLE 5-9	Rancho Los Amigos Cognitive Functioning Scale
I: No response: Total assistance	Patient appears to be in a deep sleep and is completely unresponsive to any stimuli.
II: Generalized response: Total assistance	Patient acts inconsistently and purposely to stimuli in a nonspecific manner. Responses are limited and often the same regardless of stimulus presented. Responses may be physiological changes, gross body movements, and/or vocalization.
III: Localized response: Total assistance	Patient reacts specifically but inconsistently to stimuli. Response is not directly related to the type of stimulus presented. Patient may follow simple commands, such as closing eyes or squeezing hands, in an inconsistent, delayed manner.
IV: Confused–agitated: Maximal assistance	Patient is in heightened state of activity. Behavior is bizarre and nonpurposeful relative to immediate environment. Patient does not discriminate among persons or objects and is unable to cooperate directly with treatment efforts. Verbalizations frequently are incoherent and/or inappropriate to the environment; confabulation may be present. Gross attention to environment is very brief. Patient lacks short- and long-term recall.
V: Confused–inappropriate: Maximal assistance	Patient is able to respond to simple commands fairly consistently. However, with increased complexity of commands or lack of any external structure, responses are nonpurposeful, random, or fragmented. Patient demonstrates gross attention to the environment that is highly distractible and lacks ability to focus attention on a specific task. With structure, patient may be able to converse on a social automatic level for short periods of time. The vocalization is often inappropriate and confabulatory. Memory is severely impaired. Patient often shows inappropriate use of objects; he or she may perform previously learned tasks with structure but is unable to learn new information.
VI: Confused–appropriate: Moderate assistance	Patient shows goal-directed behavior but is dependent on external input or direction. He or she follows simple directions consistently and shows carryover for relearned problems but appropriate to the situation; past memories show more depth and detail than recent memory.
VII: Automatic–appropriate: Minimal assistance with activities of daily living	Patient appears appropriate and oriented within hospital and home settings; he or she goes through daily routine automatically, but is frequently robot-like with minimal to absent confusion and shallow recall of activities. Patient shows carryover for new learning but at a decreased rate. With structure, patient is able to initiate social or recreational activities; judgment remains impaired.
VIII: Purposeful-appropriate: Standby assistance	Patient is able to recall and to integrate past and recent events and is aware of and responsive to environment. Patient shows carryover for new learning and needs no supervision once activities are learned. Patient may continue to show a decreased ability relative to premorbid abilities. Patient is able to engage in abstract reasoning, shows tolerance for stress, and demonstrates judgment in emergencies or unusual circumstances.
IX: Purposeful-appropriate: Standby assistance on request	Patient able to independently shift back and forth between tasks and completes them accurately for at least two consecutive hours. Patient initiates and carries out steps to complete familiar activities of daily living with assistance when requested. Patient is aware of and acknowledges impairments and disabilities and takes appropriate corrective action but requires stand-by assist to anticipate a problem before it occurs and take action to avoid it. Patient is able to think about consequences of decisions or actions with assistance when requested, and accurately estimates abilities. Patient also is able to self-monitor appropriateness of social interaction with stand-by assistance.
X: Purposeful, appropriate: Modified independent.	Patient able to handle multiple tasks simultaneously in all environments but may require periodic breaks. Patient able to independently initiate and carry out steps to complete familiar activities of daily living but may require more than usual amount of time and/or compensatory strategies to complete them. Patient able to accurately estimate abilities and independently adjusts to task demands. Social interaction behavior of patient is consistently appropriate.

Data from Hagen C, Malkmus D, Durham P: Rancho Los Amigos Cognitive Scale, Rancho Los Amigos Hospital, 1972

auditory, olfactory, gustatory, visual, tactile, kinesthetic, and vestibular.[161]

- Patient and family education. The family should be taught about the stages of recovery and what can be expected in the future.
- Managing the effects of abnormal tone and spasticity. A wide variety of methods are available to the therapist to treat the adverse effects of abnormal tone (refer to "Management Strategies for Specific Conditions")
- Early transition to sitting postures. As soon as medically stable, the patient should be transferred to a sitting position and out of bed to a wheelchair or chair. This transition may require the use of a tilt table.

Concussion

Concussion is caused by deformity of the deep structures of the brain, leading to widespread neurologic dysfunction that can result in impaired consciousness or coma. Concussion is considered a mild form of diffuse axonal injury.

Spinal Cord Injury

Patients with spinal cord injury (SCI) usually have permanent and often devastating neurologic deficits and disability. The extent and seriousness of the consequences depend on the location and severity of the lesion.

- Injury to the corticospinal tract or dorsal columns, respectively, results in ipsilateral paralysis or loss of sensation of light touch, proprioception, and vibration.
- Injury to the lateral spinothalamic tract causes contralateral loss of pain and temperature sensation.
- Because the anterior spinothalamic tract also transmits light touch information, injury to the dorsal columns may result in complete loss of vibration sensation and proprioception but only partial loss of light touch sensation.

> ● **Key Point** Injuries below L1 are not considered SCIs because they involve the segmental spinal nerves and/or cauda equina. Spinal injuries proximal to L1, above the termination of the spinal cord, often involve a combination of spinal cord lesions and segmental root or spinal nerve injuries.

Spinal cord injuries can be categorized as complete or incomplete. A complete cord syndrome is characterized clinically as complete loss of motor and sensory function below the level of the traumatic lesion.

> ● **Key Point** *Tetraplegia* refers to complete paralysis of all four extremities and trunk, including the respiratory muscles, and results from lesions of the cervical cord. *Paraplegia* refers to complete paralysis of all or part of the trunk and both lower extremities resulting from lesions of the thoracic or lumbar spinal cord or cauda equina.

Incomplete cord syndromes (**Table 5-10**) have variable neurologic findings with partial loss of sensory and/or motor function below the level of injury. The term *sacral sparing* refers to an incomplete lesion of the spinal cord where some of the innermost (long) tracts with the sacral fibers remain intact and innervated. Signs and symptoms of sacral sparing include sensation of the saddle area, movement of the toe flexors, and rectal sphincter contraction. A spinal cord concussion is characterized by a transient neurologic deficit localized to the spinal cord that fully recovers without any apparent structural damage. It is extremely important for clinicians and researchers to be able to accurately determine the extent of neurological impairment in terms of motor and sensory loss.

> ● **Key Point** The neurological level is defined as the most caudal level of the spinal cord with normal motor and sensory function on both the left and right sides of the body.
> - *Motor level:* The most caudal segment of the spinal cord with normal motor function bilaterally.
> - *Sensory level:* The most caudal segment of the spinal cord with normal sensory function bilaterally.
>
> For example, a patient with C5 quadriplegia has, by definition, abnormal motor and sensory function from C6 down.

Complications Associated with Spinal Cord Injury

Autonomic Dysreflexia

Autonomic dysreflexia (AD)[164–170] is a syndrome of massive imbalanced reflex sympathetic discharge occurring in patients with spinal cord injury (SCI) above the splanchnic sympathetic outflow (T5–6). The potential triggers for AD are numerous and include:

- Bladder distension
- Urinary tract infection
- Bowel distension or impaction
- Hemorrhoids
- Deep vein thrombosis
- Pulmonary emboli
- Pressure ulcers
- Ingrown toenail

AD occurs after the phase of spinal shock in which reflexes return. Below the injury, intact peripheral sensory nerves transmit impulses that stimulate

TABLE
5-10

The Incomplete SCI Syndromes

Syndrome	Description	Characteristic Findings
Anterior cord	Usually seen as a result of compression of the anterior spinal artery from bone fragments or a large disc herniation.	Manifested by complete motor paralysis (corticospinal function) and sensory anesthesia (spinothalamic function); sparing of the dorsal column (deep pressure and proprioception are only retained sensibilities of the trunk and lower extremities); greater motor loss in the legs than arms.
Posterior cord	A rare incomplete lesion with primary damage to the posterior sensory cortex and posterior columns as a result of impact injuries or a hyperextension force.	Loss of deep touch, position, and vibration below the level of the lesion, with preservation of motor function, pain, and temperature sensation. Unfortunately, the sense of proprioception is lost, which can limit the patient's potential for functional gait.
Central cord	Usually involves a cervical lesion. Most often occurs after hyperextension injury in an individual with long-standing cervical spondylosis. Injury may result both from posterior pinching of the cord by buckled ligamentum flavum or from anterior compression by osteophytes.	Greater motor weakness in the upper extremities than in the lower extremities. The pattern of motor weakness shows greater distal involvement in the affected extremity than proximal muscle weakness. Sensory loss is variable, and the patient is more likely to lose pain and/or temperature sensation than proprioception and/or vibration. Dysesthesias, especially those in the upper extremities (e.g., sensation of burning in the hands or arms), are common. Sacral sensory sparing usually exists.
Brown–Séquard	Hemisection of the spinal cord, often in the cervical region resulting in interruption of the lateral corticospinal tracts, the lateral spinal thalamic tract, and at times the posterior columns.	Interruption of the lateral corticospinal tracts resulting in ipsilateral spastic paralysis below the level of the lesion, Babinski sign ipsilateral to lesion (abnormal reflexes and Babinski sign may not be present in acute injury).
		Interruption of lateral spinothalamic tracts resulting in contralateral loss of pain and temperature sensation. This usually occurs 2–3 segments below the level of the lesion. Interruption of posterior white column resulting in ipsilateral loss of tactile discrimination, vibratory, and position sensation below the level of the lesion.
Conus medullaris syndrome	A sacral cord injury involving the most distal bulbous part of the spinal cord (conus medullaris) with or without involvement of the lumbar nerve roots.	A combination of upper motor neuron (UMN) and lower motor neuron (LMN) symptoms. Areflexia in the bladder, bowel, and to a lesser degree, lower limbs. Motor and sensory loss in the lower limbs is variable.
Cauda equina	An injury to the lumbosacral nerve roots caudal to the level of spinal cord termination. Causes include trauma, lumbar disk disease, abscess, spinal anesthesia, tumor, metastatic causes, or CNS elements, late-stage ankylosing spondylitis, or idiopathic causes.	Areflexic bowel and/or bladder, with variable motor and sensory loss in the lower limbs. Because this syndrome is a nerve root injury rather than a true SCI, the affected limbs are areflexic. This injury is usually caused by a central lumbar disk herniation.

sympathetic neurons located in the intermediolateral gray matter of the spinal cord. The inhibitory outflow above the SCI from cerebral vasomotor centers is increased, but it is unable to pass below the block of the SCI. The result is sudden elevation in blood pressure and vasodilation above the level of injury. Clinical manifestations of AD may include:

- A sudden significant rise in both systolic and diastolic blood pressures, usually associated with bradycardia.

- Profuse sweating above the level of lesion, especially in the face, neck, and shoulders
- Complaints of a headache (caused by vasodilation of pain sensitive intracranial vessels)
- Piloerection (goose bumps) above, or possibly below, the level of the lesion
- Flushing of the skin above the level of the lesion, especially in the face, neck, and shoulders
- Visual disturbances

Spinal/Neurogenic Shock

Spinal shock is defined as the complete loss of all neurologic function, including reflexes (areflexia) and rectal tone, below a specific level that is associated with autonomic dysfunction. In addition, it is characterized by hypotension, relative bradycardia, peripheral vasodilation, and hypothermia. Neurogenic shock, which may last for several days to several weeks, does not usually occur with SCI below the level of T6.

Spasticity

Spasticity is defined as velocity-dependent (resistance increases with velocity) hypertonia and hyperactive deep tendon reflexes (DTRs) resulting from hyperexcitability of the stretch reflex. Spasticity is a common sequela of an anatomic or physiologic anomaly of the CNS, specifically an injury to the corticospinal system (suprasegmental/upper motor neuron lesions).[63–65] If left untreated, spasticity can lead to the development of secondary impairment such as contracture, postural asymmetries, and deformity.

Heterotopic Ossification

Heterotopic ossification is the abnormal formation of true bone within extraskeletal soft tissues. A strong association exists between heterotopic ossification and spinal cord injury, with lesions occurring at multiple sites and showing a strong propensity to recur. The condition originates when osteoprogenitor stem cells, lying dormant within the affected soft tissues, are stimulated to differentiate into osteoblasts, beginning the process of osteoid formation, and eventually leading to mature heterotopic bone. Heterotopic ossification often begins as a painful palpable mass that gradually becomes nontender and smaller but firmer to palpation.

Orthostatic Hypotension

The communication between the brainstem and the autonomic nervous system is important for the control of the cardiovascular system and is often compromised after spinal cord injury (SCI). Orthostatic hypotension is a sign of autonomic dysfunction and dysautonomia. Upper thoracic and cervical SCI, especially complete injuries, leave individuals without the ability to control all or most of their sympathetic nervous system (SNS) function. Immediately after SCI occurs, blood pressure rises acutely. This brief response is followed by a period of decreased SNS activity because of interruption of the descending sympathetic tracts. Lack of supraspinal input develops, causing cutaneous vasodilatation, lack of sympathetic vasoconstrictor activity, and absent sympathetic input to the heart.

Pressure Ulcers

Details on pressure ulcers can be found in Chapter 8.

Deep Vein Thrombosis

Circulation in the lower extremities is decreased after SCI to about 50% to 67% of normal as a result of ANS control and decreased local blood flow.[171–174] Factors predisposing individuals with acute SCI to DVT include venous stasis secondary to muscle paralysis and transient hypercoagulable state with reduced fibrinolytic activity along with increased factor VIII activity.

Impaired Temperature Control

After damage to the spinal cord, the hypothalamus can no longer control cutaneous blood flow or amount of sweating.[175] This lack of sweating is often associated with excessive compensatory diaphoresis above the level of lesion.[175]

Respiratory Impairment

Respiratory function varies considerably, depending on the level of lesion. Between C1 and C3, phrenic nerve innervation and spontaneous respiration are significantly impaired or lost.[175]

Bladder and Bowel Dysfunction

Urinary tract infections are among the most frequent medical complications during the initial medical–rehabilitation period.[175]

Following spinal shock, one of two types of bladder conditions will develop, depending on location of the lesion:

- *Spastic or reflex (automatic) bladder*: Lesions that occur within the spinal cord above the conus medullaris.
- *Flaccid or non-reflex (autonomous) bladder*: A lesion of the conus medullaris or cauda equina.

As with the bladder, the neurogenic bowel condition that develops after spinal shock subsides are of two types:

- *Spastic or reflex (automatic) bowel:* Lesion that occurs within the spinal cord above the conus medullaris.
- *Flaccid or non-reflex (autonomous) bowel:* A lesion of the conus medullaris or cauda equina.

Sexual Dysfunction

As with bowel and bladder function, sexual capabilities are broadly divided between UMN and LMN lesions.

Physical Therapy Intervention for Neurologic Injuries

The following goals should act as guidelines in the acute care setting:

- Respiratory management (deep breathing exercises, assisted coughing, airway clearance, abdominal support) as appropriate (**Table 5-11**).
- Pain management.
- Maintenance of joint range of motion and prevention of contractures. Full range of motion exercises should be completed daily except in those areas that are contraindicated or require selective stretching. It is important to remember that patients with spinal cord injury do not require full range of motion in all joints. Some joints benefit from allowing tightness to develop in certain muscles to enhance function. For example, with tetraplegia, tightness of the lower trunk musculature will improve sitting posture by increasing trunk stability.[175]
- Selective strengthening (Table 5-11).
- Orientation to the vertical position and increased sitting tolerance. Being able to come to a sitting position from supine assists with ADLs, bed mobility, and in preparation for transfers. Seated scooting is the ability to move from side to side in the seated position.
- Independence with bed mobility as appropriate. Rolling is taught early in rehabilitation because it is essential for many ADLs, for independence in bed mobility and bed positioning, and as a building block for other mobility skills.[176] The following functional postures are important to emphasize:[176]
  - *Prone on elbows:* Used for bed positioning, rolling, and progressing to sitting positions. Also relieves pressure from posterior structures after periods of sitting or lying supine and stretches anterior hip muscles at the hips and trunk that can easily become shortened with prolonged sitting.
  - *Supine on elbows:* Used primarily to increase flexibility and mobility at the shoulder and in preparation for moving from supine to long sitting.
  - *Quadruped and tall kneeling:* Used to challenge trunk, pelvic, and lower extremity control in preparation for activities requiring upright balance and control in sitting and standing.
  - *Long sitting:* Used as the primary position during dressing and other ADLs, especially for individuals without trunk or full upper extremity control.
  - *Short sitting:* Crucial for independence with transfers, mat or bed mobility, and some ADLs and to have the arms free for functional activities.
- Independence in body handling skills (coming to sit, sitting balance, rolling, performing ischial pressure relief) as appropriate (Table 5-11). Most sources agree that pressure relief should initially be performed for 15 seconds or more, at least every 15 to 30 minutes.[176] For patients with tetraplegia at or above the C4 level, pressure relief is performed by an assistant or power system tilting or reclining a wheelchair. A variety of techniques can be used for patients with SCI at the C5–C6 level with good head and neck control and some upper-extremity function (not including triceps). These include leaning forward with the chest moving toward the thighs, and leaning sideways.[176] For individuals with functional use of the triceps, pressure relief may be performed using the seated push-up technique.[176]
- Independence in wheelchair transfers to mat, bed, car, toilet, bathtub, and floor as appropriate (Table 5-11).
- Independence in wheelchair mobility as appropriate (Table 5-11). After the initial period of skill and endurance training, an individual should be able to propel his or her wheelchair throughout an average day at the community level without creating muscle soreness or fatigue.[176] Patients should also be taught to protect themselves in the case of a fall.
- Independence in preventative measures (self skin inspection; self lower-extremity range-of-motion exercises) as appropriate (Table 5-11).

TABLE
5-11

Functional Outcomes Related to Level of Spinal Cord Injury

Level of Lesion	Neuromuscular Control	Care Needs	Functional Ability	Equipment Needs
C1–C3	Patient has: Limited head and neck movement Able to perform neck rotation (sternocleidomastoid), and neck extension (cervical paraspinals) Difficulties in speech and swallowing Total paralysis of trunk, upper and lower extremities (UE and LE)	24-hour care Patient is able to direct care needs	Patient has impaired communication and is dependent for all care needs.	Patient is dependent on ventilator. Adapted computer Bedside/portable ventilator Suction machine Specialty bed Power wheelchair Hoyer lift Reclining shower chair
C4	Patient has: Head and neck control (cervical paraspinals). Ability to shrug shoulders (upper trapezius) Inspiration capability (diaphragm) Patient lacks shoulder control (deltoids) and has paralysis of trunk, UE and LE, and an inability to cough, with low respiratory reserve	24-hour care needs Patient is able to direct care needs	Patient has some communication ability. Patient can perform assisted cough but is dependent for all care needs.	Patient may or may not be ventilator dependent. Adapted computer Bedside/portable ventilator as needed Suction machine Specialty bed Power wheelchair Hoyer lift Reclining shower chair
C5	Patient has: Shoulder control (deltoids) Elbow flexion (biceps/elbow flexors) Supinate hands (brachialis and brachioradialis) Lack of elbow extension and hand pronation Paralysis of trunk and LE	10 hours of personal care per day 6 hours of home making assistance per day	Patient needs help with equipment setup, eating, drinking, face washing, and teeth brushing. Patient needs assistance with coughing as well as bowel, bladder, and lower body hygiene. Patient is dependent for bed mobility and transfers. Patient has limited mobility and needs assistance getting into wheelchair using a Hoyer lift or stand pivot transfer.	Power and manual wheelchairs Adaptive splints/braces Page turners/computer adaptations
C6	Patient has: Wrist extension (extensor carpi ulnaris and extensor carpi radialis longus/brevis) Ability to cross arm over chest (clavicular pectoralis) Lack of elbow extension (triceps) Lack of wrist flexion Lack of hand control Paralysis of trunk and LE	6 hours of personal care per day 4 hours of homemaking assistance per day	Patient needs assistance with coughing; setup for feeding; bathing; and dressing. Independent with performing pressure relief, turning in bed, and with self-skin assessment. Patient may be independent for bowel/bladder care.	Slide board for independent transfer Manual wheelchair Adaptive equipment for driving

Level of Lesion	Neuromuscular Control	Care Needs	Functional Ability	Equipment Needs
C7	Patient has: Elbow flexion and extension (biceps/triceps) Ability to cross arm toward body (sternal pectoralis) Lack of finger function Lack of trunk stability	6 hours of personal care per day 2 hours of homemaking assistance per day	Patient can cough more effectively. Patient needs fewer adaptive aids (e.g., no adaptive equipment needed for wheelchair transfers). Patient is independent for all ADLs. Patient may need adaptive aids for bowel care.	Manual wheelchair
C8–T1	Patient has: Increased finger and hand strength Finger flexion (flexor digitorum) Finger extension (extensor communis) Thumb movement (pollices longis brevis) Ability to separate fingers (interossei)	4 hours of personal care per day 2 hours of homemaking assistance per day	Patient is independent with or without assistive devices. Patient needs assistance with complex meal prep and home management.	Manual wheelchair
T2–T6	Patient has: Normal motor function of head, neck, shoulders, arms, hands, and fingers Increased use of intercostals Increased trunk control (erector spinae)	3 hours of help with personal care and homemaking per day	Patient is independent in personal care. Patient has limited walking capability and can drive using hand controls.	Manual wheelchair Extensive bracing for walking Hand controls for driving
T7–T12	Patient has: Added motor function Increased abdominal control Increased trunk stability	2 hours of help with personal care and homemaking per day	Patient is independent. Patient has improved cough and improved balance control. Patient has limited walking capability and can drive using hand controls.	Manual wheelchair Bracing for limited walking Hand controls for driving
L2–L5	Patient has added motor function in hips and knees and is able to utilize (depending on level of lesion): L2 hip flexors (iliopsas) L3 knee extensors (quadriceps) L4 ankle dorsiflexors (tibialis anterior) L5 long toe extensors (ext hallucis longus)	May need 1 hour of help with personal care and homemaking per day	Patient is independent. Patient may walk short distances and drive using hand controls.	Manual wheelchair Braces and assistive devices for walking Hand controls for driving
S1–S5	Patient has: Ankle function (plantar flexors—gastrocnemius) Various degrees of bowel, bladder, and sexual function	No personal care or homemaking needs	Patient is independent.	Adaptive/supportive devices (needed less; patients have increased ability to walk) Manual wheelchair for distance mobility

- Identify therapeutic equipment needs.
- Gait training as appropriate (Table 5-11). In patients with complete SCI or incomplete SCI without functional ambulation skill, interventions may include bracing accompanied by instruction in alternative gait patterns.[176] The most commonly taught pattern is a two-point swing-through pattern with use of forearm crutches and bilateral knee-ankle-foot orthoses (KAFOs) with the knee joints locked in extension and the ankles locked in slight dorsiflexion.[176]
- Plan for discharge.

Syringomyelia

Syringomyelia is the development of a fluid-filled cavity or syrinx within the spinal cord[177-181] (hydromyelia is a dilatation of the central canal by CSF and may be included within the definition of syringomyelia). Although many mechanisms for syrinx formation have been postulated, the exact pathogenesis is still unknown. Syringomyelia usually progresses slowly; the course may extend over many years. The condition may have a more acute course, especially when the brainstem is affected (i.e., in syringobulbia). Syringomyelia usually involves the cervical area. Clinical manifestations include the following:

- *Dissociated sensory loss:* Syrinx interrupts the decussating spinothalamic fibers that mediate pain and temperature sensibility, resulting in loss of these sensations, while light touch, vibration, and position senses are preserved.
- *Motor changes:* Syrinx extension into the anterior horns of the spinal cord damages motor neurons (lower motor neuron) and causes diffuse muscle atrophy that begins in the hands and progresses proximally to include the forearms and shoulder girdles. Clawhand may develop.
  - Arm reflexes are diminished early in the clinical course.
  - Lower limb spasticity, which may be asymmetrical, appears with other long-tract signs, such as paraparesis, hyperreflexia, and extensor plantar responses.
- Respiratory insufficiency, which is usually related to changes in position, may occur.
- Impaired bowel and bladder functions usually occur as a late manifestation.

The presence of a syringobulbia is characterized by dysphagia, nystagmus, pharyngeal and palatal weakness, asymmetric weakness and atrophy of the tongue, and sensory loss involving primarily pain and temperature senses in the distribution of the trigeminal nerve.

Lumbar syringomyelia can occur and is characterized by atrophy of the proximal and distal leg muscles with dissociated sensory loss in the lumbar and sacral dermatomes. Lower limb reflexes are reduced or absent. Impairment of sphincter function is common.

A variety of surgical treatments have been proposed for syringomyelia, including suboccipital and cervical decompression, microsurgical lysis of any adhesions, opening of the fourth ventricular outlet and plugging of the obex, and laminectomy and syringotomy (dorsolateral myelotomy). The placement of shunts is also an option.

Cauda Equina Syndrome

Cauda equina syndrome (CES)[182-186] has been defined as low back pain, unilateral or usually bilateral sciatica, saddle sensory disturbances, bladder and bowel dysfunction, and variable lower-extremity motor and sensory loss. CES may result from any lesion that compresses the CE nerve roots.

The symptoms associated with CES include some or all of the following: low back pain; acute or chronic radiating pain; unilateral or bilateral lower-extremity motor and/or sensory abnormality; bowel and/or bladder dysfunction; saddle (perineal) anesthesia (the clinician can inquire if toilet paper feels different when wiping); bladder dysfunction (may present as incontinence, but often presents earlier as difficulty starting or stopping a stream of urine). Reflex abnormalities may be present; they typically include loss or diminution of reflexes. Hyperactive reflexes may signal spinal cord involvement and exclude the diagnosis of CES. CES is a medical emergency.

Neurodegenerative and Inflammatory Disorders

Alzheimer Disease
Alzheimer disease is discussed in Chapter 11.

Multiple Sclerosis
Multiple sclerosis (MS)[187-199] is an inflammatory demyelinating disease of the CNS. The PNS is rarely involved. MS is regarded as an autoimmune disease. Patients with MS commonly present with an individual mix of neuropsychological dysfunction, which tends to progress over years to decades. The review of systems for the PTA should concentrate on the

evidence of bladder, kidney, lung, or skin infection and irritative or obstructive bladder symptoms. Classic MS symptoms include:

- Sensory changes (i.e., paresthesias); usually an early complaint.
- Pain; most common types are trigeminal neuralgia, paroxysmal limb pain, and headache.
- Motor (e.g., muscle cramping secondary to spasticity, fatigue, and weakness) and autonomic (e.g., bladder, bowel, sexual dysfunction) spinal cord symptoms (e.g., spasticity).
- Balance and coordination deficits (e.g., Charcot triad of dysarthria, ataxia, tremor) and dizziness.
- Bowel, bladder, and sexual dysfunction.
- Constitutional symptoms, especially fatigue and dizziness.
- Subjective reports of difficulties with attention span, concentration, memory, and judgment.
- Depression and affective changes.
- Eye symptoms, including optic neuritis (i.e., inflammation, demyelination of optic nerve), and diplopia on lateral gaze.

The diagnosis of MS is made by a neurologist based on the classic presentation described above and on the identification of other neurologic abnormalities, which may be indicated by the patient history and exam. Typical findings on an MRI also help establish a diagnosis of MS.

Medical management includes identifying disease-modifying agents, and management of relapses and symptoms through the use of corticosteroids, antispasticity medications, pain medications, and medications to help alleviate fatigue, tremor, cognitive and emotional problems, and bowel and bladder problems. The physical therapy intervention is based on the impairments identified in the examination but typically includes:

- Regulation of activity level
- Relaxation and energy conservation techniques
- Normalization of tone
- Adaptive/assistive device training
- Balance activities
- Gait training
- Exercises that emphasize core stabilization and trunk control
- Patient and caregiver education

Myasthenia Gravis

Myasthenia gravis (MG)[200–211] is a relatively rare autoimmune disorder of peripheral nerves in which antibodies form against acetylcholine (ACh) nicotinic postsynaptic receptors at the myoneural junction. A reduction in the number of ACh receptors (approximately 30% of normal) results in a characteristic pattern of progressively reduced muscle strength with repeated use of the muscle and recovery of muscle strength following a period of rest. The smooth and cardiac muscles are not affected by the disease. The bulbar muscles (muscles of the throat, tongue, jaw, and face) are affected most commonly and most severely and may lead to ptosis, diplopia, blurred vision, difficulty swallowing, or dysarthria. Ptosis and diplopia are by far the most common complaints. In addition, most patients also develop some degree of intermittent generalized weakness. Most patients who present to physical therapy have an established diagnosis of MG and are already taking appropriate medications. The activity of the disease fluctuates and adjusts, so appropriate monitoring is important. Patients with MG can present with a wide range of signs and symptoms, depending on the severity of the disease. Mild presentations of MG may be associated with only subtle findings, such as ptosis, that are limited to bulbar muscles. Recovery of strength is seen after a period of rest or with application of ice to the affected muscle. Conversely, increased ambient or core temperature may worsen muscle weakness. Severe exacerbations of MG (myasthenic crisis) have a more dramatic presentation:

- The facial muscles (and jaw) may be slack, and face may be expressionless.
- The patient may be unable to support the head, which will fall onto the chest while the patient is seated.
- The voice has a nasal quality.
- The body is limp.
- The gag reflex is often absent; such patients are at risk for aspiration of oral secretions.
- The patient has respiratory distress.

● **Key Point** The most important aspect of MG for the PTA is the detection of the myasthenic crisis.

The patient's ability to generate adequate ventilation and to clear bronchial secretions are of utmost concern with severe exacerbations of MG. An inability to cough leads to an accumulation of secretions; therefore, rales, rhonchi, and wheezes may be auscultated locally or diffusely. MG is controllable with cholinesterase-inhibiting medications.

PTAs treating patients with MG are responsible for the following:

- Monitoring changes in the patient's condition for complications: vital signs, respiration, swallowing
- Maintaining or improving cardiovascular endurance without exacerbating fatigue
- Promoting independence in functional mobility skills and activities of daily living
- Teaching energy conservation techniques
- Providing psychological and emotional support
- Educating family and caregivers

Idiopathic Inflammatory Myopathies

Polymyositis (PM), dermatomyositis (DM), and inclusion body myositis (IBM) are the major members of a group of skeletal muscle diseases called the *idiopathic inflammatory myopathies*.[212-223] The specific etiology is unknown but is thought to be autoimmune. No strictly defined diagnostic criteria for PM or DM exist; however, the findings during the history and physical examination typically reveal the characteristic rash, symmetric proximal muscular weakness, elevated serum muscle enzyme levels, electromyographic evidence of myopathic abnormalities, and characteristic findings at muscle biopsy. Although IBM is classified as an inflammatory myopathy, it shows minimal evidence of inflammation. IBM is the most common inflammatory myopathy in patients older than 50 years. It presents as a distal weakness and also has distinct biopsy findings. Studies so far have not yielded significant response to treatment. In both PM and DM, immune-mediated muscle inflammation and vascular damage occur.

- In PM, the immune system is primed to act against previously unrecognized muscle antigens.
- In DM, complement-mediated damage to endomysial vessels and microvasculature of the dermis occur.

The history and clinical presentation of patients with PM or DM typically include the following:

- Symmetric proximal muscle weakness with insidious onset. Muscle tenderness on palpation may be present.

- Dysphagia.
- Aspiration, if pharyngeal and esophageal muscles are involved.
- Arthralgias.
- Functional loss. Patient may have difficulty kneeling, climbing or descending stairs, raising arms, and arising from a seated position; weak neck extensors cause difficulty holding the head up. The involvement of the pelvic girdle is usually greater than the upper-body weakness.
- Characteristic rash of face, trunk, and hands (seen in DM only). The heliotrope rash is a symmetric, confluent, purple-red, macular eruption of the eyelids and periorbital tissue. Other rashes seen with DM include erythematous nail beds and a scaly, purple erythematous papular eruption over the dorsal metacarpophalangeal and interphalangeal joints (Gottron sign).
- Congestive heart failure (CHF), arrhythmia, interstitial lung disease, pneumonia/aspiration.

The PTA treating patients with these conditions is responsible for the following:

- Monitoring changes in the patient's condition for complications: vital signs, respiration, swallowing
- Maintaining or improving cardiovascular endurance without exacerbating fatigue
- Promoting independence in functional mobility skills and activities of daily living
- Teaching energy conservation techniques
- Providing psychological and emotional support
- Educating family and caregivers

Epilepsy

A seizure is an abnormal paroxysmal discharge of cerebral neurons due to cortical hyperexcitability.[224-233] The International Classification of Seizures divides seizures into two categories: partial seizures (i.e., focal or localization-related seizures) and generalized seizures.

Partial seizures:

- Result from a seizure discharge within a particular brain region or focus, and they manifest focal symptoms
- Can generalize secondarily and result in tonic–clonic activity

A reliable history of aura identifies the seizure as partial and not generalized.

Generalized convulsive seizures are always associated with loss of consciousness. Patients may report having a prodrome, which comprises premonitory symptoms occurring hours or days before a seizure. Common prodromes include mood changes, sleep disturbances, lightheadedness, anxiety, irritability, difficulty concentrating, and, rarely, an ecstatic feeling.

The patient may have completely nonfocal findings on neurologic examination when not having seizures. Seizures typically are divided into tonic, clonic, and postictal phases.

Tonic Phase

Generalized convulsive seizures may begin with myoclonic jerks or, rarely, with absences. This stage lasts for 10 to 20 seconds. The tonic phase begins with flexion of the trunk and elevation and abduction of the elbows. Subsequent extension of the back and neck is followed by extension of arms and legs. This can be accompanied by apnea, which is secondary to laryngeal spasm. Autonomic signs are common during this phase and include increase in pulse rate and blood pressure, profuse sweating, and tracheobronchial hypersecretion. Although urinary bladder pressure rises, voiding does not occur because of sphincter muscle contraction.

Clonic Phase

The tonic stage gives way to clonic convulsive movements, in which the tonic muscles relax intermittently, lasting for a variable period of time. During the clonic stage, a generalized tremor occurs at a rate of eight tremors per second, which may slow down to about four tremors per second. This is because phases of atonia alternate with repeated violent flexor spasms. Each spasm is accompanied by pupillary contraction and dilation. The atonic periods gradually become longer until the last spasm. Voiding may occur at the end of the clonic phase as sphincter muscles relax. The atonic period lasts about 30 seconds. The patient continues to be apneic during this phase.

The convulsion, including tonic and clonic phases, lasts for 1 to 2 minutes.

Postictal State

The postictal state includes a variable period of unconsciousness during which the patient becomes quiet and breathing resumes. The patient gradually awakens, often after a period of stupor or sleep, and often is confused and exhibits some automatic behavior. Headache and muscular pain are common. The patient does not recall the seizure itself.

The role of a PTA during a seizure event is as follows:

- Protect the patient from injury and remain with the patient

- Remove any potentially harmful nearby objects and loosen restrictive clothing
- Do not restrain the limbs
- Establish an airway and prevent aspiration. Artificial ventilation should not be initiated during tonic–clonic activity

Cerebellar Disorders

Lesions to the cerebellum are associated with intention tremor, ataxia, poor coordination of trunk and extremities, athetosis (repetitive involuntary, slow, sinuous, writhing movements, which are especially severe in the hands), dysmetria (a lack of coordination of movement typified by under- or overshooting the intended position with the hand, arm, leg, or eye), balance deficits, and dysdiadochokinesia (an inability to perform rapid, alternating movements).

Ataxia–Telangiectasia

Ataxia–telangiectasia (A–T) is an autosomal recessive, complex, multisystem disorder characterized by progressive neurologic impairment, cerebellar ataxia, variable immunodeficiency with susceptibility to sinopulmonary infections, impaired organ maturation, x-ray hypersensitivity, ocular and cutaneous telangiectasia, and a predisposition to malignancy.

Friedreich Ataxia

The major pathophysiologic finding in Friedreich ataxia (FA) is a "dying back phenomena" of axons, beginning in the periphery.[234–243] The primary sites of these changes are the spinal cord (posterior columns and corticospinal, ventral, and lateral spinocerebellar tracts) and spinal roots. Onset of FA is early, with gait ataxia (both of a sensory and cerebellar type) being the usual presenting symptom. Typically, both lower extremities are affected equally. The cerebellar features of gait ataxia in FA include a wide-based gait with constant shifting of position to maintain balance. Sitting and standing are associated with titubation (nodding movement of the head and body). Attempts to correct any imbalance typically result in abrupt and wild movements. As the disease progresses, ataxia affects the trunk, legs, and arms. As the arms become grossly ataxic, both action and intention tremors may develop. Facial, buccal, and arm muscles may become tremulous and occasionally display choreiform movements. The patient may experience easy fatigability.

Patients with advanced FA may have profound distal weakness of the legs and feet, although significant weakness of the arms is rare before the patient becomes bedridden. Eventually, the patient is unable to walk because of the progressive weakness and ataxia, becoming wheelchair bound and ultimately bedridden. With further disease progression, dysarthria and dysphagia appear. Speech becomes slurred, slow, and eventually incomprehensible. Incoordination of breathing, speaking, swallowing, and laughing may result in the patient nearly choking while speaking.

The goals of a physical therapy intervention will be determined from the findings from the clinical examination but will likely include some or all of the following:

- Ensuring functional mobility and safety through assistive and adaptive equipment as appropriate. Gaining postural stability (static and dynamic) through:
  - ❑ Weight-bearing postures
  - ❑ Weight-shifting progressions with carefully graded manual resistance
  - ❑ Reaching and pointing activities
- Promoting control during small-range movements, movement transitions (e.g., sitting to standing), and reversals of movement. Improving coordination with accuracy and precision of limb movements through:
  - ❑ Eye-hand coordination exercises
  - ❑ Eye-head coordination exercises
  - ❑ Upper- and lower-extremity coordination through Frenkel exercises (**Table 5-12**)
  - ❑ Proprioceptive neuromuscular facilitation (PNF) patterns
- Activities involving reciprocal movement (e.g., gait, stationary bike)
- Standing balance and gait activities.
- Patient education regarding energy conservation techniques.

Vestibular Disorders

Dizziness is one of the most common complaints adults report to physicians, and its prevalence increases with age.[244] Dizziness is not so much a disease but a symptom of disease. The four main categories of dizziness that patients describe are:

- *Vertigo:* An illusion of motion (an illusion is a misperception of a real stimulus); represents a disorder of the vestibular proprioceptive system. Of the various causes of vertigo, benign positional vertigo (BPV) is the most common cause (see next section).
- *Near-syncope:* Caused by reduced blood flow to the entire brain. Because the head

is above the heart, the CNS has evolved a complicated neural reflex that allows the preservation of blood flow to the brain in the standing position. However, many things can interfere with this reflex. Common causes include orthostatic hypotension (anemia, volume depletion, antihypertensive medications), cardiac disease (cardiomyopathy, dysrhythmias, aortic stenosis), vasovagal episodes (or neurocardiogenic syncope), and hyperventilation (decreases P_{CO_2}, which constricts blood vessels in the brain).

- *Dysequilibrium:* Essentially a gait disorder, most often caused by cervical spondylosis. Other causes include extrapyramidal disease and cerebellar disease.
- *Psychophysiologic dizziness:* The least understood source of dizziness; thought to be due to altered central integration of sensory signals arising from normal end organs. Some patients are overfocused on the normal physiological sensations, while others (such as those with panic syndrome) may have a neurochemical imbalance.

The etiology of peripheral and central vestibular deficits includes the following: age-related multisensory deficits, strokes and vascular insufficiencies, cerebellar degeneration, acoustic neuroma, chemical and drug toxicities, benign paroxysmal positional vertigo (BPPV), motion sickness, uncompensated Ménière disease, vestibular neuritis, labyrinthitis, and head trauma.

Balance disorders are significant risk factors for falls in elderly individuals. Falls have been estimated to be the leading cause of serious injury and death in persons older than 65 years.

Vestibular Neuronitis

Vestibular neuronitis[245–252] may be described as acute, sustained dysfunction of the peripheral vestibular system with secondary nausea, vomiting, and vertigo. As this condition is not clearly inflammatory in nature, neurologists often refer to it as vestibular neuropathy. Patients usually complain of abrupt onset of severe, debilitating vertigo with associated unsteadiness, nausea, and vomiting. They often describe their vertigo as a sense that either they or their surroundings are spinning. Viral infection of the vestibular nerve and/or labyrinth is believed to be the most common cause of vestibular neuronitis. Common findings include:

TABLE 5-12	Frenkel Exercises for Coordination

Exercises for Lower Extremities

Supine position	Flex and extend each leg at hip and knee joint, with heel sliding on bed.
	Abduct and adduct each leg with knee bent, with heel sliding on bed. Repeat same with knee extended.
	Flex and extend one knee at the time with heel raised.
	Place heel upon some definite part of the opposite leg—for example, on the patella, mid-tibia, ankle, or toes.
	Slide heel from contralateral knee joint down along shin and back to knee.
	Flex and extend both legs simultaneously, holding knees and ankles together.
	Draw up one extremity while extending the other to perform reciprocal flexion and extension.
	Flex and extend one leg and simultaneously abduct and adduct the other. Reverse procedure.
Sitting position	Alternately raise each leg, then place foot firmly on a footprint on the floor.
	Glide each foot alternately over a cross marked on the floor: forward, backward, to left, to right.
	With a foot in footprint, raise heel, lift foot off floor; in this position extend and flex knee, and bring toes back to original position; bring heel down in corresponding part of footprint.
	Practice sitting down on chair: Avoid falling into chair; allow muscles of hips and knees to ease the body down. Stand in front of chair, with knee slightly flexed and body bent slightly forward. Sit down by continuing the flexion of knees, hips, and trunk.
	Practice standing up: Draw feet back until they are partly under the chair so that the whole foot can be firmly planted. Bend body forward and rise slowly, extending the knees and hips and straightening the body.
Standing position	Walk on entire foot.
	Stand on tiptoe, then on the heel of one leg.
	Walk sideways a few steps in each direction.
	Walk between two parallel bars 14 inches apart, keeping a distance of 6 inches between the feet. Avoid outward rotation of legs.
	Walk on straight line; avoid toeing out.
	Take one half step and bring other foot in apposition. Continue taking several alternate half steps. Repeat with quarter steps.
	Alternate half and quarter steps, bringing each foot in apposition after each step. Then walk by alternate half steps and quarter steps.
	Make a complete turn to the left, using left heel as a pivot. Repeat to right.
	Walk along a circle on the floor, first in one direction, then in the other.

Reaching Activities for Extremities

	Place the hand or foot on marks at different levels on the wall.
	Add marks with chalk to symbols on blackboard, e.g., change minus to plus, cross *t*, dot *i*, play tic-tac-toe.
	Place small, readily grasped objects on squares of check board that has been numbered.
	Practice writing.
	Practice drawing geometric figures.

- Vertigo may increase with head movement.
- Patient may experience spontaneous, unidirectional, horizontal nystagmus (the most significant physical finding). Fast-phase oscillations beat toward the healthy ear. Nystagmus may be positional and apparent only when the patient is gazing toward the healthy ear, or during Hallpike maneuvers (a test that determines whether vertigo is triggered by certain head movements).
- The patient tends to fall toward his or her affected side when attempting ambulation or

during Romberg tests (a test that is based on the premise that a person requires at least two of the three following senses to maintain balance while standing: proprioception, sensation, and vision).
- The affected side has either unilaterally impaired or no response to caloric stimulation.

Central Vertigo
Vertigo implies an abnormal sensation of movement or rotation of the patient or his or her environment. Central vertigo[253-259] is vertigo due to a disease originating from the central nervous system (CNS). In clinical practice, it often includes lesions of cranial nerve VIII as well. Individuals with vertigo experience hallucinations of motion of their surroundings. Central vertigo may be caused by hemorrhagic or ischemic insults to the cerebellum, the vestibular nuclei, and their connections within the brain stem. Other causes include CNS tumors, infection, trauma, and multiple sclerosis.

Physical therapy will include:

- Implementation of safety measures: sensory substitution, compensatory strategies.
- Use of assistive and adaptive equipment as appropriate.
- Vestibular rehabilitation exercises and activities:
  - Habituation training: Repetition of movement and positions that provoke dizziness and vertigo.
  - Eye exercises: Involving up and down and side to side movements of the eyes, progressing from slow to fast movements.
  - Head motions in all directions, progressing from slow to fast movements.
  - Functional mobility training, with an emphasis on turning, rapid changes of direction, and activities involving spatial and timing constraints.

Benign Positional Vertigo
Benign positional vertigo (BPV)[260-270] is caused by calcium carbonate particles called otoliths (or otoconia) that are inappropriately displaced into the semicircular canals of the vestibular labyrinth of the inner ear. Patients with BPV characteristically perceive that the room or world seems to be spinning. Symptoms of BPV are usually worse in the morning (the otoliths are more likely to clump together as the patient sleeps) and improve as the day progresses (the otoliths become more dispersed with head movement). Nausea is typically present. A history of head trauma may be present, especially in young patients with BPV. The head trauma may dislodge the otoliths off their membrane within the utricle, allowing them the opportunity to enter the semicircular canals.

Labyrinthitis
Labyrinthitis is an inflammation or dysfunction of the vestibular labyrinth (a system of intercommunicating cavities and canals in the inner ear). The syndrome is defined by the acute onset of vertigo, commonly associated with head or body movement. Vertigo often is accompanied by nausea, vomiting, or malaise.

Ménière Syndrome
Ménière syndrome,[271-273] also known as endolymphatic hydrops, is an inner ear (labyrinthine) disorder in which there is an increase in volume and pressure of the endolymph of the inner ear. It typically presents with waxing and waning hearing loss and tinnitus associated with vertigo. Patients may report an abnormal sensation of pressure or fullness in the ears. Multiple episodes may occur over a span of years, with remissions between each acute episode. Hearing loss typically occurs.

Basal Ganglia Disorders
Parkinson Disease
For details about the pathogenesis, examination, and intervention of Parkinson disease, refer to Chapter 11.

Huntington Chorea
Huntington chorea (HC),[274-276] also known as Huntington disease (HD), is an autosomal dominant inherited disease characterized by degeneration and atrophy of the basal ganglia and cerebral cortex, which results in choreiform movements and progressive dementia. The autosomal dominant trait is linked to a defect of chromosome 4 and to the gene identified as *IT-15*. Symptoms arising from a typical presentation of HC usually do not develop until a person is aged 35 years or older. By the time of diagnosis, many patients already have had children and have passed the gene to another generation. The majority of patients affected by HC present with primary complaints of involuntary movements or rigidity. In the remainder of cases, the primary presentation is one of early mental status changes that initially appear as increased irritability, moodiness, or antisocial behavior. Classic choreiform movements begin as a piano-playing motion of the fingers or as facial grimaces. As the disorder advances and involves the trunk, a characteristic dancing gait evolves. Although patients appear to be off balance, the

ability to balance is actually well preserved. Dementia develops as the disease progresses. As HC progresses, the movement disorder becomes more generalized. Eventually, the patient's gait is impaired. Rigidity and dystonia predominate in later stages of the disease in adults. In juvenile cases, rigidity and dystonia may appear as the initial symptoms. Symptoms become worse with anxiety or stress.

Medical management of HC requires a multi-disciplinary approach. Once choreiform movement begins to impair a patient's functional capacity, pharmacological intervention in the form of anti-convulsants and antipsychotics can be initiated, but the associated adverse effects can be severe. However, suppression of the movements does not result in improved function, and most patients are actually untroubled by the choreic movements.

Physical therapy intervention focuses on maximizing:

- Strength (co-activation of muscles and trunk stabilization)
- Endurance
- Balance
- Postural control
- Functional mobility
- Patient education:
  - Relaxation through biofeedback
  - Prevention of deformities and contracture through prone lying
  - Specific stretching
  - Safety with mobility
- Caregiver education regarding posture, seating, transfer training, and the use of adaptive equipment

Cranial and Peripheral Nerve Disorders

Bell's Palsy

Bell's palsy[277-282] is one of the most common neurologic disorders affecting the cranial nerves. A common theory is that Bell's palsy is an inflammation of the facial nerve (CN VII), yet other cranial nerves are probably also affected. The actual pathophysiology is unknown, although vascular, infectious, genetic, and immunologic causes have all been proposed. The most common signs and symptoms include an abrupt, unilateral, peripheral facial paresis or paralysis with no explainable reason.

Most patients recover fully from this condition in several weeks or months. Some are prescribed medications (corticosteroids and analgesics). The physical therapy intervention in these patients is typically supportive, and includes:

- Providing some form of protection for the cornea (artificial tears or temporary patching)
- Providing electrical stimulation of specific motor points of the facial muscles to maintain tone and support function
- Prescribing facial muscle exercises, such as forehead wrinkle, eyebrow raises, frowning, smiling, eye closing, cheek puffing
- Providing functional training—for example, teaching the patient to chew on one side of the mouth

Peripheral Nerve Injury

Peripheral nerve injuries[283-290] may occur due to trauma (e.g., a blunt or penetrating wound, trauma) or acute compression. The clinical appearance of an injured nerve depends on the nerve affected and the extent of the injury. The classification of nerve injury described by Seddon in 1943 comprised neurapraxia, axonotmesis, and neurotmesis. Sunderland, in 1951, expanded this classification system to five degrees of nerve injury (**Table 5-13**). A sixth-degree injury was introduced by Mackinnon to describe a mixed nerve injury that combines the other degrees of injury.

The thoracic nerves may be involved in the same types of impairments that affect other peripheral nerves. A loss of function of one or more of the thoracic nerves may produce partial or complete paralysis of the abdominal muscles and a loss of the abdominal reflexes in the affected quadrants. With unilateral impairments of the nerve, the umbilicus usually is drawn toward the unaffected side when the abdomen is tensed (Beevor sign), indicating a paralysis of the lower abdominal muscles as a result of a lesion at the level of the 10th thoracic segment. A specific syndrome called the T4 syndrome[291-293] has been shown to cause vague pain, numbness, and paresthesia in the upper extremity and generalized posterior head and neck pain.

> **● Key Point** Injury to the long thoracic nerve leads to paralysis of the serratus anterior muscle, resulting in medial scapular winging.

The long and relatively superficial course of the long thoracic nerve makes it susceptible to injury. Injury to the long thoracic nerve can occur from any of the following causes.[294-297]

- Entrapment of the fifth and sixth cervical roots as they pass through the scalenus medius muscle
- Compression of the nerve during traction to the upper extremity by the undersurface of the scapula as the nerve crosses over the second rib

TABLE 5-13	Sunderland's Nerve Injury Classification System
First-degree (neuropraxia)	A temporary conduction block with demyelination of the nerve at the site of injury. Recovery may take up to 12 weeks.
Second-degree (axonotmesis)	Wallerian degeneration distal to the level of injury and proximal axonal degeneration to at least the next node of Ranvier. Axonal regeneration occurs at the rate of 1 millimeter per day or 1 inch per month.
Third-degree	Introduced by Sunderland to describe an injury more severe than second-degree injury. Wallerian degeneration occurs. Endoneurial tubes are not intact, and regenerating axons therefore may not reinnervate.
Fourth-degree	Large area of scar at the site of nerve injury that precludes any axons from advancing distal to the level of nerve injury. Patient requires surgery to restore neural continuity.
Fifth-degree	Complete transection of the nerve. Surgery is required to restore neural continuity.

■ Compression and traction to the nerve by the inferior angle of the scapula during general anesthesia or with passive abduction of the arm

An injury to the long thoracic nerve may cause scapular winging; that is, the scapula assumes a position of medial translation and upward rotation of the inferior angle.[298,299]

● **Key Point** The radial nerve is frequently entrapped at its bifurcation in the region of the elbow, where the common radial nerve becomes the sensory branch and a deep or posterior interosseous branch.

The major disability associated with radial nerve injury is a weak grip, which is weakened because of poor stabilization of the wrist and finger joints. In addition, the patient demonstrates an inability to extend the thumb, wrist, and elbow, as well as the proximal phalanges. Pronation of the forearm and adduction of the thumb also are affected, and the wrist and fingers adopt a position termed *wrist drop*. The triceps and other radial reflexes are absent, but the sensory loss is often slight, owing to overlapping innervation.

The site of the entrapment of the radial nerve can often be determined by the clinical findings, as follows:

■ If the injury occurs at a point below the triceps innervation, the strength of the triceps remains intact.

■ If the injury occurs at a point below the brachioradialis branch, some supination is retained.

■ If the injury occurs at a point in the forearm, the branches to the small muscle groups, extensors of the thumb, extensors of the index finger, extensors of the other fingers, and extensor carpi ulnaris may be affected.

■ If the injury occurs at a point on the dorsum of the wrist, only sensory loss on the hand is affected.

● **Key Point** The clinical features of median nerve impairment, depending on the level of injury, include the following:[7]

• Paralysis is noted in the flexor–pronator muscles of the forearm, all of the superficial palmar muscles except the flexor carpi ulnaris, and all of the deep palmar muscles, except the ulnar half of the flexor digitorum profundus and the thenar muscles that lie superficial to the tendon of the flexor pollices longus.
• In the forearm, pronation is weak or lost.
• At the wrist, there is weak flexion and radial deviation, and the hand inclines to the ulnar side.
• In the hand, an ape-hand deformity can be present. This deformity is associated with:
  • An inability to oppose or flex the thumb, or abduct it in its own plane.
  • A weakened grip, especially in thumb and index finger, with a tendency for these digits to become hyperextended and the thumb adducted.
  • An inability to flex the distal phalanx of the thumb and index finger.
  • Weakness of middle finger flexion.
  • Atrophy of the thenar muscles.
• There is a loss of sensation to a variable degree over the cutaneous distribution of the median nerve, most constantly over the distal phalanges of the first two fingers.
• Pain is present in many median nerve impairments.
• Atrophy of the thenar eminence is seen early. Atrophy of the flexor–pronator groups of muscles in the forearm is seen after a few months.
• The skin of the palm is frequently dry, cold, discolored, chapped, and at times keratotic.

Herniated Lumbar Disc

A herniated disc is an intervertebral disc that bulges and protrudes posterolaterally against a nerve root. Sciatica is a set of symptoms, including pain, that may be caused by general compression and/or irritation of one of five spinal nerve roots (L4–5, S1–3) that give rise to each sciatic nerve, or by compression or irritation of the sciatic nerve. Injury to the sciatic nerve may also result from a hip dislocation, local aneurysm, or direct external trauma of the sciatic notch, the latter of which can be confused with a compressive radiculopathy of the lumbar or sacral nerve root.[304] Following are some useful clues to help distinguish the two conditions:

- Pain from radiculopathy should not significantly change with hip motion except in the case of a straight leg raise, whereas with a sciatic entrapment by the piriformis pain is accentuated with hip internal rotation and relieved by hip external rotation.
- Sciatic neuropathy produces sensory changes on the sole of the foot, whereas radiculopathy generally does not, unless there is predominant S1 involvement.
- Compressive radiculopathy below the L4 level causes palpable atrophy of the gluteal muscles, whereas a sciatic entrapment spares these muscles.
- The sciatic trunk is frequently tender from root compression at the foraminal level, whereas it is not normally tender in a sciatic nerve entrapment.[305,306]

The natural history of radiculopathy and disc herniation is not quite as favorable as for simple low back pain, but it is still excellent, with approximately 50% of patients recovering in the first 2 weeks and 70% recovering in 6 weeks.[130] Complete bed rest is not recommended in the first 4 to 6 weeks after onset of symptoms.[131,132] Surgery is often recommended after 4 to 6 weeks, if the symptoms persist, following MRI and CT scan findings.[133] The physical therapy intervention focuses on a return to normal activities as soon as possible, patient education and involvement, and therapeutic exercises. The McKenzie exercise progression can be valuable to the overall intervention strategy and, if centralization of pain occurs, a good response to physical therapy can be anticipated.[137,138] In cases of radiculopathy, the goal is to decrease radiating symptoms into the limb and, thus, to centralize the pain using specific maneuvers or positions, such as the lateral shift correction. Once this centralizing position is identified, the patient is instructed to perform these maneuvers repetitively or sustain certain positions for specific periods throughout the day.[79] In addition, the patient is instructed in a lumbar stabilization program in which neutral zone mechanics are practiced in various positions to decrease stress to the lumbosacral spine. Lumbar stabilizing exercises have been recommended to improve lumbar function in patients with low back injury so that these patients may improve their activities of daily living.[134]

The conservative intervention for mild cases of peripheral nerve injury typically includes protection of the joints, including the surrounding ligaments and tendons, activity modification, passive range of motion, and physician-prescribed NSAIDs. Splints, slings, or both may be prescribed. For example, a radial nerve injury results in a loss of wrist and finger extension, a "wrist drop." A wrist-resting splint may be used to support the hand in a neutral wrist position and place the hand in a more functional position. In patients with brachial plexus nerve injuries, particularly when C5–6 is affected, continued downward stress at the glenohumeral joint may cause the glenohumeral joint to subluxate without the muscle support of the rotator cuff muscles. A sling is helpful to unload this joint, prevent complete shoulder dislocation, and decrease pain. Night splints appear to help to reduce the nocturnal symptoms associated with carpal tunnel syndrome and allow the wrist to rest fully. Splints worn during the day are helpful only if they do not interfere with normal activity. The positioning of the splint may be significant. Ergonomic modifications can help reduce the incidence of peripheral nerve injuries and alleviate symptoms in the already symptomatic patient. Patient education is also important to avoid sustained activities and positions/postures as well as repetitive motions.

The surgical intervention for nerve injuries can involve reconstruction, nerve grafting, and nerve transfer:

- *Reconstruction:* Reconstruction of nerve continuity can be performed with direct repair. This is performed when the two ends of the nerve can be directly coapted without tension. If the repair cannot be performed without tension, nerve grafting is performed. If the adjacent joint must be flexed or extended to permit coaptation of the distal and proximal ends of the nerve, a nerve graft is used. (With wrist flexion, the median nerve can be directly repaired; if it is under tension with a wrist-neutral position, a nerve graft is used.)
- *Nerve graft:* In cases in which a gap is present between the proximal and distal end of the nerve, a nerve graft is typically used. The use of a donor nerve results in a sensory loss in the distribution of the donor nerve. This area of sensory loss becomes smaller over 1 to 3 years with collateral sprouting from the surrounding sensory nerves. In cases in which a large nerve gap is present, the sural nerve is used due to the large length of nerve graft material that can be obtained. For shorter nerve gaps, the anterior branch of the medial antebrachial cutaneous (MABC) nerve is a good nerve graft donor because the donor site scar is minimal and the resultant sensory loss is on the anterior aspect of the forearm.
- *Nerve transfer:* The concept of a nerve-to-nerve transfer permits a normal neighboring

noncritical nerve to be coapted to the distal end of the injured nerve. This is particularly useful in cases in which a large nerve gap is present and/or for proximal nerve injuries.

Following nerve surgery, the patient is sent to therapy, initially for the splint and then for exercises. Initially, the goals of therapy are to regain passive range of motion of the joints and soft tissues that have been immobilized. The patient should be instructed in exercises to maintain strength in the unaffected muscles. In the later stages, sensory and motor reeducation is recommended to maximize the outcome.

Herpes Zoster
Varicella-zoster virus infection initially produces chickenpox.[307–314] Following resolution of the chickenpox, the virus lies dormant in the dorsal root ganglia until focal reactivation along a ganglion's distribution results in herpes zoster (shingles). Herpes zoster manifests as a vesicular rash, usually in a single dermatome. Development of the rash may be preceded by paresthesias or pain along the involved dermatome. Ocular involvement and zoster keratitis may result if the ophthalmic division of the trigeminal nerve is involved. Involvement of the geniculate ganglion may produce the syndrome of Ramsay Hunt, characterized by development of pain in the ear and unilateral facial paralysis with herpetic vesicles of the external ear or tympanic membrane (without paralysis, this is termed *herpes zoster oticus*). Occasionally, Ramsay Hunt syndrome is associated with vertigo, tinnitus, and hearing disorders.

Trigeminal Neuralgia
Trigeminal neuralgia (TN), also known as tic douloureux, is a pain syndrome recognizable by patient history alone.[315–325] The condition is characterized by pain often accompanied by a brief facial spasm or tic. Pain distribution is unilateral and follows the sensory distribution of cranial nerve V, typically radiating to the maxillary (V2) or mandibular (V3) area. At times, both distributions are affected. The clinical presentation is as follows:

- Pain, which is typically unilateral and described as stabbing or shock-like, is brief and paroxysmal, but it may occur in volleys of multiple attacks. One or more branches of the trigeminal nerve (usually maxillary or mandibular) are involved.
- Activities such as shaving, face washing, or chewing often trigger an episode.

Spinal Muscular Atrophy

The spinal muscular atrophies (SMAs)[326–332] are characterized by primary degeneration of the anterior horn cells of the spinal cord and often of the bulbar motor nuclei without evidence of primary peripheral nerve or long-tract involvement. Because bulbar features are often present, the term *SMA* does not technically describe the disorder. Consequently, alternative designations, such as bulbospinal muscular atrophy, hereditary motor neuronopathy (HMN), and progressive muscular atrophy, have been used. The SMAs present with a diversity of symptoms and differ in age of onset, mode of inheritance, distribution of muscle weakness, and progression of symptoms. Additionally, atypical forms of the disease have been described, including those with associated sensory deficits, hearing loss, or arthrogryposis. Patients typically present with predominantly LMN signs that include hypotonia (i.e., loss of postural tone), flaccid weakness, decreased or absent stretch reflexes, fasciculations, and atrophy. The physical therapy role is based on the presenting impairments.

Guillain–Barré Syndrome

In its classic form, Guillain–Barré syndrome (GBS)[333–344] is an acute inflammatory demyelinating polyneuropathy characterized by progressive symmetric ascending muscle weakness, paralysis, and hyporeflexia with or without sensory or autonomic symptoms. In severe cases, muscle weakness may lead to respiratory failure, and labile autonomic dysfunction may complicate the use of vasoactive and sedative drugs. Peripheral nerves and spinal roots are the major sites of demyelination, but cranial nerves also may be involved. GBS is believed to result from an autoimmune response—the typical GBS patient presents 2 to 4 weeks after a relatively benign respiratory or gastrointestinal illness complaining of dysesthesias of the fingers and lower-extremity proximal muscle weakness. The weakness may progress over hours to days to involve the arms, truncal muscles, cranial nerves, and the muscles of respiration. The illness progresses from days to weeks. A plateau phase of persistent, unchanging symptoms then ensues, followed days later by gradual symptom improvement. Up to one-third of patients require hospitalization for cardiac monitoring, plasma exchange, and mechanical ventilation during the course of the disease. Pharmacological intervention often includes immunosuppressive and analgesic/narcotic medications. Causes of Guillain–Barré include cranial nerve involvement affecting airway maintenance and respiratory muscle paralysis.

The role of physical therapy includes:

- Helping to maintain respiratory function
- Providing pulmonary (chest) physical therapy
- Preventing indirect impairments such as:
  - Skin breakdown
  - Contractures
  - Injury to denervated muscles
  - Splinting and positioning
- Guiding muscle reeducation through active assistance and active exercise progressing to resistive exercises
- Teaching energy conservation techniques and activity pacing
- Improving cardiovascular endurance
- Implementing functional mobility and gait training progressions as appropriate

Amyotrophic Lateral Sclerosis

Amyotrophic lateral sclerosis (ALS),[345–352] commonly known as Lou Gehrig's disease, is a disease characterized by slowly progressive degeneration of upper and lower motor neurons. No single cause for ALS explains its entire pathology. Upper motor neuron involvement of spinal cord tracts results in spastic weakness of the limbs (primary lateral sclerosis). Later, spread to other motor areas produces the classic combination of upper and lower motor neuron dysfunction recognized as ALS:

- *Bulbar symptoms:* The patient's family first notices slurring of words or choking during a meal. An aspiration event or acute respiratory symptoms of air hunger occur.
- *Arm weakness:* The patient notices wrist drop interfering with his or her work performance.
- *Leg weakness:* The patient develops foot drop resulting in a fall or sprain.
- *Lower motor neuron signs:* The patient experiences weakness, atrophy, fasciculations, and depressed reflexes. Fasciculations are observed with the muscle at rest.
- *Upper motor neuron signs:* The patient experiences an upper motor neuron pattern of weakness (greatest in the extensors of the arm and flexors of the leg), spastic bulbar and limb muscles, hyperreflexia, and extensor plantar responses. A hyperreflexic jaw jerk helps to confirm upper motor neuron involvement causing dysarthria and dysphagia.

- *Ocular, sensory, or autonomic dysfunction:* These symptoms occur only very late in the disease course.
- *Respiratory impairments:* ALS is eventually fatal because of respiratory muscle weakness. Aspiration pneumonia and medical complications of immobility contribute to morbidity.

Younger patients may have a slower rate of progression. Patients with bulbar onset, particularly the lower motor neuron type, have a poorer prognosis.

The medical intervention includes the use of disease-modifying agents for symptomatic management. The physical therapy role with ALS is restorative intervention geared toward remediating or improving impairments and functional limitations. This includes:

- Maintenance of respiratory function
- Pulmonary physical therapy: airway clearance techniques, cough facilitation, breathing exercises, chess stretching, suctioning, incentive spirometry
- Prevention of indirect impairments, such as:
  - Skin breakdown
  - Contractures
  - Injury to denervated muscles
  - Splinting and positioning
- Muscle reeducation through active assistance and active exercise progressing to resistive exercises; aerobic exercises should be carefully monitored to prevent fatigue or overwork
- Energy conservation techniques and activity pacing
- Improvement or maintenance of cardiovascular endurance
- Functional training and progression; maintaining maximal functional independence
- Implementation of devices and adaptive equipment as appropriate
- Patient, family, caregiver education

Post-Polio Syndrome

Post-polio syndrome (PPS) is a condition that affects polio survivors years after recovery from an initial acute attack of the poliomyelitis virus.[353–363] PPS is mainly characterized by new weakening in muscles that were previously affected by the polio infection and in muscles that seemingly were unaffected. Symptoms usually appear earlier in patients who have very severe residual weakness, those who experience early bulbar respiratory difficulty in the acute illness, and those who were older when they contracted acute polio. The basic management principles for individuals with PPS include energy conservation and pacing one's activities. Patients usually benefit from different adaptive techniques and equipment to perform any activities of daily living. A speech therapy evaluation usually is recommended with any suggestion of swallowing problems.

Motor Learning

Motor learning is a complex set of internal processes that involve the relatively permanent acquisition and retention of a skilled movement or task through practice.[364–366]

- *Performance:* Involves acquisition of a skill
- *Learning:* Involves both acquisition and retention of a skill

Three basic types of motor tasks are involved in motor learning:[97,367]

- *Discrete:* Involves a movement with a recognizable beginning and end. For example, throwing a ball or opening a door.
- *Serial:* Involves a series of discrete movements that are combined in a particular sequence. For example, getting out of a chair when using crutches.
- *Continuous:* Involves repetitive, uninterrupted movements that have no distinct beginning and ending. Examples include walking and cycling.

> ● **Key Point** Note the following definitions:
> - *Action:* The observable outcome resulting from the performer's purposeful interaction with the environment.
> - *Movement:* The means by which action is realized.
> - *Neuromotor processes:* The organizational mechanisms within the central nervous system (CNS) that constrain and sequence movement.

A number of theories of skill acquisition have been proposed:

- Open (temporal and spatial factors in an unpredictable environment) versus closed skills (spatial factors only in a predictable environment), involving a single dimensional continuum. Using sports as an example, a closed skill could include shooting a foul shot in basketball. An example of an open skill would involve playing through a ball in soccer. Open and closed skills can be viewed as a continuum, where the perceptual and habitual nature of a task determines whether the task is open or closed.

- Gentile's taxonomy of motor tasks.[368] This two-dimensional classification system for teaching motor skills uses the concept that motor skills range from simple to complex. Gentile expanded the popular one-dimensional classification system of open and closed skills to combine the environmental context together with the function of the action (**Table 5-14**):[367,369]
  - ❑ The environmental (closed or open) context in which the task is performed. Regulatory conditions (other people, objects) in the environment may be either stationary (closed skills) or in motion (open skills).
  - ❑ The intertrial variability (absent or present) of the environment that is imposed on the task. When the environment in which a task is set is unchanging from one performance of a task to the next, intertrial variability is absent; the environmental conditions are predictable—for example, walking on just one type of surface. Intertrial variability is present when the demands change from one attempt or repetition of the task to the next—for example, walking over varying terrain.
  - ❑ The need for a person's body to remain stationary (stable) or to move (transport) during the task. Skills that require body transport are more complex than skills that require no body transport as there are more variables to consider. For example, a body transport task could include walking in a crowded shopping mall.
  - ❑ The presence or absence of manipulation of objects during the task. When a person must manipulate an object, the skill increases in

complexity because the person must do two things at once—manipulate the object correctly and adjust the body posture to fit the efficient movement of the object.

Table 5-14 illustrates Gentile's taxonomy of tasks. 1A represents the simplest task, and 4D represents the most complex task.

Stages of Motor Learning

There are three stages of motor learning:[369]

- *Cognitive:* This stage begins when the patient is first introduced to the motor task. The patient must determine the objective of the skill as well as the relational and environmental cues to control and regulate the movement. The patient is more concerned with what to do and how to do it. During this phase, the PTA should provide frequent and explicit positive feedback using a variety of forms of feedback (verbal, tactile, visual), and allow trial and error to occur within safe limits.
- *Associative:* The patient is concerned with performing and refining the skills. The important stimuli have been identified and their meaning is known. Conscious decisions about what to do become more automatic, and the patient concentrates more on the task and appears less rushed. During this phase, the PTA should begin to increase the complexity of the task, emphasize problem solving, avoid manual guidance, and vary the sequence of tasks.
- *Autonomous:* This stage is characterized by a nearly automatic kind of performance—for example, when walking occurs automatically without conscious thought. During this phase,

TABLE 5-14	Gentile's Taxonomy				
		Body Stability		Body Transport	
Environmental Context		No Object Manipulation	Object Manipulation	No Object Manipulation	Object Manipulation
Stationary regulatory conditions	No intertrial variability	1A	1B	1C	1D
	Intertrial variability	2A	2B	2C	2D
In motion regulatory conditions	No intertrial variability	3A	3B	3C	3D
	Intertrial variability	4A	4B	4C	4D

the PTA should set up a series of progressively more difficult activities the patient can do independently, such as increasing the speed, distance, and complexity of the task.

Practice and Feedback

Practice, repeatedly performing a movement or series of movements in a task, is probably the single most important variable in learning a motor skill.[367,369] The various types of practice for motor learning are outlined in **Table 5-15**. Second only to practice, feedback is considered the next most important variable that influences learning. The various types of feedback associated with motor learning are outlined in **Table 5-16**.

Theories of Neurological Rehabilitation

For theories of motor development, refer to Chapter 10.

Constraint-Induced Movement Therapy

Constraint-induced movement therapy[98–103] has been demonstrated to effect significant and large improvements in upper extremity function. Two factors that are critical to the successful outcomes achieved with this technique are:

- The concentrated and repetitive practice of the involved upper extremity.
- The restriction of movement in the uninvolved upper extremity through the use of mitts, sling, or brace so that the patient is forced to use the involved side to perform functional movements. This has the consequence of increasing the total number of movements that the involved side has to perform.

Task-Oriented Approaches

The task-oriented (functional) approaches are based on scientists' current understanding of how movement arises from the interaction between systems at the levels of the individual, the environment, and the task. Central to the functional/task-oriented approach to motor control is the idea that specific task-oriented training with extensive practice is essential to reacquiring skill and enhancing recovery.[96] This approach is sometimes referred to as the *systems approach* as

TABLE 5-15	Types of Practice for Motor Learning	
Type of Practice	**Components**	**Description**
Part versus whole	Part	A task is broken down into separate components and the individual components (usually the more difficult) are practiced. After mastery of the individual components, the components are combined in a sequence so the whole task can be practiced.
	Whole	The entire task is performed from beginning to end and is not practiced in separate components.
Blocked, random, and random-blocked	Blocked	The same task or series of tasks is performed repeatedly under the same conditions and in a predictable order—for example, consistently practicing walking in the same environment.
	Random	Slight variations of the same task are carried out in an unpredictable order. For example, a patient could practice on a variety of walking surfaces.
	Random-blocked	Variations of the same task are performed in random order, but each variation of the task is performed more than once. For example, the patient walks on a particular surface and then repeats the same task a second time before moving on to a different surface.
Physical versus mental	Physical	The movements of a task are actually performed.
	Mental (visualization, imagery)	A cognitive rehearsal of how a motor task is to be performed occurs prior to actually doing the task.

Data from Kisner C, Colby LA: Therapeutic exercise: Foundational concepts, in Kisner C, Colby LA (eds): Therapeutic Exercise: Foundations and Techniques (ed 5). Philadelphia, F. A. Davis, 2002, pp 1–36

TABLE 5-16	Types of Feedback Associated with Motor Learning

Type of Feedback	Description
Intermittent versus continuous	Intermittent: Occurs irregularly, randomly; has been shown to promote learning more effectively than continuous feedback.
	Continuous: Is ongoing. Patients improve skill acquisition more quickly during the initial stage of learning and intermittent feedback.
Immediate, delayed, and summary	Immediate: Is given directly after a task is completed; used most frequently during the cognitive (initial) stage of learning.
	Delayed: Is given after an interval of time elapses, allowing the learner to reflect on how well or poorly a task was performed. Promotes retention and generalizability of the learned skills.
	Summary: Is given about the average performance of several repetitions of the movement or task; used most frequently during the associative stage of learning.
Knowledge of performance (KP) versus knowledge of results (KR)	KP: Can be either intrinsic feedback sense during a task or immediate, post-task, extrinsic feedback (usually verbal) about the nature or quality of the performance of the motor task.
	KR: Immediate, post-task, extrinsic feedback about the outcome of the motor task.
Intrinsic	A sensory cue (proprioceptive, kinesthetic, tactile, visual, or auditory) or set of cues inherent in the execution of the motor task and that arise from within the learner and are derived from performance of the task. They may immediately follow completion of a task or may occur even before task has been completed.
Extrinsic (augmented)	Sensory cues from an external source (mechanical or from another person) that are supplemental to the intrinsic feedback but are not inherent in the execution of the task. Unlike intrinsic feedback, the clinician can control the type, timing, and frequency of extrinsic feedback.

Data from Kisner C, Colby LA: Therapeutic exercise: Foundational concepts, in Kisner C, Colby LA (eds): Therapeutic Exercise: Foundations and Techniques (ed 5). Philadelphia, F. A. Davis, 2002, pp 1–36

it views the entire body as a mechanical system with many interacting subsystems that all work cooperatively in managing internal and environmental influences. In this approach, it is assumed that normal movement emerges as an interaction among many systems, each contributing its own aspect of control. In addition, the movement is organized around a behavioral goal (using behavioral shaping techniques) and is constrained by the environment. Thus, the role of sensation in normal movement is not limited to a stimulus-response reflex mode but is essential to predictive and adaptive control of movement as well. The examination approach of this system utilizes observation of functional performance, analysis of the strategies or compensations used to accomplish tasks, and the assessment of impairments. Using this information, the clinician focuses on resolving impairments, designing and implementing an effective recovery and compensation strategies, and retraining the patient using functional activities. The functional/task-oriented approach is currently emphasized in interventions for children with neuromuscular disorders such as cerebral palsy (CP).[370]

Rood's Concept of Levels of Control

Rood's concept that sensory stimuli affect the motor response uses a series of positions and activities that go through the normal sequencing of motor development. Muscles are classified as either mobilizers or stabilizers. The development stages include:

- Mobility (reciprocal interaction)
- Stability (co-contraction)
- Controlled mobility (proximal muscles move while the distal muscles are fixed)
- Skill (proximal muscles are fixed while the distal muscles move)

Impairment-Focused Interventions

Impairment-focused training includes developmental activity training, motor training, movement pattern training, and neuromuscular education or reeducation.[96] A central concept of this approach was the use of sensory input to modify the CNS and stimulate motor output. Two of the most popular approaches include neurodevelopmental treatment (NDT) and proprioceptive neuromuscular facilitation (PNF).

Neuro Motor Development Treatment

The neuromotor development treatment (NDT) approach evolved from the work of Karl and Berta Bobath, whose work focused on the hierarchical model of neurophysiologic function. The theoretical basis for this approach is that a maturational lag in the integration of primitive postural reflexes is often found in learning-disabled children. Based on this finding, it was assumed that abnormal postural reflex activity and abnormal muscle tone was caused by the loss of central nervous system control at the brainstem and spinal cord levels. Thus the emphasis was on the inhibition/integration of primitive postural patterns, the promotion of the development of normal postural reactions, and the normalization of abnormal tone, while avoiding abnormal and compensatory patterns of movement. Current NDT theory recognizes that many different factors can contribute to the loss of motor function in patients with neurological dysfunction, including the full spectrum of sensory and motor deficits. NDT therapy emphasizes the importance of postural control in skill learning.

The NDT approach uses facilitatory, inhibitory, and reinforcement techniques:

- *Inhibition:* A technique utilized to decrease/ inhibit the capacity to initiate a movement response to altered synaptic potential. Inhibitory techniques include positioning and the use of specific movement patterns.
- *Facilitation:* A technique utilized to elicit voluntary muscular contraction through guided and assisted movement. It aims to develop normal sensory motor behavior by using the normal movement released by the prior inhibition process.
- *Reinforcement:* Reinforcement of inhibition of abnormal behavior by the repeated use and development of the released normal movement.

The other key areas of treatment of this approach include:

- The normalization of postural alignment and stability.
- The normalization of sensory/perceptual experiences.

- The resumption of normal functional activities through meaningful and goal-oriented patterns of movement.

Proprioceptive Neuromuscular Facilitation

The concept of proprioceptive neuromuscular facilitation (PNF; also termed *complex motions*) was developed by Hermann Kabat, then by Charles Sherrington, and finally by Margaret Knott and Dorothy Voss (**Table 5-17, Table 5-18**, and **Table 5-19**).

The Brunnstrom Approach: Movement Therapy in Hemiplegia

This approach is based on the hierarchical model using a combination of very precise observation of the sequential changes in motor function that typically occurred following stroke and an understanding of the reflex function of the nervous system. The Brunnstrom approach emphasizes eliciting motor behavior in the sequence in which it would occur following a stroke, using synergy patterns. Despite the fact that reinforcing synergy patterns is rarely utilized these days, except for stroke patients, Brunnstrom's very detailed and accurate observations have enabled clinicians to document patients' progress based on Brunnstrom's seven stages of recovery (**Table 5-20**).

Integrated Approach

To develop an effective treatment program for patients with motor developmental problems,[366] a number of factors must be considered:

- Variable practice within a class of movement will facilitate skill transfer to a novel condition of the constant practice.
- The practice order within a treatment session should be random or serial, rather than involving repetitive practice of one activity per treatment session. The former creates regeneration of a motor plan, which ultimately facilitates recall of the task.
- The specific tasks related to motor learning should involve functional activities and pre-gait activities (as appropriate). Functional activities include bed mobility, repositioning, and arising from the floor.

Bed mobility involves:

- Rolling to side lying
- Rolling to prone
- Scooting up in bed

TABLE 5-17	Proprioceptive Neuromuscular Facilitation Terms and Techniques

Technique	Description
Irradiation (overflow)	The spread of energy from the prime agonist to complementary agonists and antagonists within a pattern. Can occur from proximal to distal, distal to proximal, upper trunk to lower trunk (and vice versa) muscle groups, and from one extremity to another. Weaker muscle groups benefit from the irradiation they gain while working in synergy with stronger, more normal partners. Irradiation is stimulated by the clinician through the use of resistance.
Manual and maximal resistance	In PNF, the direction, quality, and quantity of resistance are adjusted to prompt a smooth and coordinate response, whether for stability (i.e., holds) or for ease, smoothness, and pace of movement. The resistance should be at an appropriate level to prompt proper irradiation and facilitate function and should be no greater than the resistance that allows full ROM to occur.
Verbal cueing	Effective verbal cues coordinate the clinician's efforts with the patient's.
Approximation and traction	Joint compression stimulates afferent nerve endings and encourages extensor muscles and stabilizing patterns (co-contraction), thereby inhibiting abnormal tone and enhancing stabilization of the proximal segment. Compression techniques can be used to prepare a joint for weightbearing. Joint traction provides a stretch stimulus and enhances movement by elongating the adjacent muscles. Traction techniques are commonly used in the presence of pain to inhibit excessive compression and facilitation of flexor muscles and mobilizing patterns. Traction techniques may also be used to help decrease spasticity.
Stretch	Stretch is frequently performed at the starting position of the pattern or movement to promote reflexive activity that is facilitating. The resulting reflex activation is then synchronized with volitional effort through verbal cues.
Timing	Describes the sequencing of movement. Timing for emphasis suggests that, to facilitate and enhance muscular response, the clinician can intentionally interrupt the normal timing sequence at specific points in the ROM to the more powerful muscle groups to obtain "overflow" to weaker muscle groups. These techniques can be performed within a limb (ipsilateral from one muscle group to another) or using overflow from one limb to contralateral limb, or trunk to limb and the techniques are typically combined with repeated contractions to the weak components, or superimposed upon normal timing in a distal to proximal sequence. Indications include weakness, incoordination.
Combination of isotonics (formerly referred to as agonist reversals)	A slow isotonic, shortening contraction through the range followed by an eccentric, lengthening contraction using the same muscle groups. Indications include weak postural muscles, inability to eccentrically control body weight during movement transitions—for example, sitting down.
Stabilizing reversals (formerly referred to as alternating isometrics)	Isometric holding is facilitated first on one side of the joint, followed by alternate holding of the antagonist muscle groups. Can be applied in any direction (anterior–posterior, medial–lateral, diagonal). Indications include instability in weight bearing and holding, poor antigravity control, weakness, ataxia.
Contract–relax (CR)	A relaxation technique usually performed at a point of limited range of motion in the agonist pattern: isotonic movement in rotation is performed followed by an isometric hold of the range-limiting muscles in the antagonist pattern against slowly increasing resistance, then voluntary relaxation, and active contraction in the newly gained range of the agonist pattern. The patient is then asked to contract the muscle(s) to be stretched (agonists).The clinician resists this contraction except for the rotary component. The patient is then asked to relax, and the clinician moves the joint further into the desired range. Indications include limitations in range of motion caused by muscle adaptive shortening, spasticity. Although primarily used as a stretching technique, due to the isometric contractions involved, some strengthening does occur.
Hold–relax (HR)	A similar technique in principle to contract–relax, except that, when the patient contracts, the clinician allows no motion (including rotation) to occur. Following the isometric contraction the patient's own contraction causes the desired movement to occur. Typically used as a relaxation technique in the acutely injured patient as it tends to be less aggressive than the contract/relax technique.

(continued)

Proprioceptive Neuromuscular Facilitation Terms and Techniques (continued)

Technique	Description
Replication (formerly referred to as hold-relax–active motion)	An isometric contraction performed in the mid- to shortened range followed by a voluntary relaxation and passive movement into the lengthened range, and resistance to an isotonic contraction through the range. May be used with patients who have an inability to initiate movement, hypotonia, weakness, and marked imbalances between antagonists.
Manual contact	A deep but painless pressure is applied through the clinician's contact to stimulate a muscle, tendon, and/or joint afferents.
Maximal resistance	Resistance is applied to stronger muscles to obtain overflow to weaker muscles. Indications include weakness, muscle imbalances.
Quick stretch	A suddenly applied motion stimulates the tendon receptors, resulting in a facilitation of motor recruitment and thus more force.
Reinforcement	The coordinated use of the major muscle groups, or other body parts, to produce a desired movement pattern. Often used to increase the stability of the proximal segments.
Repeated contractions (RC)	A unidirectional technique that involves repeated isotonic contractions induced by quick stretch. Enhanced by resistance performed to the range or part of range at the point of weakness. Indications include weakness, incoordination, muscle imbalances, lack of endurance. Facilitation of the agonist and relaxation of the antagonist.
Reversals of antagonists	Many functional tasks involve reversing movement patterns that task body balance and postural stability. For example, the reciprocal activity of the limbs in the swing compared with stance phases of walking. To facilitate static and dynamic postural ballots, reciprocal movement of the antagonistic groups is facilitated with static (isometric) or dynamic (isotonic) contractions.
Dynamic reversals of antagonists (formerly referred to as slow reversal)	The technique of dynamic reversals enhances reciprocal or reversing motions. Dynamic (isotonic) contractions of antagonistic movements are facilitated reciprocally in a range appropriate to the goal of the exercise. Indications include inability to reverse directions, muscle imbalances, weakness, incoordination, and instability.
Rhythmic initiation (RI)	Unidirectional or bidirectional voluntary relaxation followed by passive movement through increasing range of motion, followed by active-assisted contractions progressing to light tracking resistance to isotonic contractions. Indications include spasticity, rigidity, inability to initiate movement, motor learning deficits, communication deficits.
Rhythmic stabilization (RS)	The application of alternating isometric contractions of the agonist and antagonist muscles to stimulate movement of the agonist, develop stability, and relax the antagonist. Indications include instability in weight bearing and holding, poor antigravity control, weakness, ataxia. May also be used to decrease limitations in range of motion caused by adaptive muscle shortening and painful muscle splinting.
Stabilizing reversals	Alternating resistance is applied to an agonist–antagonist pair while seeking a maximal dynamic (isotonic) contraction. The technique is similar in many ways to rhythmic stabilization, but it can also be used when the patient is unable to perform a true static (isometric) contraction.
Rhythmic rotation	Voluntary relaxation combined with slow, passive, rhythmic rotation of the body or body part around a longitudinal axis and passive movement into newly gained range. Active holding in the new range is then stressed. Indications include hypertonia with limitations in functional range of motion.
Resisted progression (RP)	A stretch and tracking resistance is applied in order to facilitate progression in walking, creeping, kneel-walking, or movement transitions. Indications include impaired strength, timing, motor control, and endurance.

TABLE 5-18 — PNF Patterns for the Upper Extremities

Joint	D1 Flexion	D1 Extension	D2 Flexion	D2 Extension
Scapulothoracic	Upward rotation, abduction, (protraction) anterior elevation	Downward rotation, adduction, (retraction) posterior depression	Upward rotation, adduction, posterior elevation	Downward rotation, abduction, anterior depression
Glenohumeral	External rotation, adduction, flexion	Internal rotation, abduction, extension	External rotation, abduction, flexion	Internal rotation, adduction, extension
Elbow	Flexion	Extension	Flexion	Extension
Radioulnar	Supination	Pronation	Supination	Pronation
Wrist	Flexion, radial deviation	Extension, ulnar deviation	Extension, radial deviation	Flexion, ulnar deviation
Fingers	Flexion, adduction to the radial side	Extension, abduction to the ulnar side	Extension, abduction to the radial side	Flexion, adduction to the ulnar side
Thumb	Flexion, abduction	Extension, abduction	Extension, adduction	Flexion, abduction

TABLE 5-19 — PNF Patterns for the Lower Extremities

Joint	D1 Flexion	D1 Extension	D2 Flexion	D2 Extension
Hip	External rotation, adduction, flexion	Internal rotation, abduction, extension	Internal rotation, abduction, flexion	External rotation, adduction, extension
Knee	Flexion or extension	Extension or flexion	Flexion or extension	Extension or flexion
Ankle	Dorsi flexion	Plantar flexion	Dorsi flexion	Plantar flexion
Subtalar	Inversion	Eversion	Eversion	Inversion
Toes	Extension, abduction to the tibial side	Flexion, adduction to the fibular side	Extension, abduction to the fibular side	Flexion, adduction to the tibial side

- Transitioning from supine position to short sitting

Repositioning in a chair involves:

- Transitioning from sitting to standing
- Gaining lateral weight relief
- Gaining anterior/posterior weight relief

Arising from the floor involves:

- Pulling up on support (anterior approach)
- Pushing up (posterior support)
- Arising from the half-kneel position

Cognitive Rehabilitation

Cognitive rehabilitation is a systematic, goal-oriented treatment program designed to improve cognitive functions and functional abilities, and to increase levels of self-management and independence following neurological damage to the central nervous system. Although the specific tasks are individualized to patients' needs, treatment generally emphasizes restoring lost functions, teaching compensatory strategies to circumvent impaired cognitive functions, and improving competence in performing instrumental activities of daily living (IADLs) such as managing medications, using the telephone, and handling finances. Cognitive rehabilitation has been postulated to lead to maintenance or improvement in language, memory, and other cognitive abilities in neurologically impaired individuals. There are a number of treatment approaches to cognitive rehabilitation.[371]

TABLE 5-20	Brunnstrom's Seven Stages of Recovery from Stroke
Stage	Description
1	No volitional movement initiated.
2	The appearance of basic limb synergies. The beginning of spasticity.
3	The synergies are performed voluntarily; spasticity increases.
4	Spasticity begins to decrease. Movement patents are not dictated solely by limb synergies.
5	A further decrease in spasticity is noted with independence from limb synergy patterns.
6	Isolated joint movements are performed with coordination.
7	Normal motor function is restored.

Data from Brunnstrom S: Motor testing procedures in hemiplegia: Based on sequential recovery stages. Phys Ther. 46:357–75, 1966

Retraining Approach

Also known as the transfer of training approach, this approach is based on the assumption that a disruption in one brain region can have a negative impact on brain functioning as a whole. It focuses on the remediation of underlying skills the patient has lost. Intervention focuses on doing specifically selected perceptual exercises, such as pegboard activities, under the premise that practicing one task with particular cognitive perceptual requirements will enhance performance in other tasks with similar perceptual demands.

Restorative Cognitive Rehabilitation

Also known as the restorative approach, the restorative cognitive rehabilitation (RCR) approach is based on the theory that repetitive exercise can restore lost functions. It targets internal cognitive processes with a goal of generalizing improvements in real-world environments. Intervention techniques include auditory, visual, and verbal stimulation and practice; number manipulation; computer-assisted stimulation and practice; performance feedback; reinforcement; video feedback; and meta-cognitive procedures such as behavior modification.

Sensory Integrative Approach

This approach involves the integration of basic sensorimotor functions (tactile, proprioceptive, and vestibular) that proceed in a developmental sequence in a normal child within the context of goal-directed, meaningful activity. Some of the treatment modalities employed include rubbing or icing to provide sensory input, resistance, and weight bearing to impart proprioceptive input, and the use of spinning to provide vestibular input.

Neurofunctional Approach

The focus of this approach is on retraining real-world skills rather than on retraining specific cognitive and perceptual processes.

Compensatory Cognitive Rehabilitation

The compensatory cognitive rehabilitation (CCR) approach works toward developing external prosthetic assistance for dysfunctions. CCR does not rely on the ability to generalize learning or restore lost abilities. CCR employs visual cues, written instructions, memory notebooks, watches, beepers, computers, and other electronic devices to trigger behavior. Clinicians simplify complex tasks, capture the patient's attention, minimize distractions, and teach self-monitoring procedures. This approach encourages and reinforces an individual's remaining strengths with the goal of achieving or maintaining independence.

Management Strategies for Specific Conditions

Strategies to Manage Hypertonia

Physical and occupational therapists play important roles in the management of patients with spasticity. Essential to the management of spasticity is the avoidance of noxious stimuli, prompt intervention for urinary tract complications, proper skin care, and prevention of thrombophlebitis and heterotopic ossification.[372] Precise handling of a spastic limb is important—the clinician should use constant, firm manual contacts positioned over nonspastic areas to avoid directly stimulating spastic muscles.[26] Specific intervention techniques include:[26]

- *Prolonged icing:* The application of cold packs, with the duration variable depending on patient response.
- *Prolonged stretch:* A slow, maintained stretch, applied at maximum available lengthened range.
- *Inhibitory pressure:* Deep, maintained pressure applied across the longitudinal axis of tendons; prolonged positioning in extreme lengthened range.

- *Neutral warmth:* Retention of body heat to the application of bandage wraps, snug-fitting clothing, towel wraps, and tepid baths to the body or body parts.
- *Rhythmic rotation:* A highly effective exercise technique that can be used to reduce hypotonicity and increase range. Relaxation is achieved with slow, repeated rotation of a limb at a point where limitation is noticed. As muscles relax, the limb is slowly and gently (actively or passively) moved into the range, and as new tension is felt, the technique is repeated.[26]
- *Neuromuscular electrical stimulation (NMES):*[82] Neuromuscular electrical stimulation is the application of electrical stimuli to a group of muscles, for the purpose of muscle rehabilitation.
- *Transcutaneous electrical nerve stimulation (TENS):*[81] The use of electric current produced by a device to stimulate the nerves for therapeutic purposes.

Serial Casting

Serial casting[75–79] is a method by which a series of casts are applied to a joint to reduce contracture. Serial casting is used when traditional techniques fail and the patient is at risk for development of contractures and deformity, or demonstrates ineffective movement patterns or severe limitations in hygiene and skin care.[26] Inhibitory and ROM techniques are first used to move the limb into its fully lengthened range.[26] The cast is then applied while the limb is held at the end of the available range. The prolonged stretch (minimum of 6 hours) applied to the muscle during casting mimics the stretch applied by growing bone. Each time a cast is removed (every 5 to 7 days), the joint is further stretched to its comfortable end range and recasted.

- Conditions in which contractures commonly develop include cerebral palsy, burns, traumatic brain injury, stroke, extended periods of immobility, and spinal cord injury.
- The joints that are commonly casted include the ankles (plantarflexion contractures), knees, elbows, and wrists (flexion contractures).
- The muscles most commonly involved with contractures include the two joint muscles of the gastrocnemius, hamstrings, and finger flexors.

The materials commonly used in the fabrication of serial casts include:

- *Plaster:* Advantages include cost and time allowed to adjust the cast before it sets. Disadvantages include its heaviness.
- *Fiberglass:* Advantages include choice of colors, light weight. Disadvantages include the cost and speed of setting.
- *SoftCast:* Advantages include ease of removal, light weight, and allowance of more movement within the cast. Disadvantages include cost.

> ● **Key Point** The terms R_1 and R_2 are used with serial casting:
> - R_1: The initial end range encountered when a joint is moved quickly through its arc of motion—the functional range of motion.[80]
> - R_2: The maximal range of motion that can be achieved.[80]
>
> For example, if the goal is to achieve a functional range of 10 degrees of ankle dorsiflexion (R_1), the maximal range to cast (R_2) must be greater than 10 degrees.

Indications for serial casting include:[80]

- Less than full functional range of motion of a joint.
- Reliable patient or caregiver to monitor for swelling or color change.
- Adequate therapy, with splints or orthotics, available after casting is completed.

Contraindications for serial casting include:[26]

- Poor casting techniques, such as lack of range positioning of the limb, loose-fitting cast, or insufficient padding
- Severe heterotopic ossification
- Muscle rigidity
- Skin conditions such as open wounds, blisters, or abrasions
- Impaired circulation and edema
- Uncontrolled hypertension
- Unstable intracranial pressure
- Pathological inflammatory conditions such as arthritis or gout
- Individuals at risk for compartment syndrome or nerve impingement
- Application to individuals with long-standing contractures (longer than 6 to 12 months)

Functional Electrical Stimulation

While the short-term effect of functional electrical stimulation is to decrease spasticity, long-term use has been associated with increasing spasticity in patients with incomplete spinal cord injury and quadriplegia.

Thermotherapy and Cryotherapy

Superficial heat can reduce hypertonicity by facilitating uptake of released neurotransmitters and returning calcium to the sarcoplasmic reticulum. Cryotherapy is reported to reduce deep tendon reflexes and clonus.

Sensory Stimulation

Mechanical vibration of large muscles has been shown to reduce spasticity.

Nerve Blocks

To reduce tone in spastic muscles, a local injection with anesthetic paralytic or escharotic agent may be performed. The anatomic localization of the injection site determines which nerve and/or muscle is affected; the type of medication and its concentration, volume, and proximity to neuroactive structures determine the intensity and duration of that effect. Medications useful in nerve block procedures include local anesthetics, phenol, absolute alcohol, and botulinum toxin. Many clinicians use various combinations of treatments. The distribution of spasticity is vital in determining whether to use focal or global treatment, and in deciding which measures should be used.

Intrathecal Baclofen

Intrathecal baclofen (ITB)[373] consists of long-term delivery of baclofen to the intrathecal space. This treatment can be helpful for patients with severe spasticity affecting the lower extremities, particularly for patients whose conditions are not sufficiently relieved by oral baclofen and other oral medications.

Surgical Management

The surgical management of spasticity can be divided into orthopedic and neurosurgical procedures. Careful preoperative evaluation is important in assessing patients with spastic contractures, and treatment of each individual area must be tailored to each patient's specific problems. In the upper and lower extremities, the general goals of surgical treatment are to improve function, improve hygiene, provide pain relief, and facilitate total care of the patient.

Strategies to Manage Hypotonia

Range of Motion

Active and passive range of motion techniques applied in conjunction with proper positioning and splinting are recommended. A daily program of stretching helps restore resting length of muscle, tendon, and joint capsule and can prevent contracture.

Therapeutic Exercise

Therapeutic exercise may be applied in several forms. Neurodevelopmental techniques invoke proprioceptive neuromuscular facilitation. Active or resisted exercises are used to strengthen spastic limbs, which must include a balancing of agonist and antagonist muscle groups. Decreased spasticity and improvements in range of motion and strength have considerable implications for activities such as dressing, bathing, feeding, and grooming.

REVIEW Questions

1. In a patient with a spinal cord injury at the T12 level, which of the following would *not* be one of the expected goals in the POC?
   a. Independent control of the trunk musculature above the level of T12
   b. Good sitting balance
   c. Bowel and bladder control
   d. Ambulation without assistive device
2. The femoral nerve innervates all but which of the following muscles?
   a. Sartorius
   b. Vastus lateralis
   c. Adductor magnus
   d. Pectineus
3. A patient presents with weak quadriceps muscles with a diagnosis of a lumbar disc herniation. What other muscle has the same innervation?
   a. Sartorius
   b. Adductor magnus
   c. Biceps femoris
   d. Iliopsoas
4. You are treating a patient with a hemi-section of the spinal cord (Brown–Sequard) at the T12 level. Which of the following would you likely find?
   a. Muscle paralysis
   b. Loss of position sense
   c. Loss of pain sensation
   d. Loss of vibratory sense
5. What happens to the intracranial pressure of a patient placed in the Trendelenburg position? Does it increase or decrease?
6. Which of the following would you expect to find in a patient diagnosed with carpal tunnel syndrome?
   a. Tingling in the ulnar side of the hand and reports of pain in the hand with rest

b. Tingling in the radial side of the hand and pain in the hand at night
   c. Loss of peripheral vision
   d. Pain with elbow extension

7. Which of the following is characterized by a deep sleep from which the patient cannot be aroused?
   a. Stupor
   b. Lethargy
   c. Coma
   d. Obtundation

8. All of the following are true statements with regard to epidural hematomas, except:
   a. They are mostly venous in origin, involving the venous dural sinuses.
   b. They are most commonly caused by head trauma.
   c. They are commonly characterized by alternating CNS depression—with lethargy and confusion.
   d. They are, acutely, the most serious of the intracranial hemorrhages.

9. Myasthenia gravis is an example of a myopathy due to:
   a. Nerve injury
   b. Muscle disuse
   c. Metabolic abnormality
   d. Myoneural junction block

10. Which of the following would least likely be a causative agent in encephalitis?
    a. Polio
    b. Pneumococcus
    c. Measles
    d. Rabies

11. Which two cranial nerves arise from the midbrain?

12. Which four cranial nerves arise from the pons?

13. How many pairs of spinal nerves are there?
    a. 32
    b. 31
    c. 33
    d. 24

14. Which nerve roots commonly form the cervical plexus?

15. Which nerve roots commonly form the brachial plexus?

16. What are the three divisions of the trigeminal nerve called?

17. Which two cranial nerves have distributions in other regions besides the head and neck?

18. Which area of the brain controls the autonomic nervous system?

19. Which of the two systems, parasympathetic or sympathetic, stimulates the release of epinephrine from the adrenal medulla?

20. Which nerve innervates all but one of the intrinsic muscles of the tongue?

21. Which nerve innervates the sternocleidomastoid and the trapezius muscles?

22. An injury to which part of the brachial plexus would cause weakness of the biceps, coracobrachialis, and finger flexors?

23. An injury to which part of the brachial plexus would cause an inability to raise the arm over 90 degrees of shoulder flexion?

24. An injury to which part of the brachial plexus would cause an inability to extend the arm and perform wrist extension?

25. Which cord of the brachial plexus supplies the radial nerve?

26. What three arm muscles does the musculocutaneous nerve supply?

27. A lesion to which nerve results in a claw-hand deformity?

28. Which peripheral nerve is responsible for stimulating the muscles that produce dorsiflexion?

29. Which two nerves innervate the adductor magnus?

30. Which peripheral nerve can be trapped in the Arcade of Frohse?

31. Which peripheral nerve can be trapped between the two heads of the pronator teres?

32. Which peripheral nerve can be trapped by the ligament of Struthers?

33. Atrophy of the hypothenar eminence could indicate a lesion to which nerve?

34. A lesion to which nerve can result in an ape-hand deformity?

35. List two special tests the PT could use to help diagnose carpal tunnel syndrome.

36. Which muscles does the suprascapular nerve innervate?

37. Which nerve innervates the serratus anterior?

38. Which nerve innervates the latissimus dorsi muscle?

39. Which muscles are innervated by the superior gluteal nerve?

40. A herniated disc between the C6 and C7 vertebral levels could impinge upon which nerve root level?

41. Injury to the radial nerve in the spiral groove would result in weakness of which group of muscles?

42. Which of the following muscles is not innervated by the median nerve?
    a. Abductor pollicis brevis
    b. Flexor pollicis longus
    c. Medial heads of flexor digitorum profundus
    d. Superficial head of flexor pollicis brevis
    e. Pronator quadratus
43. Name the nerve that innervates the first lumbrical muscle in the hand.
44. A patient reports a burning sensation in the anterolateral aspect of the thigh. Dysfunction of which nerve could lead to these symptoms?
    a. Lateral cutaneous (femoral) nerve of the thigh
    b. Femoral
    c. Obturator
    d. Genitofemoral
    e. Ilioinguinal
45. The saphenous nerve supplies cutaneous sensation to the medial aspect of the leg. From which nerve does the saphenous nerve arise?
    a. Obturator
    b. Deep fibular (peroneal)
    c. Sciatic
    d. Femoral
    e. The saphenous nerve arises as a direct branch from the sacral plexus
46. An injury to the deep branch of the fibular (peroneal) nerve would result in a sensory deficit to which of the following locations?
    a. Medial side of the foot
    b. Lateral side of the foot
    c. Lateral one and one-half toes
    d. Medial border of the sole of the foot
    e. Adjacent dorsal surfaces of the first and second toes
47. A brachial plexus injury in the upper portion of the plexus produces winging of the scapula. Weakness of which of the following muscles would produce the winging observed?
    a. Long head of the triceps
    b. Supraspinatus
    c. Deltoid
    d. Pectoralis major
    e. Serratus anterior
48. Which of the following flexor muscles is not innervated by the median nerve?
    a. Flexor carpi radialis
    b. Flexor carpi ulnaris
    c. Palmaris longus
    d. Flexor digitorum superficialis
    e. Flexor pollicis longus

49. Which two muscles does the anterior interosseous branch of the median nerve innervate?
50. A birth injury that results in injury to the lower portion of the brachial plexus is referred to as:
    a. Bell palsy
    b. Erb paralysis
    c. Klumpke paralysis
    d. Saturday night palsy
    e. Tinel sign
51. The axillary nerve can occasionally be injured when it passes through which muscle?
52. The lateral ventricles of the brain drain into what structure?
53. Which arteries are connected by the anterior communicating artery in the brain?
54. Name the structure that connects the anterior intercranial division and the posterior intercranial division blood supplies of the brain.
55. In the brain, what is Wernicke's area responsible for?
56. Which structure connects the two cerebral hemispheres?
57. Which cranial nerve is responsible for chewing?
58. Which nerve supplies cutaneous sensation to the dorsum of the medial one and one-half fingers?
59. Identify six impairments or functional limitations that would warrant (or indicate the need for) a PT examination of sensory function.
60. Define the following: *arousal*, *attention*, *orientation*, and *cognition*.
61. Salutatory conduction in a nerve fiber refers to:
    a. Difference in nervous tissue conduction when the person is on a high sodium diet.
    b. Difference in nervous tissue conduction when the person is on a low sodium diet.
    c. The increased conduction velocity as the action potential jumps from node to node of Ranvier.
    d. The method by which pain transmissions are conducted.
62. Sensory perception of vibration is mediated through:
    a. Pacinian corpuscles
    b. Free nerve endings
    c. The proprioceptive receptors
    d. All the different tactile receptors
63. All of the following are false about the stretch reflex except:
    a. It is found only in primates.
    b. It may be either mono- or polysynaptic.

c. It is more easily demonstrated than any other reflex.

d. It is monosynaptic.

64. All of the following features may be found in muscle spindles except:
    a. They require a change in length as well as in the rate of change in order to fire.
    b. They demonstrate two kinds of intrafusal fibers: nuclear bag and nuclear chain fibers.
    c. They are arranged in parallel with the extrafusal fibers of the muscle itself.
    d. They are innervated by one very large, type Ia fiber that serves both fiber types.

65. True or false: Muscle spindles, under normal conditions, emit sensory nerve impulses constantly.

66. The perception of the position of the extremities in space is often referred to as:
    a. Depth perception
    b. Spatial discrimination
    c. Paresthesias
    d. Kinesthesia

67. The organ most concerned with detecting sensations relating to equilibrium is:
    a. The cochlea
    b. The cerebellum
    c. The vestibular apparatus
    d. The pinna

68. All of the following are examples of the simple stretch reflex, except:
    a. Knee-jerk
    b. Monosynaptic reflex
    c. Myotatic reflex
    d. Flexor withdrawal reflex

69. All of the following spinal functions are affected during or following spinal shock, except:
    a. Autonomic regulation of blood pressure
    b. All skeletal muscle reflexes integrated in the spinal cord
    c. The sacral reflexes for control of bladder and colon evacuation
    d. The vomiting reflex

70. The two cerebral hemispheres derive from what early embryological portion of the neural tube?
    a. Metencephalon
    b. Mesencephalon
    c. Telencephalon
    d. Diencephalon

71. Which lobe of the brain is responsible for vision and integration of visual data?

72. Which lobe of the brain is responsible for somatic sensory perception and interpretation?

73. Which lobe of the brain is responsible for memory, hearing, and comprehension of speech?

74. Which portion of the brain regulates peripheral autonomic nervous system discharges and is responsible for homeostatic mechanisms such as regulation of body temperature?
    a. Hypothalamus
    b. Thymus
    c. Thalamus
    d. The pons

75. Which of the following structures do not compose the limbic system?
    a. The parahippocampal gyrus
    b. A cingulate gyrus
    c. The uncus
    d. The corpus callosum

76. Functions of the "right brain" include all of the following except:
    a. Control of the left side of the body
    b. Tactile identification of objects
    c. Control of the right side of the body
    d. Processing of information

77. The red nucleus is involved in all of the following except:
    a. Motor movement
    b. Postural reflex patterns
    c. Blushing
    d. None of the above

78. True or false: The autonomic nervous system serves as the essential neurogenic regulatory system for homeostatic maintenance.

79. True or false: The sympathetic division maintains normal homeostasis during rest and prepares the body for stress, while the parasympathetic system returns functions to normal following stress.

80. All of the following controls are affected by the ANS except:
    a. Heart rate and blood pressure
    b. Body temperature regulation
    c. Fine motor control
    d. Sweating and salivation

81. You have been asked to use the neurodevelopmental treatment (NDT) approach with a patient recovering from stroke. Which of the following components would not be included?
    a. Facilitation of early movement in synergistic patterns followed quickly by movement patterns out of synergy.
    b. Reduction of spasticity and abnormal reflex activity through positioning and handling techniques.

   c. Facilitation of selective movement control out of synergistic patterns.

   d. Functional activities emphasizing reintegration of the hemiplegic side.

82. You have been asked by the PT to perform an adaptive equipment check for a 3-year-old boy with moderate spastic diplegia. Which of the following equipment is *not* indicated in this case?

   a. Bilateral KAFOs

   b. Prone stander

   c. AFOs to reduce tone

   d. Posterior walker

83. You are performing an intervention for an individual recovering from traumatic brain injury who demonstrates Rancho Level Cognitive Function VII. The best intervention strategy in this case would be to:

   a. Involve the patient in decision making, emphasizing safety and independent performance.

   b. Provide a high degree of environmental structure.

   c. Provide assistance for guided movements during all movement tasks.

   d. Provide maximum supervision to ensure successful performance.

84. In treating an 87-year-old resident of a community nursing home diagnosed with organic brain syndrome, Alzheimer's type, it is important to understand that he:

   a. Will likely be resistant to activity training if unfamiliar activities are used.

   b. Can usually be trusted to be responsible for his daily care needs.

   c. Is more likely to remember current experiences then past ones.

   d. Can usually be trusted with transfers and with appropriate positioning of the wheelchair.

85. During surgery to remove an apical lung tumor, the long thoracic nerve was injured. The muscle that you would expect to find weakened (3+/5) is:

   a. Serratus anterior

   b. Upper trapezius

   c. Serratus anterior

   d. Subscapularis

References

1. Martin J: Introduction to the central nervous system, in Martin J (ed): Neuroanatomy: Text and Atlas (ed 2). New York, McGraw-Hill, 1996, pp 1–32

2. Van de Graaff KM, Fox SI: Functional organization of the nervous system, in Van de Graaff KM, Fox SI (eds): Concepts of Human Anatomy and Physiology. New York, WCB/McGraw-Hill, 1999, pp 371–406

3. Waxman SG: Correlative Neuroanatomy (ed 24). New York, McGraw-Hill, 1996

4. Morgenlander JC: The autonomic nervous system, in Gilman S (ed): Clinical Examination of the Nervous System. New York, McGraw-Hill, 2000, pp 213–225

5. Bogduk N: Innervation and pain patterns of the cervical spine, in Grant R (ed): Physical Therapy of the Cervical and Thoracic Spine. New York, Churchill Livingstone, 1988

6. Fawcett DW: The nervous tissue, in Fawcett DW (ed): Bloom and Fawcett: A textbook of histology. New York, Chapman & Hall, 1984, pp 336–339

7. Chusid JG: Correlative Neuroanatomy & Functional Neurology, (ed 19). Norwalk, Conn, Appleton-Century-Crofts, 1985, pp 144–148

8. Reis FP, de Camargo AM, Vitti M, et al: Electromyographic study of the subclavius muscle. Acta Anatomica 105:284–90, 1979

9. Hoffman GW, Elliott LF: The anatomy of the pectoral nerves and its significance to the general and plastic surgeon. Ann Surg 205:504, 1987

10. Delagi EF, Perotto A: Arm, in Delagi EF, Perotto A (eds): Anatomic Guide for the Electromyographer (ed 2). Springfield, Charles C Thomas, 1981, pp 66–71

11. Sunderland S: The musculocutaneous nerve, in Sunderland S (ed): Nerves and Nerve Injuries (ed 2). Edinburgh, Churchill Livingstone, 1978, pp 796–801

12. de Moura WG, Jr.: Surgical anatomy of the musculocutaneous nerve: A photographic essay. J Reconstr Microsurg 1:291–297, 1985

13. Flatow EL, Bigliani LU, April EW: An anatomic study of the musculocutaneous nerve and its relationship to the coracoid process. Clin Orthop 244:166–171, 1989

14. Stern PJ, Kutz JE: An unusual variant of the anterior interosseous nerve syndrome: a case report and review of the literature. J Hand Surg 5:32–34, 1980

15. Hope PG: Anterior interosseous nerve palsy following internal fixation of the proximal radius. J Bone and Joint Surg 70B:280–282, 1988

16. Amadio PC, Beckenbaugh RD: Entrapment of the ulnar nerve by the deep flexor-pronator aponeurosis. J Hand Surg Am 11A:83–87, 1986

17. Hirasawa Y, Sawamura H, Sakakida K: Entrapment neuropathy due to bilateral epitrochlearis muscles: A case report. J Hand Surg Am 4:181–184, 1979

18. Chen FS, Rokito AS, Jobe FW: Medial elbow problems in the overhead-throwing athlete. J Am Acad Orthop Surgeons 9:99–113, 2001

19. Mannheimer JS, Lampe GN: Clinical Transcutaneous Electrical Nerve Stimulation. Philadelphia, F. A. Davis, 1984, pp 440–445

20. Ecker AD, Woltman HW: Meralgia paresthetica: A report of one hundred and fifty cases. J. Am. Med. Assn 110:1650–1652, 1938

21. Keegan JJ, Holyoke EA: Meralgia paresthetica: An anatomical and surgical study. J Neurosurg 19:341–345, 1962

22. Reichert FL: Meralgia paresthetica; a form of causalgia relieved by interruption of the sympathetic fibers. Surg Clin

North Am 13:1443, 1933

23. Sunderland S: Traumatized nerves, roots and ganglia: Musculoskeletal factors and neuropathological consequences, in Knorr IM, Huntwork EH (eds): The Neurobiologic Mechanisms in Manipulative Therapy. New York, Plenum, 1978, pp 137–166

24. Kenny P, O'Brien CP, Synnott K, et al: Damage to the superior gluteal nerve after two different approaches to the hip. Journal of Bone & Joint Surgery 81B:979–81, 1999

25. Ohsawa K, Nishida T, Kurohmaru M, et al: Distribution pattern of pudendal nerve plexus for the phallus retractor muscles in the cock. Okajimas Folia Anatomica Japonica 67:439–41, 1991

26. Norkin CC: Examination of gait, in O'Sullivan SB, Schmitz TJ (eds): Physical Rehabilitation (ed 5). Philadelphia, F. A. Davis, 2007, pp 317–363

27. Dommisse GF, Grobler L: Arteries and veins of the lumbar nerve roots and cauda equina. Clin Orthop 115:22–29, 1976

28. Halle JS: Neuromusculoskeletal scan examination with selected related topics, in Flynn TW (ed): The Thoracic Spine and Rib Cage: Musculoskeletal Evaluation and Treatment. Boston, Butterworth-Heinemann, 1996, pp 121–146

29. McCloskey DI: Kinesthetic sensibility. Physiol Rev 58: 763–820, 1978

30. Borsa PA, Lephart SM, Kocher MS, et al: Functional assessment and rehabilitation of shoulder proprioception for glenohumeral instability. J Sport Rehabil 3:84–104, 1994

31. Lephart SM, Warner JJP, Borsa PA, et al: Proprioception of the shoulder joint in healthy, unstable and surgically repaired shoulders. J Shoulder Elbow Surg 3:371–380, 1994

32. Lephart SM, Henry TJ: Functional rehabilitation for the upper and lower extremity. Orthop Clin North Am 26:579–592, 1995

33. Lee WA: Anticipatory control of postural and task muscles during rapid arm flexion. J Mot Behav 12:185–196, 1980

34. Skinner HB, Barrack RL, Cook SD: Age-related decline in proprioception. Clin Orthop 184:208–211, 1984

35. Barrett DS, Cobb AG, Bentley G: Joint proprioception in normal, osteoarthritic and replaced knees. J. Bone Joint Surg 73–B:53–56, 1991

36. Barrack RL, Skinner HB, Buckley SL: Proprioception in the anterior cruciate deficient knee. Am J Sports Med 17:1–6, 1989

37. Barrett DS: Proprioception and function after anterior cruciate ligament reconstruction. J Bone Joint Surg 73B: 833–837, 1991

38. Beard DJ, Kyberd PJ, Fergusson CM, et al: Proprioception after rupture of the anterior cruciate ligament: An objective indication of the need for surgery? J. Bone Joint Surg 75–B:311–315, 1993

39. Corrigan JP, Cashman WF, Brady MP: Proprioception in the cruciate deficient knee. J. Bone Joint Surg 74–B:247–250, 1992

40. Fremerey RW, Lobenhoffer P, Zeichen J, et al: Proprioception after rehabilitation and reconstruction in knees with deficiency of the anterior cruciate ligament: A prospective, longitudinal study. Journal of Bone & Joint Surgery [Br] 82:801–806, 2000

41. Voight M, Blackburn T: Proprioception and balance training and testing following injury, in Ellenbecker TS (ed): Knee Ligament Rehabilitation. Philadelphia, Churchill Livingstone, 2000, pp 361–385

42. Skinner HB, Wyatt MP, Hodgdon JA, et al: Effect of fatigue on joint position sense of the knee. J Orthop Res 4: 112–118, 1986

43. Williams GR, Chmielewski T, Rudolph KS, et al: Dynamic knee stability: Current theory and implications for clinicians and scientists. J Orthop Sports Phys Ther 31: 546–566, 2001

44. Voight ML, Cook G: Impaired neuromuscular control: Reactive neuromuscular training, in Prentice WE, Voight ML (eds): Techniques in Musculoskeletal Rehabilitation. New York, McGraw-Hill, 2001, pp 93–124

45. Berg K: Balance and its measure in the elderly: A review. Physiolother Can 41:240–246, 1989

46. Shaffer SW, Harrison AL: Aging of the somatosensory system: A translational perspective. Phys Ther. 87:193–207, 2007

47. Benjuya N, Melzer I, Kaplanski J: Aging-induced shifts from a reliance on sensory input to muscle cocontraction during balanced standing. J Gerontol A Biol Sci Med Sci. 59:166–171, 2004

48. Markus EJ, Petit TL: Neocortical synaptogenesis, aging, and behavior: Lifespan development in the motor-sensory system of the rat. Exp Neurol 96:262–278, 1987

49. Mackenzie RA, Phillips LH, 2nd: Changes in peripheral and central nerve conduction with aging. Clin Exp Neurol 18:109–116, 1981

50. Schmitz TJ: Examination of sensory function, in O'Sullivan SB, Schmitz TJ (eds): Physical Rehabilitation (ed 5). Philadelphia, F. A. Davis, 2007, pp 121–157

51. White DJ: Musculoskeletal examination, in O'Sullivan SB, Schmitz TJ (eds): Physical Rehabilitation (ed 5). Philadelphia, F. A. Davis, 2007, pp 159–192

52. Takahashi T, Ishida K, Yamamoto H, et al: Modification of the functional reach test: Analysis of lateral and anterior functional reach in community-dwelling older people. Arch Gerontol Geriatr 42:167–173, 2006

53. Schmitz TJ: Examination of coordination, in O'Sullivan SB, Schmitz TJ (eds): Physical Rehabilitation (ed 5). Philadelphia, F. A. Davis, 2007, pp 193–225

54. Lenke LG: Lenke classification system of adolescent idiopathic scoliosis: Treatment recommendations. Instr Course Lect 54:537–42, 2005

55. Lenke LG, Edwards CC, 2nd, Bridwell KH: The Lenke classification of adolescent idiopathic scoliosis: How it organizes curve patterns as a template to perform selective fusions of the spine. Spine 28:S199–207, 2003

56. Lowe T, Berven SH, Schwab FJ, et al: The SRS classification for adult spinal deformity: Building on the King/Moe and Lenke classification systems. Spine 31:S119–S125, 2006

57. Weinstein SL, Ponseti IV: Curve progression in idiopathic scoliosis. J Bone Joint Surg Am 65:447–455, 1983

58. Faber MJ, Bosscher RJ, van Wieringen PC: Clinimetric properties of the performance-oriented mobility assessment. Phys Ther 86:944–954, 2006

59. Ponseti IV, Friedman B: Prognosis in idiopathic scoliosis. J Bone Joint Surg Am 32A:381–395, 1950

60. Dutton M: The nervous system, in Dutton M (ed): Orthopedic examination, evaluation, & intervention. New York, McGraw-Hill, 2004, pp 7–19

61. Goldberg S: The four minute neurological examination. Miami, Medmaster, 1992

62. Judge RD, Zuidema GD, Fitzgerald FT: Head, in Judge RD, Zuidema GD, Fitzgerald FT (eds): Clinical Diagnosis (ed 4). Boston, Little, Brown and Company, 1982, pp 123–151

63. Legaspi O, Edmond SL: Does the evidence support the existence of lumbar spine coupled motion? A critical review of the literature. J Orthop Sports Phys Ther 37:169–178, 2007

64. Makofsky HW: Spinal Manual Therapy. Thorofare, NJ, Slack, 2003

65. Pociask FD: Electrotherapy, in Placzek JD, Boyce DA (eds): Orthopaedic Physical Therapy Secrets. Philadelphia, Hanley & Belfus, 2001, pp 60–74

66. Pressure ulcer prevention and treatment following spinal cord injury: A clinical practice guideline for health-care professionals. J Spinal Cord Med. 24 Suppl 1:S40–101, 2001

67. McCulloch JM: Wound healing and management, in Placzek JD, Boyce DA (eds): Orthopaedic Physical Therapy Secrets. Philadelphia, Hanley & Belfus, 2001, pp 171–176

68. Bluman AG: The nature of probability and statistics, in Bluman AG (ed): Elementary Statistics: A Step by Step Approach (ed 4). New York, McGraw-Hill, 2008, pp 1–32

69. Bluman AG: Organizing Data, in Bluman AG (ed): Elementary Statistics: A Step by Step Approach (ed 4). New York, McGraw-Hill, 2008, pp 33–100

70. Bluman AG: Measures of Central Tendency, in Bluman AG (ed): Elementary Statistics: A Step by Step Approach (ed 4). New York, McGraw-Hill, 2008, pp 101–176

71. Bluman AG: Probability and counting rules, in Bluman AG (ed): Elementary Statistics: A Step by Step Approach (ed 4). New York, McGraw-Hill, 2008, pp 177–242

72. Bluman AG: The normal distribution, in Bluman AG (ed): Elementary Statistics: A Step by Step Approach (ed 4). New York, McGraw-Hill, 2008, pp 281–341

73. Bluman AG: Confidence intervals and sample size, in Bluman AG (ed): Elementary Statistics: A Step by Step Approach (ed 4). New York, McGraw-Hill, 2008, pp 343–385

74. Bluman AG: Hypothesis testing, in Bluman AG (ed): Elementary Statistics: A Step by Step Approach (ed 4). New York, McGraw-Hill, 2008, pp 387–455

75. Marshall S, Teasell R, Bayona N, et al: Motor impairment rehabilitation post acquired brain injury. Brain Inj 21:133–160, 2007

76. Booth MY, Yates CC, Edgar TS, et al: Serial casting vs combined intervention with botulinum toxin a and serial casting in the treatment of spastic equinus in children. Pediatr Phys Ther 15:216–220, 2003

77. Westberry DE, Davids JR, Jacobs JM, et al: Effectiveness of serial stretch casting for resistant or recurrent knee flexion contractures following hamstring lengthening in children with cerebral palsy. J Pediatr Orthop 26:109–114, 2006

78. Singer BJ, Dunne JW, Singer KP, et al: Non-surgical management of ankle contracture following acquired brain injury. Disabil Rehabil 26:335–345, 2004

79. Stoeckmann T: Casting for the person with spasticity. Top Stroke Rehabil 8:27–35, 2001

80. Donovan E: Serial casting, in Placzek JD, Boyce DA (eds): Orthopaedic Physical Therapy Secrets. Philadelphia, Hanley & Belfus, 2001, pp 200–203

81. Goulet C, Arsenault AB, Bourbonnais D, et al: Effects of transcutaneous electrical nerve stimulation on H-reflex and spinal spasticity. Scand J Rehabil Med 28:169–176, 1996

82. Vodovnik L, Bowman BR, Hufford P: Effects of electrical stimulation on spinal spasticity. Scand J Rehabil Med 16:29–34, 1984

83. Gillette PD: Exercise in aging and disease, in Placzek JD, Boyce DA (eds): Orthopaedic Physical Therapy Secrets. Philadelphia, Hanley & Belfus, 2001, pp 235–242

84. Thompson LV: Iatrogenic effects, in Kaufmann TL (ed): Geriatric Rehabilitation Manual. New York, Churchill Livingstone, 1999, pp 318–324

85. Wiater JM: Functional anatomy of the shoulder, in Placzek JD, Boyce DA (eds): Orthopaedic Physical Therapy Secrets. Philadelphia, Hanley & Belfus, 2001, pp 243–248

86. Wee AS: Correlation between the biceps brachii muscle bulk and the size of its evoked compound muscle action potential. Electromyogr Clin Neurophysiol 46:79–82, 2006

87. Tiberio D, Hinkebein JR: Foot orthoses and shoe design, in Placzek JD, Boyce DA (eds): Orthopaedic Physical Therapy Secrets. Philadelphia, Hanley & Belfus, 2001, pp 455–462

88. Nelson AJ: Functional ambulation profile. Phys Ther 54:1059–1065, 1974

89. Ganji S, Peters G, Frazier E: Alpha-coma: clinical and evoked potential studies. Clin Electroencephalogr 18:103–113, 1987

90. Schmitz TJ: Examination of the environment, in O'Sullivan SB, Schmitz TJ (eds): Physical Rehabilitation (ed 5). Philadelphia, F. A. Davis, 2007, pp 401–467

91. Lee RE, Booth KM, Reese-Smith JY, et al: The Physical Activity Resource Assessment (PARA) instrument: Evaluating features, amenities and incivilities of physical activity resources in urban neighborhoods. Int J Behav Nutr Phys Act 2:13, 2005

92. Keysor J, Jette A, Haley S: Development of the home and community environment (HACE) instrument. J Rehabil Med 37:37–44, 2005

93. Oliver R, Blathwayt J, Brackley C, et al: Development of the Safety Assessment of Function and the Environment for Rehabilitation (SAFER) tool. Can J Occup Ther 60:78–82, 1993

94. Shumway-Cook A, Patla A, Stewart AL, et al: Assessing environmentally determined mobility disability: self-report versus observed community mobility. J Am Geriatr Soc 53:700–704, 2005

95. Shumway-Cook A, Patla A, Stewart A, et al: Environmental components of mobility disability in community-living older persons. J Am Geriatr Soc 51:393–398, 2003

96. O'Sullivan SB: Strategies to improve motor function, in O'Sullivan SB, Schmitz TJ (eds): Physical Rehabilitation (ed 5). Philadelphia, F. A. Davis, 2007, pp 471–522

97. Schmidt R, Lee T: Motor control and learning (ed 4). Champaign, IL, Human Kinetics, 2005

98. Hoare B, Wasiak J, Imms C, et al: Constraint-induced movement therapy in the treatment of the upper limb in children with hemiplegic cerebral palsy. Cochrane Database Syst Rev CD004149, 2007

99. Wu CY, Chen CL, Tsai WC, et al: A randomized controlled trial of modified constraint-induced movement

therapy for elderly stroke survivors: changes in motor impairment, daily functioning, and quality of life. Arch Phys Med Rehabil 88:273–278, 2007

100. Boake C, Noser EA, Ro T, et al: Constraint-induced movement therapy during early stroke rehabilitation. Neurorehabil Neural Repair 21:14–24, 2007

101. Mark VW, Taub E, Morris DM: Neuroplasticity and constraint-induced movement therapy. Eura Medicophys 42:269–284, 2006

102. Morris DM, Taub E, Mark VW: Constraint-induced movement therapy: Characterizing the intervention protocol. Eura Medicophys 42:257–268, 2006

103. Smania N: Constraint-induced movement therapy: An original concept in rehabilitation. Eura Medicophys 42:239–240, 2006

104. Passat N, Ronse C, Baruthio J, et al: Magnetic resonance angiography: From anatomical knowledge modeling to vessel segmentation. Med Image Anal 10:259–274, 2006

105. Schmitz TJ: Locomotor training, in O'Sullivan SB, Schmitz TJ (eds): Physical Rehabilitation (ed 5). Philadelphia, F. A. Davis, 2007, pp 523–560

106. Starr JA: Chronic pulmonary dysfunction, in O'Sullivan SB, Schmitz TJ (eds): Physical Rehabilitation (ed 5). Philadelphia, F. A. Davis, 2007, pp 561–588

107. Man SF, McAlister FA, Anthonisen NR, et al: Contemporary management of chronic obstructive pulmonary disease: clinical applications. JAMA 290:2313–2316, 2003

108. Wilson GE: A comparison of traditional chest physiotherapy with the active cycle of breathing in patients with chronic supurative lung disease. Eur Respir J 8:171S, 1995

109. Eaton T, Young P, Zeng I, et al: A randomized evaluation of the acute efficacy, acceptability and tolerability of flutter and active cycle of breathing with and without postural drainage in non-cystic fibrosis bronchiectasis. Chron Respir Dis 4:23–30, 2007

110. Phillips GE, Pike SE, Jaffe A, et al: Comparison of active cycle of breathing and high-frequency oscillation jacket in children with cystic fibrosis. Pediatr Pulmonol 37:71–75, 2004

111. Lapin CD: Airway physiology, autogenic drainage, and active cycle of breathing. Respir Care 47:778–785, 2002

112. Thompson CS, Harrison S, Ashley J, et al: Randomised crossover study of the Flutter device and the active cycle of breathing technique in non-cystic fibrosis bronchiectasis. Thorax 57:446–448, 2002

113. Di Salvo G, Pergola V, Ratti G, et al: Atrial natriuretic factor and mitral valve prolapse syndrome. Minerva Cardioangiol 49:317–325, 2001

114. Grimes K: Heart disease, in O'Sullivan SB, Schmitz TJ (eds): Physical Rehabilitation (ed 5). Philadelphia, F. A. Davis, 2007, pp 589–641

115. Molloi S, Wong JT: Regional blood flow analysis and its relationship with arterial branch lengths and lumen volume in the coronary arterial tree. Phys Med Biol 52:1495–1503, 2007

116. Yildirim A, Soylu O, Dagdeviren B, et al: Cardiac resynchronization improves coronary blood flow. Tohoku J Exp Med 211:43–47, 2007

117. Carabello BA: Understanding coronary blood flow: the wave of the future. Circulation 113:1721–1722, 2006

118. Tanaka N, Takeda K, Nishi S, et al: A new method for measuring total coronary blood flow using the lithium dilution method. Osaka City Med J 51:11–18, 2005

119. Mittal N, Zhou Y, Linares C, et al: Analysis of blood flow in the entire coronary arterial tree. Am J Physiol Heart Circ Physiol 289:H439–46, 2005

120. Reijnen MM, Disselhoff BC, Zeebregts CJ: Varicose vein surgery and endovenous laser therapy. Surg Technol Int 16:167–174, 2007

121. Well DS, Meier JM, Mahne A, et al: Detection of age-related changes in thoracic structure and function by computed tomography, magnetic resonance imaging, and positron emission tomography. Semin Nucl Med 37:103–119, 2007

122. Myers K, Fris R, Jolley D: Treatment of varicose veins by endovenous laser therapy: assessment of results by ultrasound surveillance. Med J Aust 185:199–202, 2006

123. Peden E, Lumsden A: Radiofrequency ablation of incompetent perforator veins. Perspect Vasc Surg Endovasc Ther 19:73–77, 2007

124. Clarke M, Hpewell S, Juszczak E, et al: Compression stockings to prevent deep vein thrombosis in long-haul airline passengers. Int J Epidemiol 35:1410–1411; discussion 1411, 2006

125. Attia J, Hatala R, Cook DJ, et al: Does this adult patient have acute meningitis? JAMA 282:175–181, 1999

126. DeFaria Yeh D, Freeman MW, Meigs JB, et al: Risk factors for coronary artery disease in patients with elevated high-density lipoprotein cholesterol. Am J Cardiol 99:1–4, 2007

127. Boekholdt SM, Sandhu MS, Day NE, et al: Physical activity, C-reactive protein levels and the risk of future coronary artery disease in apparently healthy men and women: The EPIC-Norfolk prospective population study. Eur J Cardiovasc Prev Rehabil 13:970–976, 2006

128. Schooling CM, Lam TH, Leung GM: Effect of obesity in patients with coronary artery disease. Lancet 368:1645; author reply 1645–1646, 2006

129. Orchard TJ, Costacou T, Kretowski A, et al: Type 1 diabetes and coronary artery disease. Diabetes Care 29:2528–2538, 2006

130. Ludvig J, Miner B, Eisenberg MJ: Smoking cessation in patients with coronary artery disease. Am Heart J 149:565–572, 2005

131. Lee CS, Lu YH, Lee ST, et al: Evaluating the prevalence of silent coronary artery disease in asymptomatic patients with spinal cord injury. Int Heart J 47:325–330, 2006

132. Bauman WA, Spungen AM, Raza M, et al: Coronary artery disease: Metabolic risk factors and latent disease in individuals with paraplegia. Mt Sinai J Med 59:163–168, 1992

133. Pepine CJ, Kowey PR, Kupfer S, et al: Predictors of adverse outcome among patients with hypertension and coronary artery disease. J Am Coll Cardiol 47:547–551, 2006

134. Graner M, Syvanne M, Kahri J, et al: Insulin resistance as predictor of the angiographic severity and extent of coronary artery disease. Ann Med 39:137–144, 2007

135. Ask the doctors. I recently read that patients with coronary artery disease ought to have their blood pressure reduced to less than 120/80. I thought 120/80 was normal

blood pressure, so why would you want blood pressure to be lower than normal? Heart Advis 10:8, 2007

136. Sadeghian S, Darvish S, Salimi S, et al: Metabolic syndrome: Stronger association with coronary artery disease in young men in comparison with higher prevalence in young women. Coron Artery Dis 18:163–168, 2007

137. Turhan S, Tulunay C, Gulec S, et al: The association between androgen levels and premature coronary artery disease in men. Coron Artery Dis 18:159–162, 2007

138. Lundberg GD: A new aggressive approach to screening and early intervention to prevent death from coronary artery disease. Med Gen Med 8:22, 2006

139. Ahmed A, Lefante CM, Alam N: Depression and nursing home admission among hospitalized older adults with coronary artery disease: A propensity score analysis. Am J Geriatr Cardiol 16:76–83, 2007

140. de Carvalho T, Curi AL, Andrade DF, et al: Cardiovascular rehabilitation of patients with ischemic heart disease undergoing medical treatment, percutaneous transluminal coronary angioplasty, and coronary artery bypass grafting. Arq Bras Cardiol 88:72–78, 2007

141. Winsor T, Hyman C: A Primer of Peripheral Vascular Diseases. Philadelphia, Lea & Febiger, 1965

142. DeTurk WE: Exercise and the intolerant heart. Clin Management 12:67–73, 1992

143. Jones GL: Upper extremity stress fractures. Clin Sports Med 25:159–174, xi, 2006

144. Moon BS, Price CT, Campbell JB: Upper extremity and rib stress fractures in a child. Skeletal Radiol 27:403–405, 1998

145. Maitra AK: The hanging head method for the treatment of acute wry neck. Arch Emerg Med 8:71, 1991

146. Banerjee A: The hanging head method for the treatment of acute wry neck. Arch Emerg Med 7:125, 1990

147. Fukazawa R, Ikegam E, Watanabe M, et al: Coronary artery aneurysm induced by kawasaki disease in children show features typical senescence. Circ J 71:709–715, 2007

148. Agha A, Phillips J, Thompson CJ: Hypopituitarism following traumatic brain injury (TBI). Br J Neurosurg 21:210–216, 2007

149. Kokiko ON, Hamm RJ: A review of pharmacological treatments used in experimental models of traumatic brain injury. Brain Inj 21:259–274, 2007

150. Zehtabchi S, Sinert R, Soghoian S, et al: Identifying traumatic brain injury in patients with isolated head trauma: are arterial lactate and base deficit as helpful as in polytrauma? Emerg Med J 24:333–335, 2007

151. Hartl R: Back to basics, or the evolution of traumatic brain injury management since Scipione Riva-Rocci. Crit Care Med 35:1196–1197, 2007

152. Irdesel J, Aydiner SB, Akgoz S: Rehabilitation outcome after traumatic brain injury. Neurocirugia (Astur) 18:5–15, 2007

153. Teasell R, Bayona N, Lippert C, et al: Post-traumatic seizure disorder following acquired brain injury. Brain Inj 21:201–214, 2007

154. Scherer M: Gait rehabilitation with body weight-supported treadmill training for a blast injury survivor with traumatic brain injury. Brain Inj 21:93–100, 2007

155. Pressman HT: Traumatic brain injury rehabilitation: Case management and insurance-related issues. Phys Med Rehabil Clin N Am 18:165–174, viii, 2007

156. Young JA: Pain and traumatic brain injury. Phys Med Rehabil Clin N Am 18:145–163, vii–viii, 2007

157. Yen HL, Wong JT: Rehabilitation for traumatic brain injury in children and adolescents. Ann Acad Med Singapore 36:62–66, 2007

158. Chua KS, Ng YS, Yap SG, et al: A brief review of traumatic brain injury rehabilitation. Ann Acad Med Singapore 36:31–42, 2007

159. Ducrocq SC, Meyer PG, Orliaguet GA, et al: Epidemiology and early predictive factors of mortality and outcome in children with traumatic severe brain injury: Experience of a French pediatric trauma center. Pediatr Crit Care Med 7:461–467, 2006

160. Chesnut RM: The evolving management of traumatic brain injury: Don't shoot the messenger. Crit Care Med 34:2262; author reply 2262–2263, 2006

161. Fulk GD: Traumatic brain injury, in O'Sullivan SB, Schmitz TJ (eds): Physical Rehabilitation (ed 5). Philadelphia, F. A. Davis, 2007, pp 895–935

162. de Jong LD, Nieuwboer A, Aufdemkampe G: Contracture preventive positioning of the hemiplegic arm in subacute stroke patients: A pilot randomized controlled trial. Clin Rehabil. 20:656–667, 2006

163. Chatterton HJ, Pomeroy VM, Gratton J: Positioning for stroke patients: A survey of physiotherapists' aims and practices. Disabil Rehabil. 23:413–421, 2001

164. Osgood SL, Kuczkowski KM: Autonomic dysreflexia in a parturient with spinal cord injury. Acta Anaesthesiol Belg 57:161–162, 2006

165. Wu KP, Lai PL, Lee LF, et al: Autonomic dysreflexia triggered by an unstable lumbar spine in a quadriplegic patient. Chang Gung Med J 28:508–511, 2005

166. Adiga S: Further lessons in autonomic dysreflexia. Arch Phys Med Rehabil 86:1891; author reply 1891, 2005

167. Sullivan-Tevault M: Autonomic dysreflexia in spinal cord injury. Emerg Med Serv 34:79–80, 85, 2005

168. Jacob C, Thwaini A, Rao A, et al: Autonomic dysreflexia: The forgotten medical emergency. Hosp Med. 66:294–296, 2005

169. Bycroft J, Shergill IS, Chung EA, et al: Autonomic dysreflexia: A medical emergency. Postgrad Med J 81:232–235, 2005

170. Taylor AG: Autonomic dysreflexia in spinal cord injury. Nurs Clin North Am 9:717–725, 1974

171. Prayaga S: Asian Indians and coronary artery disease risk. Am J Med 120:e15; author reply e19, 2007

172. Cay S, Metin F, Korkmaz S: Association of renal functional impairment and the severity of coronary artery disease. Anadolu Kardiyol Derg 7:44–48, 2007

173. Sbarsi I, Falcone C, Boiocchi C, et al: Inflammation and atherosclerosis: The role of TNF and TNF receptors polymorphisms in coronary artery disease. Int J Immunopathol Pharmacol 20:145–154, 2007

174. Pamukcu B, Oflaz H, Onur I, et al: Clinical relevance of aspirin resistance in patients with stable coronary artery disease: A prospective follow-up study (PROSPECTAR). Blood Coagul Fibrinolysis 18:187–192, 2007

175. Fulk GD, Schmitz TJ, Behrman AL: Traumatic spinal cord injury, in O'Sullivan SB, Schmitz TJ (eds): Physical Rehabilitation (ed 5). Philadelphia, F. A. Davis, 2007, pp 937–996

176. Spangler LL: Nonprogressive spinal cord disorders, in Cameron MH, Monroe LG (eds): Physical Rehabilitation: Evidence-Based Examination, Evaluation, and Intervention. St. Louis, MO, Saunders/Elsevier, 2007, pp 538–579

177. Greitz D: Unraveling the riddle of syringomyelia. Neurosurg Rev 29:251–263; discussion 264, 2006

178. Milhorat TH: Classification of syringomyelia. Neurosurg Focus 8:E1, 2000

179. Pearce JM: Syringes and syringomyelia. Eur Neurol 54:243, 2005

180. Todor DR, Mu HT, Milhorat TH: Pain and syringomyelia: A review. Neurosurg Focus 8:E11, 2000

181. Wollman DE: Syringomyelia: An uncommon cause of myelopathy in the geriatric population. J Am Geriatr Soc 52:1033–1034, 2004

182. Ahn UM, Ahn NU, Buchowski JM, et al: Cauda equina syndrome secondary to lumbar disc herniation: a meta-analysis of surgical outcomes. Spine 25:1515–1522, 2000

183. Brown KL: Cauda equina syndrome. Implications for the orthopaedic nurse in a clinical setting. Orthop Nurs 17:31–35; quiz 36–37, 1998

184. Kennedy JG, Soffe KE, McGrath A, et al: Predictors of outcome in cauda equina syndrome. Eur Spine J 8:317–322, 1999

185. Orendacova J, Cizkova D, Kafka J, et al: Cauda equina syndrome. Prog Neurobiol 64:613–637, 2001

186. Small SA, Perron AD, Brady WJ: Orthopedic pitfalls: Cauda equina syndrome. Am J Emerg Med 23:159–163, 2005

187. Hennessey JV, Westrick E: Coronary artery disease and cerebrovascular disease prevention in diabetes mellitus: Early identification and aggressive modification of risk factors. Med Health R I 81:350–352, 1998

188. Sukhija R, Aronow WS, Yalamanchili K, et al: Prevalence of coronary artery disease, lower extremity peripheral arterial disease, and cerebrovascular disease in 110 men with an abdominal aortic aneurysm. Am J Cardiol 94:1358–1359, 2004

189. Ness J, Aronow WS: Prevalence of coronary artery disease, ischemic stroke, peripheral arterial disease, and coronary revascularization in older African-Americans, Asians, Hispanics, whites, men, and women. Am J Cardiol 84:932–933, A7, 1999

190. White LJ, McCoy SC, Castellano V, et al: Effect of resistance training on risk of coronary artery disease in women with multiple sclerosis. Scand J Clin Lab Invest 66:351–355, 2006

191. Steffens DC, O'Connor CM, Jiang WJ, et al: The effect of major depression on functional status in patients with coronary artery disease. J Am Geriatr Soc 47:319–322, 1999

192. Londahl M, Katzman P, Nilsson A, et al: A prospective study: hyperbaric oxygen therapy in diabetics with chronic foot ulcers. J Wound Care 15:457–459, 2006

193. Mathieu D: Role of hyperbaric oxygen therapy in the management of lower extremity wounds. Int J Low Extrem Wounds 5:233–235, 2006

194. Koetters KT: Hyperbaric oxygen therapy. J Emerg Nurs 32:417–419, 2006

195. Lin LC, Yau G, Lin TF, et al: The efficacy of hyperbaric oxygen therapy in improving the quality of life in patients with problem wounds. J Nurs Res 14:219–227, 2006

196. Fonder MA, Mamelak AJ, Lazarus GS, et al: Occlusive wound dressings in emergency medicine and acute care. Emerg Med Clin North Am 25:235–242, 2007

197. Burd A: Evaluating the use of hydrogel sheet dressings in comprehensive burn wound care. Ostomy Wound Manage 53:52–62, 2007

198. Fleck CA: Innovative dressings improve wound care management. Mater Manag Health Care 16:24–26, 28, 2007

199. Ovington LG: Advances in wound dressings. Clin Dermatol 25:33–38, 2007

200. Leaper DJ: Silver dressings: their role in wound management. Int Wound J 3:282–294, 2006

201. O'Donnell TF, Jr., Lau J: A systematic review of randomized controlled trials of wound dressings for chronic venous ulcer. J Vasc Surg 44:1118–1125, 2006

202. Shreenivas S, Magnuson JS, Rosenthal EL: Use of negative-pressure dressings to manage a difficult surgical neck wound. Ear Nose Throat J 85:390–391, 2006

203. Attinger CE, Janis JE, Steinberg J, et al: Clinical approach to wounds: Debridement and wound bed preparation including the use of dressings and wound-healing adjuvants. Plast Reconstr Surg 117:72S–109S, 2006

204. Jones V, Grey JE, Harding KG: Wound dressings. BMJ 332:777–780, 2006

205. Wicker P: Wound dressings. Br J Theatre Nurs 2:22–25, 1992

206. Willey T: Use a decision tree to choose wound dressings. Am J Nurs 92:43–46, 1992

207. Gomez R, Cancio LC: Management of burn wounds in the emergency department. Emerg Med Clin North Am 25:135–146, 2007

208. Prelack K, Dylewski M, Sheridan RL: Practical guidelines for nutritional management of burn injury and recovery. Burns 33:14–24, 2007

209. Khan N, Malik MA: Presentation of burn injuries and their management outcome. J Pak Med Assoc 56:394–397, 2006

210. Abdi S, Zhou Y: Management of pain after burn injury. Curr Opin Anaesthesiol 15:563–567, 2002

211. DeSanti L: Pathophysiology and current management of burn injury. Adv Skin Wound Care 18:323–332; quiz 332–334, 2005

212. Papini R: Management of burn injuries of various depths. BMJ 329:158–160, 2004

213. Hettiaratchy S, Papini R: Initial management of a major burn: II—assessment and resuscitation. BMJ 329:101–103, 2004

214. Hettiaratchy S, Papini R: Initial management of a major burn: I—overview. BMJ 328:1555–7, 2004

215. Bishop JF: Burn wound assessment and surgical management. Crit Care Nurs Clin North Am 16:145–177, 2004

216. Montgomery RK: Pain management in burn injury. Crit Care Nurs Clin North Am 16:39–49, 2004

217. Danks RR: Burn management. A comprehensive review of the epidemiology and treatment of burn victims. JEMS 28:118–139; quiz 140–41, 2003

218. Sheridan RL: Airway management and respiratory care of the burn patient. Int Anesthesiol Clin 38:129–145, 2000

219. Hui AC, Wong SM, Leung T: Prognosis of polymyositis and dermatomyositis. Clin Rheumatol 26:92, 2007

220. Bronner IM, van der Meulen MF, de Visser M, et al: Long-term outcome in polymyositis and dermatomyositis. Ann Rheum Dis 65:1456–1461, 2006

221. Rhee JS, Matthews BA, Neuburg M, et al: The skin cancer index: Clinical responsiveness and predictors of quality of life. Laryngoscope 117:399–405, 2007

222. Telfer NR: Skin cancer: prevalence, prevention and treatment. Clin Med 6:622; author reply 623, 2006

223. Gloster HM, Jr., Neal K: Skin cancer in skin of color. J Am Acad Dermatol 55:741–760; quiz 761–764, 2006

224. Honda KS: HIV and skin cancer. Dermatol Clin 24:521–530, vii, 2006

225. Information from your family doctor: Checking yourself for signs of skin cancer. Am Fam Physician 74:819–820, 2006

226. Information from your family doctor. Melanoma: A type of skin cancer. Am Fam Physician 74:813–814, 2006

227. Dixon A: Skin cancer in patients with multiple health problems. Aust Fam Physician 35:717–718, 2006

228. Sharpe G: Skin cancer: prevalence, prevention and treatment. Clin Med 6:333–634, 2006

229. Thomas DR: Prevention and management of pressure ulcers. Mo Med 104:52–57, 2007

230. Evans J, Stephen-Haynes J: Identification of superficial pressure ulcers. J Wound Care 16:54–56, 2007

231. McNees P, Meneses KD: Pressure ulcers and other chronic wounds in patients with and patients without cancer: A retrospective, comparative analysis of healing patterns. Ostomy Wound Management 53:70–78, 2007

232. Stewart TP, Magnano SJ: Burns or pressure ulcers in the surgical patient? Adv Skin Wound Care 20:74, 77–78, 80 passim, 2007

233. Camfield P, Camfield C: The office management of epilepsy. Semin Pediatr Neurol 13:201–207, 2006

234. Whitney J, Phillips L, Aslam R, et al: Guidelines for the treatment of pressure ulcers. Wound Repair Regen 14:663–679, 2006

235. Dini V, Bertone M, Romanelli M: Prevention and management of pressure ulcers. Dermatol Ther 19:356–364, 2006

236. Rycroft-Malone J, McInnes L: The prevention of pressure ulcers. Worldviews Evid Based Nurs 1:146–149, 2004

237. Effective methods for preventing pressure ulcers. J Fam Pract 55:942, 2006

238. Benbow M: Guidelines for the prevention and treatment of pressure ulcers. Nurs Stand 20:42–44, 2006

239. Cullum N, Nelson EA, Nixon J: Pressure ulcers. Clin Evid:2592–2606, 2006

240. Reddy M, Gill SS, Rochon PA: Preventing pressure ulcers: A systematic review. Jama 296:974–984, 2006

241. Baranoski S: Pressure ulcers: a renewed awareness. Nursing 36:36–41; quiz 42, 2006

242. Gschwandtner ME, Ambrozy E, Maric S, et al: Microcirculation is similar in ischemic and venous ulcers. Microvasc Res 62:226–235, 2001

243. Jeter KF, Tintle TE: Rethinking ischemic ulcers: From etiology to treatment outcome. Prog Clin Biol Res 365:45–54, 1991

244. Sloane PD, Coeytaux RR, Beck RS, et al: Dizziness: State of the science. Ann Intern Med. 134:823–832, 2001

245. Gacek RR: The pathology of facial and vestibular neuronitis. Am J Otolaryngol 20:202–210, 1999

246. Gacek RR, Gacek MR: Vestibular neuronitis. Am J Otol 20:553–554, 1999

247. Gacek RR, Gacek MR: Vestibular neuronitis: a viral neuropathy. Adv Otorhinolaryngol 60:54–66, 2002

248. Imate Y, Sekitani T, Okami M, et al: Central disorders in vestibular neuronitis. Acta Otolaryngol Suppl 519:204–205, 1995

249. Ishikawa K, Edo M, Togawa K: Clinical observation of 32 cases of vestibular neuronitis. Acta Otolaryngol Suppl 503:13–15, 1993

250. Lumio JS, Aho J: Vestibular neuronitis. Ann Otol Rhinol Laryngol 74:264–270, 1965

251. Ogata Y, Sekitani T, Shimogori H, et al: Bilateral vestibular neuronitis. Acta Otolaryngol Suppl 503:57–60, 1993

252. Tahara T, Sekitani T, Imate Y, et al: Vestibular neuronitis in children. Acta Otolaryngol Suppl 503:49–52, 1993

253. Baloh RW: Differentiating between peripheral and central causes of vertigo. Otolaryngol Head Neck Surg 119:55–59, 1998

254. Baloh RW: Differentiating between peripheral and central causes of vertigo. J Neurol Sci 221:3, 2004

255. Buttner U, Helmchen C, Brandt T: Diagnostic criteria for central versus peripheral positioning nystagmus and vertigo: a review. Acta Otolaryngol 119:1–5, 1999

256. Drozd CE: Acute vertigo: peripheral versus central etiology. Nurse Pract 24:147–148, 1999

257. Frederic MW: Central vertigo. Otolaryngol Clin North Am 6:267–285, 1973

258. Williams D: Central vertigo. Trans Med Soc Lond 74:15–19, 1958

259. Williams DJ: Central vertigo. Proc R Soc Med 60:961–964, 1967

260. Di Girolamo S, Ottaviani F, Scarano E, et al: Postural control in horizontal benign paroxysmal positional vertigo. Eur Arch Otorhinolaryngol 257:372–375, 2000

261. Dornhoffer JL, Colvin GB: Benign paroxysmal positional vertigo and canalith repositioning: Clinical correlations. Am J Otol 21:230–233, 2000

262. Furman JM, Cass SP: Benign paroxysmal positional vertigo. N Engl J Med 341:1590–1596, 1999

263. Herdman SJ, Blatt PJ, Schubert MC: Vestibular rehabilitation of patients with vestibular hypofunction or with benign paroxysmal positional vertigo. Curr Opin Neurol 13:39–43, 2000

264. Hilton M, Pinder D: Benign paroxysmal positional vertigo. BMJ 326:673, 2003

265. Karlberg M, Hall K, Quickert N, et al: What inner ear diseases cause benign paroxysmal positional vertigo? Acta Otolaryngol 120:380–385, 2000

266. Kentala E, Pyykko I: Vertigo in patients with benign paroxysmal positional vertigo. Acta Otolaryngol Suppl 543:20–22, 2000

267. Kovar M, Jepson T, Jones S: Diagnosing and treating benign paroxysmal positional vertigo. J Gerontol Nurs 32:22–27; quiz 28–29, 2006

268. Mosca F, Morano M: Benign paroxysmal positional vertigo, incidence and treatment. Ann Otolaryngol Chir Cervicofac 118:95–101, 2001

269. Solomon D: Benign Paroxysmal Positional Vertigo. Curr Treat Options Neurol 2:417–428, 2000

270. von Brevern M, Lempert T: Benign paroxysmal positional vertigo. Arch Neurol 58:1491–1493, 2001

271. Gussen R: Meniere syndrome. Compensatory collateral venous drainage with endolymphatic sac fibrosis. Arch Otolaryngol 99:414–418, 1974

272. Haubrich WS: Meniere of Meniere's syndrome. Gastroenterology 114:1150, 1998

273. Lee H, Yi HA, Lee SR, et al: Drop attacks in elderly patients secondary to otologic causes with Meniere's syndrome or non-Meniere peripheral vestibulopathy. J Neurol Sci 232:71–76, 2005

274. Karagol U, Deda G, Kukner S, et al: Early-onset Huntington chorea. Eur J Pediatr 154:752–753, 1995

275. Lanska DJ: George Huntington and hereditary chorea. J Child Neurol 10:46–48, 1995

276. Tolosa ES, Sparber SB: Huntington chorea. Arch Neurol 34:58–59, 1977

277. Patient information. Bell's palsy. J Fam Pract 52:160, 2003

278. Managing Bell's palsy. Drug Ther Bull 44:49–53, 2006

279. Cederwall E, Olsen MF, Hanner P, et al: Evaluation of a physiotherapeutic treatment intervention in "Bell's" facial palsy. Physiother Theory Pract 22:43–52, 2006

280. Holland J: Bell's palsy. Clin Evid 1745–1750, 2006

281. Hutchinson M: The management of Bell's palsy. Ir Med J 98:165, 2005

282. Salinas R: Bell's palsy. Clin Evid 8:1301–1304, 2002

283. Burnett MG, Zager EL: Pathophysiology of peripheral nerve injury: A brief review. Neurosurg Focus 16:E1, 2004

284. Costa J, Henriques R, Barroso C, et al: Upper limb tremor induced by peripheral nerve injury. Neurology 67:1884–1886, 2006

285. Duff SV: Impact of peripheral nerve injury on sensorimotor control. J Hand Ther 18:277–291, 2005

286. Hirate H, Sobue K, Tsuda T, et al: Peripheral nerve injury caused by misuse of elastic stockings. Anaesth Intensive Care 35:306–307, 2007

287. Mohler LR, Hanel DP: Closed fractures complicated by peripheral nerve injury. J Am Acad Orthop Surg 14:32–37, 2006

288. Reyes O, Sosa I, Kuffler DP: Promoting neurological recovery following a traumatic peripheral nerve injury. P R Health Sci J 24:215–223, 2005

289. Tomaino MM: Upper extremity peripheral nerve injury. Am J Orthop 34:60–61, 2005

290. Winfree CJ: Peripheral nerve injury evaluation and management. Curr Surg 62:469–476, 2005

291. McGuckin N: The T 4 syndrome, in Grieve GP (ed): Modern Manual Therapy of the Vertebral Column. New York, Churchill Livingstone, 1986, pp 370–376

292. DeFranca GG, Levine LJ: The T 4 syndrome. J Manip Physiol Ther 18:34–37, 1995

293. Grieve GP: Thoracic musculoskeletal problems, in Boyling JD, Palastanga N (eds): Grieve's Modern Manual Therapy of the Vertebral Column (ed 2). Edinburgh, Churchill Livingstone, 1994, pp 401–428

294. Gozna ER, Harris WR: Traumatic winging of the scapula. J Bone Joint Surg 61A:1230–1233, 1979

295. Kauppila LI: The long thoracic nerve: Possible mechanisms of injury based on autopsy study. J Shoulder Elbow Surg 2:244–248, 1993

296. Kauppila LI, Vastamaki M: Iatrogenic serratus anterior paralysis: Long-term outcome in 26 patients. Chest 109:31–34, 1996

297. Sunderland S: Nerves and Nerve Injuries. Edinburgh, E & S Livingstone, 1968

298. Post M: Orthopaedic Management of Neuromuscular Disorders, in Post M, Bigliani LU, Flatow EL, et al (eds): The Shoulder: Operative Technique. Baltimore, Williams and Wilkins, 1998, pp 201–234

299. Kuhn JE, Plancher KD, Hawkins RJ: Scapular winging. J Am Acad Orthop Surgeons 3:319–325, 1995

300. Warfel BS, Marini SG, Lachmann EA, et al: Delayed femoral nerve palsy following femoral vessel catheterization. Arch Phys Med Rehabil 74:1211–1215, 1993

301. Hardy SL: Femoral nerve palsy associated with an associated posterior wall transverse acetabular fracture. J Orthop Trauma 11:40–42, 1997

302. Papastefanou SL, Stevens K, Mulholland RC: Femoral nerve palsy: An unusual complication of anterior lumbar interbody fusion. Spine 19:2842–2844, 1994

303. Fealy S, Paletta GA, Jr: Femoral nerve palsy secondary to traumatic iliacus muscle hematoma: course after nonoperative management. J Trauma-Injury Infect Crit Care 47:1150–1152, 1999

304. Sogaard I: Sciatic nerve entrapment: case report. J Neurosurg 58:275–276, 1983

305. Robinson DR: Pyriformis syndrome in relation to sciatic pain. Am J Surg 73:355–358, 1947

306. Resnick D: Diagnosis of bone and joint disorders. Philadelphia, Saunders, 1995

307. Heald PW: Current treatment practice of herpes zoster. Expert Opin Pharmacother 2:1283–1287, 2001

308. Leung AK, Robson WL, Leong AG: Herpes zoster in childhood. J Pediatr Health Care 20:300–303, 2006

309. Miller GG, Dummer JS: Herpes simplex and varicella zoster viruses: Forgotten but not gone. Am J Transplant 7:741–747, 2007

310. Morrow T: Herpes zoster vaccine brings relief for the elderly. Manag Care 15:57–58, 2006

311. Raza N, Dar NR, Ejaz A: Simultaneous onset of herpes zoster in a father and son. J Ayub Med Coll Abbottabad 18:64–65, 2006

312. Sauerbrei A, Wutzler P: Herpes simplex and varicella-zoster virus infections during pregnancy: Current concepts of prevention, diagnosis and therapy. Part 2: Varicella-zoster virus infections. Med Microbiol Immunol 196:95–102, 2007

313. Thyregod HG, Rowbotham MC, Peters M, et al: Natural history of pain following herpes zoster. Pain 128:148–156, 2007

314. Volpi A, Gatti A, Serafini G, et al: Clinical and psychosocial correlates of acute pain in herpes zoster. J Clin Virol 38:275–279, 2007

315. Bagheri SC, Farhidvash F, Perciaccante VJ: Diagnosis and treatment of patients with trigeminal neuralgia. J Am Dent Assoc 135:1713–1717, 2004

316. Bennetto L, Patel NK, Fuller G: Trigeminal neuralgia and its management. BMJ 334:201–205, 2007

317. Cheshire WP: Trigeminal neuralgia: diagnosis and treatment. Curr Neurol Neurosci Rep 5:79–85, 2005

318. Cheshire WP, Jr.: Trigeminal neuralgia. Curr Pain Headache Rep 11:69–74, 2007

319. Ecker AD: The cause of trigeminal neuralgia. Med Hypotheses 62:1023, 2004

320. El Gammal T, Brooks BS: Trigeminal neuralgia. Radiology 231:284, 2004

321. Liu JK, Apfelbaum RI: Treatment of trigeminal neuralgia. Neurosurg Clin N Am 15:319–34, 2004

322. Rozen TD: Trigeminal neuralgia and glossopharyngeal neuralgia. Neurol Clin 22:185–206, 2004

323. Scrivani SJ, Mehta N, Mathews ES, et al: Clinical criteria for trigeminal neuralgia. Oral Surg Oral Med Oral Pathol Oral Radiol Endod 97:544; author reply 544–545, 2004

324. Zakrzewska JM: Trigeminal neuralgia. Clin Evid:1490–1498, 2003

325. Zakrzewska JM, Lopez BC: Trigeminal neuralgia. Clin Evid:1599–1609, 2003

326. Briese M, Esmaeili B, Sattelle DB: Is spinal muscular atrophy the result of defects in motor neuron processes? Bioessays 27:946–957, 2005

327. Iannaccone ST, Smith SA, Simard LR: Spinal muscular atrophy. Curr Neurol Neurosci Rep 4:74–80, 2004

328. Muthukrishnan J, Varadarajulu R, Mehta SR, et al: Distal spinal muscular atrophy. J Assoc Physicians India 51:1113–1115, 2003

329. Scheffer H: Spinal muscular atrophy. Methods Mol Med 92:343–358, 2004

330. Wang HY, Ju YH, Chen SM, et al: Joint range of motion limitations in children and young adults with spinal muscular atrophy. Arch Phys Med Rehabil 85:1689–93, 2004

331. Wirth B, Brichta L, Hahnen E: Spinal muscular atrophy and therapeutic prospects. Prog Mol Subcell Biol 44:109–132, 2006

332. Yap SH: Spinal muscular atrophy. Int J Obstet Anesth 12:237, 2003

333. Bartell JC, Hayney MS: In the spotlight: Guillain-Barre syndrome. J Am Pharm Assoc (Wash DC) 46:104–106, 2006

334. Chaudhuri A: Guillain-Barre syndrome. Lancet 367:472–473; author reply 473–474, 2006

335. Cosi V, Versino M: Guillain-Barre syndrome. Neurol Sci 27 Suppl 1:S47–51, 2006

336. Douglas MR, Winer JB: Guillain-Barre syndrome and its treatment. Expert Rev Neurother 6:1569–1574, 2006

337. Gurwood AS, Drake J: Guillain-Barre syndrome. Optometry 77:540–546, 2006

338. Kashyap AS, Anand KP, Kashyap S: Guillain-Barre syndrome. Lancet 367:472; author reply 473–474, 2006

339. Kuwabara S: Guillain-barre syndrome. Curr Neurol Neurosci Rep 7:57–62, 2007

340. Logullo F, Manicone M, Di Bella P, et al: Asymmetric Guillain-Barre syndrome. Neurol Sci 27:355–359, 2006

341. Saxena AK: Guillain-Barre syndrome. Lancet 367:472; author reply 473–474, 2006

342. Shahar E: Current therapeutic options in severe Guillain-Barre syndrome. Clin Neuropharmacol 29:45–51, 2006

343. Tsang RS, Valdivieso-Garcia A: Pathogenesis of Guillain-Barre syndrome. Expert Rev Anti Infect Ther 1:597–608, 2003

344. van Doorn PA, Jacobs BC: Predicting the course of Guillain-Barre syndrome. Lancet Neurol 5:991–993, 2006

345. Logroscino G, Armon C: Amyotrophic lateral sclerosis: A global threat with a possible difference in risk across ethnicities. Neurology 68:E17, 2007

346. Kurt A, Nijboer F, Matuz T, et al: Depression and anxiety in individuals with amyotrophic lateral sclerosis : epidemiology and management. CNS Drugs 21:279–291, 2007

347. Grossman AB, Woolley-Levine S, Bradley WG, et al: Detecting neurobehavioral changes in amyotrophic lateral sclerosis. Amyotroph Lateral Scler 8:56–61, 2007

348. Hardiman O, Greenway M: The complex genetics of amyotrophic lateral sclerosis. Lancet Neurol 6:291–292, 2007

349. Lederer CW, Santama N: Amyotrophic lateral sclerosis: The tools of the trait. Biotechnol J, 2007

350. Pozza AM, Delamura MK, Ramirez C, et al: Physiotherapeutic conduct in amyotrophic lateral sclerosis. Sao Paulo Med J 124:350–354, 2006

351. Shoesmith CL, Strong MJ: Amyotrophic lateral sclerosis: Update for family physicians. Can Fam Physician 52:1563–1569, 2006

352. Aguilar JL, Echaniz-Laguna A, Fergani A, et al: Amyotrophic lateral sclerosis: All roads lead to Rome. J Neurochem 2007

353. Postpolio syndrome. J Indian Med Assoc 98:24–25, 2000

354. Carlson M, Hadlock T: Physical therapist management following rotator cuff repair for a patient with postpolio syndrome. Phys Ther 87:179–192, 2007

355. Dalakas M: Postpolio syndrome. Curr Opin Rheumatol 2:901–907, 1990

356. Gevirtz C: Managing postpolio syndrome pain. Nursing 36:17, 2006

357. Hodges DL, Kumar VN: Postpolio syndrome. Orthop Rev 15:218–222, 1986

358. Howard RS: Poliomyelitis and the postpolio syndrome. Bmj 330:1314–1318, 2005

359. Moskowitz E: Postpolio syndrome. Arch Phys Med Rehabil 68:322, 1987

360. Nollet F, de Visser M: Postpolio syndrome. Arch Neurol 61:1142–1144, 2004

361. Owen RR: Postpolio syndrome and cardiopulmonary conditioning. West J Med 154:557–558, 1991

362. Sliwa J: Postpolio syndrome and rehabilitation. Am J Phys Med Rehabil 83:909, 2004

363. Winters R: Postpolio syndrome. J Am Acad Nurse Pract 3:69–74, 1991

364. Winstein CJ, Knecht HG: Movement science and its relevance to physical therapy. Phys Ther. 70:759–762, 1990

365. Winstein CJ: Knowledge of results and motor learning—implications for physical therapy. Phys Ther. 71:140–149, 1991

366. Winstein CJ: Motor learning considerations in stroke rehabilitation, in Duncan PW, Badke MB (eds): Stroke Rehabilitation: the Recovery of Motor Control. Chicago, Yearbook Medical Publishers, 1987, pp 109–134

367. Kisner C, Colby LA: Therapeutic exercise: Foundational concepts, in Kisner C, Colby LA (eds): Therapeutic Exercise: Foundations and Techniques (ed 5). Philadelphia, F. A. Davis, 2002, pp 1–36

368. Gentile AM: Skill acquisition: Action, movement, and neuromotor processes, in Carr J, Shepherd R (eds): Movement science: Foundations for physical therapy in rehabilitation. Gaithersburg, MD, Aspen, 2000, pp 111–187

369. Magill RA: Motor learning and control: Concepts and applications (ed 8). New York, McGraw-Hill, 2007

370. Clayton-Krasinski D, Klepper S: Impaired neuromotor development, in Cameron MH, Monroe LG (eds): Physical Rehabilitation: Evidence-Based Examination, Evaluation, and Intervention. St Louis, MO, Saunders/Elsevier, 2007, pp 333–366

371. Unsworth CA: Cognitive and perceptual dysfunction, in O'Sullivan SB, Schmitz TJ (eds): Physical Rehabilitation (ed 5). Philadelphia, F. A. Davis, 2007, pp 1149–1188

372. Parziale JR, Akelman E, Herz DA: Spasticity: Pathophysiology and management. Orthopedics 16:801–811, 1993

373. Vanek ZF, Menkes JH: Spasticity, Available at: http://www.emedicine.com/neuro/topic706.htm, 2005

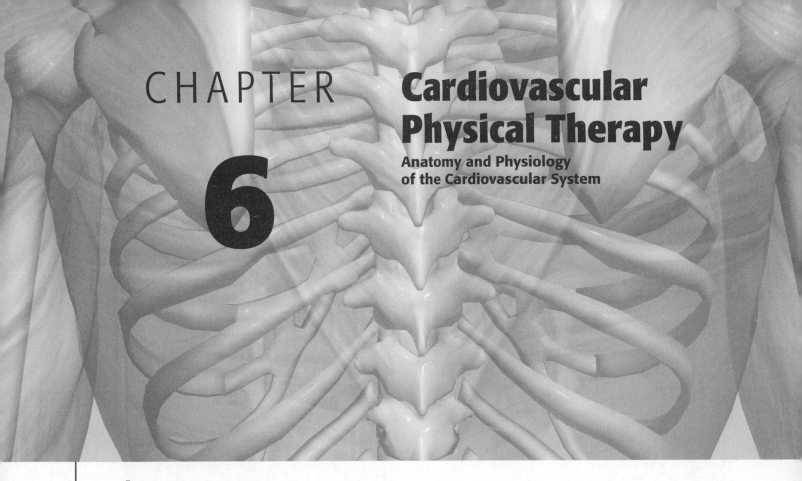

CHAPTER 6

Cardiovascular Physical Therapy

Anatomy and Physiology of the Cardiovascular System

Peripheral Circulation

The aorta receives blood directly from the left ventricle of the heart via the aortic valve (**Table 6-1**). With the exception of pulmonary and umbilical arteries, and their corresponding veins, arteries carry oxygenated blood away from the heart and deliver it to the body via arterioles and capillaries, where nutrients and gasses are exchanged; afterward, venules and veins carry deoxygenated blood back to the heart. Pulmonary arteries carry oxygen deficient blood that has just returned from the body to the lungs, where carbon dioxide is exchanged for oxygen.

> ● **Key Point** The hemoglobin (Hb) molecule is the primary transporter of oxygen in mammals and many other species. The normal level of hemoglobin is 12 to 16 grams per deciliter for women and 13.5 to 18 grams per deciliter for men. The pulse oximeter is an electronic device that measures the degree of saturation of hemoglobin with oxygen (Sao_2). Normal oxygen saturation levels are between 96% and 100%. In general, saturation levels below 90% are considered significant and warrant additional testing and the potential need for administration of supplemental oxygen.[1]

Though not considered true arteries, the capillaries play an important role in the circulatory system. The specific role of the capillaries varies according to location:

- In the lungs, carbon dioxide is exchanged for oxygen.
- In the tissues, oxygen and carbon dioxide and nutrients and wastes are exchanged.
- In the kidneys, wastes are released to be eliminated from the body.
- In the intestine, nutrients are picked up and wastes released.

TABLE 6-1   Segments and Branches of the Aorta

Segment of Aorta	Arterial Branch	General Region or Organ Served
Ascending portion of aorta	Right and left coronary aa.	Heart
Aortic arch	Brachiocephalic trunk	
	• Right common carotid a.	Right side of head and neck
	• Right subclavian a.	Right shoulder and right upper extremity
	Left common carotid a.	Left side of head and neck
	Left subclavian a.	Left shoulder and left upper extremity
Thoracic portion of aorta	Pericardial aa.	Pericardium of heart
	Posterior intercostal aa.	Intercostal and thoracic muscles, and pleurae
	Bronchial aa.	Bronchi of lungs
	Superior phrenic aa.	Superior surface of diaphragm
	Esophageal aa.	Esophagus
Abdominal portion of aorta	Inferior phrenic aa.	Inferior surface of diaphragm
	Celiac trunk	
	• Common hepatic a.	Liver, upper pancreas, and duodenum
	• Left gastric a.	Stomach and esophagus
	• Splenic a.	Spleen, pancreas, and stomach
	Superior mesenteric a.	Small intestine, pancreas, cecum, appendix, ascending colon, and transverse colon
	Suprarenal aa.	Adrenal (suprarenal) glands
	Lumbar aa.	Muscles and spinal cord of lumbar region
	Renal aa.	Kidneys
	Gonadal aa.	
	• Testicular aa.	Testes
	• Ovarian aa.	Ovaries
	Inferior mesenteric a.	Transverse colon, descending colon, sigmoid colon, and rectum
	Common iliac aa.	
	• External iliac aa.	Lower extremities
	• Internal iliac aa.	Genital organs and gluteal muscles

Abbreviations: aa., arteries; a., artery

Data from Van de Graaff KM, Fox SI: Circulatory system, in Van de Graaff KM, Fox SI (eds): Concepts of Human Anatomy and Physiology. New York, WCB/McGraw-Hill, 1999, pp 610–691

Lymphatic System

The lymphatic system is a network of strategically placed lymph nodes connected by a substantial network of lymphatic vessels, which act as the immune system's circulatory system. This system transports lymph, but unlike the circulatory system, it has no pump.

● **Key Point**   The lymphatic system has four major purposes:

- To return proteins, lipids, and water from the interstitium to the intravascular space.
- To act as a safety valve for fluid overload and to help keep edema from forming.
- To maintain the homeostasis of the extracellular environment.
- To cleanse the interstitial fluid and provide a blockade to the spread of infection or malignant cells in the lymph nodes.

As lymph fluid moves more centrally, the diameter of lymph vessels increases. Larger lymph collectors, known as trunks or ducts, handle these larger volumes of lymph fluid.

> ● **Key Point** The majority of the lymph produced by the body in a 24-hour period (2 to 4 liters) returns to the left venous angle via the thoracic duct.

All substances transported by the lymph pass through at least one lymph node, which filters out and destroys foreign substances before the fluids return to the bloodstream. In the lymph nodes, white blood cells can collect, interact with one another and antigens, and create immune responses to foreign substances. Once through the lymph node, lymph then travels from lymphatic capillaries to lymphatic vessels to ducts to the left subclavian vein.

> ● **Key Point** Edema and lymphedema are not synonymous. *Edema* is an increase of water in the interstitial space, which results from immobility, chronic venous insufficiency, hypoproteinuria, cardiac insufficiencies, or pregnancy. *Lymphedema* arises from a mechanical insufficiency that arises in an area, when lymph collectors sustain functional and structural damage resulting in the accumulation of hydrophilic proteins in the tissues.

The Heart and Circulation

The Heart

In the human body, the heart is normally situated slightly to the left of the sternum. Cardiac striated muscle fibers, called *myocardium*, have numerous mitochondria and can work continuously without fatigue.

> ● **Key Point** Cardiac muscle has a myogenic origin (an integral source of contraction), whereas skeletal (striated) muscle has a neurogenic source for contraction (its motor nerve supply).

> ● **Key Point** Cardiac landmarks include:
> • *Apex:* Located at the fifth intercostal space at the midclavicular line. The apex of the heart is the blunt point at the inferior tip of the left ventricle.
> • *Base:* Located at the second intercostal space behind the sternum on the posterior aspect of the heart.

> ● **Key Point** Note the following definitions:
> • *Pericardium:* Fibrous protective sac that encloses the heart.
> • *Epicardium:* Inner layer of the pericardium.
> • *Myocardium:* Heart muscle, the major portion of the heart.
> • *Endocardium:* Smooth lining of the inner surface and cavities of the heart.

Heart Chambers and Valves

The heart consists of four chambers (Figure 6-1), the two upper atria (singular: atrium) and the two lower ventricles. Blood is pumped through the heart chambers aided by four heart valves.

> ● **Key Point** Valves are flap-like structures that allow blood to flow in one direction. The heart has two kinds of valves, atrioventricular and semilunar.

Right Atrium

The right atrium (RA) receives blood from the systemic circulation via the superior vena cava (refer to Figure 6-1), which drains the upper part of the body, and the inferior vena cava, which drains the lower part of the body. The coronary sinus is an additional venous return into the right atrium, receiving blood from the heart itself. Blood passes from the right atrium into the right ventricle via the right atrioventricular (AV) valve (also known as the tricuspid valve because three triangular leaflets, or cusps, form it).

> ● **Key Point** The AV valves are held in position by chordae tendineae, which in turn are secured to the ventricular wall by the papillary muscles. The papillary muscles serve to maintain approximation of the valve leaflets during contraction of the ventricles. The chordae tendineae prevent the valves from everting when the ventricles contract, thereby stopping any back flow of blood.

Right Ventricle

The right ventricle (RV) receives blood from the RA. The ventricular contraction causes the right atrioventricular valve to close and the oxygen-depleted blood to leave the right ventricle via the pulmonary trunk to the lungs. The blood then enters the capillaries of the right and left pulmonary arteries, where gaseous exchange takes place and the blood releases carbon dioxide into the lung cavity and picks up oxygen. The oxygenated blood then flows through pulmonary veins to the left atrium.

> ● **Key Point**
> • The blood that is pumped to the pulmonary trunk passes through the pulmonary valve (also called the pulmonary semilunar valve), which lies at the base of the pulmonary trunk and serves to prevent blood from leaking back into the right ventricle.
> • *Semilunar valves* are half-moon-shaped flaps of endocardium and connective tissue reinforced by fibers that prevent the valves from turning inside out. Their main function is to prevent the back flow of blood from the aorta and pulmonary arteries into the ventricles when the heart relaxes between beats. They comprise the pulmonary valve and the aortic valve (see "Left Ventricle" section).

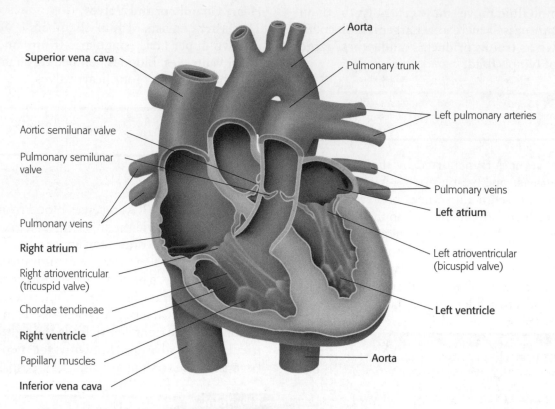

Aorta

Superior vena cava

Pulmonary trunk

Left pulmonary arteries

Aortic semilunar valve

Pulmonary semilunar valve

Pulmonary veins

Left atrium

Pulmonary veins

Right atrium

Left atrioventricular (bicuspid valve)

Right atrioventricular (tricuspid valve)

Chordae tendineae

Left ventricle

Right ventricle

Papillary muscles

Aorta

Inferior vena cava

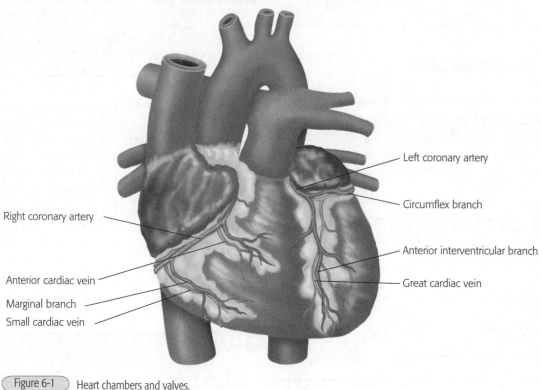

Left coronary artery

Circumflex branch

Right coronary artery

Anterior interventricular branch

Anterior cardiac vein

Great cardiac vein

Marginal branch

Small cardiac vein

Figure 6-1 Heart chambers and valves.

Left Atrium

The left atrium (LA) receives the oxygenated blood from the lungs via four pulmonary veins (two left and two right pulmonary veins). From the LA the blood passes through the mitral (bicuspid) valve to enter the left ventricle.

> **● Key Point** When the left ventricle is relaxed, the mitral valve is open, allowing blood to flow from the atrium into the ventricle; when the left ventricle contracts, the mitral valve closes, preventing the back flow of blood into the atrium.

Left Ventricle

The left ventricle (LV), which forms most of the diaphragmatic side of the heart, receives blood from the LA.

> **● Key Point** The majority of heart diseases primarily affect the LV (i.e., ischemia, infarction, cardiomyopathy, heart failure).[2] When the RV is involved, it will be documented within the medical records based on findings from diagnostic testing, such as echocardiogram (ECG) imaging or cardiac catheterization.[2]

The LV is much more muscular than the right because it has to pump blood around the entire body against considerable vascular pressure (the RV, in contrast, needs to pump blood only to the lungs, so it requires less muscle). The aortic valve allows blood to flow from the LV into the aorta and then closes to prevent blood from leaking back into the LV.

> **● Key Point** A septum (also known as the fiber skeleton of the heart) divides the right atrium and ventricle from the left atrium and ventricle, preventing blood from passing between them.

> **● Key Point** The closing of the valves produces the familiar beating sounds of the heart, commonly referred to as the "lub-dub" sound—due to the closing of the semilunar and atrioventricular valves.

Coronary Circulation and the Cardiac Cycle

The blood supply to the heart itself (coronary circulation) is supplied by the left and right coronary arteries, which branch off directly from the aorta near the aortic valve (sinus of Valsalva).[3–7]

> **● Key Point** The coronary arteries receive the majority of their blood flow during diastole, unlike the other arteries of the body, which are perfused during systole.[2]

Right Coronary Artery

The right coronary artery (RCA) originates above the right cusp of the aortic valve, where it is known as the conus artery. The RCA supplies blood to the right ventricle and 25% to 35% of the left ventricle.

Left Coronary Artery

The left coronary artery (LCA) arises from the aorta above the left cusp of the aortic valve. It typically bifurcates into the left anterior descending artery and supplies 45% to 55% of the left ventricle.

> **● Key Point** Coronary artery disease (CAD) is linked to myocardial ischemia (angina pectoris) and to myocardial infarction (MI). As cardiac muscle is strictly aerobic, the myocardium begins to deteriorate if the blood flow is occluded for more than 8 to 12 beats.

The veins involved in the coronary circulation function in parallel to, and in balance with, the arterial system.

> **● Key Point** The coronary sinus is the main drainage channel of venous blood from the myocardium. It functions to empty the venous blood from the myocardium into the right atrium.

Cardiac Cycle

Every single beat of the heart involves a sequence of interrelated events known as the cardiac cycle (Figure 6-2). The cardiac cycle consists of three major stages:

- The *atrial systole* consists of the contraction of the atria. This contraction occurs during the last third of diastole and complete ventricular filling.
- The *ventricular systole* consists of the contraction of the ventricles and flow of blood into the circulatory system.
- The *complete cardiac diastole* involves relaxation of the atria (atrial diastole) and ventricles (ventricular diastole) in preparation for refilling with circulating blood.

Electrical Conduction System of the Heart

The electrical conduction system of the heart relies on specialized conduction tissue, which relays electrical impulses in the myocardium.

Sinoatrial Node

The sinoatrial (SA) node, the main pacemaker of the heart, is located at the junction of the superior vena cava and right atrium. Under normal conditions, the SA node spontaneously generates an electrical impulse that is propagated to (and stimulates) the myocardium, causing a contraction.

I. Ventricular Filling

A. This process begins when ventricular pressure falls below atrial pressure.

B. The first phase is the period of rapid ventricular filling (a).

    1. This is the initial flow upon opening of the AV valves.

C. The second phase is called diastasis.

    1. In this phase all contractions of the heart have stopped; the cardiac muscle is relaxed.

    2. The ventricles are still being filled with blood as it flows from the great veins through the atria into the ventricles.

    3. By the end of this phase, approximately 70% of the blood that enters the ventricles has done so.

D. The third phase is the period of atrial systole.

    1. The sinoatrial (SA) node fires, sending an action potential across the atria.

    2. The atria are contracting in response to this action potential (atrial systole), ejecting more blood into the ventricles (b).

    3. Only about 30% of the blood that enters the ventricles does so during atrial systole.

II. Ventricular Systole

A. The action potential now passes through the atrioventricular (AV) bundle into the bundle branches and spreads throughout the ventricles.

B. In response to this, the myocardium of the ventricles begins to contract.

C. This elevates the ventricular pressure.

D. When ventricular pressure exceeds atrial pressure, the AV valves close, causing the first heart sound "lubb."

E. This begins the period of isovolumetric contraction, the period in which the AV valves are closed, the semilunar valves are closed, the ventricles are continuing to contract, and no blood is being pumped (c).

F. The ejection period begins when ventricular pressure exceeds arterial pressure. When this happens, the semilunar valves open and blood is ejected from the ventricles into the aorta and the pulmonary trunk. During the ejection period, slightly more than half of the volume of blood contained in the ventricles is ejected (d).

III. Ventricular Diastole

A. The action potential has now passed through the ventricles, and they are starting to relax, entering ventricular diastole.

B. As the ventricles relax, ventricular pressure begins to fall.

C. When ventricular pressure falls below arterial pressure, the semilunar valves close, causing the second heart sound "dupp."

D. The period of isovolumetric relaxation is the period in which the AV valves are closed, the semilunar valves are closed, the ventricles are continuing to relax, and no blood is being pumped (e).

E. This period continues until the ventricular pressure falls below the atrial pressure, at which time the AV valves open and the ventricular filling stage begins.

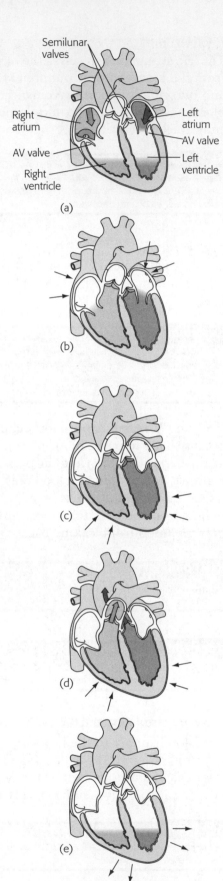

Figure 6-2 The cardiac cycle.

Atrioventricular Node

The atrioventricular (AV) node, located at the junction of the right atrium and the right ventricle, functions as a critical delay in the conduction system. Without this delay, the atria and ventricles would contract at the same time, and blood would not flow effectively from the atria to the ventricles. The distal portion of the AV node is known as the bundle of His. The bundle of His splits into two branches. These two bundle branches taper out to produce numerous Purkinje fibers, which are the specialized conducting tissue of the ventricles and which stimulate individual groups of myocardial cells to contract.

Chemical and Physical Influences on the Heart

Although the heart is designed to continue to beat according to the rhythm set by the spontaneous depolarization of the resting membrane potential of the SA node, both sympathetic and vagus (parasympathetic) nerve (cranial nerve X) fibers to the heart can modify the rate of this spontaneous depolarization.

Bainbridge Reflex

The Bainbridge reflex is the result of stimulation of mechanoreceptors located within the right atrial myocardium. The stimulation occurs because of an increase in pressure and stretch (distension) of the right atrium caused by an increase in venous return. Vasomotor centers of the medulla respond by increasing the sympathetic input and thus the heart rate, or by decreasing the sympathetic input and heart rate on those occasions when the heart is beating too rapidly.

Hemodynamics

Hemodynamics concerns the physical factors governing blood flow within the circulatory system.

- *Stroke volume (SV)*: The amount of blood pumped out by the left ventricle of the heart with each beat. The heart does not pump all the blood out of the ventricle—normally, only about two-thirds.
- *Cardiac output (CO)*: The amount of blood discharged by each ventricle (not both ventricles combined) per minute, usually expressed as liters per minute. Factors that influence CO include venous pressure, heart rate (HR), and left ventricular contractility.[2] CO is calculated by multiplying stroke volume (SV) by HR. For example, if each ventricle has a rate of 72 beats per minute and ejects 70 milliliters with each beat, the cardiac output equals 72 beats per minute × 0.07 liters per beat = 5.0 liters per minute.
- *Cardiac index*: A valuable diagnostic and prognostic tool when treating patients with pulmonary hypertension (PH). Calculated as cardiac output (liters) per unit time (minutes) divided by body surface area (m²); normally calculated in liters per minute per square meter. Normal cardiac index ranges between 2.5 and 40.0 liters per minute per meter.

Normal Exercise Response

A *metabolic equivalent unit* (MET) is defined as the energy expenditure for sitting quietly, talking on the phone, or reading a book, which, for the average adult, approximates 3.5 ml of oxygen uptake per kilogram of body weight per minute (3.5 mL O_2/kg/min)—1.2 kcal/min for a 70-kilogram individual) (see Chapter 12). An increase in V_{O_2} occurs with an increase in external workload. There is a direct, almost linear relationship between HR and external workload (intensity). Therefore, if a physical therapy intervention requires an increase in systemic oxygen consumption expressed as an increase in either MET levels, kcal, L/O_2, or ml/O_2 per kg of body weight per minute, then HR also should increase.[2]

> **● Key Point** The magnitude at which the HR increases with increasing workloads is influenced by many factors, including age, fitness level, type of activity being performed, presence of disease, medications, blood volume, and environmental factors such as temperature, humidity, and altitude. Failure of the heart rate to increase with increasing workloads (*chronotropic incompetence*) should be of concern, even if the patient is taking beta blockers for an abnormal heart rhythm.[2]

In the normal heart, as workload increases:

- Stroke volume (SV) increases linearly up to 50% of aerobic capacity, after which it increases only slightly. Factors that influence the magnitude of change in SV include ventricular function, body position, and exercise intensity.
- Cardiac output (CO) increases linearly with workload because of the increases in HR and SV in response to increasing exercise intensity. Factors that influence the magnitude of change in CO include age, posture, body size, presence of disease, and level of physical conditioning.

Blood Pressure

Blood pressure (BP), a product of CO and peripheral vascular resistance, is defined as the pressure exerted by the blood on the walls of the blood vessels, specifically arterial blood pressure (the pressure in the large arteries).

> **● Key Point** *Valsalva maneuver*, an attempt to exhale forcibly with the glottis, nose, and mouth closed, typically occurs during isometric exercise.[1] This results in:
> - An increase in intrathoracic pressure with an accompanying collapse of the veins of the chest wall.
> - A decrease in blood flow to the heart, and a decreased venous return.
> - A drop in arterial blood pressure.
>
> When the breath is released, the intrathoracic pressure decreases, and venous return is suddenly reestablished as an *overshoot* mechanism to compensate for the drop in blood pressure. This causes a marked increase in heart rate and arterial blood pressure.[1]

> **● Key Point** *Orthostatic hypotension* is a decrease in BP below normal (a systolic blood pressure decrease of at least 20 mm Hg or a diastolic blood pressure decrease of at least 10 mm Hg within 3 minutes of standing) to the point where the pressure is not adequate for normal oxygenation of the tissues when assuming an upright position.[10]

Regulation of Blood Pressure

The CNS regulatory site for BP is the vasomotor center, which is located bilaterally in the lower pons and upper medulla. The vasomotor center mediates sympathetic and vagal inputs and is influenced by neural impulses arising in the baroreceptors, chemoreceptors, hypothalamus, cerebral cortex, and skin.

Baroreceptor (Pressoreceptor) Reflex

Baroreceptors, located in the walls of the aortic arch and carotid sinus, are activated by either pressure or stretch receptors located within the internal carotid (carotid sinus) and aortic arch. Because these receptors are more responsive to constantly changing pressure than to sustained constant pressure, they play a key role in the short-term adjustment of blood pressure. Adjustments are made in the mean arterial pressure by facilitating a compensatory decrease in cardiac output (CO) and peripheral vascular resistance (PVR).[2]

Increased BP results in a decrease in sympathetic activation of the heart, arterioles, and veins, and an increase in parasympathetic stimulation: Vasodilation of peripheral blood vessels/decrease in blood pressure.

Decreased BP results in a decreased firing of the arterial baroreceptors, resulting in an increase in sympathetic activation of the heart, veins, and arterioles, and a decrease in parasympathetic activity of the heart: Vasoconstriction of peripheral blood vessels/increase in blood pressure.

Renin–Angiotensin System

The renin–angiotensin system (RAS) is generally known for its long-term adjustment of blood pressure. The RAS allows the kidney to compensate for loss in blood volume or drops in blood pressure by activating an endogenous vasoconstrictor known as angiotensin II.

> **● Key Point** Medications called *afterload reducers* (e.g., ACE inhibitors, angiotensin receptor blockers) block the effects of the renin–angiotensin system, thereby reducing both preload and afterload.[2]

Aldosterone Release

Aldosterone, a steroid hormone, is released from the adrenal gland in response to either high serum potassium levels or if angiotensin II is present. This hormone increases the excretion of potassium by the kidneys, while increasing sodium retention. Since sodium is the main ion that determines the amount of fluid in the blood vessels by osmosis, aldosterone will increase fluid retention and thus, indirectly, blood pressure.

Measurement of Blood Pressure

Arterial Pressure

Blood pressure values, measured with a sphygmomanometer, are usually given in millimeters of mercury (mm Hg). The manual method of measuring blood pressure (BP) is commonly used by the PTA. While listening with a stethoscope placed over the brachial artery at the elbow, the clinician slowly inflates the blood pressure cuff until the sound of the artery is completely occluded. At this point, the clinician slowly releases the pressure in the cuff. At the point when the clinician begins to hear a "whooshing" or pounding sound (called the first Korotkoff sound— see the following), the pressure reading (systolic) is noted. The cuff pressure is further released until no sound can be heard (fifth Korotkoff sound). This is the diastolic blood pressure.

> **● Key Point** *Korotkoff sounds* are the sounds that medical personnel listen for when they are taking blood pressure. Korotkoff described five phases of sounds:
>
> 1. The first clear, rhythmic tapping sound that gradually increases in intensity. This represents the highest pressure in the arterial system during ventricular contraction and is recorded as the systolic pressure. The clinician should be alert for the presence of an auscultatory gap, especially in patients with hypertension.[1] An auscultatory gap is the temporary disappearance of sound normally heard over the brachial artery between phase 1 and phase 2 and may cover a range of as much as 40 mm Hg.[1] Not identifying this gap may lead to an underestimation of systolic pressure and overestimation of diastolic pressure.[1]
> 2. A murmur or swishing sound heard as the artery widens and more blood flows through the artery. This sound is heard for most of the time between the systolic and diastolic pressures.
> 3. Sounds become crisp, more intense, and louder.
> 4. The sound is distinct, with abrupt muffling, soft blowing quality. At pressures within 10 mm Hg above the diastolic blood pressure (in children less than 13 years old, pregnant women, and patients with high cardiac output or peripheral vasodilation), the muffling sound should be used to indicate diastolic pressure, but both muffling (phase 4) and disappearance (phase 5) should be recorded.
> 5. The last sound that is heard, traditionally recorded as diastolic blood pressure.

Traditionally, the systolic blood pressure is taken to be the pressure at which the first Korotkoff sound is first heard, and the diastolic blood pressure reading is taken at the point at which the fourth Korotkoff sound is just barely audible. However, there has recently been a move toward the use of the fifth Korotkoff sound (i.e., silence) as the diastolic blood pressure, as this has been felt to be more reproducible.[11–16]

In pregnancy a fifth phase may not be identifiable, in which case the fourth is used.[17–19]

> **● Key Point** *Systolic pressure* is the pressure exerted on the brachial artery when the heart is contracting.[10] *Diastolic pressure* is the pressure exerted on the brachial artery during the relaxation phase of the heart contraction.[10]

> **● Key Point** The values for resting blood pressure in adults are:
>
> - *Normal:* Systolic blood pressure <120 mm Hg and diastolic blood pressure <80 mm Hg
> - *Pre-hypertension:* Systolic blood pressure 120–139 mm Hg or diastolic blood pressure 80–90 mm Hg
> - *Stage 1 hypertension:* Systolic blood pressure 140–159 mm Hg or diastolic blood pressure 90–99 mm Hg
> - *Stage 2 hypertension:* Systolic blood pressure ≥ 160 mm Hg or diastolic blood pressure ≥ 100 mm Hg
>
> The normal values for resting blood pressure in children are:
>
> - *Systolic:* Birth to one month 60 to 90; up to three years of age 75 to 130; over 3 years of age 90 to 140
> - *Diastolic:* Birth to one month 30 to 60; up to three years of age 45 to 90; over 3 years of age 50 to 80

> **● Key Point** *White coat hypertension* (WCH), also known as the white coat effect or isolated office hypertension, is the presence of higher BP when measured in the physician's office than at other times.[20–22] Whether WCH is a benign phenomenon or carries increased cardiovascular risk is still not known.

Venous Pressure

Venous pressure (VP) is the blood pressure in a vein. Measurement of pressures in the venous system and the pulmonary vessels plays an important role in intensive care medicine but requires invasive techniques.

Relevance of Blood Pressure to Rehabilitation

Typically, systolic BP rises rapidly and diastolic pressure rises slightly during the first few minutes of aerobic exercise, and then both level off.[23,24] With resistance training, systolic BP rises more dramatically within the first few minutes. High-level resistance training can cause rises in systolic BP that can be harmful for individuals with preexisting hypertension or heart disease, and therefore, loads should be kept lower in such patients. Aerobic exercise performed with the arms produces a greater rise in systolic and diastolic BP than lower-extremity exercise performed at the same intensity (as measured by percentage of maximal oxygen uptake).

Although exercise causes an acute increase in BP during the first few minutes, regular submaximal aerobic and resistance training do not cause long-term increases in resting BP but rather result in lowered BP for 2 to 3 hours after exercise, lowered resting BP, and blunting of the BP response to this form of exercise.

Pulse

The pulse results from pressure waves moving through the blood vessels. The term *pulse* is often used, although incorrectly, to denote the frequency of the heartbeat, usually measured in beats per minute (bpm). The pulse rate (or frequency) is the number of pulsations (peripheral pulse waves) per minute.

● **Key Point** The pulse is usually an accurate measure of heart rate. However, in certain cases, including arrhythmias, the heart rate can be (much) higher than the pulse rate. In these cases, the heart rate should be determined by auscultation of the central pulse at the heart apex (fifth interspace, midclavicular vertical line, also known as the apical pulse or point of maximal impulse [PMI]). The pulse deficit (difference between heart beats and pulsations at the periphery) is determined by simultaneous palpation at the radial artery and auscultation at the heart apex.

The peripheral pulse is commonly taken by palpating the radial artery at the wrist. Sometimes the pulse cannot be taken at the wrist; it can also be taken at the elbow (brachial artery), at the neck against the carotid artery (carotid pulse), in the inguinal region (femoral artery), behind the knee (popliteal artery), or in the foot (dorsalis pedis or posterior tibial arteries).

● **Key Point** The carotid artery should be palpated gently to avoid stimulating the baroreceptors, which can provoke severe bradycardia or even stop the heart in some sensitive patients. Also, the clinician should avoid palpating both of a person's carotid arteries at the same time, to avoid a risk of fainting or brain ischemia.

To take a peripheral pulse, the clinician's fingers must be placed near the artery and pressed gently against a firm structure, usually a bone, in order to feel the pulse. One should avoid using the thumb when taking a pulse because the thumb has its own pulse, which can interfere with detecting the patient's pulse. In a healthy individual, the pulse rhythm is regular and indicates that the time intervals between pulse beats are essentially equal. The clinician should palpate for 15 seconds and multiply by 4 with regular rhythm (evenly spaced beats), one minute with regularly irregular (regular pattern overall with "skipped" beats) or irregularly irregular (chaotic, no real pattern) rhythm (**Table 6-2**).

TABLE 6-2	Normal and Abnormal Pulses

Type	Description
Normal	The pulse is smooth and regular.
Large, bounding	The pulse feels strong and bounding. Causes include: • Increased stroke volume • Decreased peripheral resistance • Complete heart block • Decrease compliance of the aortic walls, as in aging or atherosclerosis
Bisferiens	An increased arterial pulse. Causes include: • Aortic regurgitation • Combined aortic stenosis and regurgitation
Pulsus alterans	The pulse alternates in amplitude from beat to beat even though the rhythm is basically regular. Usually indicates left ventricular failure.
Bigeminal	May masquerade as pulsus alternans. Caused by a normal beat alternating with a premature contraction.
Paradoxical	A palpable decrease in the pulse amplitude on quiet inspiration. Typically associated with pericardial tamponade, constrictive pericarditis, and obstructive lung disease.

Data from Schmitz TJ: Vital Signs, in O'Sullivan SB, Schmitz TJ (eds): Physical Rehabilitation (ed 5). Philadelphia, F. A. Davis, 2007, pp 81–120

● **Key Point**
• The normal adult heart rate is 70 bpm, with a range of 60 to 80 bpm.
• A rate of greater than 100 bpm is referred to as *tachycardia*.
• A rate of less than 60 bpm is referred to as *bradycardia*.
• The normal rate for a newborn is 120 bpm (range 70 to 170 bpm).
• *Arrhythmia* or *dysrhythmia* refers to an irregular rhythm in which pulses are not evenly spaced.[1]

● **Key Point** The ease of palpability of a pulse is dictated by the patient's blood pressure. If his or her systolic blood pressure is:
• Below 90 mm Hg, the radial pulse will not be palpable.
• Below 80 mm Hg, the brachial pulse will not be palpable.
• Below 60 mm Hg, the carotid pulse will not be palpable. Since systolic blood pressure rarely drops that low, the lack of a carotid pulse usually indicates death.

The pulse quality and rate are influenced by a number of factors, including the age of the patient, patient gender, the force of contraction, the volume and viscosity of blood, the diameter and elasticity of vessels, patient emotions, the amount of exercise performed prior to testing, medications, systemic or local temperature, and hormones.

> **● Key Point** To grade a peripheral pulse, the following scales may be used:
>
> *0–3 Scale*
> 0 Absent
> 1+ Weak/thready pulse
> 2+ Normal
> 3+ Bounding
>
> *Pulse Amplitude*
> 0 Absent
> 1+ Barely palpable
> 2+ Normal
> 3+ Moderately increased
> 4+ Markedly increased, aneurysmal

Examination of Heart Sounds

Auscultation is the process of listening for sound within the body. To examine the heart sounds, the clinician places a stethoscope directly on the chest using the recognized auscultation landmarks and notes the intensity and quality of the heart sounds produced by the closing of the AV and semilunar valves ("lub-dub").

- The "lub," or first sound (S1), is produced with the normal closure of the AV valves (mitral and tricuspid valves) at the onset of systole.
- The "dub," or second sound (S2), is produced with the normal closure of the semilunar valves (aortic and pulmonary) at the onset of diastole.

> **● Key Point** Rarely, there may be a third heart sound (S3), called a *ventricular gallop*, that occurs at the beginning of diastole after S2. The third heart sound is benign in youth, some trained athletes, and sometimes in pregnancy, but if it re-emerges later in life it may signal cardiac problems like a failing left ventricle, as in dilated congestive heart failure (CHF).
>
> A rare fourth heart sound (S4) is sometimes audible in healthy children and again in trained athletes, but when audible in an adult it is called an *atrial gallop*. The sound occurs at the end of diastole and immediately before S1. It is a sign of a pathologic state, usually a failing left ventricle, but it can also be heard in other conditions, such as restrictive cardiomyopathy.

Examination of the Heart Rhythm

The most accurate way to examine heart rhythm is to use an electrocardiogram (ECG). A typical ECG tracing of a normal heartbeat consists of a P wave, a QRS complex, and a T wave.

> **● Key Point** Twelve-lead ECG provides information about rate, rhythm, conduction, areas of ischemia and infarct, hypertrophy, and electrolyte imbalances. An ECG is constructed by measuring electrical potential between 12 different points of the body using a galvanometer. The 12 leads measure the average electrical activity generated by the summation of the action potentials of the heart at a particular moment in time.

P Wave

The P wave is the electrical signature of the current that causes atrial contraction. Both the left and right atria contract simultaneously. Its relationship to QRS complexes determines the presence of a heart block.[8]

> **● Key Point**
> - The shape of the P waves may indicate atrial problems.
> - Irregular or absent P waves may indicate arrhythmia.

> **● Key Point** The normal sinus rhythm consists of:
> - A P wave at a rate of 60 to 100 per minute
> - A QRS rate of 60 to 100 per minute
> - A P wave before every QRS complex
> - A regular P–P interval
> - A regular R-R interval

QRS Complex

The QRS complex corresponds to the current that causes contraction of the left and right ventricles. Abnormalities in the QRS complex may indicate bundle branch block (when wide), ventricular origin of tachycardia, ventricular hypertrophy, or other ventricular abnormalities.

> **● Key Point**
> - Very wide and deep Q waves indicate myocardial infarction that involves the full depth of the myocardium and has left a scar.
> - The R and S waves represent contraction of the myocardium itself.
> - The T wave represents the repolarization of the ventricles.

> **● Key Point** The ST segment connects the QRS complex and the T wave. It can be depressed in ischemia and elevated in myocardial infarction, and it upslopes with digoxin use. T wave abnormalities may indicate electrolyte disturbance, such as hyperkalemia and hypokalemia.

- *R-R interval:* A regular rhythm has equally sized spaces between all intervals. An intermittently irregular rhythm is generally regular with occasional disruptions (for example, extra beats). A regularly irregular rhythm has a cyclical pattern of varying R-R intervals. An irregularly irregular rhythm has no recurring pattern; R-R intervals vary in an inconsistent manner.
- *QT interval:* The QT interval is measured from the beginning of the QRS complex to the end of the T wave. A normal QT interval is usually about 0.40 seconds.
- *P-R interval:* The P-R interval is measured from the P wave to the QRS complex. It is usually 0.12 to 0.20 seconds (3 to 5 small boxes). A prolonged P-R indicates a slowing of conduction from the SA node into the AV junction and defines a first-degree (atrioventricular) heart block, while a shortening of the P-R indicates increased AV conduction or an atrial impulse that does not originate in the SA node.

In order to calculate the heart rate from an ECG strip, the clinician should multiply the number of QRS complexes in a 6-second strip (most ECG paper has markers every 1, 3, or 6 seconds) by 10 (chart speed = 25 mm/sec). Estimate the portion of the R-R interval when only a portion of one is contained at the end of 6 seconds. Alternatively, the clinician can divide 300 by the number of whole or partial large boxes between two consecutive R waves.

Cardiac Rhythms and Arrhythmias

Cardiac rhythms are generally named by the beat that initiates conduction to the ventricles and the rate (**Table 6-3**). For example, sinus bradycardia is a slow rate originating in the SA node, a junctional (or nodal) rhythm is a normal rate originating in the AV junction, and ventricular tachycardia is a rapid rhythm originating in the ventricles. Extra waves or complexes signify myocardial irritability, with the problem being atrial, junctional, and/or ventricular.

TABLE 6-3 ECG Characteristics of Abnormal Cardiac Rhythms

Rhythm	Description	ECG Characteristic
Sinus bradycardia	A heart rate < 60 bpm	P wave rate < 60/min QRS rate < 60/min
Sinus tachycardia	A heart rate > 100 bpm	P wave rate < 100/min QRS rate < 100/min
Premature atrial contraction (PAC)	Originate from areas of irritable, sometimes ischemic, myocardium that form the wall of the atrium. PACs are generally not as important as premature ventricular contractions: the loss of adequate filling and contraction of the atria associated with PACs are not as hemodynamically disruptive as premature contractions within the ventricles.	P-QRS occur earlier P wave may be abnormal in shape/configuration QRS is normal P-R interval may be altered Incomplete compensatory pause
Atrial fibrillation (A. fib)	Atrial fibrillation is characterized by multiple ectopic foci, or firing at random throughout the cardiac cycle with no single, unified wave of depolarization in the atria, and thus no organized myocardial contraction.	Absence of P waves; fibrillatory base line Fibrillatory rate > 350/min Irregular R-R interval QRS rate < P wave rate
Ventricular tachycardia	A run of three or more PVCs occurring sequentially; very rapid rate (150 to 200 bpm); may occur paroxysmally (abrupt onset); usually the result of an ischemic ventricle.	QRS rate > 100/min, regular (refer to ideoventricular rhythm for other characteristics)
Ventricular fibrillation (V. fib)	Chaotic activity of ventricle originating from multiple foci resulting in a pulseless, emergency situation requiring emergency medical treatment: cardiopulmonary resuscitation (CPR), defibrillation, medications.	Coarse waviness of baseline Fine waviness of baseline No visible QRS complexes
Premature ventricular contraction (PVC)	A premature beat arising from the ventricle; occurs occasionally in the majority of the normal population.	QRS duration > 0.10 sec T wave is opposite polarity of QRS Complete compensatory pause

The severity of an arrhythmia is related to the location, frequency, and number of sites where extra beats are initiated.

Heart Blocks

Heart blocks occur when conduction from the SA node to the AV node gets altered, usually at the level of the AV node. Heart blocks are graded by levels of severity, from first degree, to second degree, to third degree. A third-degree block is a complete heart block and usually requires the insertion of an artificial pacemaker.

> **● Key Point** Note the following definitions:
> - *Bigeminy:* Premature beats alternating regularly with normal beats. Bigeminy is either atrial or ventricular bigeminy, depending upon whether the alternating regular premature beats are atrial or ventricular. Bigeminy is generally considered pathological, especially when symptomatic. Because the premature beats alternate regularly, bigeminy generally sounds like a regularly irregular heart rhythm. Bigeminy can be associated with hypoxia, ischemia, acute myocardial infarction, and medication overdose.
> - *Trigeminy:* A type of premature ventricular contraction (PVC) pattern. The PVC follows very two normal QRS complexes. Possible causes are electrolyte imbalances, hypoxia, ischemia, acute myocardial infarction, and medication toxicity.

Exercise Tolerance Testing

Exercise tolerance testing (also known as graded exercise testing or stress test) is an important diagnostic and prognostic tool for assessing the ability of the cardiovascular system to accommodate increasing Vo_2 in patients with suspected or known ischemic heart disease. The patient exercises through stages of increasing workloads, expressed in units of oxygen—L/min, ml O_2/kg /min, kcal, or metabolic equivalents (METs).[2]

> **● Key Point** The two major goals of exercise testing are to detect the presence of ischemia and determine the functional aerobic capacity of the individual.[2]

During the test, an electrocardiogram machine or a Holter monitor (**Table 6-4**) can be used to provide a continuous record of the heart rate, and the 12-lead electrocardiogram is recorded intermittently. The aim of the exercise is for the patient to achieve his or her maximum predicted heart rate. Numerous protocols for exercise tests and other tests (Table 6-4) have been devised to assess cardiac responses to increased workloads.

Borg Rating of Perceived Exertion Scale

In exercise testing, the Borg Rating of Perceived Exertion (RPE) scale measures perceived exertion and can be used to document the patient's exertion during a test. The original scale introduced by Borg[25] rated exertion on a scale of 6 to 20, but a more recent one designed by Borg included a category (C) ratio (R) scale, the Borg CR10 Scale® (refer to Table 3-1). This scale is specifically used in clinical diagnosis of breathlessness and dyspnea, chest pain, angina, and musculoskeletal pain.

Basic Life Support/ Cardiopulmonary Resuscitation

Cardiopulmonary resuscitation (CPR) involves a series of procedures to create artificial circulation through rhythmic pressing on the patient's chest by the rescuer to manually pump blood through the heart, called chest compressions, and can also involve the rescuer exhaling into the patient (or using a device) to ventilate the lungs, called artificial respiration. Before starting CPR, check:

- Is the person conscious or unconscious?
- If the person appears unconscious, tap or shake his or her shoulder and ask loudly, "Are you OK?"
- Check the pulse for 10 seconds.
- If the person doesn't respond and two people are available, one should call 911 or the local emergency number and one should begin CPR. If you are alone and have immediate access to a telephone, call 911 before beginning CPR—unless you think the person has become unresponsive because of suffocation (such as from drowning). In this special case, perform CPR for one minute and then call 911.
- If an automatic external defibrillator (AED) is immediately available, deliver one shock if instructed by the device, then begin CPR. Check the heart rate rhythm every 2 minutes and reuse the defibrillator if no rhythm is detected.

> **● Key Point** Think CAB: chest compressions, airway, and breathing.

TABLE 6-4	Cardiac Diagnostic Testing and Monitoring

Test	Description
Holter monitor	A small, portable, battery-powered ECG machine worn by a patient to record heartbeats on tape over a period of 24 to 48 hours during normal activities. At the end of the time period, the monitor is returned to the physician's office so the tape can be read and evaluated.
Exercise gated blood pool scan, exercise MUGA, or exercise radionuclide angiography	A nuclear scan to see how the heart wall moves and how much blood is expelled with each heartbeat, just after the patient has walked on a treadmill or ridden on a stationary bike. *Resting First Pass*: The scan taken while the patient is at rest to measure the percentage of blood going through the heart with each beat. *Exercise First Pass:* The scan taken while the patient is exercising to measure the percentage of blood going through the heart with each beat.
Event recorder	A small, portable, battery-powered machine used by a patient to record ECG over a long period of time. Patients may keep the recorder for several weeks. Each time symptoms are experienced, the patient presses a button on the recorder to record the ECG sample. As soon as possible, this sample is transmitted to the physician's office by telephone hookup for evaluation.
Thallium scans or myocardial perfusion scans	*Resting SPECT thallium scan or myocardial perfusion scan:* A nuclear scan given while the patient is at rest that may reveal areas of the heart muscle that are not getting enough blood. *Exercise Thallium Scan or Myocardial Perfusion Scan:* A nuclear scan given while the patient is exercising that may reveal areas of the heart muscle that are not getting enough blood. *Persantine Thallium Scan or Myocardial Perfusion Scan:* A nuclear scan given to a patient who is unable to exercise to reveal areas of the heart muscle that are not getting enough blood. Chemicals injected include dipyridamole thallium (thallium-201, a potent vasodilator) and dobutamine.
Positron emission tomography (PET) scan	A nuclear scan that gives information about the flow of blood through the coronary arteries to the heart muscle.
PET F-18 FDG (fluorodeoxyglucose) scan	A glucose scan sometimes done immediately after the PET scan to determine if heart muscle has permanent damage.
Radionuclide angiography	Red blood cells tagged with a radionuclide are injected into the blood; ventricular wall motion can be evaluated and the ejection fraction determined; abnormal blood flow with valve and congenital defects also can be detected; techniques include gated-pool equilibrium studies and first-pass techniques.
Technetium 99m scanning (hotspot imaging)[1]	Technetium 99m injected into the blood is taken up by damaged myocardial tissue; this identifies and localizes acute myocardial infarctions. This radioisotope is readily available, and its short half-life reduces handling problems and patient exposure.
Thallium-201 myocardial perfusion imaging (cold spot imaging)[1]	Thallium-201 injected into the blood at peak exercise; scanning identifies ischemic and infarcted myocardium, which does not take up thallium-201; used to diagnose coronary artery disease and perfusion particularly when ECG is equivocal.
Cardiac catheterization	The passage of a tiny tube into heart via blood vessels with the introduction of a contrast medium into coronary arteries that is then visualized with cinefluoroscopy to evaluate narrowing or occlusion of arteries. 1. Provides information about anatomy of heart and great vessels, ventricular function, cardiac output, and abnormal wall movement. 2. Allows determination of intracardiac, transvalve, pulmonary artery pressures, ejection fraction (EF), and blood gas pressures.

Data from Rothstein JM, Roy SH, Wolf SL: Vascular Anatomy, Cardiology, and Cardiac Rehabilitation, The Rehabilitation Specialists Handbook. Philadelphia, F. A. Davis, 1991, pp 548–550

Chest Compressions

1. Place the heel of one hand over the center of the person's chest, between the nipples. Place your other hand on top of the first hand. Keep your elbows straight and position your shoulders directly above your hands.

2. Use your upper body weight (not just your arms) as you push straight down on (compress) the chest at least 2 inches (approximately 5 centimeters). Push hard and fast at a rate of at least 100 compressions a minute. Allow for a complete recoil of the chest in between compressions.

3. After 30 compressions, tilt the head back and lift the chin up to open the airway. Prepare to give two rescue breaths. Pinch the nose shut and breathe into the mouth for one second. If the chest rises, give a second rescue breath. If the chest doesn't rise, repeat the head-tilt, chin-lift maneuver and then give the second rescue breath. That's one cycle. If someone else is available, ask that person to give two breaths after you do 30 compressions. If you're not trained in CPR and only feel comfortable performing chest compressions, skip rescue breathing and continue chest compressions at a rate of 100 compressions a minute until medical personnel arrive.

4. If the person has not begun moving after five cycles (about 2 minutes) and an automatic external defibrillator (AED) is available, apply it and follow the prompts. Administer one shock, and then resume CPR—starting with chest compressions—for two more minutes before administering a second shock. If you're not trained to use an AED, a 911 operator may be able to guide you in its use. Use pediatric pads, if available, for children ages 1 to 8. Do not use an AED for babies younger than age 1.

Airway: Clear the Airway

Minimize the time away from compressions to 10 seconds.

1. Put the person on his or her back on a firm surface.

2. Kneel next to the person's neck and shoulders.

3. Open the person's airway using the head-tilt, chin-lift maneuver. Put your palm on the person's forehead and gently tilt the head back. Then with the other hand, gently lift the chin forward to open the airway.

4. Check for normal breathing, taking no more than 5 or 10 seconds. Look for chest motion, listen for normal breath sounds, and feel for the person's breath on your cheek and ear. Gasping is not considered to be normal breathing. If the person isn't breathing normally and you are trained in CPR, begin mouth-to-mouth breathing. If you believe the person is unconscious from a heart attack and you haven't been trained in emergency procedures, skip mouth-to-mouth rescue breathing and proceed directly to chest compressions.

Breathing: Breathe for the Person

Rescue breathing can be mouth-to-mouth breathing or mouth-to-nose breathing if the mouth is seriously injured or can't be opened.

1. With the airway open (using the head-tilt, chin-lift maneuver), pinch the nostrils shut for mouth-to-mouth breathing and cover the person's mouth with yours, making a seal.

2. Prepare to give two rescue breaths. Give the first rescue breath—lasting one second—and watch to see if the chest rises. If it does rise, give the second breath. If the chest doesn't rise, repeat the head-tilt, chin-lift maneuver and then give the second breath.

3. Begin chest compressions to restore circulation.

> ● **Key Point** Continue CPR until there are signs of movement or until emergency medical personnel take over. CPR is generally continued, usually in the presence of advanced life support (such as from EMS providers), until the patient regains a heartbeat or is declared dead.

Performing CPR on a Child

The procedure for giving CPR to a child age 1 through 8 is essentially the same as that for an adult. The differences are as follows:

- If you're alone, perform five cycles of compressions and breaths on the child—this should take about two minutes—before calling 911 or your local emergency number or using an AED.

- Use only one hand to perform heart compressions. The depth of the compression should be one third the anteroposterior (AP) diameter of the chest (about 2 inches).

- Breathe more gently.

- Use the same compression-breath rate as is used for adults: 30 compressions followed by two breaths. This is one cycle. Following the two breaths, immediately begin the next cycle of compressions and breaths.

- After five cycles (about 2 minutes) of CPR, if there is no response and an AED is available, apply it and follow the prompts. Use pediatric pads if available. If pediatric pads aren't available, use adult pads.

Continue until the child moves or help arrives.

Performing CPR on an Infant

Most cardiac arrests in babies occur from lack of oxygen, such as from drowning or choking. If you know the baby has an airway obstruction, clear the airway. If you don't know why the baby isn't breathing, perform CPR. To begin, examine the situation. Stroke the baby and watch for a response, such as movement, but don't shake the baby. If there's no response, follow the CAB procedures below and time the call for help as follows:

- If you're the only rescuer and CPR is needed, do CPR for 2 minutes—about five cycles—before calling 911 or your local emergency number.
- If another person is available, have that person call for help immediately while you attend to the baby.

Chest Compressions

1. Imagine a horizontal line drawn between the baby's nipples. Place two fingers of one hand just below this line, in the center of the chest.
2. Gently compress the chest to about one-third to one-half the depth of the chest (about 1 to 2 inches).
3. Count aloud as you pump in a fairly rapid rhythm. You should pump at a rate of at least 100 compressions a minute.
4. Give two breaths after every 30 chest compressions.

Airway

1. Place the baby on his or her back on a firm, flat surface, such as a table. The floor or ground also will do.
2. Gently tip the head back by lifting the chin with one hand and pushing down on the forehead with the other hand.
3. In no more than 10 seconds, put your ear near the baby's mouth and check for breathing: Look for chest motion, listen for breath sounds, and feel for breath on your cheek and ear.
   If the infant isn't breathing, begin mouth-to-mouth rescue breathing immediately. Compressions-only CPR doesn't work for infants.

Breathing

1. Cover the baby's mouth and nose with your mouth.
2. Prepare to give two rescue breaths. Use the strength of your cheeks to deliver gentle puffs of air (instead of deep breaths from your lungs) to slowly breathe into the baby's mouth one time, taking one second for the breath. Watch to see if the baby's chest rises. If it does, give a second rescue breath. If the chest does not rise, repeat the head-tilt, chin-lift maneuver and then give the second breath.
3. If the baby's chest still doesn't rise, examine the mouth to make sure no foreign material is inside. If the object is seen, sweep it out with your finger. If the airway seems blocked, perform first aid for a choking baby.
4. Begin chest compressions to restore blood circulation.

Diagnostic Tests

Left Heart Catheterization/Coronary Angiogram

This procedure involves insertion of a catheter into a major artery (often the femoral or radial artery) and advancing at retrograde through the aorta until it reaches the left ventricle.[2] The catheter may then proceed into the LV and is used to measure hemodynamic pressures during systole and diastole to examine LV function (ejection fraction). The angiogram component involves injecting a radiopaque dye into the the ostium of each coronary artery, observing blood flow through each of the arteries to determine the presence of lesions or blood flow obstructions.[2]

Duplex Ultrasonography Duplex

Ultrasonography is the study of choice for the evaluation of venous insufficiency syndromes. Color-flow duplex imaging uses the Doppler information to color code a two-dimensional sonogram. On the image, red indicates flow in one direction (relative to the transducer), and blue indicates flow in the other direction. With the latest-generation machines, the shade of the color may reflect the flow velocity (in the Doppler mode) or the flow volume (in the power Doppler mode).

Magnetic Resonance Venography

Magnetic resonance venography (MRV) is the most sensitive and specific test for the assessment of deep and superficial venous disease in the lower legs and pelvis, areas not accessible with other modalities. MRV is particularly useful because it can help in the detection of previously unsuspected nonvascular causes of leg pain and edema when the clinical presentation erroneously suggests venous insufficiency or venous obstruction.

Direct Contrast Venography

Direct contrast venography is a labor-intensive and invasive imaging technique. In most centers, duplex sonography has replaced this direct contrast venography in the routine evaluation of venous disease.

Physiologic Tests of Venous Function

Physiologic tests of venous function are important in assessing the cause and severity of venous insufficiency. The physiologic parameters most often measured are the venous refilling time (VRT), the maximum venous outflow (MVO), and the calf muscle pump ejection fraction (MPEF).

Doppler Ultrasound

This technique uses an ultrasonic oscillator connected to earphones. The Doppler probe is placed over a large vessel, and an ultrasound signal is given transcutaneously. Movement of blood causes an audible shift in signal frequency. Ultrasound is useful in locating nonpalpable pulses and measuring systolic BP in extremities.

● **Key Point** The *ankle-brachial index* (ABI) is a test that measures arterial perfusion using Doppler. The patient is positioned supine, and blood pressures are measured in both upper extremities (using the brachial arteries) and lower extremities (using the dorsal pedis and tibialis posterior artery). The highest lower-extremity systolic pressure is divided by the brachial systolic pressure and represented as a ratio. The following scale is used:

1.0 Normal
0.5–0.9 Arterial occlusion/impairment with wound healing/ therapeutic exercise beneficial
<0.5 Severe arterial occlusion/poor to no wound healing/exercise is unrealistic
A ratio of 0.9 at rest or 0.85 after exercise indicates peripheral artery disease.

Air Plethysmography

Air plethysmography (APG) makes use of a pneumatic device calibrated to measure patency of the venous system. The technique is as follows:

1. The cuff of the device, which is inflated around the calf, is attached to a pressure transducer and microprocessor.

2. The cuff occludes venous return and permits arterial inflow. The recorder registers increasing volume using the cuff, returning to baseline with cuff deflation.

3. The clinician performs comparison tests with patient sitting, standing, and up on tiptoes.

Chest Radiograph

A chest radiograph can help to determine the presence of lung fluid abnormalities and the overall shape and size of the heart.

Myocardial Perfusion Imaging

Myocardial perfusion imaging is used to diagnose and evaluate ischemic heart disease and myocardial infarction.

Continuous Hemodynamic Monitoring

Performed with a Swan–Ganz catheter inserted through vessels into the right side of the heart, the technique measures central venous pressure (CVP), pulmonary artery pressure (PA), and pulmonary capillary wedge pressures (PCWP).

Echocardiography

Echocardiography is a technique invloving the use of ultrasonic sound waves to create a moving picture of the heart.

Laboratory Tests and Values

Enzyme Studies

Cardiac enzyme studies measure the levels of the enzymes troponin (TnI, TnT) and creatine phosphokinase (CPK) in the blood (**Table 6-5** and **Table 6-6**). Elevated troponin levels may indicate an injury to

TABLE 6-5	Troponin Lab Values
Normal	TnI: Less than 0.3 micrograms per liter (µg/L) TnT: Less than 0.1 µg/L
Abnormal	Elevated troponin may be present with an injury to the myocardium. Blood levels of troponin typically rise within 4 to 6 hours after a heart attack, reach their highest levels within 10 to 24 hours, and fall to normal levels within 10 days.

TABLE 6-6	Creatine Phosphokinase Blood Levels			
Related Physiology	Increased Values	Decreased Values	Reference Range Example
An enzyme found predominantly in the heart, brain, and skeletal muscle. Aids in protein catabolism. Can be separated into subunits or isoenzymes, each derived from a specific tissue. CPK-BB = brain CPK-MB = cardiac CPK-MM = skeletal muscle	BB: brain injury, severe shock, renal failure, and widespread metastases MB: myocardial infarction, postcardiac surgery, muscular dystrophies, and polymyositis MM: trauma, muscular dystrophy, dermatomyositis, hypothyroidism, and seizures Total CPK: severe hypokalemia, carbon monoxide poisoning, seizures, and pulmonary and cerebral infarctions	Not typically seen	Total CPK: Less than 30

the myocardium. Creatine phosphokinase (CPK) is an enzyme found predominantly in the heart, brain, and skeletal muscle. It aids in protein catabolism and can be separated into subunits or isoenzymes, each derived from a specific tissue: brain (BB), cardiac (MB), or skeletal muscle (MM)

Lipid Profile

A lipid profile refers to a group of tests ordered together to help determine coronary risk based on target levels. The lipid profile includes total cholesterol, high-density lipoprotein (HDL) cholesterol (often called "good" cholesterol), LDL-cholesterol (often called "bad" cholesterol), and triglycerides. An LDL/HDL ratio is sometimes also included.

● **Key Point** The values listed below can be used as a general guide.

Cholesterol:
Desirable: <200
Borderline: 200–230
High risk: >240

High-Density Lipoprotein (HDL):
Low risk (negative risk factor): >60
Moderate risk: 35–60
High risk: <35

Low-Density Lipoprotein (LDL):
<100 indicates heart disease or diabetes
101–159 indicates there may be multiple risk factors
>160 indicates low risk of heart disease and diabetes

Triglycerides:
Desirable: <165

LDL/HDL Ratio:
Low risk: 0.5–3.0
Moderate risk: 3.0–6.0
High risk: >6.0

Cellular Blood Elements

The various laboratory tests for leukocytes/white blood cells (WBC) and erythrocytes/red blood cells are outlined in **Table 6-7**.

Cardiovascular Conditions

Risk Factors for Cardiac Pathology

Risk factors jointly accepted by the American Heart Association and the American College of Cardiology are divided into major independent risk factors and other risk factors:

Major Independent Risk Factors

- Cigarette smoking
- Hypertension
- Hypercholesterolemia (elevated serum total and LDL cholesterol)
- Low serum HDL cholesterol
- Diabetes mellitus
- Advancing age

Other Risk (Predisposing) Factors

- Obesity: body mass index (BMI) of greater than or equal to 30 kilograms
- Abdominal obesity: waist girth of greater than 100 centimeters
- Physical inactivity
- Family history of premature coronary heart disease
- Ethnic characteristics
- Psychosocial factors

elevation of the head of the bed, dangling one extremity over the edge of the bed, progressive sitting on the edge of the bed with active lower extremity exercise, deep breathing, and progressive sitting out of bed with the lower extremities progressed to a dependent position.[29] Elastic stockings should be worn over the lower extremities.[29] Elevating the head of the bed by 5 to 20 degrees during sleep is also recommended.[29]

Peripheral Vascular Disease

In venous insufficiency states, venous blood escapes from its normal antegrade path of flow and refluxes backward down the veins into an already congested leg. Venous insufficiency syndromes are caused by valvular incompetence in the high-pressure deep venous system, low-pressure superficial venous system, or both.

Deep Venous Insufficiency

Deep venous insufficiency occurs when the valves of the deep veins are damaged as a result of deep venous thrombosis (DVT)—see "Deep Vein Thrombophlebitis." There are no valves to prevent deep system reflux, so the hydrostatic venous pressure in the lower extremity increases dramatically. This condition is often referred to as a *post-phlebitic syndrome.*

Superficial Venous Insufficiency

Superficial venous incompetence is the most common form of venous disease. In superficial venous insufficiency, the deep veins are normal, but venous blood escapes from a normal deep system and flows backward through dilated superficial veins in which the valves have failed. Over time, the incompetent superficial veins become visibly dilated and tortuous, at which point they are recognized as varicose veins.

Interventions for Venous Insufficiency

Graduated Compression

Graduated compression is the cornerstone of the modern treatment of venous insufficiency. Properly fitted gradient compression stockings provide 30–40 or 40–50 mm Hg of compression at the ankle, with gradually decreasing compression at more proximal levels of the leg. This amount of gradient compression is sufficient to restore normal venous flow patterns in many or most patients with superficial venous reflux and to improve venous flow, even in patients with severe deep venous incompetence.

The compression gradient is extremely important because nongradient stockings or high-stretch elastic bandages (e.g., ACE wraps) may cause a tourniquet effect, with worsening of the venous insufficiency. Antiembolic stockings do not provide sufficient compression to improve the venous return from the legs. No patient with symptoms due to venous insufficiency should be without gradient compression hose, which can be prescribed by a physician. The prescription should specify one pair of gradient compression hose with a 30–40 mm Hg gradient that is calf-high (or thigh-high with waist attachment or pantyhose style), with refills as needed.

Venoablation

All methods of venoablation are effective. Once the overall volume of venous reflux is reduced below a critical threshold by any mechanism, venous ulcerations heal, and patient symptoms are resolved.

Endovenous Laser Therapy

Endovenous laser therapy (EVLT),[30–32] a newer procedure, is performed by passing a laser fiber from the knee to the groin and then delivering laser energy along the entire course of the vein. Destruction of the vascular wall is followed by fibrosis of the treated vessel. EVLT has demonstrated excellent early (4-year) results and an extremely low rate of complications, but the duration of follow-up is not yet long enough to provide information about midterm and long-term results.

Radiofrequency Ablation

Radiofrequency ablation (RFA)[33] is a relatively new procedure that has a low rate of complications. It has produced excellent results that have been confirmed after several years of follow-up. RFA is performed by passing a special radiofrequency (RF) catheter from the knee to the groin and by heating the vessel until thermal injury causes shrinkage. The process is repeated every few centimeters along the course of the vein. Initial thermal injury is followed by fibrosis of the treated vessel.

Physical Therapy

Regular exercise using a walking program for those with claudication helps develop collateral circulation and improves walking tolerance. Treadmill exercise (35 to 50 minutes, 3 to 4 times per week) has been reviewed as another treatment with a number of positive outcomes, including reduction in cardiovascular events and improved quality of life. In addition, non-weight-bearing exercises such as swimming and stationary cycling can supplement a walking program.

Thrombophlebitis

Microscopic thrombosis is a normal part of the dynamic balance of hemostasis. There are two types of venous thrombosis: superficial vein thrombophlebitis and deep vein thrombophlebitis. Superficial vein thrombophlebitis and deep vein thrombophlebitis share the same pathophysiology, pathogenesis, and risk factors.

Superficial Vein Thrombophlebitis

Superficial vein thrombophlebitis may occur spontaneously or as a complication of medical or surgical interventions. Patients with superficial thrombophlebitis often give a history of a gradual onset of localized tenderness, followed by the appearance of an area of erythema along the path of a superficial vein. Graduated compression stockings have been proven effective in the prophylaxis of thromboembolism and are also effective in preventing progression of thrombus in patients who already have superficial phlebitis or actual DVT and PE.[34-37]

Deep Vein Thrombophlebitis

Deep venous thrombosis (DVT) and its sequela, pulmonary embolism, are the leading causes of preventable in-hospital mortality in the United States.[38] Increased potential for DVT include:

- *Genetic:* Causes include antithrombin C deficiency, protein C deficiency, and protein S deficiency.
- *Acquired:* Common in postoperative and postpartum patients, as well as patients on prolonged bed rest; causes include immobilization, long flights, severe trauma, cancer, congestive heart failure, obesity, and prior thromboembolism.

● **Key Point** Patients who undergo total hip arthroplasty or total knee arthroplasty are at high risk for DVT. If no prophylaxis is used, DVT occurs in 40% to 80% of these patients, and the proximal DVT occurs in 15% to 50%.[39]

Prophylaxic treatment of DVT includes medication (heparin, warfarin, aspirin, and dextran) and the use of mechanical modalities, such as external pneumatic compression devices and compression stockings.

● **Key Point** In the event of a suspected DVT the PTA should hold the therapeutic interventions and inform the physician. The patient should be positioned in to avoid bearing weight on the involved lower extremity.

Congestive Heart Failure

Congestive heart failure (CHF) occurs when the heart fails to pump blood at a rate required by the metabolizing tissues. CHF can be subdivided into systolic (left heart) and diastolic (right heart) dysfunction, both of which result in a decrease in stroke volume.

- *Systolic (impaired emptying of the heart) failure:* A decrease in stroke volume, which leads to activation of peripheral and central baroreflexes and chemoreflexes that are capable of eliciting marked increases in sympathetic nerve activity. This in turn produces a temporary improvement in systolic blood pressure and tissue perfusion. Signs and symptoms of left-sided heart failure include progressive severity of (1) exertional dyspnea, (2) orthopnea (shortness of breath while lying flat), (3) paroxysmal nocturnal dyspnea, (4) dyspnea at rest, and (5) pulmonary edema.
- *Diastolic (insufficient filling of the heart) failure:* An altered relaxation of the ventricle (due to delayed calcium uptake and delayed calcium efflux) occurs in response to an increase in ventricular afterload (pressure overload). This impaired relaxation of the ventricle leads to impaired diastolic filling of the left ventricle and a decrease in stroke volume. Signs and symptoms of right-sided heart failure include ascites, congestive hepatomegaly, and anasarca (generalized edema).

● **Key Point** The central hemodynamic characteristics of heart failure that contribute to exercise intolerance include:[40-42]
- Abnormal pressures within the heart
- Reduced left ventricular ejection fraction
- Reduced cardiac output
- Increased pulmonary capillary wedge pressure
- Increased production of angiotensin II, which increases heart rate, impairs cardiac filling, and increases coronary vasoconstriction and peripheral vascular resistance

Treatment focuses on improving the symptoms and preventing the progression of the disease. Reversible causes of the heart failure are also addressed (e.g., infection, alcohol ingestion, anemia, arrhythmia, hypertension). A patient diagnosed with CHF may be referred to physical therapy for generalized conditioning. Physical therapy goals include improving exercise tolerance, typically with a walking program, improving strength, and improving overall function and participation in activities of daily living.

Cor Pulmonale

Cor pulmonale,[43-47] a form of right-sided heart failure that is not congestive in nature, is defined as an alteration in the structure and function of the right ventricle caused by a primary disorder of the respiratory system. Pulmonary hypertension (see Chapter 7) is the common link between lung dysfunction and the heart in cor pulmonale. Cor pulmonale can develop secondary to a wide variety of cardiopulmonary disease processes.

> ● **Key Point** Although cor pulmonale commonly has a chronic and slowly progressive course, acute onset or worsening cor pulmonale with life-threatening complications can occur.

Clinical manifestations of cor pulmonale are generally nonspecific. The patient may complain of fatigue, exertional dyspnea, exertional chest pain, and syncope with exertion—symptoms reflecting a relative inability to increase cardiac output during exercise with a subsequent drop in the systemic arterial pressure.

Cardiomyopathy

Cardiomyopathy is part of a group of conditions affecting the heart muscle itself so that the fibers involved with contraction and relaxation of the myocardial muscle are impaired. Causes include coronary artery disease (CAD; discussed below), valvular disorders, hypertension, congenital defects, and pulmonary vascular disorders.

Valvular Disease

Heart problems that occur secondary to impairment of the valves may be caused by infection such as endocarditis, congenital deformity, or disease. Three types of valve deformities may affect aortic, mitral, tricuspid, or pulmonary valves: stenosis, insufficiency, or prolapse.

- *Mitral stenosis:* A sequela of rheumatic heart disease that primarily affects women.
- *Mitral regurgitation (insufficiency):* Many causes, but involvement of the mitral valve accounts for approximately 50% of all cases of heart disease. Other causes include infective endocarditis, dilated cardiomyopathy, rheumatic disease, collagen vascular disease, rupture of the chordae tendineae, and, rarely, cardiac tumors.[48]
- *Mitral valve prolapse (floppy valve syndrome, Barlow syndrome):* Characterized by a slight variation in shape or structure of the mitral valve. Prolapse has an unknown etiology, although there may be a genetic component.
- *Aortic stenosis:* A disease of aging most commonly caused by progressive valvular calcification.
- *Aortic regurgitation (insufficiency):* Used to occur secondary to rheumatic fever; antibiotics have reduced the number of rheumatic-related cases. Nonrheumatic causes include congenital defects, infective endocarditis, and hypertension, or it may occur secondary to aortic dissection.
- *Tricuspid stenosis and regurgitation:* Usually occurs in people with severe mitral valve disease.

Arrhythmias

Arrhythmias are a group of conditions that affect the cardiac nervous system. Arrhythmias are usually classified according to their origin (ventricular or supraventricular [atrial]), pattern (fibrillation or flutter), or the speed or rate at which they occur (tachycardia or bradycardia). Causes include congenital defects, hypertrophy of the heart muscle fibers, valvular heart disease, and degeneration of conducted tissue.

Coronary Artery Disease

Coronary artery disease (CAD) is a complex disease involving a narrowing of the lumen of one or more of the arteries that encircle and supply the heart, resulting in ischemia to the myocardium. Injury to the endothelial lining of arteries, an inflammatory reaction, thrombosis, calcification, and hemorrhage all contribute to arteriosclerosis or scarring of an artery wall. The clinical symptoms of CAD include any symptoms that may represent cardiac ischemia, such as an ache, pressure, pain, other discomfort, or possibly just decreased activity tolerance due to fatigue, shortness of breath, or palpitations.

Atherosclerosis

Atherosclerosis primarily affects the lower extremities. When the arteries of the heart are affected it is referred to as coronary artery disease (CAD) or coronary heart disease (CHD); when the arteries to the brain are affected cerebrovascular disease (CVD) develops.[49]

Angina Pectoris

Angina pectoris[50] is the result of myocardial ischemia caused by an imbalance between myocardial blood supply and oxygen demand, which causes myocardial cells to switch from aerobic to anaerobic metabolism, with a progressive impairment of metabolic, mechanical, and electrical functions.

> **● Key Point** Most patients with angina pectoris complain of retrosternal chest discomfort rather than frank pain. The former is usually described as a pressure, heaviness, squeezing, burning, or choking sensation. Anginal pain may be localized primarily in the epigastrium, back, neck, or jaw. Typical locations for radiation of pain are the arms, shoulders, and neck (C8–T4 dermatomes). Typically, exertion, eating, exposure to cold, or emotional stress precipitate angina. Episodes typically last for approximately 1 to 5 minutes and are relieved by rest or by taking nitroglycerin.

Myocardial Infarction

Myocardial infarction (MI)[51] is the rapid development of myocardial necrosis caused by a critical imbalance between the oxygen supply and demand of the myocardium. This usually results from plaque rupture with thrombus formation in a coronary vessel, resulting in an acute reduction of blood supply to a portion of the myocardium.

- *Atherosclerotic causes:* The most common cause of MI. Plaque rupture with subsequent exposure of the basement membrane results in platelet aggregation, thrombus formation, fibrin accumulation, hemorrhage into the plaque, and varying degrees of vasospasm. MI occurs most frequently in persons older than 45 years.
- *Nonatherosclerotic causes:* Include coronary vasospasm as seen in variant (Prinzmetal) angina and in patients using cocaine and amphetamines, coronary emboli from sources such as an infected heart valve, occlusion of the coronaries due to vasculitis, or other causes leading to mismatch of oxygen supply and demand, such as acute anemia from GI bleeding.

Signs and symptoms of MI include:

- Chest pain, typically described as tightness, pressure, or squeezing, located across the anterior precordium. Pain may radiate to the jaw, neck, arms, back, and epigastrium. The left arm is affected more frequently; however, pain may be felt in both arms.
- Dyspnea, which may accompany chest pain or occur as an isolated complaint (especially in an elderly person or a diabetic patient).
- Nausea and/or abdominal pain with or without vomiting often are present in infarcts involving the inferior or posterior wall.
- Anxiety.
- Lightheadedness with or without syncope.
- Cough.

- Diaphoresis.
- Wheezing.
- Denial (many people do not accept that they are having an MI).

> **● Key Point** As many as half of MIs are clinically silent in that they do not cause the classic symptoms. This is particularly true with elderly patients and those with diabetes who may have particularly subtle presentations—complaints of fatigue, syncope, or weakness. The elderly may also present with only altered mental status.

Physical therapy intervention typically begins once the patient is stable and involves progressing the patient through a cardiac rehabilitation program (see "Cardiac Rehabilitation").

Inflammatory Conditions of the Heart

Myocarditis, pericarditis, and infective endocarditis are all inflammatory conditions of the heart.

Myocarditis

Myocarditis is a relatively uncommon inflammatory condition of the muscular walls of the heart (*myocardium*), usually the result of bacterial or viral infection. Other possible causes include chest radiation for treatment of malignancy, sarcoidosis, and drugs such as lithium and cocaine.[48]

Pericarditis

Pericarditis is most commonly drug-induced or associated with an autoimmune disease (e.g., connective tissue disorders such as systemic lupus erythematosus [SLP], rheumatoid arthritis), with post-myocardial infarction, with renal failure, after open-heart surgery, and after radiation therapy.[48]

Infective Endocarditis

Infective endocarditis is an infection (frequently caused by bacteria—streptococci or staphylococci) of the endocardium, including the heart valves. Can occur at any age, but rarely occurs in children. Rheumatic fever is a form of endocarditis caused by streptococcal group A bacteria.

Surgical Interventions for Cardiovascular Conditions

Heart Valve Surgery

Surgery on defective heart valves is sometimes necessary in cases of mitral valve regurgitation. Surgical options include:

- Mitral valve reconstruction with mitral annuloplasty, quadratic segmental resection, shortening of the elongated chordae, or posterior leaflet resection.

- Mitral valve replacement with either a mechanical valve (requiring lifelong anticoagulation) or a bioprosthetic porcine valve.

Percutaneous Transluminal Coronary Angioplasty

Percutaneous transluminal coronary angioplasty (PTCA) encompasses a variety of procedures used to treat patients with diseased arteries of the heart. Typically, PTCA is performed by threading a slender balloon-tipped catheter under fluoroscopy from an artery in the groin to a trouble spot in an artery of the heart. Once positioned correctly inside the lumen, the balloon is inflated, compressing the plaque and dilating the narrowed coronary artery, resulting in improved coronary blood flow, improved left ventricular function, and anginal relief. There are at present no guidelines for when a patient may resume aerobic training following this procedure. Conventional wisdom, however, favors waiting approximately 2 weeks to allow the inflammatory process resulting from the intervention an appropriate time to subside.[2]

Coronary Artery Bypass Graft

Coronary artery bypass graft (CABG) surgery is a procedure that allows a circumvention of an obstructed coronary artery using a healthy heart or vein taken from the patient's chest, leg, or arm (e.g., saphenous vein, internal mammary artery). Coronary artery bypass graft surgery often is the treatment of choice for patients with severe coronary artery disease (characterized by three or more diseased arteries with impaired function in the left ventricle). Physical therapy intervention following this procedure should address any soft tissue impairments that may be affected by the incision to maintain appropriate flexibility and postures, with an awareness that patients often indicate soreness and/or discomfort around the donor site.[2] Some surgeons choose to limit upper extremity flexibility exercises during the 4 to 6 weeks following surgery while the sternum is healing.

Cardiac Transplantation

Cardiac transplantation,[52] the procedure by which a failing heart is replaced with another heart from a suitable donor, is a widely accepted therapy for the treatment of end-stage congestive heart failure. A ventricular assist device (VAD) is a mechanical pump that helps a heart that is too weak to pump

blood through the body. It is sometimes referred to as a "bridge to transplant" since it can help a patient survive until a heart transplant can be performed. A cardiac allograft can be sewn in a heterotopic or orthotopic position:

- *Heterotopic:* Usually restricted to only those patients with severe pulmonary hypertension due to inherent problems (e.g., pulmonary compression of the recipient, difficulty obtaining endomyocardial biopsy, need for anticoagulation).
- *Orthotopic:* Involves excision of the recipient's heart above the atrioventricular valves and replacement with the donor heart using either the classic Shumway–Lower technique or as a bicaval anastomosis. The graft includes the sinus node so that a sinus rhythm is possible after transplantation; however, some patients need lifelong pacing.

● **Key Point** Because the transplanted heart is denervated, it can respond to cardiovascular influences by humoral mechanisms but not by sympathetic or parasympathetic nerve stimulation.

Immunosuppression is started soon after surgery. Long-term immunosuppression usually is maintained with cyclosporine, azathioprine, and prednisone.

Transmyocardial Revascularization

Transmyocardial revascularization (TMR) is a new laser surgery designed to improve myocardial oxygenation, eliminate or reduce angina, and improve cardiovascular function in those patients who are not candidates for bypass surgery or angioplasty. The surgeon makes an incision over the left breast to expose the heart and then, using a laser, interjects a strong energy pulse into the left ventricle, vaporizing the ventricular muscle and creating a transmural channel with a 1-millimeter diameter. The precise physiologic mechanism for the efficacy of TMR is not thoroughly understood.

Cardiac Rehabilitation

Cardiac rehabilitation provides many benefits for patients. The most important benefits are:[53]

- Improved exercise tolerance
- Control of symptoms
- Improvement in the blood levels of lipids

- Beneficial effect on body weight
- Possible improvement with high blood pressure
- Reduction in smoking
- Improved psychosocial well-being
- Reduction of stress
- Enhanced social adjustment and functioning
- Return to work
- Reduced mortality

Cardiac rehabilitation has to be both comprehensive and individualized at the same time. The goals of a cardiac rehabilitation program can be separated into short- and long-term goals.

Short-Term Goals

Short-term goals of cardiac rehabilitation include the following:

- "Reconditioning" sufficient for resumption of customary activities
- Limiting the physiologic and psychological effects of heart disease
- Decreasing the risk of sudden cardiac arrest or reinfarction
- Controlling the symptoms of cardiac disease

Long-Term Goals

Long-term goals of cardiac rehabilitation include the following:

- Identification and treatment of risk factors
- Stabilizing or even reversing the atherosclerotic process
- Enhancing the psychological status of the patient

Phases of Cardiac Rehabilitation

Cardiac rehabilitation programs can be stratified into four phases.[54,55]

Phase 1

This phase occurs in the hospital inpatient department, starting in the cardiac intensive care unit (CICU) and continuing through the step-down phase (approximately 24 days). This program includes a visit by a member of the cardiac rehabilitation team (cardiac nurse, exercise specialist, PT/PTA, occupational therapist, dietitian, and social worker), education regarding the disease and its recovery process, personal encouragement, and inclusion of family members in classroom group meetings. In the coronary care unit, assisted range of motion exercises can be initiated within the first 24 to 48 hours. Low-risk patients should be encouraged to sit in a bedside chair and begin to perform self-care activities (e.g.,

shaving, oral hygiene, sponge bathing). Early mobilization programs are designed for uncomplicated patients with acute MI in order to progressively increase activity levels in three areas—active exercises, activities of daily living, and educational activities with the goal of early return to independence. On transfer to the step-down unit, patients should try to sit up, stand, and walk in their rooms in the beginning. Subsequently, they should start to walk in the hallway at least twice daily either for certain specific distances or as tolerated without unduly pushing them or holding them back. Standing heart rate and blood pressure should be obtained followed by 5 minutes of warm-up or stretching. Walking, often with assistance, is resumed with a target heart rate of less than 20 beats above the resting heart rate, and RPE under 14. Starting with 5 to 10 minutes of walking each day, exercise time gradually can be increased to up to 30 minutes daily. Team members should incorporate in the discharge planning an appropriate emphasis on secondary prevention through risk factor modification and therapeutic lifestyle changes (TLC), such as smoking cessation, lipid management, weight management, and stress management. They must also ensure that phase 1 patients get referred to appropriate local, convenient, and comprehensive phase 2 programs.

Phase 1.5: Post-Discharge Phase

This phase begins after the patient returns home from the hospital. Team members check the patient's medical status and continuing recovery and should offer reassurance and education about risk-reduction strategies as the patient regains health and strength. This phase of recovery includes low-level exercise and physical activity and instruction about changes for resumption of an active and satisfying lifestyle. After 2 to 6 weeks of recovery at home, the patient is ready to start cardiac rehabilitation phase 2.

Phase 2: Supervised Exercise

The patients who have completed hospitalization and 2 to 6 weeks of recovery at home can begin phase 2 of their cardiac rehabilitation program. This subacute phase is designed to allow the heart muscle time to heal and to progress the patient to full resumption of activities of daily living. During this phase, patients are allowed to return to work and are advised to commence a walking or biking program.

Physician and cardiac rehabilitation staff members formulate the level of exercise to meet an individual patient's needs. Exercise treatments usually are scheduled 3 times a week at the rehabilitation facility. Constant medical supervision is provided, including monitoring through exercise electrocardiograms (ECGs) as well as supervision by a nurse and exercise specialist. Patients are gradually weaned from continuous monitoring of vital signs to spot checks and self-monitoring. Risk factor modification, activity pacing, and energy conservation are emphasized. For example, in addition to exercise, counseling, and education about stress management, smoking cessation, nutrition, and weight loss are also incorporated. This phase of rehabilitation may last 3 to 6 months.

Phase 3: Maintenance

Phase 3 of cardiac rehabilitation is a maintenance program designed to continue for the patient's lifetime. The exercise sessions usually occur 3 times a week. ECG monitoring usually is not necessary. Activities should consist of the type of exercises the patient enjoys, such as walking, bicycling, or jogging. The main goal of phase 3 is to promote habits that lead to a healthy and satisfying lifestyle. Phase 3 programs do not usually require medical or nursing supervision. In fact, most patients participate in "phase 3" equivalent exercises at facilities in the community (e.g., YMCA/YWCA, Gold's Gym, Life-Style Fitness). Entrance into this phase begins with the performance of a maximum, symptom-limited exercise test, the results of which are used to write an exercise prescription. During this phase, patients exercise at 65% to 85% of their maximum heart rate. Three main components of an exercise program are as follows:

- *Frequency:* The minimum frequency for exercising to maintain or improve cardiovascular fitness is 3 times weekly.
- *Time:* Patients usually need to allow 30 to 60 minutes for each session, which includes a warm-up of at least 10 minutes.
- *Intensity:* The intensity prescribed is in relation to one's target heart rate. Aerobic conditioning is emphasized in the first few weeks of exercise. Strength training is introduced later. The Borg scale of rate of perceived exertion (RPE) is used. Patients usually should exercise at an RPE of 13 to 15.

REVIEW Questions

1. The term *cardiac output* refers to the amount of blood pumped by the heart
   a. During any 24-hour period
   b. Relative to body mass
   c. Relative to respiratory rate
   d. In one minute
2. What is the function of the pulmonary arteries?
3. Which component of blood is the primary transporter of oxygen in mammals and many other species?
4. In the heart, what is the function of the AV node?
5. On which side of the heart is the tricuspid valve?
6. From which arteries does the heart receive its own blood supply?
7. Which of the four chambers of the heart receives blood from the systemic circulation via the superior vena cavae?
8. What causes the first heart sound (lub)?
9. The tricuspid and mitral valves differ from the semilunar valves in that the latter
   a. Are subjected to more stress and pressure
   b. Are located within the heart
   c. Do not have attachments to papillary muscles
   d. Have attachments to papillary muscles
10. The state of the cardiac chamber during its period of contraction is known as:
    a. Syncope
    b. Diastole
    c. Systole
    d. None of the above
11. The clinical signs and symptoms of severe heart failure include all of the following except:
    a. Hypertrophy
    b. Resultant congestive heart failure
    c. Lower than normal cardiac output
    d. Higher than normal cardiac output
12. The heart sounds heard by using a stethoscope over the anterior surface of the chest are associated primarily with:
    a. A combination of the respiratory intake plus the heartbeat
    b. Contraction of the ventricles
    c. Contractions of the atria
    d. Opening and closing of the four major heart valves
13. What is the function of the chordae tendineae?
14. True or false: Cardiac tissue has the ability to depolarize spontaneously; to contract without external nervous stimulation.
15. Which of the following is the normal conduction pathway for muscular contraction of the heart to follow?
    a. Left ventricle, right ventricle, atrium
    b. Right atrium, left atrium, ventricles

c. Left atrium, right atrium, ventricles

d. Right ventricle, left ventricle, atrium

16. All of the following are involved with peripheral circulation except:
    a. Arteries
    b. Capillaries
    c. Veins
    d. Sinuses

17. At what part of the cardiac cycle do the coronary arteries receive the majority of their blood flow?

18. All of the following are signs and symptoms associated with atherosclerosis except:
    a. Systolic pressure
    b. Little or no increase in diastolic pressure
    c. Large increase in pulse pressure
    d. No appreciable change in mean pressure

19. The specialized receptors lying in the carotid sinus and the aortic arch involve all of the following except:
    a. Mechanoreceptors
    b. Pressoreceptors
    c. Baroreceptors
    d. Chemoreceptors

20. Active forces that contribute to lymphatic flow include all of the following except:
    a. Skeletal muscle function
    b. Negative intrathoracic pressure
    c. Lymphatic valves
    d. Cardiac function

21. What effect does the Bainbridge reflex have?

22. Factors promoting venous return to the heart during exercise include all of the following except:
    a. Comparative ease of flow from arteries to veins through dilated skeletal muscle arterioles
    b. Increase in venous tone
    c. Increased respiratory movements
    d. Decreased peristalsis

23. Edema may be defined as or the following except:
    a. Brawny or indurated
    b. Excess fluid in the interstitial space
    c. Acquired or congenital
    d. Excess fluid in the intercellular space

24. Clinical signs and symptoms of congestive heart failure include:
    a. Orthopnea
    b. Cyanosis
    c. Pitting edema
    d. All of the above

25. Hypertrophy of the left ventricle of the heart is associated with:
    a. Aortic stenosis
    b. Mitral stenosis
    c. Pulmonary stenosis
    d. None of the above

26. The clinical features of right ventricular hypertrophy in congestive half failure do not include which of the following?
    a. Cyanosis
    b. Dyspnea
    c. Edema of the lower extremities
    d. Ascites

27. Which of the following cardiovascular disorders causes hypertrophy of the left ventricle?
    a. Pulmonary hypertension
    b. Systemic hypotension
    c. Stenosis of the mitral valves
    d. Stenosis of the aortic valves

28. Which of the following clinical features of congestive heart failure would not be attributable to right ventricular failure?
    a. Pulmonary edema
    b. Increase in venous pressure
    c. Peripheral edema
    d. Congestion of the liver

29. The most frequent area of involvement for myocardial infarction is in the:
    a. Right ventricle
    b. Right atrium
    c. Left ventricle
    d. Left atrium

30. A disease involving the aorta and its large branches is called:
    a. Arteriosclerosis
    b. Atherosclerosis
    c. Arteriolosclerosis
    d. Venosclerosis

31. The P wave of an ECG corresponds to which of the following?
    a. Mitral depolarization
    b. Atrial depolarization
    c. Mitral repolarization
    d. Atrial repolarization

32. The T wave of an ECG is generated by:
    a. Atrial repolarization
    b. Atrial depolarization
    c. Ventricular repolarization
    d. Ventricular depolarization

33. Intermittent claudication in the lower extremities suggests:
    a. Still disease

    b. Raynaud disease

    c. Buerger disease

    d. Pott disease

34. Acute bacterial endocarditis may develop from:

    a. Gonococci

    b. Pneumococci

    c. Streptococci

    d. All of the above

35. The closure of the mitral valve occurs when:

    a. Left atrial pressure equals left ventricular pressure

    b. Left ventricular pressure exceeds left atrial pressure

    c. Left atrial pressure exceeds aortic pressure

    d. Left atrial pressure exceeds left ventricle pressure

36. One of the early symptoms of mitral stenosis is:

    a. Palpitations

    b. Angina

    c. Chest pain

    d. Dyspnea with exertion

37. What is the normal resting blood pressure for adults?

38. Describe the classic triad for the pathogenesis of venous thrombosis.

39. Where do most deep vein thromboses (DVT) originate?

40. When do most postoperative DVTs occur?

41. What is the most serious complication of DVT?

42. What prophylactic measures are recommended to prevent DVT?

43. What are the signs and symptoms of pulmonary thromboembolism?

References

1. Schmitz TJ: Vital Signs, in O'Sullivan SB, Schmitz TJ (eds): Physical Rehabilitation (ed 5). Philadelphia, F. A. Davis, 2007, pp 81–120

2. Grimes K: Heart disease, in O'Sullivan SB, Schmitz TJ (eds): Physical Rehabilitation (ed 5). Philadelphia, F. A. Davis, 2007, pp 589–641

3. Molloi S, Wong JT: Regional blood flow analysis and its relationship with arterial branch lengths and lumen volume in the coronary arterial tree. Phys Med Biol 52:1495–1503, 2007

4. Yildirim A, Soylu O, Dagdeviren B, et al: Cardiac resynchronization improves coronary blood flow. Tohoku J Exp Med 211:43–47, 2007

5. Carabello BA: Understanding coronary blood flow: the wave of the future. Circulation 113:1721–1722, 2006

6. Tanaka N, Takeda K, Nishi S, et al: A new method for measuring total coronary blood flow using the lithium dilution method. Osaka City Med J 51:11–18, 2005

7. Mittal N, Zhou Y, Linares C, et al: Analysis of blood flow in the entire coronary arterial tree. Am J Physiol Heart Circ Physiol 289:H439–446, 2005

8. Cahalin LP: Cardiovascular Evaluation, in DeTurk WE, Cahalin LP (eds): Cardiovascular and pulmonary physical therapy: An evidence-based approach. New York, McGraw-Hill, 2004, pp 273–324

9. Van de Graaff KM, Fox SI: Circulatory system: Cardiac output and blood flow, in Van de Graaff KM, Fox SI (eds): Concepts of Human Anatomy and Physiology. New York, WCB/McGraw-Hill, 1999, pp 655–691

10. Bailey MK: Physical examination procedures to screen for serious disorders of the low back and lower quarter, in Wilmarth MA (ed): Medical Screening for the Physical Therapist. Orthopaedic Section Independent Study Course 14.1.1 La Crosse, Wisconsin, Orthopaedic Section, APTA, 2003, pp 1–35

11. O'Sullivan J, Allen J, Murray A: The forgotten Korotkoff phases: How often are phases II and III present, and how do they relate to the other Korotkoff phases? Am J Hypertens 15:264–268, 2002

12. Venet R, Miric D, Pavie A, et al: Korotkoff sound: The cavitation hypothesis. Med Hypotheses 55:141–146, 2000

13. Weber F, Anlauf M, Hirche H, et al: Differences in blood pressure values by simultaneous auscultation of Korotkoff sounds inside the cuff and in the antecubital fossa. J Hum Hypertens 13:695–700, 1999

14. Paskalev D, Kircheva A, Krivoshiev S: A centenary of auscultatory blood pressure measurement: A tribute to Nikolai Korotkoff. Kidney Blood Press Res 28:259–263, 2005

15. Perloff D, Grim C, Flack J, et al: Human blood pressure determination by sphygmomanometry. Circulation 88:2460–2470, 1993

16. Strugo V, Glew FJ, Davis J, et al: Update: Recommendations for human blood pressure determination by sphygmomanometers. Hypertension 16:594, 1990

17. Higgins JR, Walker SP, Brennecke SP: Re: Which Korotkoff sound should be used for diastolic blood pressure in pregnancy? Aust N Z J Obstet Gynaecol 38:480–481, 1998

18. Likeman RK: Re: Which Korotkoff sound should be used for diastolic blood pressure in pregnancy? Aust N Z J Obstet Gynaecol 38:479–480, 1998

19. Franx A, Evers IM, van der Pant KA, et al: The fourth sound of Korotkoff in pregnancy: A myth. Eur J Obstet Gynecol Reprod Biol 76:53–59, 1998

20. Huber MA, Terezhalmy GT, Moore WS: White coat hypertension. Quintessence Int 35:678–679, 2004

21. Chung I, Lip GY: White coat hypertension: Not so benign after all? J Hum Hypertens 17:807–809, 2003

22. Alves LM, Nogueira MS, Veiga EV, et al: White coat hypertension and nursing care. Can J Cardiovasc Nurs 13:29–34, 2003

23. Peterson BK: Vital signs, in Cameron MH, Monroe LG (eds): Physical Rehabilitation: Evidence-Based Examination, Evaluation, and Intervention. St Louis, MO, Saunders/Elsevier, 2007, pp 598–624

24. DeTurk WE, Cassady SL: Essentials of Exercise Physiology, in DeTurk WE, Cahalin LP (eds): Cardiovascular

and Pulmonary Physical Therapy: An Evidence-Based Approach. New York, McGraw-Hill, 2004, pp 35–72

25. Borg GAV: Perceived exertion as an indicator of somatic stress. Scand J Rehabil Med 2:92–98, 1970

26. Winsor T, Hyman C: A Primer of Peripheral Vascular Diseases. Philadelphia, Lea & Febiger, 1965

27. Nauer K A: Acute dissection of the aorta: a review for nurses. Crit Care Nurs Quarterly 23:20–27, 2000

28. McKnight JT, Adcock BB: Paresthesias: A practical diagnostic approach. Am Fam Phys 56:2253–2260, 1997

29. Gillette PD: Exercise in aging and disease, in Placzek JD, Boyce DA (eds): Orthopaedic Physical Therapy Secrets. Philadelphia, Hanley & Belfus, 2001, pp 235–242

30. Reijnen MM, Disselhoff BC, Zeebregts CJ: Varicose vein surgery and endovenous laser therapy. Surg Technol Int 16:167–174, 2007

31. Schmedt CG, Meissner OA, Hunger K, et al: Evaluation of endovenous radiofrequency ablation and laser therapy with endoluminal optical coherence tomography in an ex vivo model. J Vasc Surg 2007

32. Myers K, Fris R, Jolley D: Treatment of varicose veins by endovenous laser therapy: Assessment of results by ultrasound surveillance. Med J Aust 185:199–202, 2006

33. Peden E, Lumsden A: Radiofrequency ablation of incompetent perforator veins. Perspect Vasc Surg Endovasc Ther 19:73–77, 2007

34. Clarke M, Hpewell S, Juszczak E, et al: Compression stockings to prevent deep vein thrombosis in long-haul airline passengers. Int J Epidemiol 35:1410–1411; discussion 1411, 2006

35. Ali A, Caine MP, Snow BG: Graduated compression stockings: Physiological and perceptual responses during and after exercise. J Sports Sci 25:413–419, 2007

36. Compression stockings: How hosiery can help circulation and leg swelling. Mayo Clin Womens Healthsource 10:6, 2006

37. Graduated compression stockings: Prevention of postoperative venous thromboembolism is crucial. Am J Nurs 106:72AA–DD, 2006

38. Motsch J, Walther A, Bock M, et al: Update in the prevention and treatment of deep vein thrombosis and pulmonary embolism. Curr Opin Anaesthesiol 19:52–58, 2006

39. Garmon RG: Pulmonary embolism: incidence, diagnosis, prevention, and treatment. J Am Osteopath Assoc 85:176–185, 1985

40. Rees K, Taylor RS, Singh S, et al: Exercise based rehabilitation for heart failure. Cochrane Database Syst Rev 3, 2004

41. Pina IL, Daoud S: Exercise and heart failure. Minerva Cardioangiol 52:537–546, 2004

42. Pina IL, Apstein CS, Balady GJ, et al: Exercise and heart failure: A statement from the American Heart Association Committee on exercise, rehabilitation, and prevention. Circulation 107:1210–1225, 2003

43. Budev MM, Arroliga AC, Wiedemann HP, et al: Cor pulmonale: An overview. Semin Respir Crit Care Med 24:233–244, 2003

44. Weitzenblum E: Chronic cor pulmonale. Heart 89:225–230, 2003

45. Lehrman S, Romano P, Frishman W, et al: Primary pulmonary hypertension and cor pulmonale. Cardiol Rev 10:265–278, 2002

46. Romano PM, Peterson S: The management of cor pulmonale. Heart Dis 2:431–437, 2000

47. Missov ED, De Marco T: Cor Pulmonale. Curr Treat Options Cardiovasc Med 2:149–158, 2000

48. Goodman CC: The cardiovascular system, in Goodman CC, Boissonnault WG, Fuller KS (eds): Pathology: Implications for the Physical Therapist (ed 2). Philadelphia, Saunders, 2003, pp 367–476

49. Roffe C: Aging of the heart. Br J Biomed Sci 55:136–148, 1998

50. Alaeddini J, Alimohammadi B: Angina Pectoris, Available at: http://www.emedicine.com/med/topic133.htm, 2006

51. Fenton DE, Stahmer S: Myocardial infarction, Available at: http://www.emedicine.com/EMERG/topic327.htm, 2006

52. Mancini MC, Gangahar DM: Heart transplantation, Available at: http://www.emedicine.com/med/topic3187.htm, 2006

53. de Carvalho T, Curi AL, Andrade DF, et al: Cardiovascular rehabilitation of patients with ischemic heart disease undergoing medical treatment, percutaneous transluminal coronary angioplasty, and coronary artery bypass grafting. Arq Bras Cardiol 88:72–78, 2007

54. Certo CM, DeTurk WE, Cahalin LP: History of cardiopulmonary rehabilitation, in DeTurk WE, Cahalin LP (eds): Cardiovascular and pulmonary physical therapy. New York, McGraw-Hill, 2004, pp 3–14

55. Vibhuti NS, Schocken DD: Cardiac rehabilitation, Available at: http://www.emedicine.com/pmr/topic180.htm, 2006

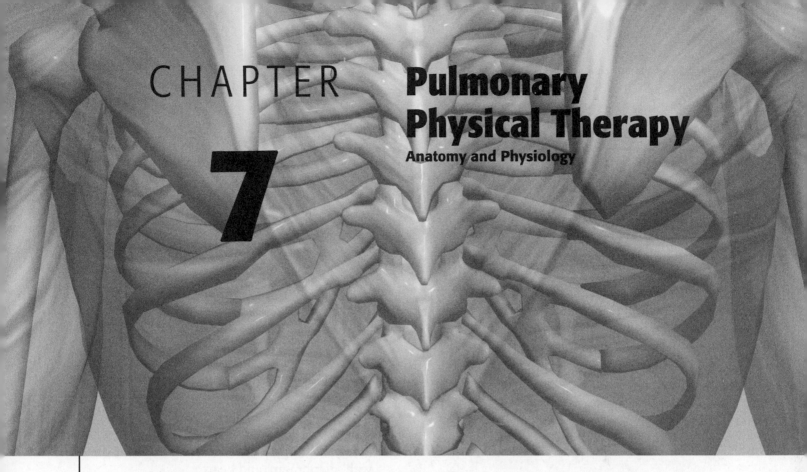

CHAPTER 7

Pulmonary Physical Therapy
Anatomy and Physiology

The pulmonary or respiratory system is contained within a cage-like structure. The sternum, 12 pairs of ribs, the clavicle, and the vertebrae of the thoracic spine form the thoracic cage.

Rib Cage

The rib cage is formed by 12 pairs of ribs, each different from the others in size, width, and curvature, although they share some common characteristics:

- Ribs 1–7 are considered to be *true ribs* and have a single anterior costochondral attachment to the sternum. Approximately 32 structures attach to the first rib and body of T1.
- Ribs 8–10 are referred to as *false ribs* because they share costochondral attachments before attaching anteriorly to the sternum.
- Ribs 11 and 12 are termed *floating* or *costovertebral ribs* because they have no anterior attachment with the sternum.

Posteriorly, the 12 pairs of ribs articulate with the thoracic vertebrae. The orientation of the joint axes of the thoracic vertebrae determines the type of rib movement:

- *Upper ribs:* Primarily in an anterior and posterior direction (pump handle)
- *Lower ribs:* Primarily in the medial–lateral direction (bucket handle)

Attached to the entire interior of the thoracic cage is a thin sheet of cells, the pleura, which folds back on itself to form two completely enclosed sacs that cover the lungs.

> **● Key Point** The primary function of the respiratory system is to exchange gases between tissue, the blood, and the environment so that arterial blood oxygen, carbon dioxide, and pH levels remain within specific limits throughout many different physiological limits.[1] The pulmonary system also plays a number of other roles, including contributing to temperature homeostasis via evaporative heat loss from the lungs, and filtering, humidifying, and warming or cooling the air to body temperature.[1] This process protects the remainder of the respiratory system from damage caused by dry gases or harmful debris.[1]

> **● Key Point** Note the following definitions:
> - *Ventilation:* The movement of air through the conducting airways.
> - *Respiration:* A term used to describe the gas exchange within the body.
> - *External respiration:* The exchange of gases between the atmosphere and the blood.
> - *Internal respiration:* The exchange of gases between the blood and the cells of the body.
> - *Anatomic dead space:* The volume of gas contained in the conducting airways. It is decreased by reduction of the size of the airways, as occurs with bronchoconstriction or a tracheostomy.
> - *Alveolar dead space:* The volume of gas in areas of "wasted ventilation"—alveoli that are ventilated but poorly or underperfused.
> - *Physiological dead space:* The total volume of gas that is not involved in gas exchange. It represents the sum of the anatomic dead space and alveolar dead space. In health, this represents only about 30% of the tidal volume. In contrast, in patients with nonuniform structural abnormalities of the lung, 60% to 70% of each tidal volume may be composed of dead-space volume.

The respiratory system is arranged basically like an upside-down tree that can be divided into two main portions:[1]

- *The conducting portion:* Includes the upper airways, the lower airway (trachea, bronchi and the bronchioles).
- *The respiratory portion:* Includes the terminal portion of the bronchial tree and alveoli, the site of gas exchange. The gases readily move by diffusion through the alveoli into the pulmonary capillaries.

> **● Key Point** The transitional zone, consisting of the respiratory bronchioles, separates the conducting and respiratory portions.

Lungs

The lungs lie within the thoracic cavity, on either side of the mediastinum. The most superior aspect of each lung is called its apex.

- *Right lung:* Divided into three lobes
- *Left lung:* Divided into two lobes

> **● Key Point** Surface tension, created by the presence of the interface between air in the alveoli and the watery alveolar tissue, is responsible for much of the lung's elastic recoil. A chemical called *surfactant* maintains surface tension at an optimal level.[2] Because no surfactant is produced until about the eighth month in utero, premature babies are sometimes born with lungs that lack sufficient surfactant, and their alveoli are collapsed as a result.[2] This condition is called *respiratory distress syndrome* (RDS) or *hyaline membrane disease* (see Chapter 10). Even under normal conditions, the first breath of life is a difficult one because the newborn must overcome great surface tension forces in order to inflate his or her partially collapsed pulmonary alveoli. The transpulmonary pressure required for the first breath is 15 to 20 times that required for subsequent breaths.[2]

Pleurae

The pleurae are a pair of dual-layered sacs that stabilize the lungs and separate them from the chest wall, diaphragm, and heart.[2]

- *Parietal pleura:* The pleura that lines the inside of the thoracic cage, diaphragm, and the mediastinal border of the lung, and the great vessels in the superior mediastinum.
- *Visceral pleura:* The pleura that covers the outer surface of the lung, including the fissure lines.
- *Pleural cavity:* The potential space between the two pleura that is supplied by a small amount of pleural fluid that serves to hold the parietal and visceral pleurae together during ventilation while reducing friction between the lungs and the thoracic wall.[3]

Muscles of Respiration

The Diaphragm

The diaphragm, innervated by the phrenic nerve, is the primary muscle of inspiration, with the ribs serving as levers. When the diaphragm contracts it descends over the abdominal contents, flattening the dome, which causes the lower ribs to move outward, resulting in protrusion of the abdominal wall. In addition, the contracting diaphragm causes a decrease in intrathoracic pressure, which pulls air into the lungs.[3]

Intercostal Muscles

The muscles of the thoracic cage include the 11 internal and external intercostals, which connect one rib to the next and serve to elevate the ribs and increase thoracic volume:[3]

- The external intercostals function to elevate the ribs and to increase thoracic volume.
- The internal intercostals function to lower the ribs, thereby decreasing thoracic volume.

Accessory Muscles of Inspiration

The accessory muscles of inspiration are used when a more rapid or deep inhalation is required, or in disease states.

> ● **Key Point** The accessory muscles of inspiration include the scalenes and sternocleidomastoid; the levator costarum; and the trapezius, pectorals, and serratus anterior.

Pulmonary System Physiology and Testing

Volumes and Capacities

There are four primary lung volumes:

- *Tidal volume (TV):* Volume of gas inhaled or exhaled during a normal respiration. The average adult TV is 500 mL (range = 300–800 mL).
- *Inspiratory reserve volume (IRV):* The additional air that can be inhaled after a normal tidal breath in.
- *Expiratory reserve volume (ERV):* The amount of additional air that can be breathed out after normal expiration (about 1–1.5 L for the average adult).
- *Residual volume (RV):* The volume of gas that remains in the lungs after ERV has been exhaled.

The four volumes can be combined to form four capacities (**Table 7-1**).

Flow Rates

Flow rate measurements reflect the degree of obstruction or narrowing of the airways. The measurements are abnormal in obstructive disorders, such as chronic obstructive pulmonary disease and asthma.

- *Forced expiratory volume in one second (FEV$_1$):* The amount of air exhaled during the first second. In healthy individuals, FEV$_1$ is 83% of vital capacity (VC).

- *Forced expiratory volume in two seconds (FEV$_2$):* The amount of air exhaled during the first second. In healthy individuals, FEV$_2$ is 94% of vital capacity (VC).
- *Forced expiratory volume in three seconds (FEV$_3$):* The amount of air exhaled during the first three seconds. In healthy individuals, FEV$_3$ is 97% of vital capacity (VC).

Mechanics of Breathing

Normal, quiet inspiration results from muscle contraction—the inspiratory muscles (diaphragm and intercostal muscles) contract, expanding the chest wall and lowering the diaphragm. During relaxed breathing, expiration is essentially a passive process.[4]

Controls of Ventilation

The rate and depth of respiration are regulated by two control systems—the automatic and the voluntary mechanisms—that usually interact with each other.[4] Normal cyclic breathing is controlled by the respiratory centers in the dorsal region of the medulla, which are influenced by centers in the pons, and by chemoreceptors.[1]

TABLE 7-1	**Terms Used to Describe Lung Capacities**
Term	Definition
Inspiratory capacity (IRV+TV)	The amount of air that can be inhaled after a normal expiration. The average adult inspiratory capacity is 3000–4000 mL.
Vital capacity (IRV+TV+ERV)	The three volumes of air that are under volitional control, inspiratory reserve volume, expiratory reserve volume, and tidal volume, conventionally measured as a forced expiratory vital capacity (FVC). The average adult vital capacity is 4000–5000 mL.
Functional residual capacity (ERV+RV)	The amount of air that resides in the lungs after a normal resting tidal exhalation.
Total lung capacity (IRV+TV+ERV+RV)	The total amount of air the lungs can hold (approximately 5 L).

Data from Van de Graaff KM, Fox SI: Respiratory system, in Van de Graaff KM, Fox SI (eds): Concepts of Human Anatomy and Physiology. New York, WCB/McGraw-Hill, 1999, pp 728–777

- *Central chemoreceptors:* Monitor the carbon dioxide levels of both the arterial blood and cerebrospinal fluid.[1]
- *Peripheral chemoreceptors:* Located in the carotid and aortic bodies.[1]

Chemoreceptor input to the brainstem modifies the rate and depth of breathing at an efficient level. Of the two respiratory gases, carbon dioxide is the most tightly controlled.[1]

> ● **Key Point** Three chemical levels in particular play a critical role in controlling respiration: the blood acid-base balance (pH—the concentration of free-floating hydrogen ions within the body), the partial pressure of carbon dioxide within the arterial blood bicarbonate ($Paco_2$), and the amount of bicarbonate ions within the arterial blood (Hco_3-).

> ● **Key Point**
> • The normal range for arterial pH is 7.36 to 7.44. Acidosis refers to an arterial pH below 7.35, and alkalosis refers to an arterial pH above 7.5.
> • The normal range of Pco_2 is 40 mm Hg. A rise in Pco_2, called hypercapnia, is caused by hypoventilation. Conversely, hyperventilation results in a fall in Pco_2, hypocapnea.

The terms used to describe blood oxygen and carbon dioxide levels are as follows:

- *Hypoxemia:* A lower than normal oxygen content or Po_2 in arterial blood.
- *Hypoxia:* A lower than normal oxygen content or Po_2 in the lungs, blood, or tissues. This is a more general term than hypoxemia. Tissues can be hypoxic, for example, even though there is no hypoxemia (as when the blood flow is occluded).

- *Hypercapnia (hypercarbia):* An increase in the Pco_2 of systemic arteries to above 40 mm Hg. Usually this occurs when the ventilation is inadequate for a given metabolic rate (*hypoventilation*).

Gas Exchange

Respiratory gas exchange[1] takes place in the alveoli, by a process of diffusion. Alveoli are small evaginations of the repiratory bronchioles, alveolar ducts, and alveolar sacs. The alveolar wall consists of two thin layers of epithelial cells spread over a layer of connective tissue that is particularly suited for gas exchange. Oxygen enters the blood from the alveolar air; carbon dioxide enters the alveolar air from the blood. If the fractional concentration of oxygen in a dry gas mixture is 21%, the partial pressure exerted by the oxygen is 21% of the total pressure (Figure 7-1). The total pressure of ambient (*atmospheric*) air is the barometric pressure. At sea level this is 1 atmosphere (atm), or 760 mm Hg.

> ● **Key Point** The barometric pressure determines the total pressure of the air in the respiratory passages and the alveoli when the respiratory system is at rest

Alveolar air is a mixture of nitrogen, oxygen, carbon dioxide, and water vapor. The concentrations and consequently the partial pressures of these gases in the alveolar air differ considerably from their concentrations in the ambient air. In ambient air, the water vapor content (humidity) is variable.

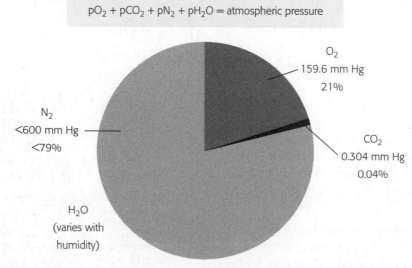

$pO_2 + pCO_2 + pN_2 + pH_2O =$ atmospheric pressure

O_2
159.6 mm Hg
21%

CO_2
0.304 mm Hg
0.04%

N_2
<600 mm Hg
<79%

H_2O
(varies with humidity)

Figure 7-1   Partial pressure of gases.

As air travels through the nasal passages and upper airways, it is warmed to 37°C and it becomes completely saturated with water vapor.[5] At body temperature, water vapor exerts a pressure of 47 mm Hg (P_{H_2O}). In order to represent accurately the partial pressures presented to the lung for gas exchange (i.e., after warming and humidification), P_{H_2O} is first subtracted from the barometric pressure. Thus, for inspired, tracheal gases at sea level: $P_{O_2} = 0.21 \times (760 - 47)$ mm Hg = 150 mm Hg.[5]

The concentration of oxygen in the alveoli (about 14%) is much less than in ambient air (21%). Although the oxygen supply to the alveolar is periodically renewed during inspiration, oxygen is constantly removed from the alveolar air by the blood. The average partial pressure of oxygen in alveolar air (P_{aO_2}) at sea level is about 100 mm Hg. There is a negligible amount of carbon dioxide in ambient air and significant amounts (about 5.6%) in alveolar air because carbon dioxide is constantly being added to the alveolar air by the blood. During normal breathing the average partial pressure of alveolar carbon dioxide (P_{aCO_2}) is 40 mm Hg.

The values for alveolar gas pressures are basically the resultant of only two variables, both of which depend upon the integrity of the pulmonary and circulatory systems:

- The relative magnitudes of the alveolar ventilation
- The oxygen consumption and carbon dioxide production

When liquid is exposed to a gas mixture, as pulmonary capillary blood is to alveolar air, the molecules of each gas diffuse between air and liquid until the pressure of the dissolved molecules equals the partial pressure of that gas in the gas mixture.

The diffusion pathway between air and red blood cells consist of both tissue and blood. The tissue barrier, which is extremely thin, is made up of the surfactant lining the alveolus, the alveolar epithelium, the interstitial tissue, and the capillary endothelium.

The blood entering the pulmonary capillaries has come from the tissues and therefore has a high P_{CO_2} (46 mm Hg) and a low P_{O_2} (40 mm Hg). As it passes through the pulmonary capillaries, the blood is separated from the alveolar air by the tissue barrier, which allows for the net diffusion of oxygen into the blood and carbon dioxide into the alveoli, which causes the capillary blood oxygen levels to rise and the carbon dioxide levels to fall. Once the alveolar and capillary partial pressures become equal, the net diffusion of these gases ceases.

Gas Transport

After the diffusion of oxygen from the alveolar air into the blood, oxygen is transported by the blood to the tissue capillaries.[1] Capillaries are tiny blood vessels composed of a single layer of flattened endothelial cells that allow blood to be in close contact with tissues.

When the hemoglobin is 100% saturated with oxygen, each molecule is capable of combining with four molecules of oxygen.

Carbon dioxide is transported from the tissues to the lungs by way of the red blood cells. Carbon dioxide is carried by the blood in three forms:[2]

- Approximately 1/10 of the total blood carbon dioxide is dissolved in plasma.
- Approximately 1/5 of the total blood carbon dioxide is carried attached to an amino acid in hemoglobin called carbaminohemoglobin.
- Most of the carbon dioxide carried by the blood is in the form of bicarbonate.

Intrapulmonary Shunt

For ideal gas exchange, equal volumes of fresh air entering the alveoli should come into contact with equal volumes of blood flowing through the alveolar capillaries.[1] In other words, alveolar ventilation ($\dot{V}_A$) should match the pulmonary blood flow ($\dot{Q}$). The relationship of the two flows is the ventilation perfusion ratio, or the $\dot{V}/\dot{Q}$ ratio. In the ideal matching of equal volumes of gas and blood, the ratio would be 1. However, when one is considering the lungs as a whole, the ratio is 0.8. Usually the $\dot{V}/\dot{Q}$ ratio is considered for various areas of the lungs and not for the lungs as a whole. Alveolar ventilation and blood flow vary independently throughout the lung. In an upright person, blood flow is less than ventilation at the lung apex because some of the capillaries are compressed (i.e., the $\dot{V}/\dot{Q}$ ratio is high). At the base of the lung, ventilation is three times greater but blood flow is 10 times greater than that of the apex (the $\dot{V}/\dot{Q}$ ratio is low).

In areas of the lung with low $\dot{V}/\dot{Q}$ ratios, the renewal of the alveolar oxygen supply is sufficient to oxygenate adequately the blood flowing through the pulmonary capillaries. The end-capillary blood is not fully oxygenated. This is termed a *physiological intrapulmonary shunt*. The poorly oxygenated blood from these areas mixes with blood from other, better-ventilated areas. In healthy patients, the percentage of intrapulmonary shunt is less than 10%. The protective reflex that attempts to limit intrapulmonary shunt is *hypoxic pulmonary vasoconstriction* (HPV); alveolar hypoxia leads to vasoconstriction of the perfusing vessel. This partially corrects the regional $\dot{V}/\dot{Q}$ mismatch by improving P_{aO_2} at the expense of increasing pulmonary vascular resistance.

Exercise Tolerance Tests

Refer to Chapter 6.

Sputum Analysis

Clinical analysis of a sputum sample can reveal important information:

Color

- Red (blood)
- Pink (pulmonary edema)
- White or clear (may indicate chronic cough or cystic fibrosis or chronic bronchitis)
- Yellow (an improving infection)
- Brown/rust (pneumonia)
- Greenish-brown (acute infection)
- Gray (abscess)

Consistency

- Thin—patient is often less sick
- Moderately thick—patient is often slightly more sick than the patient with thin consistency of sputum

- Thick—patient is often more sick than the patient with thin or moderately thick consistency of sputum

Smell

- No striking smell—patient is often less sick
- Foul smell—patient is often sicker

Arterial Blood Gas

An arterial blood gas (ABG) test measures the levels of oxygen and carbon dioxide in the blood to determine the effectiveness of alveolar ventilation. Values are expressed as the partial pressure of the gas. An ABG measures:

- *Partial pressure of oxygen* (PaO_2): The oxygen level (normally at 105 mm Hg in the alveoli) indicates how well oxygen is able to move from the airspace of the lungs into the blood.
- *Partial pressure of carbon dioxide* ($PaCO_2$): The carbon dioxide level (normally 37–43 mm Hg) indicates how well carbon dioxide is able to move out of the blood into the airspace of the lungs and out with exhaled air.
- *pH*: The pH is a measure of hydrogen (H^+) in blood that indicates the acid or base (alkaline) nature of blood. A pH of less than 7 is acidic, and a pH greater than 7 is called basic (alkaline). The pH of blood is usually close to 7.4. A pH less than 7.2 is indicative of severe acidemia, whereas a pH greater than 7.6 is indicative of severe alkalemia. A determination can be made as to whether the change in pH level is the result of a metabolic or respiratory condition (see Chapter 1) and the state of compensation (if uncompensated the pH level is abnormal but the HCO_3 and $PaCO_2$ levels are normal):
  - *Respiratory acidosis (hypercapnea)*: PCO_2 increases and is compensated by metabolic alkalosis (HCO_3 increases).
  - *Respiratory alkalosis (hypocapnea)*: PCO_2 decreases and is compensated by metabolic acidosis (HCO_3 decreases).
  - *Metabolic acidosis (hypokalemia)*: HCO_3 decreases and is compensated by respiratory alkalosis (PCO_2 decreases).
  - *Metabolic alkalosis (hyperkalemia)*: HCO_3 increases and is compensated by respiratory acidosis (PCO_2 increases).
- *Bicarbonate* (HCO_3): Buffers are chemical substances that keep the pH of blood within a normal range. Bicarbonate is the most important buffer in the blood. Bicarbonate saturation levels, controlled chiefly by the kidneys, are normally at 22–28 mmoles/liter.
- *Oxygen content* (O_2CT) *and oxygen saturation* (O_2Sat) *values.* Like the PaO_2, these values provide information about the amount of oxygen in the blood.

Pulmonary Pathology

One of the most common subjective reports of patients with pulmonary disorders is dyspnea.[6] Dyspnea can be evaluated using a variety of different methods, including listening to the breathing cycle using a stethoscope (there are six to eight auscultatory sites on the posterior chest and four to six sites on the anterior chest) and observing the breathing patterns. The abnormal breath sounds and breathing patterns are outlined in **Table 7-2** and **Table 7-3**, respectively. The following are considered normal breath sounds:

- *Bronchial:* Consist of a full inspiratory and expiratory phase, with the inspiratory phase usually being louder. They are normally heard over the trachea and larynx but may also be heard over the hilar region in individuals that are breathing hard (e.g., after exercise). Bronchial sounds heard over the thorax suggest lung consolidation and pulmonary disease (pulmonary consolidation results in improved transmission of breath sounds originating in the trachea and primary bronchi that are then heard at increased intensity over the thorax).
- *Bronchovesicular:* Consist of a full inspiratory phase with a shortened and softer expiratory phase. They are normally heard over the hilar region but should be quieter than the tracheal breath sounds. Increased intensity of bronchovesicular sounds is most often associated with increased ventilation or pulmonary consolidation.
- *Vesicular:* Consist of a quiet, wispy inspiratory phase followed by a short, almost silent expiratory phase that is heard over the periphery of the lung field. These sounds are the result of attenuation of breath sounds produced in the bronchi at the hilar region of the lungs. An increased intensity may be associated with pulmonary consolidation.

TABLE 7-2	Abnormal Breath Sounds
Sound	**Description**
Crackles	Crackles are discontinuous, explosive, "popping" sounds that are heard when an obstructed airway suddenly opens and the pressures on either side of the obstruction suddenly equilibrate. Crackles, which imply either accumulation of fluid secretions or exudate within airways or inflammation and edema in the pulmonary tissue, can be heard during inspiration when intrathoracic negative pressure results in opening of the airways or on expiration when thoracic positive pressure forces collapsed or blocked airways open.
Wheezes	Continuous musical tones that can be classified as either high- or low-pitched wheezes and which result as a collapsed airway lumen gradually opens during inspiration or gradually closes during expiration. Wheezes imply decreased airway lumen diameter due to either thickening of reactive airway walls or collapse of airways caused by pressure from surrounding pulmonary disease.
Stridor	Intense continuous monophonic wheezes that tend to be accentuated during inspiration when extrathoracic airways collapse due to lower internal lumen pressure. Stridor indicates upper airway obstruction.
Rhonchi	Abnormal dry, leathery sounds heard in the lungs that indicate inflammation of the bronchial tubes.

TABLE 7-3	Abnormal Breathing Patterns
Pattern	**Description**
Cheyne–Stokes	Characterized by alternating periods of apnea and hyperpnea. Over a period of one minute, a 10- to 20-second episode of apnea or hypopnea is observed, followed by respirations of increasing depth and frequency. The cycle then repeats itself. Cheyne–Stokes occurs in congestive heart failure, encephalitis, cerebral circulatory disturbances, and drug overdose, manifesting as a lesion of the bulbar center of respiration.
Kussmaul's breathing	Rhythmic gasping with normal or reduced frequency associated with severe diabetic or renal acidosis or coma.
Hyperventilation	Rapid breathing, often caused by anxiety.
Biot (ataxic) breathing	Breathing that is irregular in timing and depth. It is indicative of meningitis or medullary lesions.
Apneustic breathing	Characterized by a post-inspiratory pause. The usual cause of apneustic breathing is a pontine lesion.
Paradoxical respiration	A pattern of breathing in which the abdominal wall is sucked in during inspiration (it is usually pushed out). Paradoxical respiration is due to paralysis of the diaphragm.
Sleep apnea	Sleep apnea is defined as the cessation of breathing during sleep. There are three different types of sleep apnea: • *Obstructive:* Characterized by repetitive pauses in breathing during sleep due to the obstruction and/or collapse of the upper airway (throat), usually accompanied by a reduction in blood oxygen saturation and followed by an awakening to breathe. • *Central:* A neurological condition causing cessation of all respiratory effort during sleep, usually with decreases in blood oxygen saturation. • *Mixed:* A combination of the previous two.

A normal breathing pattern consists of an outward upper- and lower-chest wall motion during inspiration and inward upper- and lower-chest wall motion during expiration.

> **● Key Point** Chest wall excursion can be measured at three anatomical sites using a tape measure. The three anatomical sites include the sternal angle of Louis on the sternum (at the second rib), the xiphoid process, and a midpoint between the xiphoid process and the umbilicus. The difference between the resting position and the position of full inspiration, measured at the base of the lungs, should be between 2 and 3 inches.

Respiration rate is the number of breaths taken each minute (a breath is one inhalation and one exhalation). The rate is usually measured when a person is at rest and simply involves counting the number of breaths for one minute by counting how many times the chest rises. Normal respiration rates for an adult person at rest range from 15 to 20 breaths per minute (the normal rate for a newborn is between 30 and 60 breaths per minute). Respiration rates over 25 breaths per minute or under 12 breaths per minute (when at rest) may be considered abnormal. The expirations are normally approximately twice as long as the inspirations. The opposite occurs in conditions such as chronic obstructive pulmonary disease (COPD).

Risk Factors for Pulmonary Disorders

Risk factors for pulmonary dysfunction are based on pathology:

- *Obstructive lung disease:* Smoking, occupational exposure to irritants or allergens (e.g., asbestos, chemicals), residing in locations with high levels of air pollution, premature birth—bronchopulmonary dysplasia, emphysema, asthma, bronchitis, bronchiectasis, and cystic fibrosis.
- *Restrictive lung disease:* Occupational exposure to irritants or allergens (e.g., asbestos, chemicals), cardiovascular disorders (e.g., pulmonary edema from heart failure, pulmonary emboli), neuromuscular disorders (e.g., spinal cord injury, cerebrovascular accident, Guillain–Barré, muscular dystrophy), musculoskeletal disorders (e.g., scoliosis, ankylosing spondylitis), integumentary disorders (marked burns to thorax, scleroderma), past oncologic disorder treated with chemotherapy or radiation therapy, trauma (e.g., crush injuries), surgical pain or scarring, obesity, pregnancy, and premature births—hyaline membrane disease.

Obstructive Diseases

Chronic Obstructive Pulmonary Disease

Chronic obstructive pulmonary disease (COPD) is a generic term that refers to lung diseases that result in air trapping in the lungs, causing hyperinflation of the lungs and a barrel chest deformity.[7] COPD is characterized by airway narrowing, parenchymal destruction, and pulmonary vascular thickening. COPD can be subdivided into:

- *Nonseptic obstructive pulmonary diseases:* Include such diseases as asthma, chronic bronchitis, emphysema, and α_1 antitrypsin (α_1 ATD) deficiency.
- *Septic obstructive pulmonary diseases:* Include cystic fibrosis and bronchiectasis.

At the onset, there is minimal shortness of breath, but as the disease progresses patients with COPD may eventually require supplemental oxygen and may have to rely on mechanical respiratory assistance. The medical management of chronic pulmonary disease includes smoking cessation, pharmacological agents, and the use of supplemental oxygen. An absolute indication for use of long-term oxygen therapy is an arterial partial pressure of oxygen (PaO_2) of 55 mm Hg or less, which correlates with an SaO_2 of 88% or less.[8]

Nonseptic Obstructive Pulmonary Diseases
Asthma

Asthma is a chronic pulmonary disease, characterized by reversible obstruction to airflow within the lungs, which is caused by increased reaction of the airways to various stimuli. An asthma episode is a series of events that result in narrowed airways. These include: swelling of the lining, tightening of the muscle, and increased secretion of mucus in the airway. Although the breathing problems associated with asthma usually happen in "episodes," the inflammation underlying asthma is continuous. Triggers include:

- Respiratory infections, colds
- Cigarette smoke
- Allergic reactions to such allergens as pollen, mold, animal dander, feather, dust, food, and cockroaches
- Indoor and outdoor air pollutants, including ozone
- Vigorous exercise (exercise-induced asthma)

- Exposure to cold air or sudden temperature change
- Excitement/stress
- Over-the-counter medications (aspirin)

The classic symptoms of asthma are episodic wheezing (due to bronchoconstriction), dyspnea, chest pain, facial distress, and usually a nonproductive cough.[9] Asthma can be a life-threatening disease if not properly managed. The first intervention for asthma is prevention, including smoking cessation and minimizing exposure to stimulants that precipitate an asthmatic episode. The goal of pharmacotherapy is to provide relief of symptoms and prevent complications and/or progression with a minimum of side effects.[10] Asthma medications help reduce underlying inflammation in the airways and relieve or prevent symptomatic airway narrowing. Control of inflammation should lead to reduction in airway sensitivity and help prevent airway obstruction. Establishment of a routine exercise program is also important.[7]

Chronic Bronchitis
Chronic bronchitis is a clinical diagnosis—a persistent productive cough that produces sputum for more than three months per year for at least two consecutive years in the absence of another definable medical cause.[7] Chronic bronchitis produces inflammation and eventual scarring of the lining of the bronchial tubes. Patients are sometimes referred to as *blue bloaters*. Presenting symptoms include:[11,12]

- Patient may be obese
- Chronic cough with frequent clearing of the throat
- Low-grade fever
- Increased mucus
- Shortness of breath (dyspnea on exertion)
- Use of accessory muscles for breathing
- Coarse rhonchi and wheezing may be heard on auscultation
- Signs of right heart failure (i.e., cor pulmonale), such as edema and cyanosis

Medical management includes supplemental oxygen therapy, antiviral medications, and corticosteroids to suppress the inflammatory process.[7] Bronchodilators may be utilized for the management of bronchospasm.[7]

Emphysema
Emphysema is a long-term, progressive disease of the lung in which the tissues necessary to support the physical shape and function of the lungs are destroyed. Emphysema begins insidiously with the destruction of the elastin protein within the alveoli of the lungs, the walls of which become thin and fragile. As the alveoli are destroyed, the lungs are able to transfer increasingly less oxygen to the bloodstream, causing shortness of breath/hyperinflation, and compensatory changes of the chest wall. Hyperinflation causes shortening of the inspiratory muscles and flattening of the diaphragm with loss of sarcomeres.[7] The end result is a loss of diaphragmatic excursion and a decline in the mechanical effectiveness of the diaphragm and other respiratory muscles to support the increased demand of ventilation.[13] Patients are sometimes referred to as *pink puffers*. Signs and symptoms of emphysema include:

- Barrel chest (enlarged anterior–posterior dimension), with an increased rib angle.
- Chronic cough and sputum production; will vary and depend on the infectious history of the patient.
- Diminished breath sounds and wheezing.
- Shortness of breath, especially with exertion (dyspnea on exertion) assisted by pursed lips and use of accessory respiratory muscles, the latter of which may be hypertrophied through overuse).
- Heart sounds appear very distant.
- Emaciation in later stages of the disease; patient may adopt the tripod sitting position.

The primary cause of emphysema is the smoking of cigarettes. In some cases it may be due to alpha 1–antitrypsin deficiency (see next section). Other causes of emphysema include exposure to air pollution, lower respiratory infections, secondhand smoke, or other chemicals and toxins. Diagnosis is made by pulmonary function tests, chest x-ray (reveals hyperinflation with flattened diaphragm, decreased vascular markings, and possibly enlargement of the right side of the heart), along with the patient's history and physical examination.

There are a number of medical interventions for emphysema:

- Smoking cessation
- Pharmacology (e.g., bronchodilators, anticholinergic drugs, corticosteroids)
- Long-term oxygen therapy, including the use of BiPAP ventilation
- Bullectomy (a *bulla* is a large airspace that is the result of destruction of the parenchyma and no longer participates in gas exchange or diffusion)

- Lung volume reduction surgery
- Lung transplantation (single or double) (for patients with end-stage disease who have maximized medical intervention)

Physical therapy intervention is based on the severity of the disease and can include general exercise in endurance training (while monitoring the patient's oxygen saturation using pulse oximetry), patient education on posture and energy conservation techniques, ventilatory muscle strengthening, airway secretion clearance, breathing exercises including pursed lip breathing, and chest wall exercises.

α_1 Antitrypsin Deficiency

Antitrypsin deficiency (ATD) is a condition caused by the inherited deficiency of a protein called α_1-antitrypsin (AAT) or alpha 1–protease inhibitor. AAT is an enzyme produced by the liver that counterbalances degradation of tissue caused by the protolytic enzyme protease.[7] Symptoms of AAT deficiency usually begin before the age of 50 years, with a mean onset of 46 years.[14] The primary significance of ATD is the premature development of emphysema, occurring in the third or fourth decade of life.[14] Shortness of breath and decreased exercise capacity are typically the first symptoms.[15] Smoking significantly increases the severity of emphysema in AAT-deficient individuals.[14] Most of the available treatment protocols are consistent with the treatments for emphysema with bronchodilators, corticosteroids, cessation of smoking, and preventative vaccinations.[7] Pulmonary rehabilitation and supplemental oxygen therapy also are effective.[7]

Septic Obstructive Pulmonary Diseases

Cystic Fibrosis

More details on cystic fibrosis can be found in Chapter 10.

Bronchiectasis

Bronchiectasis is the permanent dilation of the bronchi caused by the destruction of the muscular and elastic properties of the lung.[7] It is characterized by inflamed airways that are full of purulent sputum.[16] When the body is unable to get rid of mucus, mucus becomes stuck and accumulates in the airways, leading to the weakening and widening of the passages. The weakened passages can become scarred and deformed, allowing more mucus and bacteria to accumulate, resulting in a cycle of infection and destruction. There are three types of bronchiectasis that describe the severity of the condition:

- *Cylindrical:* Most common and refers to the slight widening of the respiratory passages. This type can be reversed and may be seen after acute bronchitis.
- *Varicose:* Bronchial walls have both extended and collapsed portions.
- *Cystic:* Most severe type; involves irreversible ballooning of the bronchi.

Symptom severity varies widely from patient to patient, and occasionally a patient is asymptomatic. Symptoms of bronchiectasis include coughing (worse when lying down), persistent production of large volumes of secretions, recurrent hemoptysis, shortness of breath, abnormal chest sounds (crackles, rhonchi, and pleural rubs), weakness, weight loss, and fatigue.[16] With infections the mucus may be discolored, foul smelling, and may contain blood. When the underlying disease in the obstructive process is emphysema or cystic fibrosis, there will be a barrel chest and an obstructive pattern on the pulmonary function tests.[7] The diagnosis can be confirmed with a chest x-ray, breathing tests, sputum culture, or a computed tomography (CT) scan.[16] The principal treatment for bronchiectasis involves management of the underlying disease, which commonly includes the use of antibiotics, corticosteroids, and bronchodilators.[7] Nutritional support, supplemental oxygen, pulmonary hygiene, and patient education are also key components.[7] Surgical resection of the lung tissue that is the source of recurrent infections or hemoptysis may be an effective treatment plan to minimize recurrent exacerbations and further loss of lung function.[7,17] Lung transplants are also an option for severe cases.[17]

Infectious and Inflammatory Diseases

Bronchiolitis

Details on bronchiolitis can be found in Chapter 10.

Pneumonia

Pneumonia is an inoculation of the respiratory tract by infectious organisms that leads to an acute inflammatory response of the alveoli and terminal airspaces in response to invasion by an infectious agent.[18–27] A large variety of organisms cause pneumonia. Bacterial, viral, mycoplasmal, chlamydial, fungal, and mycobacterial infections are relatively common.

The typical clinical presentation for pneumonia includes fever and a productive cough with sputum production that is usually yellowish-green or rust-colored.[7] Fatigue, weight loss, dyspnea, and tachycardia may also be present, depending on the extent of the disease.[7] Identifying the infectious agent is the most valuable piece of information in managing a complicated pneumonia. Several diagnostic studies are available:

- Sputum culture
- Bronchoscopy, which is most useful in immunocompromised patients or patients who are severely ill
- Blood culture, which is rarely positive in the presence of pneumonia
- Lung aspirate
- Thoracentesis, which is performed for diagnostic and therapeutic purposes in children with pleural effusions
- Serology
- Radiography, the primary imaging study used to confirm the diagnosis of pneumonia

Once the diagnosis of pneumonia is made, antibiotics are chosen based on the likely organism, bearing in mind the age of the patient, the history of exposure, the possibility of resistance, and other pertinent history.

Mycobacterium Tuberculosis

Pulmonary tuberculosis (TB) is a contagious bacterial infection caused by *Mycobacterium tuberculosis* (*M. tuberculosis*).[29–33] The lungs are primarily involved, but the infection can spread to other organs.

Examination of the lungs by stethoscope can reveal crackles (Table 7-2). Enlarged or tender lymph nodes may be present in the neck or other areas. Fluid may be detectable around a lung. Clubbing of the fingers or toes may be present. Confirmatory tests may include:

- Chest x-ray
- Sputum cultures
- Tuberculin skin test; the Mantoux skin test (intradermal inoculation of 5 TU of purified protein derivative) should be read 48 to 72 hours after placement
- Bronchoscopy
- Thoracentesis
- Chest CT
- Interferon (IFN)–gamma blood test; this type of test looks for an immune response to proteins produced by *M. tuberculosis*
- Biopsy of the involved tissue (typically lungs, pleura, or lymph nodes)

The goal of the intervention is to cure the infection with antitubercular drugs. Daily oral doses of multiple drugs are continued until culture results show the drug sensitivity of the mycobacterial infection. Hospitalization may be indicated to prevent the spread of the disease to others until the contagious period has been resolved with drug therapy. All healthcare workers must follow the guidelines for isolation precautions (Chapter 1) to prevent transmission of TB both for themselves and their patients. This is especially important for the PTA treating aged, immunocompromised, or, chronically ill individuals.

Restrictive Lung Disease

Restrictive lung disease is a grouping of diseases with differing etiologies that result in difficulty in expanding the lungs and a reduction in lung volume.[34]

Interstitial Lung Disease/Pulmonary Fibrosis

Interstitial lung disease (ILD), also referred to as idiopathic pulmonary fibrosis and interstitial pulmonary fibrosis, is a general term that includes a variety of chronic lung disorders.

The initial injury appears to damage the alveolar and epithelial cells. The damage causes inflammatory cells to release cytokines, tumor necrosis factor, and platelet-derived growth factor.

The inflammatory chemicals result in smooth muscle proliferation, degradation of the alveoli, and the proliferation of fibroblasts and collagen deposition.[35] Fibrosis, or scarring of the lung tissue, results in permanent loss of that tissue's ability to transport oxygen.

An insidious onset of breathlessness and a nonproductive cough can be the first symptoms of these diseases. The patient may also complain of systemic symptoms of low-grade fever, malaise, arthralgias, weight loss, and clubbing of the fingers and toenails.[35] Specific tests include bronchoalveolar lavage (BAL), a test performed during bronchoscopy that permits removal and examination of cells from the lower respiratory tract and open lung biopsy.

Systemic Sclerosis

Systemic sclerosis (SSc), which is characterized by alterations of the microvasculature, disturbances of the immune system, and by massive deposition of collagen, is a clinical disorder that affects the connective tissue of the skin and internal organs such as the gastrointestinal tract, lungs, heart, and kidneys.[36,37] Arthritis, often resembling rheumatoid arthritis at the onset, is the initial symptom in 66% of SSc patients, often preceding the typical skin changes.[37] Contractures are generally dermatogenic due to sclerotic changes of the overlying skin or surrounding connective tissue.[37] Neurological manifestations include peripheral neuropathy with reduction in the conduction velocity.[38] Hematological abnormalities are mostly related to renal disease, microangiopathic hemolytic anemia, or bleeding gastrointestinal teleangiectasias.[39]

Chest Wall Disease or Injury

Environmental and Occupational Diseases

Pneumoconiosis

Coal worker's pneumoconiosis (CWP) can be defined as the accumulation of coal dust in the lungs and the tissue's reaction to its presence—the dust is engulfed by alveolar and interstitial macrophages.[40] The phagocytosed coal particles are transported by macrophages up the mucociliary elevator and are expelled in the mucus or through the lymphatic system.[41] When this system becomes overwhelmed, the dust-laden macrophages accumulate in the alveoli and may trigger an immune response.[41,42]

Hypersensitivity Pneumonitis

Hypersensitivity pneumonitis (HP), also called extrinsic/external allergic alveolitis, is a complex syndrome caused by sensitization to repeated inhalation of dusts containing organic antigens.[43,44] These dusts can be derived from a variety of sources, such as dairy and grain products, animal dander and protein, wood bark, and water reservoir vaporizers.[45–47] Based on the length and intensity of exposure and subsequent duration of illness, clinical presentations of HP are categorized as acute, subacute (intermittent), and chronic progressive.[47]

- *Acute HP:* Acute HP is a nonprogressive and intermittent inflammatory response to an inciting agent. Symptoms often resolve spontaneously within 12 hours to several days upon cessation of exposure. Patients abruptly develop fever, chills, malaise, cough, chest tightness, dyspnea, headache, and malaise.[43]
- *Subacute (intermittent) HP:* Patients may gradually develop a productive cough, dyspnea, fatigue, anorexia, and weight loss. Symptoms may be present in patients who experience repeated acute attacks.
- *Chronic HP:* Along with symptoms presented in the acute and subacute phases, these individuals also present with progressive dyspnea, significant fatigue, and weakness.

Parenchymal Disorders

Atelectasis

Atelectasis, defined as diminished volume affecting all or part of a lung, is a common pulmonary complication in patients following thoracic and upper abdominal procedures.[48–50] General anesthesia and surgical manipulation lead to atelectasis by causing diaphragmatic dysfunction and diminished surfactant activity.[48–50] Several types of atelectasis exist; each has a characteristic radiographic pattern and etiology. Atelectasis is divided physiologically into obstructive and nonobstructive causes.

- *Obstructive atelectasis:* The most common type; results from reabsorption of gas from the alveoli when communication between the alveoli and the trachea is obstructed. Causes of obstructive atelectasis include foreign body, tumor, and mucous plugging.
- *Nonobstructive atelectasis:* Can be caused by loss of contact between the parietal and visceral pleurae, compression, loss of surfactant, and replacement of parenchymal tissue by scarring or infiltrative disease.

Rapid bronchial occlusion with a large area of lung collapse causes pain on the affected side, sudden onset of dyspnea, and cyanosis. Hypotension, tachycardia, fever, and shock may also occur.[48,49] Slowly developing atelectasis may be asymptomatic or may cause only minor symptoms. Middle lobe syndrome is often asymptomatic, although irritation in the right middle and right lower lobe bronchi may cause a severe, hacking, nonproductive cough.[48,49]

Clinical findings show dullness to percussion over the involved area and diminished or absent breath sounds. Chest excursion in the area is reduced or absent. The trachea and the heart are deviated toward the affected side. Confirmation is achieved through lab studies and imaging (chest radiographs and CT scans). Atelectasis of a significant size results in hypoxemia as measured on arterial blood gas determinations. Arterial blood gas evaluation shows that despite hypoxemia, the Pa_{CO_2} level is usually normal or low as a result of the increased ventilation.[48,49]

Treatment of acute atelectasis, including postoperative lung collapse, requires removal of the underlying cause. Prevention of further atelectasis involves placing the patient in such a position that the uninvolved side is dependent to promote increased drainage of the affected area and intermittent manual positive airway pressure,[51] and encouraging the patient to cough and to breathe deeply.[52]

Acute Respiratory Distress Syndrome

Acute respiratory distress syndrome (ARDS) is the presence of pulmonary edema in the absence of volume overload or depressed left ventricular function.[53] ARDS occurs in children as well as adults.

The condition originates from a number of insults involving damage to the alveolocapillary membrane with subsequent fluid accumulation within the airspaces of the lung.[53] Histologically, these changes have been termed *diffuse alveolar damage.*[53] Damage to the surfactant-producing type II cells and the presence of protein-rich fluid in the alveolar space disrupt the production and function of pulmonary surfactant, leading to microatelectasis and impaired gas exchange.[54] Mild tachypnea may be the only manifestation.[55,56]

Physical Therapy Intervention for Restrictive Lung Diseases

The physical therapy intervention for restrictive lung disease is based on severity of the condition. However, there are a number of common goals, including maximizing gas exchange and functional capacity. Specific interventions may include:

- Patient education on body mechanics, energy conservation techniques, and posture
- Diaphragm and ventilatory muscle strengthening
- Breathing exercises
- Coughing techniques
- Airway secretion clearance techniques

Pulmonary Oncology

The lung is a very common site for metastasis from tumors in other parts of the body. Ninety percent to 95% of cancers of the lung are thought to arise from the epithelial, or lining, cells of the bronchi and bronchioles; for this reason lung cancers are sometimes called *bronchogenic carcinomas.*[57] Cancers can also arise from the pleura (the thin layer of tissue that surrounds the lungs); such cancers are called *mesotheliomas* (the mesothelium is a protective lining that covers most of the body's internal organs). Rarely, cancers arise from supporting tissues within the lungs—for example, blood vessels.[57] Causes of lung cancer include:[57–60]

- *Smoking:* The incidence of lung cancer is strongly correlated with cigarette smoking, with about 90% of lung cancers arising as a result of tobacco use. Pipe and cigar smoking can also cause lung cancer, although the risk is not as high as with cigarette smoking.
- *Passive smoking:* Passive smoking, the inhalation of tobacco smoke from other smokers

sharing living or working quarters, is an established risk factor for the development of lung cancer. Research has shown that nonsmokers who reside with a smoker have a 24% increase in risk for developing lung cancer when compared with other nonsmokers.

- *Asbestos fibers:* These fibers can persist for a lifetime in lung tissue following exposure to asbestos. Cigarette smoking drastically increases the chance of developing an asbestos-related lung cancer in exposed workers.
- *Radon gas:* A natural, chemically inert gas that is a natural decay product of uranium. Radon gas can travel up through soil and enter homes through gaps in the foundation, pipes, drains, or other openings. As with asbestos exposure, concomitant smoking greatly increases the risk of lung cancer with radon exposure.
- *Familial predisposition:* Numerous studies have shown that lung cancer is more likely to occur in both smoking and nonsmoking relatives of those who have had lung cancer than in the general population.
- *Lung diseases:* The presence of certain diseases of the lung, notably chronic obstructive pulmonary disease (COPD), is associated with a slightly increased risk (four to six times the risk of a nonsmoker) for the development of lung cancer even after the effects of concomitant cigarette smoking are excluded.
- *Prior history of lung cancer:* Survivors of lung cancer have an increased risk of developing another lung cancer.

Symptoms of lung cancer are varied dependent upon where and how widespread the tumor, and include:[57,60]

- No symptoms. In up to 25% of people who get lung cancer, the cancer is first discovered on a routine chest radiograph or CT scan.
- Symptoms related to the cancer, such as cough, shortness of breath, wheezing, chest pain, and coughing up blood (*hemoptysis*). If the cancer has invaded nerves, for example, it may cause shoulder pain that travels down the outside of the arm (called *Pancoast syndrome*).
- Symptoms related to metastasis. Lung cancer that has spread to the bones may produce excruciating pain at the sites of bone involvement. Cancer that has spread to the brain may cause a number of neurologic symptoms that may include blurred vision, headaches, seizures, or weakness or loss of sensation in parts of the body.
- Nonspecific symptoms, including weight loss, weakness, and fatigue.

Treatment for lung cancer can involve surgical removal of tumor, chemotherapy, or radiation therapy as well as combinations of these methods. The decision about which treatments will be appropriate for a given individual must take into account the localization and extent of the tumor as well as the overall health status of the patient. As with other cancers, therapy may be prescribed that is intended to be curative (removal or eradication of a cancer) or palliative (measures that are unable to cure a cancer but can reduce pain and suffering). The prognosis of lung cancer refers to the chance for recovery and is dependent upon the localization and size of the tumor, the presence of symptoms, the type of lung cancer, and the overall health status of the patient.[61–64]

Pulmonary Vascular Disease

Pulmonary Embolism and Infarct

Pulmonary embolism (PE), which is closely linked to the presence of deep vein thrombosis, blood clots, or thrombus in the peripheral venous system, is a common and potentially lethal disease.[65] Unfortunately, the diagnosis is often missed because patients with PE present with nonspecific signs and symptoms. The diagnosis of PE should be sought actively in patients with respiratory symptoms (dyspnea, pleuritic chest pain, hemoptysis) unexplained by an alternate diagnosis, especially when a patient has risk factors, which include recent surgery, immobility (venous stasis), or a hypercoagulable state.[65] Immediate full anticoagulation is mandatory for all patients suspected to have DVT or PE.[65]

● **Key Point** The prognosis of patients suffering from PE is dependent on the size of the PE, its impact on the cardiopulmonary system, and the immediacy of medical care.[7]

Pulmonary Hypertension

The normal mean pressure within the pulmonary arterial system is less than 15 mm Hg. Pulmonary hypertension[66–69] can be defined as a mean pulmonary arterial pressure greater than 25 mm Hg at rest, and greater than 30 mm Hg during exercise. Pulmonary hypertension is normally classified as primary or secondary:

- *Primary pulmonary hypertension (PPH):* A rare disease that predominantly affects women in their mid-30s, but children may also be affected.
- *Secondary pulmonary hypertension (PAH):* Can be the sequela of congenital heart defect, collagen vascular disease, lung disease with hypoxia, thrombembolic disease, and left heart failure.

Most patients present with nonspecific symptoms. Shortness of breath is typically the first symptom and is usually attributed to physical deconditioning by both patient and physician. The gold standard for diagnosing and documenting the severity of pulmonary hypertension is heart catheterization.[7] Although there is no cure for PPH, many medical advances have improved quality of life and prolonged survival.[7] Beyond the advances in medical treatment, the options of surgical intervention have also improved, with lung transplantation being the most common surgical intervention for PPH and for many patients with PAH.[7]

Pulmonary Edema

Pulmonary edema is defined as an abnormal accumulation of fluid in the extravascular components of the lungs, usually as a manifestation of congestive heart failure (CHF).[70] Pulmonary edema results in an increase in lung fluid secondary to leakage from pulmonary capillaries into the interstitium and alveoli of the lung. The clinical presentation of pulmonary edema does not depend on the underlying cause. The patient could present with acute or subacute onset of dyspnea, orthopnea, tachypnea, restlessness, crackles, and eventually peripheral cyanosis with hypoxemia.[71] The medical interventions for pulmonary edema include diuretics, medications to support cardiac function and blood pressure, and corticosteroids to minimize the inflammatory response.

Pleural Diseases and Disorders

Pneumothorax

A pneumothorax refers to a collection of gas in the pleural space resulting in collapse of the lung on the affected side. Two major types exist:

- *Tension pneumothorax:* A life-threatening condition caused by air within the pleural space

that is under pressure, displacing mediastinal structures and compromising cardiopulmonary function. The condition results from any lung parenchymal or bronchial injury that acts as a one-way valve and allows free air to move into an intact pleural space but prevents the free exit of that air. The positive pressure used with mechanical ventilation therapy can cause air trapping. As pressure within the intrapleural space increases, the heart and mediastinal structures are pushed to the contralateral side. The mediastinum impinges on and compresses the contralateral lung, resulting in hypoxia, decreased venous return, decreased cardiac output, hypotension, and, ultimately, in hemodynamic collapse and death, if untreated.

- *Traumatic pneumothorax:* Results from blunt or penetrating injury that disrupts the parietal or visceral pleura. Mechanisms include injuries secondary to medical or surgical procedures.

The signs and symptoms produced by a pneumothorax depend on the size and the underlying pulmonary disease. If the pneumothorax is small and there is no underlying pulmonary disease, the patient may be asymptomatic. The most common symptom is acute dyspnea. Failure to recognize a tension pneumothorax and to have a needle decompression performed likely results in rapid clinical deterioration and cardiac arrest. A more aggressive treatment approach is chemical pleurodesis, the placement of a chemical, talc, or tetracycline into the pleural space to adhere to visceral pleura to parietal pleura.[7]

Pleural Effusion

Pleural effusion is an excessive collection of fluid within the pleural space. Large amounts of fluid can cause difficulty in expanding one or both lungs when breathing, causing respiratory distress.

> ● **Key Point** *Pleurisy*, also called pleuritis, occurs when the pleura that lines the chest cavity and surrounds each of the lungs becomes inflamed. An infected pleural effusion is called an *empyema*. An empyema can develop if the pleural infusion is not treated or is not responsive to treatment.

There are many causes of pleural effusion, including infectious disease, cancer, collagen vascular disease, trauma, gastrointestinal disease, and reaction to drugs such as methotrexate penicillin.

The most common symptom is dyspnea, which may be due to the underlying cause, such as a blood clot in the lungs or pneumonia, or it may be due to the chest pain caused by breathing. This condition often is diagnosed on the history and observation alone. In addition, the clinician can detect a decrease in chest expansion, a dullness on percussion, diminished breath sounds over the effusion, and a "friction rub" (sounds like the crunching sound of walking on very dry snow) during breathing using a stethoscope. A chest x-ray will be positive for the presence of a fluid collection and distortion of the dome of the diaphragm if at least 300 mL is in the space.[7] If the patient is symptomatic, the fluid can be drained either by thoracentesis or by placement of a pigtail catheter or chest tube. The prognosis is dependent on the underlying disease.[72]

Physical Therapy Intervention

Physical therapy interventions for pulmonary conditions can be broadly classified into primary prevention and secondary intervention, although it must be remembered that both of these categories are linked by physiologic, epidemiologic, and clinical elements.

- *Primary prevention:* The prevention of a pulmonary disease from developing, even among individuals with risk factors (Preferred Practice Pattern 6A in the *Guide to Physical Therapy*).
- *Secondary intervention:* Aimed at reducing symptoms and/or slowing the progression of a pulmonary disease.

Patients requiring secondary intervention have:

- Impaired aerobic capacity/endurance associated with deconditioning (Preferred Practice Pattern 6B in the *Guide to Physical Therapy*)
- Impaired ventilation, respiration/gas exchange, and aerobic capacity/endurance associated with airway clearance dysfunction (Preferred Practice Pattern 6C)
- Impairments/ventilatory pump dysfunction or failure (Preferred Practice Pattern 6E)
- Impaired ventilation and respiration/gas exchange associated with respiratory failure (Preferred Practice Pattern 6F)
- Impaired ventilation, respiration/gas exchange, and aerobic capacity/endurance associated with respiratory failure in the neonate (Preferred Practice Pattern 6G)

Preferred Practice Patterns 6D and 6H are covered in Chapter 6.

The goals of a pulmonary physical intervention include:[73]

- Increased understanding of patient and family of disease process, expectations, goals, and outcomes
- Increased cardiovascular endurance
- Improved independence in airway clearance
- Increased control of energy expenditure
- Increased strength, power, and endurance of peripheral muscles
- Enhanced performance of physical tasks related to community and work integration
- Promote independence in activities of daily living (ADLs)
- Reduce risks of secondary impairments
- Promote self-management of symptoms
- Improve functional capacity

Physical Therapy Associated with Primary Prevention, Risk Reduction, and Deconditioning

Multiple physical therapy interventions may be used to improve ventilation, respiration, and aerobic capacity.

Therapeutic Exercise

Therapeutic exercise for patients with a pulmonary disorder can help to increase aerobic endurance, improve functional capacity, and promote independence in ADLs. Aerobic endurance enhances physical function and health status and improves physiologic response to increased oxygen demand.[74] In addition, aerobic exercise strengthens muscles, reduces bone loss during weight-bearing exercises, enhances the processing of free fatty acids and glucose, and improves skill and coordination. Aerobic exercise is characterized by the use of large muscle groups activated in a rhythmic fashion over time. Examples include walking, swimming, cycling, dancing, and jogging.

● **Key Point** Preparation for any aerobic exercise program requires determining the degree and type of monitoring needed to preserve the patient's safety.

Flexibility exercises can also be incorporated to enhance chest wall expansion and promote healthy postures. For example, trunk rotations with the pelvis stabilized enhances chest wall expansion.[74] Strength training also is an important consideration. Abdominal strengthening (or an abdominal binder in cases when the abdominal muscles cannot provide the necessary support for the abdominal contents needed for passive exhalation) can be used when abdominal muscles are too weak to provide an effective cough. Breathing exercises can be incorporated into the strength training by having the patient exhale during the lift part of the exercise.

Body mechanics and postural stabilization training have two potential benefits for the patient with airway clearance dysfunction and COPD:

- Reducing general body work
- Reducing the work of breathing and diminishing the effects of dyspnea

Breathing exercises also are important (see "Breathing Strategies and Exercises for Airway Clearance").

Functional Training
Functional training for the patient with a pulmonary disorder involves a combination of instruction in energy conservation during daily activities, and an exercise prescription based on the results of an exercise tolerance test. Simple activities like walking on level ground, getting out of a chair, or dressing are used initially and then progressed to more energy-consuming activities like climbing stairs. As appropriate, an evaluation of the home environment should include a review of daily activities. For example, on which level are bathrooms and bedrooms located? How many stairs are there to enter the house? Do the stairs have handrails? Where are the laundry facilities located? How accessible is the kitchen for demands on breathing? Is there a gas stove or an electric? (There are safety concerns when using oxygen.)[74]

Physical Therapy Associated with Airway Clearance Dysfunction
Breathing Strategies and Exercises for Airway Clearance
The goals of breathing retraining include:[66–69, 75–78]

- To improve overall ventilation and respiration
- To decrease accumulation of secretions and prevent complications
- To decrease the work of breathing
- To improve the efficiency of coughing
- To strengthen the respiratory muscles
- To improve chest wall mobility

Forced Expiratory Technique
The forced expiratory technique (FET) is based on optimal airflow and avoidance of the cough to prevent premature airway collapse and to improve

secretion mobilizations and airway clearance. The patient is instructed to take a medium breath (to mid lung volume) and then tighten the abdominal muscles firmly while huffing (expiring forcibly but with an open glottis), without contracting the throat muscles. The huff should be maintained long enough to mobilize and remove distal bronchial secretions without stimulating a spasmodic cough. The sound should be breathy and the mouth should be in the shape of an "O." The important part of this technique is the 15 to 30 seconds of relaxation with gentle diaphragmatic breathing following one or two huffs.

Active Cycle of Breathing Technique
The active cycle of breathing technique is an independent, easy-to-learn, and easy-to-teach technique for conditions such as cystic fibrosis. It combines the FET, bronchial drainage, and manual techniques.[79] The technique includes a 15- to 30-second breathing control (diaphragmatic breathing) phase, thoracic expansion exercises, a repeat of the breathing control phrase, a repeat of the thoracic expansion exercises, and then the FET technique and huffing to clear secretions from the smaller to the larger airways. The patient assumes a bronchial drainage position and focuses on a quiet breathing pattern using the lower rib cage area without upper chest movement during the thoracic expansion phases. This technique has been demonstrated to be as effective as postural drainage, percussion, and shaking.[80]

Autogenic Drainage
Autogenic drainage is an independent airway clearance technique used to sense peripheral secretions and clear them. Intensive training in the technique is necessary before it can be used effectively. Because the technique utilizes some of the same theories as active cycle of breathing, the bronchioles and alveoli should be fully developed to get the full benefit. The patient is instructed to breathe out through an O-shaped mouth and to listen during inhalation and exhalation for noises indicative of secretions, such as high-pitched wheezes, gurgling, or popping sounds. The timing and pitch of the sounds give clues as to where the secretions may be located. For example, sounds that are heard initially on inhalation and which are lower in pitch are most likely to be the result of secretions in the larger airways. These airways must be cleared with huffs or coughs prior to continuation of the technique. The keys to this technique are airflow and volume control, suppression of the cough until secretions are mobilized,

inspiratory hold at the end of inhalation to equalize air across alveoli, and most importantly, patience. The patient sits upright with a minimum of distractions in the room. This technique can be broken down into three phases:

- *Unstick phase:* After a brief period of diaphragmatic breathing, the patient exhales to a low lung volume and breathes at a normal tidal volume at that low lung volume to effect peripheral secretions.
- *Collect phase:* As the patient becomes aware of secretions in the small airways, breathing becomes a bit deeper (at mid lung volumes) to effect the mobilization of the secretions proximally into the middle airways.
- *Evacuation phase:* At this point, breathing becomes deeper (from mid to high lung volumes). The patient is asked to suppress coughing until it cannot be avoided. This phase enables secretions to accumulate in central airways and then be evacuated by huffing or a cough, using minimal effort.

The above steps, which correspond to the area of retained secretions, are repeated until all secretions are removed from the airways.

Assisted Cough/Huff Techniques
The huff or forced expiratory technique was explained previously. The assisted cough can be employed independently or with the help of an assistant. The technique can be as simple as placing a pillow over an incision to help splint the area, or as dynamic as using a manual technique at the time of the cough (see Key Point). Four types of manual assistance can be used: costophrenic (hand placement), abdominal thrust, anterior chest compression, and a counter rotation assist.[81] The amount of force used by the compression is dependent upon patient tolerance and abdominal sensation. The cough is best performed using a flexed posture.

> **● Key Point** To perform the manual assisted cough, the patient is positioned in supine. The clinician places both hands flat against the patient's upper abdomen directly below the xiphoid process. After taking a deep breath, the patient is instructed to cough two to three times. With each cough the clinician applies manual pressure inwardly and superiorly.

Segmental Breathing
Segmental breathing uses a combination of manual cues and breathing control to enhance mobilization of secretions and improve ventilation to specific areas of the chest wall. Facilitation or inhibition of a specific segment is controlled using hand placement and verbal cues to enhance breathing coordination. During the technique the patient is asked to breathe in against the resistance of the clinician's hands. Segmental breathing is inappropriate in cases of intractable hypoventilation.

Diaphragmatic Breathing
Diaphragmatic breathing (lower rib cage breathing) involves using a tactile cue such as a hand, which is placed over the lower rib cage. On inhalation, the hand on the lower rib cage should rise, indicating air filling the lungs, and there should be little movement occurring at the upper chest. Initially, diaphragmatic breathing can be made easier with the bed declined 30 degrees at the head. To apply resistance, manual contact can be used, or the clinician can place a 5- to 10-pound sandbag over the patient's abdomen.

Pursed-Lip Breathing
Pursed-lip breathing is accomplished by breathing into the nose to a count of "1, 2" and out via pursed lips to a count of "1, 2, 3, 4." Pursed-lip breathing prolongs the expiratory phase, slows the respiratory rate, increases the excretion of carbon dioxide, and improves airflow by delaying small airway closure.

Paced Breathing
Paced breathing uses a combination of pursed-lip breathing and diaphragmatic breathing performed at the normal 1:2 ratio of inspiration to expiration during functional activities. The patient is instructed to take a breath into the nose and walk two steps to a count of "1, 2," followed by an exhalation to a count of "1, 2, 3, 4" while walking the next four steps.

Stacking Breaths
The technique of stacking breaths (called inflation-hold) is used in situations when the volume of air a patient can inhale is limited. The technique involves taking a small to moderate-sized breath and adding it to two or three additional sip-like breaths to increase inspiratory volume, thereby decreasing atelectasis, moving air behind the secretions, and increasing inspiratory volume to enhance a huff or cough.

Glossopharyngeal breathing (GPB) is a form of stacking breaths that is used with patients who cannot breathe independently due to weak inspiratory muscles. GPB requires cranial nerves V, VII, and IX through XII to be intact. The technique involves the use of the glottis (throat) to add to an inspiratory effort by projecting (gulping) boluses of air into the lungs.

The glottis closes with each "gulp." One breath usually consists of six to nine gulps of 40 to 200 milliliters each. During the training period the efficiency of GPB can be monitored by spirometrically measuring the milliliters of air per gulp, gulps per breath, and breaths per minute. GPB is rarely useful in the presence of an indwelling tracheostomy tube. It cannot be used when the tube is uncapped as it is during tracheostomy intermittent positive-pressure ventilation (IPPV), and even when capped, the gulped air tends to leak around the outer walls of the tube and out the stoma as airway volumes and pressures increase during the GPB air stacking process. The safety and versatility afforded by GPB are key reasons to eliminate tracheostomy in favor of noninvasive aids.

Sustained Maximal Inspiration

Sustained maximal inspiration is a technique used to increase inhaled volume, sustain or improve alveolar inflation, and maintain or restore functional residual capacity. The patient is asked to inspire slowly through the nose or pursed lips to the point of maximal inspiration. The maximal inspiration is held for three seconds and then the volume is passively exhaled.

Inspiratory Muscle Trainers

Inspiratory muscle trainers function by loading the muscles of inspiration using a series of graded aperture openings. The trainers are appropriate for patients with decreased compliance, decreased intrathoracic volume, resistance to airflow, or an alteration in the length-tension relationship of the ventilatory muscles, and for any patient who has decreased strength of the respiratory muscles.

Bronchial Drainage

Bronchial drainage[82–84] or postural drainage utilizes the shape and direction of the lung segments to drain the uppermost segment of the lung by placing the individual in gravity-enhancing postures or positions. The contraindications for postural drainage are as follows:[85]

- Esophageal reflux
- Hemoptysis
- Dyspnea
- Orthopnea
- Bruising/rib fractures/flail chest
- Coagulopathy
- Cardiac arrhythmias
- Desaturation/hemodynamic decompensation
- Large pleural effusion
- Bronchospasm

- Spinal instability
- Recent burn grafts
- Osteopenia/osteoporosis
- Pain
- Risk for injury to caregiver and/or recipient
- Nausea and vomiting
- Untreated pneumothorax
- Increased intracranial pressure
- Recent thoracic surgery
- Indwelling venous catheter
- Feeding tubes

Nine positions can be used to drain all of the segments of the lung, although it may not be necessary to use all nine positions (**Table 7-4**). These positions may need to be modified under certain conditions.

Chest Percussion

Chest percussion is a technique involving the application of a cupped hand to a specific area of the chest wall in a rhythmic manner to loosen secretions. The technique may be done concurrently with a drainage position to enhance secretion mobilization. The area to be percussed is covered with a lightweight cloth to avoid erythema. The duration of percussion depends on the patient's needs and tolerance—the guideline is 3 to 5 minutes per postural drainage position. The force applied is sufficient to cause the patient's voice to quiver.

Shaking/Vibration

Shaking/vibration, commonly used following percussion, is a rhythmic technique applied to the rib cage throughout exhalation to hasten the removal of secretions from the tracheobronchial tree. This technique is commonly applied following percussion in the appropriate postural drainage position. As the patient exhales, the clinician makes a downward motion and a vibrating motion while maintaining full contact of the hands on the chest wall. The duration of the shaking depends on the patient's needs, tolerance, and clinical improvement—the guideline is five to seven trials of shaking.[34]

Medical Management of Respiratory Failure

Medical interventions for respiratory failure can provide supportive measures, mechanical ventilation, and supplemental O_2.

Supplemental Oxygen

Supplemental oxygen[86] is indicated when the patient can sustain sufficient work of breathing (WOB)

TABLE
7-4

Bronchial Drainage Positions

Lobe	Segment	Position and Technique
Upper	Apical	The child sits on the flat drainage table and leans back on a pillow at a 30-degree angle against the clinician. The clinician percusses and vibrates over the muscular area between the collarbone and the top of the shoulder blade on both the left and right sides.
	Anterior	The child lies on his or her back on a flat table. The clinician stands at the patient's head and percusses and vibrates between the collarbone and nipple on both the left and right sides of the chest.
	Posterior	The child sits on the edge of a flat table and leans forward over a folded pillow at a 30-degree angle. The clinician stands behind the child and percusses and vibrates on the upper back on the left and right sides of the chest.
	Left lingula	The foot of the table is elevated 14 inches (about 15 degrees). The child lies head down on the right side and rotates 1/4 turn backward. A pillow may be placed behind the child (from shoulder to hip) and the child may flex his or her knees. The clinician percusses and vibrates just outside the left nipple area. For females with tenderness around the breasts, the clinician should percuss and vibrate with the heel of hand under the armpit with the fingers extended forward beneath the breasts.
Middle (right middle)		The foot of the table is elevated 14 inches (about 15 degrees). The child lies head down on the right side and rotates 1/4 turn backward. A pillow may be placed behind the child (from shoulder to hip) and the child may flex his or her knees. The clinician percusses and vibrates just outside the right nipple area. For females with tenderness around the breasts, the clinician should percuss and vibrate with the heel of hand under the armpit with the fingers extended forward beneath the breasts.
Lower	Superior: left and right	The child lies on his or her abdomen on a flat table with two pillows under the hips. The clinician percusses and vibrates over the middle part of the back at the bottom of the scapular blade on both the left and right side of the spine while making sure not to percuss or vibrate over the spine.
	Lateral basal: left and right	The foot of the table is elevated 18 inches (about 30 degrees). The child lies on his or her left side, head down, and leans 1/4 turn forward toward the table. The child can flex his or her upper leg over a pillow for support. The clinician percusses and vibrates over the uppermost portion of the lower ribs to drain the right side. To drain the left side, the child lies on his or her right side in the same position and the clinician percusses and vibrates over the uppermost portion of the lower left ribs.
	Anterior basal: left and right	The foot of the table is elevated 18 inches (about 30 degrees). The child lies on his or her right side with the head down and a pillow behind the back. The clinician percusses and vibrates over the lower ribs on the left side of the chest, as shown in the diagram. To drain the right side of the chest, the child lies on his or her left side with the head down and a pillow behind the back. The clinician percusses and vibrates over the lower ribs on the right side of the chest.
	Posterior basal: left and right	The foot of the table is elevated 18 inches (about 30 degrees). The child lies on his or her abdomen, head down, with a pillow under the hips. The clinician percusses and vibrates on both the left and right sides of the spine, making sure not to percuss or vibrate over the spine or lower ribs.

to maintain ventilation independently but cannot maintain adequate levels of oxygenation. All oxygen delivery systems consist of a supply source and a delivery device. The amount of time a portable O_2 gas tank will depend on its size, how full it is, and the flow rate. O_2 tank sizes are letter coded.

Mechanical Ventilation

Mechanical ventilation[86] is used to support breathing of patients with respiratory insufficiency or those who cannot sustain the necessary work of breathing independently. A mechanical ventilator substitutes for or assists the patient's ventilatory pump to allow breathing to occur. When examining a patient who is using a ventilator, the clinician should note the route of intubation, mode of ventilation, rate setting, tidal volume, amount of positive end expiratory pressure (PEEP), pressure support, and the F_{IO_2}.

Special Considerations for Certain Patient Populations

Neurologic

In treating patients with neurological issues, the clinician needs to consider the following:

- *Subarachnoid hemorrhage:* The clinician should avoid activities involving incentive spirometry and forced coughing so as not to increased intracranial pressure (ICP).
- *Traumatic brain injury:* To minimize the risk of increasing the ICP, the clinician should avoid activities involving the Valsalva maneuver, coughing and suctioning, and postural drainage.

Spinal Cord Injury

Common spinal cord injuries affect physical therapy intervention for pulmonary issues. Clinicians need to consider the limitations of each condition.

Paraplegia

Paraplegia, primarily caused by injury to T1 to T5, leads to weakened and/or absent abdominal, intercostal, and erector spinae muscles as well as a slight decrease in anterior and lateral expansion. These impairments result in a moderate decrease in chest expansion and vital capacity, decreased ability to build up intrathoracic and intra-abdominal pressures, and decreased cough effectiveness.[87]

Tetraplegia

The capabilities of tetraplegic patients will depend on the area of the spine that is injured:

- Patients who have a lesion at C5–C8, are missing the aforementioned muscles and experience weakened pectoralis, serratus anterior, and scalenes. They have a marked decrease in anterior expansion, upper and lower; a marked decrease in lateral expansion; and a slight decrease in posterior expansion. These impairments result in significant decrease in chest expansion and vital capacity, FEV, and cough effectiveness.
- Patients who have a lesion at C5–T1 can rely on both diaphragmatic and cervical muscles for breathing.
- Patients who have a lesion at C4 are missing the aforementioned muscles and have weakened scalenes and diaphragm. There is a marked decrease in anterior and lateral chest expansion and slight decrease in inferior and superior expansion. These impairments result in the previously mentioned limitations, but they are more pronounced, and a decrease in tidal volume is possible. These patients may need mechanical ventilation.
- Patients who have a lesion at C3–C1 are missing the aforementioned muscles, and the last of the remaining accessory muscles are weakened and/or absent. All planes of chest expansion are severely limited. These impairments result in the previously mentioned limitations, with a significant decrease in tidal volume. Most patients will require mechanical ventilation 20 to 24 hours per day.
- Patients with a lesion at the C2–C3 levels can only rely on pharyngeal and laryngeal muscles for breathing, so only glossopharyngeal breathing exercises are appropriate.

Physical therapy intervention goals for the patient with a spinal cord injury include the following:

- Increase/maintain chest expansion in all planes of respiration
- Increase vital capacity and tidal volume where indicated
- Improve cough effectiveness
- Increase coordination and eccentric control of the diaphragm for improved phonation
- Balance the use of diaphragm and accessory muscles to minimize the work of breathing
- Increase coordination of breathing with functional activities
- Increase the patient's and/or family's ability to maintain good bronchial hygiene

Medical and Surgical Intervention for Pulmonary Disorders

Possible medical and surgical interventions for pulmonary disorders include the following:

- *Lobectomy:* The removal of a lobe, or section, of the lung performed to prevent the spread of cancer to other parts of the lung or other parts of the body, as well as to treat patients with such noncancerous diseases as chronic obstructive pulmonary disease (COPD).
- *Segmentectomy:* The removal of a segment of the lung. The procedure has several variations and many names, including segmental resection, wide excision, lumpectomy, tumorectomy, quadrantectomy, and partial mastectomy.
- *Pneumonectomy (or pneumectomy):* The removal of a lung most commonly performed to excise a tumor. Other indications for lobectomy include solitary pulmonary nodule, and bronchiectasis where other forms of treatment have failed, particularly if it is localized and recurrent hemoptysis is present.
- *Pleurectomy:* Excision of the pleura; the most common surgery employed to manage patients with diffuse mesothelioma.
- *Thoracotomy:* Surgical incision of the chest wall, used primarily as a diagnostic tool when other procedures have failed to provide adequate diagnostic information.
- *Segmental resection or wedge resection*: A resection is the removal of a part of the lung, often in order to remove a tumor. Wedge resection is removal of a wedge-shaped portion of lung tissue.
- *Volume reduction surgery:* Used to help relieve shortness of breath and increase tolerance for exercise in patients with chronic obstructive pulmonary disease, such as emphysema.

REVIEW Questions

1. The site of gaseous exchange in the pulmonary system is:
   a. The trachea
   b. The bronchi
   c. The alveoli
   d. The bronchioles

2. Which of the two bronchi is the longest?
3. What is the term used to describe the movement of air through the conducting airways?
4. What is the most superior aspect of each lung called?
5. Which of the two lungs has three lobes?
6. The primary muscle(s) of respiration is/are the:
   a. Intercostals
   b. Latissimus dorsi
   c. Diaphragm
   d. Abdominals
7. True or false: Surface tension is responsible for much of the lung's elastic recoil
8. The importance of surfactant is in its:
   a. Ability to promote lung tissue growth in keeping with chest development of the child.
   b. Ability to lower the surface tension of the water molecules on the alveolar surface.
   c. Ability to dissolve or wash out debris that passes the cilia.
   d. All of the above.
9. What is the name given to potential space between the two pleura that is supplied by a small amount of pleural fluid that serves to hold the parietal and visceral pleurae together?
10. The anatomic dead space is defined as the:
    a. Pulmonary area with the least blood supply.
    b. Area occupied by the conducting airways that does not permit gas exchange.
    c. Portion of the pulmonary tree that is inelastic and does not alter its size with either inspiration or expiration.
    d. None of the above.
11. What is the physiological dead space?
12. The amount of air that can be forcibly exhaled at the end of the normal respiration is known as:
    a. Tidal volume
    b. Functional residual capacity
    c. Expiratory reserve volume
    d. Vital capacity
    e. Residual volume
13. The maximum amount of air that can be moved in and out during a single breath is known as:
    a. Tidal volume
    b. Functional residual capacity
    c. Expiratory reserve volume
    d. Vital capacity
    e. Residual volume

14. The amount of air that enters or leaves the lungs during a single resting breath is known as:
    a. Tidal volume
    b. Functional residual capacity
    c. Expiratory reserve volume
    d. Vital capacity
    e. Residual volume

15. The total amount of air remaining in the lungs after a resting expiration is known as:
    a. Tidal volume
    b. Functional residual capacity
    c. Expiratory reserve volume
    d. Vital capacity
    e. Residual volume

16. The total amount of air remaining in the lungs after a forced expiration is known as:
    a. Tidal volume
    b. Functional residual capacity
    c. Expiratory reserve volume
    d. Vital capacity
    e. Residual volume

17. True or false: Expiration is essentially a passive process.

18. All of the following factors determine the extent to which oxygen will combine with hemoglobin except:
    a. The P_{O_2} of the blood
    b. Tissue temperature
    c. The pH of the blood
    d. The P_{CO_2} levels of the blood

19. Where are the neurogenic mechanisms that control respiration located?
    a. In the bronchi
    b. At the bifurcation of the carotid arch
    c. In the alveoli
    d. In the reticular substance of the medulla and pons

20. Of the two respiratory gases, oxygen and carbon dioxide, which is the most tightly controlled by the body?

21. Where are the peripheral chemoreceptors located?

22. What is the normal range for arterial pH?

23. The maximum amount of air that can be contained in the lungs after a maximum inspiration is called:
    a. Vital capacity
    b. Total lung capacity
    c. Residual volume
    d. Inspiratory capacity

24. The amount of air inhaled or exhaled with each breath is known as:
    a. Total lung capacity
    b. Tidal volume
    c. Vital capacity
    d. Inspiratory capacity

25. Which of the following is known as the amount of air left in the lungs after a forced exhalation?
    a. Tidal volume
    b. Total lung capacity
    c. Residual volume
    d. Functional capacity

26. True or false: Low breathing frequencies are commonly observed in the individual with a restrictive lung disease.

27. True or false: Most of the carbon dioxide carried by the blood is in the form of bicarbonate.

28. In the ideal matching of equal volumes of gas and blood, the $\dot{V}/\dot{Q}$ ratio should be what value?

29. What condition do you suspect in an individual with spontaneous attacks of wheezing and dyspnea who is otherwise usually free of these symptoms?
    a. Pulmonary emphysema
    b. Acute bronchitis
    c. Chronic bronchitis
    d. Bronchial asthma

30. You are treating a pulmonary patient who states he has a daily cough and increased sputum over the past few years. What condition would you suspect this patient to have?
    a. Bronchial asthma
    b. Pulmonary emphysema
    c. Chronic bronchitis
    d. Acute bronchitis

31. All of the following are physical signs associated with emphysema except:
    a. Increased respiratory rate
    b. Decreased resonance to percussion over the lung fields
    c. Increased AP diameter of the chest
    d. Use of excess to muscles of respiration during breathing

32. A disease characterized by dilation of bronchi and bronchioles is:
    a. Endocarditis
    b. Spondylitis
    c. Bronchiectasis
    d. Emphysema

33. A disease in which the air spaces distal to the terminal bronchioles are dilated beyond their normal size is called:
   a. Endocarditis
   b. Mitral valve prolapse
   c. Bronchiectasis
   d. Emphysema

34. All of the following diseases make up the entity known as chronic obstructive pulmonary disease except:
   a. Chronic bronchitis
   b. Pulmonary emphysema
   c. Acute bronchitis
   d. Bronchial asthma

35. Which abnormal breathing pattern is characterized by alternating periods of apnea and hyperpnea?

References

1. Shaffer TH, Wolfson MR, Gault JH: Respiratory Physiology, in Irwin S, Tecklin JS (eds): Cardiopulmonary Physical Therapy (ed 2). St. Louis, Mosby, 1990, pp 217–244

2. Van de Graaff KM, Fox SI: Respiratory system, in Van de Graaff KM, Fox SI (eds): Concepts of Human Anatomy and Physiology. New York, WCB/McGraw-Hill, 1999, pp 728–777

3. Collins SM, Cocanour B: Anatomy of the Cardiopulmonary System, in DeTurk WE, Cahalin LP (eds): Cardiovascular and Pulmonary Physical Therapy: an Evidence-Based Approach. New York, McGraw-Hill, 2004, pp 73–94

4. Schmitz TJ: Vital Signs, in O'Sullivan SB, Schmitz TJ (eds): Physical Rehabilitation (ed 5). Philadelphia, F. A. Davis, 2007, pp 81–120

5. Morgan BJ, Dempsey JA: Physiology of the Cardiovascular and Pulmonary Systems, in DeTurk WE, Cahalin LP (eds): Cardiovascular and Pulmonary Physical Therapy: An Evidence-Based Approach. New York, McGraw-Hill, 2004, pp 95–122

6. Cahalin LP: Pulmonary Evaluation, in DeTurk WE, Cahalin LP (eds): Cardiovascular and pulmonary physical therapy: An evidence-based approach. New York, McGraw-Hill, 2004, pp 221–269

7. Wells C: Pulmonary Pathology, in DeTurk WE, Cahalin LP (eds): Cardiovascular and pulmonary physical therapy: An evidence-based approach. New York, McGraw-Hill, 2004, pp 151–188

8. Man SF, McAlister FA, Anthonisen NR, et al: Contemporary management of chronic obstructive pulmonary disease: clinical applications. JAMA 290:2313–2316, 2003

9. Grimfeld A, Just J: Clinical characteristics of childhood asthma. Clin Exp Allergy 28 Suppl 5:67–70; discussion 90–91, 1998

10. Kemp JP: Comprehensive asthma management: Guidelines for clinicians. J Asthma 35:601–620, 1998

11. Chang AB, Masters IB, Everard ML: Re: membranous obliterative bronchitis: A proposed unifying model. Pediatr Pulmonol 41:904; author reply 905–906, 2006

12. Wang JS, Tseng HH, Lai RS, et al: Sauropus androgynus-constrictive obliterative bronchitis/bronchiolitis—histopathological study of pneumonectomy and biopsy specimens with emphasis on the inflammatory process and disease progression. Histopathology 37:402–410, 2000

13. Poole DC, Sexton WL, Farkas GA, et al: Diaphragm structure and function in health and disease. Med Sci Sports Exerc 29:738–754, 1997

14. Stoller JK: Clinical features and natural history of severe alpha 1-antitrypsin deficiency. Roger S. Mitchell Lecture. Chest 111:123S–128S, 1997

15. Schwaiblmair M, Vogelmeier C: Alpha 1-antitrypsin: Hope on the horizon for emphysema sufferers? Drugs Aging 12:429–440, 1998

16. Jones A, Rowe BH: Bronchopulmonary hygiene physical therapy in bronchiectasis and chronic obstructive pulmonary disease: A systematic review. Heart Lung 29:125–135, 2000

17. Mysliwiec V, Pina JS: Bronchiectasis: The 'other' obstructive lung disease. Postgrad Med 106:123–126, 128–131, 1999

18. Coughlin AM: Combating community-acquired pneumonia. Nursing 37:64hn1–3, 2007

19. Clark JE, Donna H, Spencer D, et al: Children with pneumonia: How do they present and how are they managed? Arch Dis Child 29:29, 2007

20. Parienti JJ, Carrat F: Viral pneumonia and respiratory sepsis: Association, causation, or it depends? Crit Care Med 35:639–640, 2007

21. Hospital-acquired pneumonia. J Hosp Med 1:26–27, 2006

22. Community-acquired pneumonia. J Hosp Med 1:16–17, 2006

23. Flaherty KR, Martinez FJ: Nonspecific interstitial pneumonia. Semin Respir Crit Care Med 27:652–658, 2006

24. Lynch JP, 3rd, Saggar R, Weigt SS, et al: Usual interstitial pneumonia. Semin Respir Crit Care Med 27:634–651, 2006

25. Leong JR, Huang DT: Ventilator-associated pneumonia. Surg Clin North Am 86:1409–1429, 2006

26. Agusti C, Rano A, Aldabo I, et al: Fungal pneumonia, chronic respiratory diseases and glucocorticoids. Med Mycol 44 Suppl:207–211, 2006

27. Scannapieco FA: Pneumonia in nonambulatory patients: The role of oral bacteria and oral hygiene. J Am Dent Assoc 137 Suppl:21S-25S, 2006

28. Medina-Walpole AM, Katz PR: Nursing home-acquired pneumonia. J Am Geriatr Soc 47:1005–1015, 1999

29. Richeldi L: Rapid identification of *Mycobacterium* tuberculosis infection. Clin Microbiol Infect 12 Suppl 9:34–36, 2006

30. Yoshinaga Y, Kanamori T, Ota Y, et al: Clinical characteristics of *Mycobacterium* tuberculosis infection among rheumatoid arthritis patients. Mod Rheumatol 14:143–148, 2004

31. Johnson R, Streicher EM, Louw GE, et al: Drug resistance in *Mycobacterium* tuberculosis. Curr Issues Mol Biol 8:97–111, 2006

32. Rotert R: Case of the month. Mycobacterium tuberculosis. Jaapa 19:70, 2006
33. Sterling TR, Haas DW: Transmission of Mycobacterium tuberculosis from health care workers. N Engl J Med 355:118–121, 2006
34. Starr JA: Chronic pulmonary dysfunction, in O'Sullivan SB, Schmitz TJ (eds): Physical Rehabilitation (ed 5). Philadelphia, F. A. Davis, 2007, pp 561–588
35. Nicod LP: Recognition and treatment of idiopathic pulmonary fibrosis. Drugs 55:555–562, 1998
36. Ong VH, Brough G, Denton CP: Management of systemic sclerosis. Clin Med 5:214–219, 2005
37. Haustein UF: Systemic sclerosis-scleroderma. Dermatol Online J 8:3, 2002
38. Casale R, Buonocore M, Matucci-Cerinic M: Systemic sclerosis (scleroderma): An integrated challenge in rehabilitation. Arch Phys Med Rehabil 78:767–773, 1997
39. Steen VD: Treatment of systemic sclerosis. Am J Clin Dermatol 2:315–325, 2001
40. Tang WK, Lum CM, Ungvari GS, et al: Health-related quality of life in community-dwelling men with pneumoconiosis. Respiration 73:203–208, 2006
41. Attfield MD, Kuempel ED: Pneumoconiosis, coalmine dust and the PFR. Ann Occup Hyg 47:525–529, 2003
42. Chong S, Lee KS, Chung MJ, et al: Pneumoconiosis: Comparison of imaging and pathologic findings. Radiographics 26:59–77, 2006
43. Lacasse Y, Cormier Y: Hypersensitivity pneumonitis. Orphanet J Rare Dis 1:25, 2006
44. Kurup VP, Zacharisen MC, Fink JN: Hypersensitivity pneumonitis. Indian J Chest Dis Allied Sci 48:115–128, 2006
45. Navarro C, Mejia M, Gaxiola M, et al: Hypersensitivity pneumonitis : A broader perspective. Treat Respir Med 5:167–179, 2006
46. Klote M: Hypersensitivity pneumonitis. Allergy Asthma Proc 26:493–495, 2005
47. Churg A, Muller NL, Flint J, et al: Chronic hypersensitivity pneumonitis. Am J Surg Pathol 30:201–208, 2006
48. Igarashi A, Amagasa S, Oda S, et al: Pulmonary atelectasis manifested after induction of anesthesia: A contribution of sinobronchial syndrome? J Anesth 21:66–68, 2007
49. Duggan M, Kavanagh BP: Atelectasis in the perioperative patient. Curr Opin Anaesthesiol 20:37–42, 2007
50. Wong AY, Fung LN: Pulmonary atelectasis following spinal anaesthesia for caesarean section. Anaesth Intensive Care 34:687–688, 2006
51. Schulz-Stubner S, Rickelman J: Intermittent manual positive airway pressure for the treatment and prevention of atelectasis. Eur J Anaesthesiol 22:730–732, 2005
52. Westerdahl E, Lindmark B, Eriksson T, et al: Deep-breathing exercises reduce atelectasis and improve pulmonary function after coronary artery bypass surgery. Chest 128:3482–3488, 2005
53. Hudson LD, Steinberg KP: Epidemiology of acute lung injury and ARDS. Chest 116:74S–82S, 1999
54. Luh SP, Chiang CH: Acute lung injury/acute respiratory distress syndrome (ALI/ARDS): The mechanism, present strategies and future perspectives of therapies. J Zhejiang Univ Sci B 8:60–69, 2007
55. Singh N: AIP or ARDS? Not just semantics. Crit Care 10:423, 2006
56. Bautin A, Khubulava G, Kozlov I, et al: Surfactant therapy for patients with ARDS after cardiac surgery. J Liposome Res 16:265–272, 2006
57. Collins LG, Haines C, Perkel R, et al: Lung cancer: Diagnosis and management. Am Fam Physician 75:56–63, 2007
58. Crevenna R, Marosi C, Schmidinger M, et al: Neuromuscular electrical stimulation for a patient with metastatic lung cancer: A case report. Support Care Cancer 14:970–973, 2006
59. Godtfredsen NS, Prescott E, Osler M: Effect of smoking reduction on lung cancer risk. JAMA 294:1505–1510, 2005
60. Buccheri G, Ferrigno D: Lung cancer: Clinical presentation and specialist referral time. Eur Respir J 24:898–904, 2004
61. Hotta K, Fujiwara Y, Matsuo K, et al: Recent improvement in the survival of patients with advanced nonsmall cell lung cancer enrolled in phase III trials of first-line, systemic chemotherapy. Cancer 6:6, 2007
62. Stewart DJ, Chiritescu G, Dahrouge S, et al: Chemotherapy dose-response relationships in non-small cell lung cancer and implied resistance mechanisms. Cancer Treat Rev 2:2, 2007
63. Barros JA, Valladares G, Faria AR, et al: Early diagnosis of lung cancer: The great challenge. Epidemiological variables, clinical variables, staging and treatment. J Bras Pneumol 32:221–227, 2006
64. Sugimura H, Nichols FC, Yang P, et al: Survival after recurrent nonsmall-cell lung cancer after complete pulmonary resection. Ann Thorac Surg 83:409–417; discussion 417–418, 2007
65. Alexander P, Giangola G: Deep venous thrombosis and pulmonary embolism: Diagnosis, prophylaxis, and treatment. Ann Vasc Surg 13:318–327, 1999
66. Placidi G, Cornacchia M, Polese G, et al: Chest physiotherapy with positive airway pressure: A pilot study of short-term effects on sputum clearance in patients with cystic fibrosis and severe airway obstruction. Respir Care 51:1145–1153, 2006
67. Boitano LJ: Management of airway clearance in neuromuscular disease. Respir Care 51:913–922; discussion 922–924, 2006
68. McIlwaine M: Physiotherapy and airway clearance techniques and devices. Paediatr Respir Rev 7:S220–S222, 2006
69. Kendrick AH: Airway clearance techniques in cystic fibrosis. Eur Respir J 27:1082–1083, 2006
70. Gluecker T, Capasso P, Schnyder P, et al: Clinical and radiologic features of pulmonary edema. Radiographics. 19:1507–1531; discussion 1532–1533, 1999
71. Zwischenberger JB, Alpard SK, Bidani A: Early complications: Respiratory failure. Chest Surg Clin N Am 9:543–564, viii, 1999
72. Parfrey H, Chilvers ER: Pleural disease: Diagnosis and management. Practitioner 243:412, 415–421, 1999
73. Downs AM, Bishop-Lindsay KL: Physical therapy associated with airway clearance dysfunction, in DeTurk WE, Cahalin LP (eds): Cardiovascular and Pulmonary Physical Therapy: An Evidence-Based Approach. New York, McGraw-Hill, 2004, pp 463–489

74. Cohen M, Michel TH: Cardiopulmonary symptoms in physical therapy practice. New York, Churchill Livingstone, 1988

75. Panitch HB: Airway clearance in children with neuromuscular weakness. Curr Opin Pediatr 18:277–281, 2006

76. Alison JA: Clinical trials of airway clearance techniques. Chron Respir Dis 1:123–124, 2004

77. Flume PA: Airway clearance techniques. Semin Respir Crit Care Med 24:727–736, 2003

78. Tecklin JS: Airway clearance dysfunction, in Cameron MH, Monroe LG (eds): Physical Rehabilitation: Evidence-Based Examination, Evaluation, and Intervention. St. Louis, MO, Saunders/Elsevier, 2007, pp 642–668

79. Eaton T, Young P, Zeng I, et al: A randomized evaluation of the acute efficacy, acceptability and tolerability of flutter and active cycle of breathing with and without postural drainage in non-cystic fibrosis bronchiectasis. Chron Respir Dis 4:23–30, 2007

80. Wilson GE: A comparison of traditional chest physiotherapy with the active cycle of breathing in patients with chronic supurative lung disease. Eur Respir J 8:171S, 1995

81. Massery M, Frownfelter D: Facilitating airway clearance with cough techniques, in Frownfelter D, Dean E (eds): Principles and Practice of Cardiopulmonary Physical Therapy (ed 3). Philadelphia, Mosby-Yearbook, 1996, pp 367–382

82. Spero K: Chest physical therapy. Rehab Manag 15:10, 2002

83. Oberle GM: Chest physical therapy (CPT). Rehab Manag 15:10, 2002

84. Thomas J, Cook DJ, Brooks D: Chest physical therapy management of patients with cystic fibrosis: A meta-analysis. Am J Respir Crit Care Med 151:846–850, 1995

85. Downs AM, Bishop Lindsay KL: Physical therapy associated with airway clearance dysfunction, in DeTurk WE, Cahalin LP (eds): Cardiovascular and pulmonary physical therapy: An evidence-based approach. New York, McGraw-Hill, 2004, pp 463–490

86. Dekerlegand J, Cahalin LP, Perme C: Respiratory failure, in Cameron MH, Monroe LG (eds): Physical Rehabilitation: Evidence-Based Examination, Evaluation, and Intervention. St. Louis, MO, Saunders/Elsevier, 2007, pp 689–717

87. Massery M, Cahalin LP: Physical therapy associated with ventilatory pump dysfunction and failure, in DeTurk WE, Cahalin LP (eds): Cardiovascular and Pulmonary Physical Therapy: An Evidence-Based Approach. New York, McGraw-Hill, 2004, pp 593–646

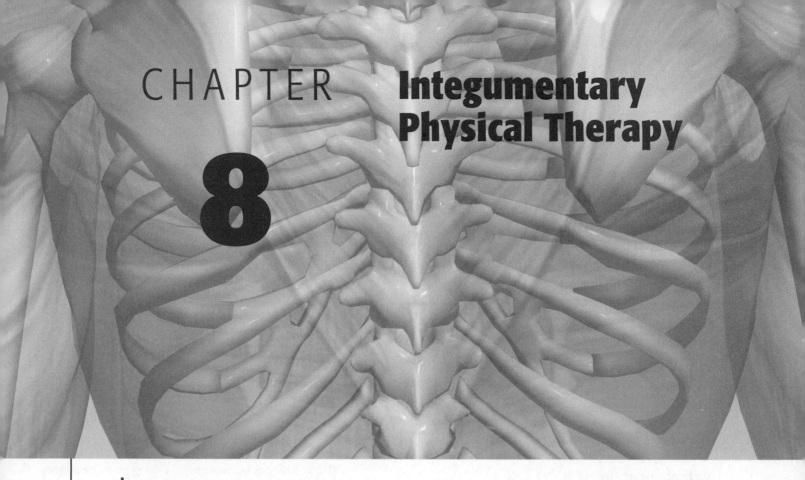

CHAPTER 8 — Integumentary Physical Therapy

Overview

The integumentary system consists of the dermal and epidermal layers of the skin, hair follicles, nails, sebaceous glands, and sweat glands. The integument, or skin, is the largest organ system of the body, constituting 15% to 20% of the body weight.[1]

> **● Key Point** Key functions of the skin include:
> - Protection against injury or invasion
> - Secretion of oils that lubricate the skin
> - Maintenance of homeostasis: fluid balance, regulation of body temperature
> - Excretion of excess water, urea, and salt via sweat
> - Maintenance of body shape
> - Providing cosmetic appearance and identity
> - Vitamin D synthesis
> - Providing cutaneous sensation via receptors in the dermis

Anatomically, the skin consists of two distinct layers of tissue: the epidermis and the dermis. A third layer involved in the anatomical consideration of the skin is the subcutaneous fat cell layer directly under the dermis and above muscle fascial layers.[1]

Epidermis

The epidermis serves as the superficial, protective layer. All but the deepest layers of the epidermis are composed of dead cells, which contain no blood vessels. The epidermis contains five layers in the lips, palms, and soles (four layers elsewhere). From bottom to top the layers are named:

- Stratum basale, a single layer of cells in contact with the dermis
- Stratum spinosum

- Stratum granulosum
- Stratum lucidum, which exists only in the lips, palms and soles
- Stratum corneum, which provides the skin its waterproof characteristic and serves the role of protection from infection

Dermis

The dermis, considered the "true" skin because it contains blood vessels, lymphatics, nerves, collagen, and elastic fibers, is deeper and thicker than the epidermis.[1] The dermis also contains sebaceous and sweat glands.

> **● Key Point** The interface between the epidermis and the dermis is termed the *rete peg region*. This area consists of an extensive series of epidermal–dermal ridges and valleys that serve to increase the surface area between the epidermis and the dermis.[1] These ridges act as the reservoir of skin and are needed to overcome fictional forces that skin is exposed to in daily activity.[1] It is the lack of these ridges in the healed burn wound that results in blisters from abrasion and poor adherence of the new epidermal tissue when it comes in contact with clothing or other surfaces.[1]

Pathology of the Skin

Injury to the skin can occur in a number of ways:

- *Abrasion:* A wearing away of the upper layer of skin as a result of applied friction force.
- *Contusion:* Caused when blood vessels are damaged or broken as the result of a direct blow to the skin.
- *Ecchymosis:* Skin discoloration caused by the escape of blood into the tissues from ruptured blood vessels.
- *Hematoma:* A localized collection of blood, usually clotted, in a tissue or organ.
- *Excoriation:* Lesion of traumatic nature with epidermal loss in a generally linear shape.
- *Laceration:* An injury involving penetration of the skin, in which the wound is deeper than the superficial skin level.
- *Penetrating wound:* A wound accompanied by disruption of the body surface that extends into the underlying tissue or into a body cavity.
- *Petechiae:* Tiny red spots in the skin that do not blanch when pressed upon. They result from red blood leaking from capillaries into the skin (intradermal hemorrhages). Petechiae are less than 3 millimeters in diameter.
- *Puncture:* A wound made by a pointed object (like a nail).

- *Ulcer:* A lesion on the surface of the skin or the surface of the mucous membrane, produced by the sloughing of inflammatory, necrotic tissue.

An *exudate* is any fluid that filters from the circulatory system into lesions or areas of inflammation. Various types of exudate exist:

- *Serous:* Presents as clear, light color with a thin, watery consistency. Serous exudate is considered to be normal in a healthy healing wound.
- *Sanguinous:* Presents as red with a thin, watery consistency. Appears to be red due to the presence of blood or maybe brown if allowed to dehydrate. May be indicative of new blood vessel growth or the disruption of blood vessels.
- *Serosanguinous:* Presents as light red or pink, with a thin, watery consistency. Can be normal in a healthy healing wound.
- *Seropurulent:* Presents as opaque, yellow, or tan color, with a thin, watery consistency. Seropurulent exudate may be an early warning sign of an impending infection.
- *Purulent:* Presents as yellow or green color with a thick, viscous consistency. This type of exudate is generally an indicator of wound infection.

Wounds to the skin can be described using the Red–Yellow–Black system (**Table 8-1**).

Patient Education

Patient education plays a critical role in the intervention and prevention of integumentary disorders. The clinician should determine those activities, positions, and postures that produce or reduce trauma to skin and the level of safety awareness that the patient

TABLE 8-1	Red–Yellow–Black System
Color	**Wound Description**
Red	Healthy, pink granular tissue with absence of necrotic tissue.
Yellow	Adherent fibrinous exudates and debris (moist yellow slough) are present.
Black	Black, thick eschar (dried necrotic tissue), firmly adhered, is present.

Data from Cozzell J: The new red, yellow, black color code. Am J Nurs 10:1014, 1989

demonstrates during functional activities. In addition, the following should be addressed:

- The likelihood of future trauma to the skin.
- Enhanced disease awareness, implementing healthy behaviors.
- Mechanisms of pressure ulcer development. These include assistive, adaptive, protective, orthotic, or prosthetic devices that produce or reduce skin trauma.
- Avoidance of prolonged positions.
- Safety awareness during self-care and during use of devices and equipment.
- Importance of ongoing activities/exercise program.
- Daily, comprehensive skin inspection, paying particular attention to bony prominences.
- Avoidance of harsh soaps, known irritants, temperature extremes, and exacerbating factors or triggers.
- Avoidance of restrictive clothing and tight-fitting shoes and socks.
- Incontinence management strategies.
- Enhancing activities of daily living, ensuring functional mobility and safety.
- Use of pressure-relieving devices.
- Enhancement of self-management of symptoms.
- Edema management through leg/arm elevation and muscle-pumping exercises, and compression therapy to facilitate the movement of excess fluid from the extremity. Therapies include:
  - ❏ Compression wraps: elastic or tubular bandages.
  - ❏ Compression stockings, e.g., Jobst.
  - ❏ Compression pump therapy.
- Review of medications. The following medications can have a negative effect on wound repair: nonsteroidal anti-inflammatories, corticosteroids, immunosuppressives, anticoagulants, and prostaglandins.

Eczema and Dermatitis

Eczema and *dermatitis* are terms that are often used interchangeably to describe a superficial inflammation of the skin caused by a recent exposure, allergic sensitization, or generally determined idiopathic factors. May be classified as:

- Acute: erythema, edema, vesiculation
- Subacute

- Chronic: mild erythema, scaliness, lichenification (thickening of the epidermis with exaggeration of normal skin lines), with or without hyperpigmentation

Exogenous (Contact) Dermatitis

Dermatitis follows some form of contact. Various types exist:

- *Irritant contact dermatitis:* Direct chemical contact (acids or alkalis) or physical action on the skin. Not immunologic. Reaction can be elicited in all individuals.
- *Allergic contact dermatitis:* A form of cell-mediated response. The hypersensitivity is based on a specific immunologic alteration requiring an incubation period of several days. Re-exposure to allergen causes dermatitis that appears 8 to 96 hours after exposure.

Endogenous (Constitutional) Dermatitis

Various types of endogenous dermatitis exist:

- *Atopic:* Increased susceptibility to atopic diseases—for example, asthma, hay fever, urticaria, allergic conjunctivitis, and systemic drug allergy. There is increased production of IgE antibodies. The skin is inherently irritable (sensitive) and dry with low threshold for itching. Itching leads to scratching and lichenification.
- *Seborrheic dermatitis:* Associated with excessive sebaceous secretion (seborrhea) and usually localized in the areas of greatest sebaceous activity. Onset is during the first few month of life and at puberty. Lesions consist of subacute dermatitis covered by greasy scales. Dandruff is a form of seborrheic dermatitis. This dermatitis is frequently associated with acne, and in adults can last for a lifetime.
- *Rosacea:* A chronic, benign, but obvious facial disorder of middle-aged and older people (the cheeks, nose, and chin have a rosy appearance marked by a reddened skin), which is often considered as a form of acne. No known causal factor has been identified, but the condition has often been linked with gastrointestinal disturbances.

Bacterial Infections

Normally the skin harbors a variety of bacterial flora, including the major pathogenic varieties of staphylococci and streptococci. The degree of pathogenicity depends on the invasiveness and toxicity of the specific organisms, the integrity of the skin, and the immune and cellular defenses of the host. Bacterial infections typically enter through portals in the skin—for example, abrasions or puncture wounds, or through the respiratory tract.

Bacterial Infections Localized to Hair

All of these infections are caused by *Staphylococcus aureus*, coagulase positive.

- *Folliculitis:* Infection of the most superficial part of the hair follicle—a pustule pierced by hair
- *Furuncle:* Painful infection of the whole length of the hair follicle
- *Carbuncle:* Infection of a group of follicles (grouped furuncles)

Generalized Bacterial Skin Infections

Types of generalized bacterial skin infections include the following:

- *Impetigo contagiosum:* Mainly an epidermal reaction and thus the most superficial. Caused by beta-hemolytic streptococci (*Streptococcus pyogenes*), *Staphylococcus aureus*, or both.
- *Echthyma:* Affects epidermis and dermis (ulcerated impetigo). Bacteriolobially similar to impetigo.
- *Cellulitis (includes erysipelas):* Affects dermis and subcutis. Caused mainly by beta-hemolytic streptococcus.

Viral Infections

Viral infections are contagious; observe standard precautions.The following are common viral infections of the integumentary system.

Herpes Simplex

Herpes simplex viruses (HSVs) are ubiquitous, extremely host-adapted pathogens that can cause a wide variety of illnesses. Two types exist: type 1 (HSV-1) and type 2 (HSV-2). HSV-1 is transmitted chiefly by contact with infected saliva, whereas HSV-2 is transmitted sexually or from a mother's genital tract infection to her newborn. The clinical course of the disease depends upon the age and immune status of the host, the anatomic site of involvement, and the antigenic type of the virus. Both HSV-1 and HSV-2 can cause similar genital and orofacial primary infections after contact with infectious secretions.

Herpes Zoster (Shingles)

More details on herpes zoster can be found in Chapter 5.

Plantar Warts

Plantar warts (verrucae) are hyperkeratotic lesions on the plantar surface. Human papillomavirus (HPV), usually of type 1, 2, or 4, causes plantar warts. HPV attacks the epidermal layers through direct contact. The warts tend to develop over areas of pressure such as the heel and ball of the foot. Although they are generally self-limited, plantar warts should be treated (with topical keratinolytic and cauterizing agents) to lessen symptomatology, decrease duration, and reduce transmission.

Fungal Infections (Tinea)

The *dermatophytes* are a group of fungi (*ringworm*) that invade the dead keratin of skin, hair, and nails. Dermatophytosis (*tinea*) is a fungal infection caused by dermatophytes. Several species of dermatophytes infect humans; these belong to the *Epidermophyton*, *Microsporum*, and *Trichophyton* genera. The infection may spread from person to person (*anthropophilic*), animal to person (*zoophilic*), or soil to person (*geophilic*). Clinically, tinea infections are classified according to the body region involved.

Fungal infections may be treated with topical agents (e.g., creams, lotions, solutions, powders, sprays) or with oral antifungals in extensive or recalcitrant disease. Topical therapy is ineffective in treating tinea of the hair and nails. Transmission is person to person or animal to person; observe standard precautions.

Parasitic Infections

Parasitic infections are caused by insect and animal contacts. Transmission is person to person, and it can be sexually transmitted. Avoid direct contact and observe standard precautions. Common parasitic infections include:

- *Scabies:* A highly contagious skin eruption caused by a parasite (female mite) that can burrow into the skin, causing inflammation, intense pruritus, and itching. Scabies is treated with excavation of the mite using a needle or scalpel blade, or with a scabicide containing permethrin or lindane.

- *Pediculosis (lousiness):* An infestation of a common parasite that can affect the head, body, and genital area that is transmitted from one person to another, usually on shared personal items such as combs, clothes, or furniture.

There are three major types of pediculosis:

- *Pediculus humanus var. capitis (head louse):* Transmitted through personal contact or through shared hairbrushes or combs.
- *Pediculus corporis (clothes louse):* Generally found in the seams of the infected individual's clothing.
- *Pediculus pubis (crab louse):* Usually transmitted by sexual contact. Treatment involves using a special soap or shampoo containing permethrin.

Melanin Pigmentary Disorders

Hypo- and Depigmentation Disorders

Pityriasis Alba
Pityriasis alba is common in young children. Lesions consist of hypopigmented macules with powdery scales. The face is commonly affected. Patients are usually asymptomatic, and the condition gradually disappears with age.

Vitiligo
Vitiligo is a genetic disease, most probably with an autoimmune etiology. It may be associated with autoimmune disorders such as thyroid diseases, pernicious anemia, Addison disease, diabetes mellitus, alopecia areata. Histologic examination shows a marked absence of melanocytes. Vitiligo is usually localized (though it may become generalized). It has scattered or confluent depigmented macules, with more over friction areas. In general, it follows a protracted course.

Idiopathic Guttate Hypomelanosis
Idiopathic guttate hypomelanosis is characterized by porcelain-white macules, usually 2 to 6 millimeters in diameter. It is of unknown etiology, but it is believed that sun exposure may play a role. The lesions are commonly present on the legs and to a lesser extent on the forearms.

.Postinflammatory Hypopigmentation
Hypopigmented macules commonly follow resolution of inflammatory skin disease such as eczema and psoriasis. These lesions are generally self-limiting.

Hyperpigmentation

Freckles
Freckles (*ephilides*) are common in individuals with red or blonde hair and blue eyes. Freckles appear on light-exposed skin and increase in number, size, and depth of pigmentation during summer.

Neurofibromatosis (von Recklinghausen Disease)
The cutaneous features of this disease include macular hyperpigmentation (cafe-au-lait patches) and neurofibromata. Clinical patterns include multiple neural tumors anywhere on the body. The presence of one or two is not diagnostic in the absence of other signs of the disease, but if six or more patches are present, the probability of neurofibromatosis is high. Bone, intracranial, and gastrointestinal (GI) lesions and symptoms may be identified. While pigmentary changes may occur at birth, the tumor formation is most aggressive during puberty.

Melasma (Choasma)
Melasma is a blotchy hypermelanosis of exposed areas that occurs most often on the face, mainly cheeks, forehead, and moustache area, usually in women. It is commonly seen in pregnancy. A similar type of pigmentation may be induced by oral contraceptives. Photosensitization to cosmetics, especially perfumes, may play a role.

Benign Dermatoses

Psoriasis
Psoriasis is one of the most common dermatoses. It appears as a chronic, bilaterally symmetric, erythematous, plaquelike lesion with a silvery scale covering. The lesions classically are located over the extensor surfaces, including the elbows, knees, back, and scalp. Psoriasis is occasionally associated with other systemic illnesses, particularly psoriatic arthritis, which occurs in approximately 5% to 10% of patients with psoriasis.

Systemic Sclerosis
A diffuse and chronic connective tissue disease that causes fibrosis of the skin, joints, blood vessels, and internal organs. It has the following characteristics:

- It is classified according to the degree and extent of skin thickening.
- There are two distinct types: systemic and localized.

- It is of unknown etiology, but it may be an acquired disease triggered by bacteria (mycoplasma) or an autoimmune mechanism.
- Altered vascular function includes increased vasospasm, reduced vasodilatory capacity, and increased adhesiveness of the blood vessels to platelets and lymphocytes.
- It has three recognized stages: edematous, sclerotic, and atrophic, although not all people pass through all the stages.

Discoid Lupus Erythematosus

Discoid lupus is a chronic, relatively common dermatitis with clinical presentation more common in women than in men. It presents with erythematous plaques that vary from an atrophic to hyperkeratotic appearance in the region of the face, scalp, neck, extremities, and trunk.

Autoimmune Skin Disorders

Scleroderma

Scleroderma, also known as progressive systemic scleroderma, describes two distinct diseases: localized scleroderma and systemic scleroderma.[2–9] Localized scleroderma is primarily a cutaneous disease. Systemic sclerosis is a multisystem connective tissue disease. The etiology of both of these diseases is not known. There are two main subsets of systemic sclerosis: limited scleroderma (the old CREST syndrome) and diffuse scleroderma. Raynaud phenomenon is present in almost all patients with scleroderma. Scleroderma has no cure. Medical treatment is primarily pharmacologic (antihypertensives, corticosteroids). The physical therapy intervention should emphasize preventing any loss of range of motion and functional activites, focusing on bed mobility, transfers, and walking. Modalities such as moist heat or paraffin may prove therapeutic.

Polymyositis

Polymyositis (PM), dermatomyositis (DM), and inclusion body myositis (IBM) are the major members of a group of skeletal muscle diseases called the idiopathic inflammatory myopathies.[10–15] PM and DM have many shared clinical features. Both are inflammatory myopathies that present as symmetric muscle weakness that develops over weeks to months. Although classified as an inflammatory myopathy, IBM shows minimal evidence of inflammation. Characteristic rash of face, trunk, and hands is seen in DM only. The heliotrope rash is a symmetric, confluent, purple-red, macular eruption of the eyelids and periorbital tissue. Edema may also be present. Other rashes seen with DM include erythematous nail beds and a scaly, purple erythematous papular eruption over the dorsal metacarpophalangeal and interphalangeal joints (Gottron sign).

Skin Cancer

Skin cancers are the most prevalent form of cancer, eventually affecting nearly all white people older than 65 years of age.[16–25] Skin cancer can be discussed using three broad categories: benign, premalignant, and malignant.

Benign Tumors

Seborrheic Keratosis

Seborrheic keratosis (SK) is a common benign tumor in advanced and middle-aged persons. It is typically a raised papular lesion of variable color from light to dark brown. SKs may be smooth or wartlike with visible pitting. Common sites include the face, trunk, and extremities.

Acrochordon

Acrochordon also is known as skin tag, fibroepithelial polyp, fibroma molle, and fibroepithelial papilloma. These lesions have been observed to follow warts, SKs, and inflammatory skin conditions. Acrochordons occasionally are associated with pregnancy, diabetes mellitus, and intestinal polyposis syndromes. They tend to be located in the intertriginous areas of the axilla, groin, and inframammary regions as well as in the low cervical area along the collar line.

Keratinous Cyst

A keratinous cyst also is known as sebaceous cyst, wen, atheroma, or steatoma. Two essential types have been identified:

- *Epidermoid or epidermal inclusion cyst:* The most common type, representing approximately 90% of keratinous cysts. Epidermoid cysts appear as firm, round, mobile, flesh-colored to yellow or white subcutaneous nodules of variable size.
- *Pilar or trichilemmal cyst:* Derived from the outer root sheath of the hair follicle; the second most common keratinizing cyst on the scalp. Pilar cysts present as smooth, movable swellings in the scalp.

Nevus

The definition of a nevus can be expanded to include any congenital lesion that is circumscribed to well defined. The term also occasionally has been used as a synonym for mole. A mole is defined as a shapeless mass. Most nevi appear between the ages of 2 to 60 years and have a predictable evolution. They rarely undergo activation or malignant degeneration. Nevi tend to be more common on the head, neck, and trunk. However, a great deal of variability exists with regard to size, shape, and even amount of hair present.

Premalignant Tumors

Actinic keratosis, also known as solar keratosis and senile keratosis, refers to lesions that are rough-appearing, scaly, erythematous papules or plaques. The lesions occur on exposed surfaces (e.g., face, hands, ears, neck, legs, thorax) of blue- or green-eyed middle-aged persons with fair skin and a history of chronic sun exposure. The color of the lesions may be red, yellow, brown, or gray. The most important attribute is its premalignant potential—almost 50% of skin cancer cases begin as actinic keratosis lesions.

Malignant Tumors

Basal Cell Carcinoma

Basal cell carcinoma is the most common cutaneous malignancy in humans. These tumors typically appear on sun-exposed skin, are slow growing, and rarely metastasize. Many types of basal cell carcinoma have been described, including nodular, superficial, infiltrating, morpheic, pigmented, basal-squamous, adenoid, cystic, keratotic, and fibroepithelioma. The classic description is of a small, well-defined nodule with a translucent, pearly border with overlying telangiectasias. Coloration varies with melanin content and the presence of areas of necrosis. Risk factors include sun exposure, x-ray exposure, chronic ulcers, immunosuppression, xeroderma pigmentosa, and Bowen disease. Neglected tumors can lead to significant local destruction and even disfigurement.

Bowen Disease

Bowen disease is also known as *carcinoma in situ* and *squamous intraepidermoid neoplasia*. Lesions involve predominantly skin unexposed to the sun (i.e., protected skin). The lesions are scaly, crusted, erythematous plaques—a persistent, brown to reddish-brown scaly plaque with well-defined margins.

Squamous Cell Carcinoma

Squamous cell carcinoma is the second most common form of skin cancer. Frequently arises on the sun-exposed skin of middle-aged and elderly individuals. General risk factors include age older than 50 years, male sex, fair skin, geography (closer to the equator), exposure to UV light (high cumulative dose), exposure to chemical carcinogens (e.g., arsenic, tar), exposure to ionizing radiation, and chronic immunosuppression. Tumors often manifest as small, firm nodules with indistinct margins or plaques. The surface may have various irregularities ranging from smooth to verruciform to ulcerated. Skin coloration is often brown to tan. Scaling, bleeding, and crusting may also occur. Typically, squamous cell carcinoma is locally invasive.

Dermatofibroma Protuberans

Dermatofibroma protuberans is a low-grade dermal sarcoma. Typically, the lesion occurs as a painless subcutaneous mass after a history of trauma. The lesion grows slowly; however, if left unattended, it can become quite large and have multiple nodules. This malignancy typically has lateral spread, but it can also invade deeper structures and may ulcerate. It is generally reddish blue. Metastasis is unlikely but has been reported.

Merkel Cell Carcinoma

Merkel cell carcinoma is an aggressive cutaneous neoplasm observed in sun-exposed areas. Older patients with long-term solar exposure are at greatest risk. The tumor originates in the dermis and appears as a pinkish nodule that enlarges by invading deeper structures.

Kaposi Sarcoma

Kaposi sarcoma is a spindle-cell tumor thought to be derived from endothelial cell lineage. Kaposi sarcoma (KS) can occur in several different clinical settings:

- *Epidemic AIDS-related KS:* Occurs in patients with advanced HIV infection and is the most common presentation of KS.
- *Immunocompromised KS:* Can occur following solid-organ transplantation or in patients receiving immunosuppressive therapy.
- *Classic KS:* Typically occurs in elderly men of Mediterranean and Eastern European background. Classic KS usually carries a protracted and indolent course.
- *Endemic African KS:* Occurs in men who are HIV seronegative in Africa and may carry an indolent or aggressive course.

Melanoma

Melanoma is a malignancy of pigment-producing cells (*melanocytes*) located predominantly in the skin, but also found in the eyes, ears, GI tract, and oral and genital mucous membranes. A changing mole is the most common warning sign for melanoma. Variation in color and/or an increase in diameter, height, or asymmetry of borders of a pigmented lesion are noted by more than 80% of patients with melanoma at the time of diagnosis.

● **Key Point** The pneumonic ABCDE (**A**symmetry, **B**order irregularity, **C**olor variegation, **D**iameter, **E**volving) is an easy way to remember those factors associated with skin cancer. Symptoms such as bleeding, itching, ulceration, and pain in a pigmented lesion are less common but warrant an evaluation.

| Ulcers

Pressure Ulcers

The terms *pressure ulcer* and *decubitus ulcer* are often used interchangeably.[26–38] Because the common denominator of all such ulcerations is pressure, *pressure ulcer* is the better term to describe this condition. Pressure ulcers result from sustained or prolonged pressure at levels greater than the level of the capillary-filling pressure on the tissue (approximately 32 mm Hg), leading to localized ischemia and/or tissue necrosis. Most pressure ulcers are avoidable through anticipation and avoidance of conditions that promote them. Prevention of pressure ulcers involves multiple members of the healthcare team. The groups of patients most susceptible include elderly individuals, those who are neurologically impaired, and those who are acutely hospitalized. Pressure against the skin over a bony prominence (**Table 8-2**) increases the risk for the development of necrosis and ulceration. Other contributing factors to pressure ulcers include shear, friction, heat, maceration (softening associated with excessive moisture), medication, malnutrition, and muscle atrophy. Risk factors associated with ulcers include:

- *Emaciation:* Bony prominences should be protected and pressure distributed equally over large surface areas. Use of pressure distribution equipment such as wheelchair cushions, custom mattresses, and alternating pressure mattress pads is advocated. Patients should avoid movements that rub, drag, or scratch the skin.
- *Immobilization:* Patients should be turned every 2 hours when in bed, and weight shifting should occur every 15 to 20 minutes when seated.

- *Decrease in activity level:* Regular cardiovascular exercise should be recommended. It will contribute to a gradual buildup of skin tolerance for new activities, equipment, and positions.
- *Diabetes and other circulatory disorders:* Regular skin inspections should occur.
- *Incontinence:* Good bowel and bladder care is paramount with immediate cleansing after episode of incontinence, and there should be current cleansing and drying of skin at least once daily. The skin should be inspected for areas of redness in both morning and night.
- *Decreased mental status.*

Pressure ulcers are graded using a four-stage system (**Table 8-3**).

● **Key Point** The term *Marjolin ulcer* is used to describe a cancer arising from any site of chronic inflammation. Ninety percent of Marjolin ulcers develop from burn scars.[39,40] Other sites include stasis ulcers and decubitus ulcers.

Arterial Insufficiency (Ischemic) Ulcers

As their name suggests, these are ulcers that develop from arterial insufficiency and ischemia as a result of atherosclerotic disease of large-sized and medium-sized arteries, such as aortoiliac and femoropopliteal atherosclerosis.[41,42] Arterial insufficiency ulcers are common in the diabetic population due to a number of metabolic abnormalities, including high low-density lipoprotein (LDL) and very low-density lipoprotein (VLDL) levels, elevated plasma fibrinogen levels, and increased platelet adhesiveness. Arterial ulcers are noted most often on the distal aspects of the feet but may occur more proximally, depending on the location of the occluded artery. These ulcers have a punched-out appearance with a pale granulation base. Patients who are symptomatic may present with intermittent claudication, ischemic pain at rest, non-healing ulceration of the foot, or frank ischemia of the foot. Signs frequently associated with arterial ulcers include a loss of hair on the extremity, poor capillary refill in the toes, and brittle nails. Intervention focuses on cleansing the ulcer, resting, reducing risk factors, and providing limb protection. Patient education emphasizes:

- Washing and drying feet thoroughly
- Inspecting legs and feet daily
- Avoiding unnecessary leg elevation
- Wearing appropriately sized shoes with clean, seamless socks

TABLE 8-2 Bony Prominences Associated with Pressure Ulcers

Supine	Prone	Sidelying	Seated
Occiput	Forehead	Ears	Spine of scapula
Spine of scapula	Anterior portion of the acromion process	Lateral portion of acromion process	Vertebral spinous processes
Inferior angle of scapula	Anterior head of humerus	Lateral head of humerus	Ischial tuberosities
Vertebral spinous processes	Sternum	Lateral epicondyle of humerus	
Medial epicondyle of humerus	Anterior superior iliac spine	Greater trochanter	
Posterior iliac crest	Patella	Head of fibula	
Sacrum	Dorsum of foot	Lateral malleolus	
Coccyx		Medial malleolus	
Heel			

- Using bandages as necessary and avoiding any unnecessary pressure
- Avoiding using heating pads or soaking feet in hot water

Neuropathic Ulcers

A neuropathic ulcer is a secondary complication associated with a combination of ischemia and neuropathy, such as that which occurs with diabetes.[43–50]

The pathophysiology of diabetic peripheral neuropathy is multifactorial but results in a loss of sensation in the foot. Unnoticed excessive heat or cold, pressure from a poorly fitting shoe, or damage from a blunt or sharp object inadvertently left in the shoe may cause blistering and ulceration. These factors, combined with poor arterial inflow, confer a high risk of limb loss on the patient with diabetes. Neuropathic ulcers are frequently found in those areas

TABLE 8-3 National Pressure Ulcer Advisory Panel (NPUAP) Pressure Ulcers Stages

Stage	Characteristics	Preferred Practice Pattern According to the *Guide*
I	An observable pressure-related alteration of intact skin whose indicators as compared with an adjacent or opposite area of the body may include changes in skin color, skin temperature (warm or cool), tissue consistency (firm or boggy), and/or sensation (pain, itching).	7B: Impaired integumentary integrity associated with superficial skin involvement
II	A partial-thickness skin loss that involves the epidermis and/or dermis. The ulcer is superficial and presents clinically as an abrasion, a blister, or shallow crater.	7C: Impaired integumentary integrity associated with partial thickness skin involvement and scar formation
III	A full-thickness skin loss that involves damage or necrosis of subcutaneous tissue that may extend down to, but not through, underlying fascia. The ulcer presents clinically as a deep crater with or without undermining adjacent tissue.	7D: Impaired integumentary integrity associated with full-thickness skin involvement and scar formation
IV	A full-thickness skin loss with extensive destruction, tissue necrosis or damage to muscle, and bone or supporting structures (e.g., tendon, joint capsule). Undermining or sinus tracts may be present.	7E: Impaired integumentary integrity associated with skin involvement extending into fascia, muscle, or bone and scar formation

Data from Pressure ulcer prevention and treatment following spinal cord injury: A clinical practice guideline for health-care professionals. J Spinal Cord Med 24 Suppl 1:S40–101, 2001; and American Physical Therapy Association: Guide to Physical Therapist Practice (ed 2). Phys Ther 81:1–746, 2001

that are most subjected to weight bearing, such as the heel, plantar metatarsal head areas, the tips of the most prominent toes (usually the first or second), and the tips of hammer toes. Ulcers also occur over the malleoli because these areas commonly are subjected to trauma.

● **Key Point** Charcot deformity, characterized by fracture as a result of repetitive trauma without splinting or allowing for repair, is seen commonly in patients with advanced stages of diabetic neuropathy. Initial signs often mimic cellulitis. A common finding in diabetic patients with early Charcot changes is a strong pulse with associated diffuse erythema.

Neuropathic ulcers are typically well defined by a prominent callus rim. The wound has good granulation tissue and little or no drainage. Patients rarely report pain with neuropathic ulcers in part due to diminished sensation. Pedal pulses are most often diminished or absent. The distal limb may appear to be shiny and appear somewhat cool to touch. The wound skin often appears to be dry or cracked. The Wagner Ulcer Grade Classification Scale is commonly used as an assessment instrument for diabetic foot ulcers (**Table 8-4**).[51,52]

TABLE 8-4	The Wagner Ulcer Grade Classification Scale

Grade	Description
0	No open lesion but may possess pre-ulcerative lesions; healed ulcers; presence of bony deformity
1	Superficial ulcer not involving subcutaneous tissue
2	Deep ulcer with penetration through the subcutaneous tissue; potentially exposing bone, tendon, ligament, or joint capsule
3	Deep ulcer with osteitis, abscess, or osteomyelitis
4	Gangrene of digit
5	Gangrene of foot requiring disarticulation

Data from Gul A, Basit A, Ali SM, et al: Role of wound classification in predicting the outcome of diabetic foot ulcer. J Pak Med Assoc 56:444–447, 2006; and Oyibo SO, Jude EB, Tarawneh I, et al: A comparison of two diabetic foot ulcer classification systems: The Wagner and the University of Texas wound classification systems. Diabetes Care 24:84–88, 2001

Venous Insufficiency Ulcers

Venous insufficiency syndromes are caused by valvular incompetence in the high-pressure deep venous system, low-pressure superficial venous system, or both.[53–57] The poor clearance of lactate, carbon dioxide, and other products of cellular respiration also contribute to the development of the syndrome. Untreated venous insufficiency in the deep or superficial system causes a progressive syndrome involving pain, swelling, skin changes, and eventual tissue breakdown. Most venous ulcers are caused by venous reflux that is purely or largely confined to the superficial venous system. Only a minority are caused by chronic DVT or by valvular insufficiency in the deep veins. Venous ulcers typically are located over the medial malleolus area. They tend to be irregular in shape and possess a good granulation base. The most common subjective symptoms are leg aching, swelling, cramping, heaviness, and soreness, which are improved by walking or by elevating the legs.

Intervention focuses on cleansing the ulcer and applying compression to control the edema. Patient education emphasizes:

- Elevating the ulcer above the heart when resting or sleeping
- Attempting active exercise including frequent range of motion
- Inspecting legs and feet daily
- Wearing appropriately sized shoes with clean, seamless socks
- Using bandages as necessary and avoiding scratching or other forms of direct contact

Wound Care

The four primary principles of wound care are:

1. *Wound cleansing:* The removal of loose cellular debris, devitalized tissue, metabolic wastes, bacteria, and topical agents that retard wound healing. The wound is cleansed initially and then at each dressing change.
2. *Management of edema:* Moisture levels in the wound should be balanced to optimize healing and prevent the excessive accumulation of fluid.

● **Key Point** Proper hydration and adequate perfusion facilitate the formation of granulation tissue and epithelial cell migration.

3. *Reduction of necrosis:* Targets harnessing endogenous systems (enzymes) to remove necrotic tissue in conjunction with dressings and debridement technologies (see "Selective and Nonselective Debridement"). Harsh soaps, alcohol-based products, or harsh antiseptic agents should be avoided because they may erode the skin and create an imbalance in the hydration of the wound.

4. *Control of microorganism level (bioburden management):* Aimed at reducing wound-bed microorganism levels through facilitating the body's normal immune response and using cleansing/debridement technologies and appropriate topical or systemic antimicrobials.

Wound Dressings

Ideally, a dressing should create a moist environment without permitting maceration or desiccation.[58–68] Two terms are used when describing dressings:

- *Occlusion:* Refers to the ability of a dressing to transmit moisture, vapor, or gases from the wound bed to the surrounding air. Occlusive dressings are completely impermeable, while nonocclusive dressings are completely permeable. The following dressings are arranged from most occlusive to nonocclusive: Hydrocolloids, hydrogels, semipermeable foam, semipermeable film, impregnated gauze, alginates, and traditional gauze.
- *Moisture:* Dressings can be classified according to the ability to retain moisture. The following list of dressings is arranged from most moisture retentive to least moisture retentive: alginates, semipermeable foam, hydrocolloids, hydrogels, semipermeable films.

The following section describes the most common types of dressing, their indications, advantages, and disadvantages.

Hydrocolloids

These dressings, containing gel-forming polymers such as gelatin with a strong film or foam adhesive backing, are generally designed to be left in place for several days to a week, depending on the quantity of exudate expressed by the wound. The dressings vary in permeability, thickness, and transparency and are designed to absorb exudate by swelling into a gel-like mass. The dressing, which can vary from being occlusive to semipermeable, anchors to intact skin surrounding the wound rather than to the actual wound itself.

Indications for this type of dressing include partial- and full-thickness wounds. The dressings can also be used effectively with granular or necrotic wounds.

Advantages of hydrocolloids include:

- Provide a moist environment with a waterproof surface that offers protection from microbial contamination
- Enable autolytic debridement, while providing moderate absorption
- Do not require a secondary dressing

Disadvantages include:

- May traumatize surrounding intact skin upon removal and tend to roll in areas of excessive friction
- Cannot be used on infected wounds

Fiber Dressings

Fiber dressings are composed of carboxymethylcellulose and draw fluid directly into the cellulose fibers. The gelling action is both immediate and nonreversible and the fluid remains in a gel state, which minimizes chances of periwound maceration.[69] Fiber dressings are excellent for highly exudative wounds such as venous insufficiency ulcers.[69]

Foam Dressings

These dressings are composed from a hydrophilic (highly absorbent) polyurethane base. The dressings are hydrophilic at the wound contact surface, but hydrophobic on the outer surface. The dressings, which come in sheets or pads with varying degrees of thickness, allow exudate to be absorbed into the foam through the hydrophilic layer.

Indications for this type of dressing include partial- and full-thickness wounds with varying levels of exudate. They can also be used as secondary dressings over amorphous hydrogels.

Advantages of foam dressings include:

- Provide a moist environment for wound healing
- Provide prophylactic protection and cushioning
- Encourage autolytic debridement, while providing moderate absorption

Disadvantages include:

- Lack of transparency, which makes inspection of wound difficult
- Tendency to roll in areas of excessive friction

Hydrogels

These dressings consist of variable amounts of water and variable amounts of gel-forming materials. Indications for this type of dressing include superficial and partial thickness wounds (e.g., abrasions, pressure ulcers) that have minimal drainage, and wounds that are prone to desiccation and in dry climates where dehydration is more of a problem. Hydrogel dressings also help to soften hard eschar and promote autolytic or mechanical debridement. Rather than absorb drainage, hydrogels are moisture retentive.

Advantages of hydrogels include:

- Provide a moist environment for wound healing
- Enable autolytic debridement

Disadvantages include:

- Dressings may dehydrate
- Cannot be used on wounds with significant drainage

Semipermeable Film

These dressings are thin membranes made from transparent polyurethane coated with water-resistant adhesives that are permeable to vapor and oxygen, but are generally impermeable to large molecule bacteria. They are highly elastic, and allow easy visual inspection of the wound since they are transparent.

Indications for this type of dressing include superficial wounds (scalds, abrasions) or partial-thickness wounds with minimal drainage.

Advantages of semipermeable film include:

- It provides a moist environment for wound healing, while allowing autolytic debridement.
- It allows visualization of the wound.
- It is resistant to shearing and frictional forces.

Disadvantages include:

- Excessive accumulation of exudate can result in periwound maceration.
- It cannot be used on infected wounds.

Gauze

Gauze dressings are manufactured from yarn or thread and are the most readily available dressings used in an inpatient environment. Impregnated gauze involves the addition of various materials such as antimicrobials.

Indications for this type of dressing include infected or noninfected wounds of any size. The dressings can be used for wet-to-wet, wet-to-moist, or wet-to-dry debridement.

Advantages of gauze include:

- It can be used alone or in combination with other dressings or topical agents.
- The number of layers can be modified to accommodate for changing wound status.

Disadvantages include:

- Frequent dressing changes are required.
- Gauze carries an increased infection rate compared with occlusive dressings.

Alginates

Alginate dressings consist of calcium salt of alganic acid, which is extracted from brown algae and kelp. Allogeneic dressings are based on the interaction of calcium ions in the dressing and the sodium ions in the wound exudate. The interaction with the wound exudate creates a gel-like substance that aids in moist wound healing. Because alginate dressings provide an excellent avenue for exudate absorption, they require a secondary dressing.

Indications for the dressings include partial- and full-thickness draining wounds, such as pressure wounds or venous insufficiency ulcers, and on infected wounds due to the likelihood of excessive drainage.

Advantages of alginates include:

- They have a high absorptive capacity.
- They enable autolytic debridement.
- They can be used on infected or uninfected wounds.

Disadvantages include:

- They may require frequent dressing changes based on level of exudates.

Other categories of dressings have evolved to deal with the unique characteristics of the complicated/infected acute wound and the biochemical changes inherent in the chronic wound.

Silver Dressings

Silver dressings have evolved due to the increasing prevalence of antibiotic-resistant organisms and the fact that lower concentrations of silver are required for microbial control. Occlusive to semiocclusive technologies and absorptive materials can be combined with silver to provide a dressing with multiple functions. Silver dressings may be broadly categorized according to silver levels. *High-content silver dressings* may provide enhanced microbial control, but they appear to inhibit epithelialization. *Lower-content silver dressings* may not provide the same level of microbial control but do not inhibit epithelialization. All silver dressings or preparations release ionic silver that is thought to interfere with microbial respiratory enzymes, protein synthesis, and DNA replication.

Cadexomer Iodine Dressings

Cadexomer iodine dressings provide a slow, timed release of active iodine to the wound bed as wound fluid is absorbed by the iodine–polymer complex. Sustained release of iodine from this polymer optimizes its antimicrobial effects while preventing the accumulation of active iodine in tissues at levels toxic to wound-bed cells. Toxicity studies have not demonstrated any local or systemic adverse effects.

Polyhexamethylene Biguanide

Polyhexamethylene biguanide (PHMB) has bidirectional fluid-handling properties (can absorb or hydrate the wound bed) and uses 0.3% PHMB as the antimicrobial constituent. PHMB is a broad-spectrum antimicrobial dressing that donates fluid to dry areas of the wound, as well as absorbs fluid from overly hydrated areas.

Wound–Matrix Dressings

These dressings enhance the function of the extracellular tissue matrix and the cells that reside there. Collagen-based dressings in powder, dried matrices, alginate, hydrogel, and hydrocolloid formulations have evolved to provide support for fibroblast migration and function and growth-factor binding. These collagen-based dressings act as temporary scaffolding for cells and are reabsorbed or removed as the wound heals.

Negative Pressure Wound Therapy

Negative pressure wound therapy (NPWT) is a topical treatment used as an adjunct to wound healing to facilitate wound closure in acute surgical wounds as well as with more challenging, slow-to-heal wounds. It involves the application of negative pressure to the wound bed. NPWT consists of a wound dressing (changed every 12 hours for infected wounds; 48 hours or longer for clean wounds), a drainage tube inserted into the dressing, occlusive transparent film, and a connection to a vacuum source, which supplies the negative pressure. NPWT has been shown to reduce edema in a wound bed, decrease bacterial colonization, stimulate angiogenesis, and draw wound edges together.[70–74]

Debridement

> ● **Key Point** Wound debridement can be accomplished in a number of ways:
> - *Mechanically:* Whirlpool, pulsatile lavage, other forms of spray irrigation, and the traditional wet-to-dry dressing.
> - *Surgically:* Performed by a physician with the patient anesthetized. Sharp debridement removes necrotic tissue by means of a scalpel or other sharp instrument with the patient alert.
> - *Chemically:* The use of enzymes or other topical agents, such as Dakin's solution (diluted bleach).
> - *Autolytically:* The body does its own cleaning. This type of debridement is the least traumatic to healthy tissue but may take longer than enzymes or more invasive forms of debridement.

Selective Debridement

Selective debridement involves removing only nonviable (necrotic or infected) tissues from the wound, as these can interfere with wound healing. The goals of wound debridement include:

- Allow for the examination of the ulcer and determination of the extent of wound
- Decrease bacterial concentration in wound; improve wound healing
- Decrease spreading infection—i.e., cellulitis or sepsis

Selective debridement is most often performed by:

- *Sharp debridement:* Requires the use of the scalpel, scissors, and forceps to selectively remove devitalized tissues, foreign materials, or debris.
- *Enzymatic debridement:* Refers to the topical application of enzymes to the surface of necrotic tissue. Enzymatic debridement can be used on infected and uninfected wounds with necrotic tissue.
- *Autolytic debridement:* Refers to the removal of nonviable tissue using the body's own mechanisms combined with semipermeable films, hydrocolloids, hydrogels, and alginates.

Nonselective Debridement

Nonselective, or mechanical, debridement involves removing both viable and nonviable tissues from the wound using wet-to-dry dressings, wound irrigation, and hydrotherapy.

Factors Influencing Wound Healing

A number of factors can contribute to the rate and degree of wound healing:

- *Age:* A decreased metabolism in older adults tends to decrease the overall rate of wound healing.
- *Illness:* Compromised medical status such as cardiovascular disease may significantly delay healing. This often results secondary to diminished oxygen and nutrients at the cellular level.
- *Infection:* An infected wound will impact essential activity associated with wound healing, including fibroblast activity, collagen synthesis, and phagocytosis.
- *Lifestyle:* Regular physical activity results in increased circulation that enhances wound healing. Lifestyle choices such as smoking negatively impact wound healing by limiting the blood's oxygen-carrying capability.
- *Medication:* There are a variety of pharmacological agents that can negatively impact wound healing. Medications falling into this category include steroids, anti-inflammatory drugs, heparin, antineoplastic agents, and oral contraceptives. Undesirable physiological effects include delayed collagen synthesis, reduced blood supply, and decreased tensile strength of connective tissues.

Scar Management

General intervention guidelines for scar management include:

- Massage of the area using cream twice per day (once the wound is completely healed)
- Use of sun block and vitamin E cream on the scar
- Use of silicone gel (softens scar)
- Pressure garments
- Ultrasound and/or electrical stimulation treatment

Therapeutic Exercise

Therapeutic exercise for scar management should include:

- Strengthening and range of motion exercises
- Aerobic conditioning
- Body mechanics, postural awareness training
- Gait, locomotion, and balance training
- Aquatic therapy

Functional Training

Functional training for scar management should cover:

- Activity of daily living training (basic and instrumental)
- Activity pacing and energy conservation; stress management
- Skin and joint protection techniques
- Instruction in safe use of assistive and adaptive devices
- Prescription, application, and training in use of orthotic, protective, or supportive devices

Manual Lymphatic Drainage

Manual lymphatic drainage (MLD) involves light, rhythmical massage that aids the body in collecting and moving lymphatic fluid. Theoretically, MLD plays a key role in delivering nutrients, antibodies, and other immune constituents to the tissue cells of the body and removing debris such as toxins, cell waste, and dead particles, which are then cleansed by clusters of lymph nodes. Once instructed in the techniques, the patient can perform a simplified version of MLD at home, called *simple lymphatic drainage* (SLD).

Electrotherapeutic Modalities

The following therapeutic modalities will help with lymphatic drainage:

- *Electrical muscle stimulation:* Involves a high-volt pulsed current.[69] Numerous controlled studies have demonstrated the benefits of high-volt galvanic stimulation in augmenting wound healing, particularly in the management of pressure sores. The standard treatment is 45 minutes to 1 hour in length, and the stimulus is delivered at a frequency of 100 pulses per second at a submotor motor intensity (enough to produce a tingling paresthesia). Polarity of the active electrode plays an important role. The positive electrode (anode) should be placed over the wound when debridement or epithelialization is the objective.[69] The negative pole (cathode) is used to stimulate production of granulation tissue or to promote antimicrobial or anti-inflammatory effects.[69] Typically the wound is filled loosely with saline-moistened gauze, and an aluminum foil electrode (smaller than the moistened gauze so that no portion of the foil comes in contact with intact skin), connected to an alligator clip lead wire, is used for conductivity.

- *Transcutaneous electrical nerve stimulation (TENS):* An electric current device with settings that can provide pain relief (see Chapter 13).
- *Cold laser:* Also referred to as low-level cold laser, lower-level infrared laser, or monochromatic infrared photo energy. This therapy, which uses light in the infrared spectrum, has been promoted for augmenting wound healing[75] and reversing the symptoms of peripheral neuropathy in individuals with diabetes.[76–78]

Physical Agents and Modalities

The following physical agents and modalities are used to treat pressure ulcers:

- *Sound agents:* Ultrasound, phonophoresis.
- *Hydrotherapy:* Aquatic therapy, Whirlpool tanks.
  - Indicated for ulcers with large amounts of exudate, slough, and necrotic tissue.
  - Increases circulation; assists in debridement of wounds or removal of dressings. Attention must be directed to the intensity, duration, and temperature of the treatment. Turbine power should be reduced to the lowest setting to avoid wound trauma.
  - Various whirlpool additives have been used over the years in wound care; however, no substantial body of research supports their use.[69]
  - With conditions such as venous insufficiency, which are complicated by limb dependency and warm water, whirlpool treatment should be used with caution, keeping water temperatures at nonthermal levels (<100°F).[69]
  - Whirlpool should be discontinued when ulcer is clean.
- *Light agents:* Ultraviolet.
- *Mechanical modalities:* Compression therapies.

Nonphysical Therapy Interventions

Surgery

Surgery is indicated for excising ulcers, enhancing vascularity and resurfacing wound (grafts), and preventing sepsis and osteomyelitis. It may be indicated for stages III and IV ulcers.

Hyperbaric Oxygen Therapy

In hyperbaric oxygen therapy (HBO),[79–82] the patient breathes 100% oxygen in a sealed, full-bodied chamber with elevated atmospheric pressure (between 2.0 and 2.5 atm absolute, ATA). Hyper-oxygenation reverses tissue hypoxia and facilitates wound healing due to enhanced solubility of oxygen in the blood. It is contraindicated in untreated pneumothorax and some antineoplastic medications (e.g., doxorubicin, disulfiram, cisplatin, mafenide acetate).

Burns

Burn injuries are classified by the depth of skin tissue involved. The amount of skin destruction is based on temperature and length of time the tissue is exposed to heat.

Superficial Burn

This type of burn, also referred to as an epidermal burn, causes cell damage only to the epidermis. Characteristics include:

- Tissue is red, erythematous, and often painful.
- Tissue blanches with pressure.
- Tissue damage is minimal and healing is spontaneous.

Sunburn is a classic example of this type of burn. This depth of burn correlates to Practice Pattern 7B, Impaired Integumentary Integrity Associated with Superficial Skin Involvement, in the *Guide to Physical Therapist Practice*.[83]

Superficial Partial-Thickness Burn

This type of burn involves damage through the epidermis and into the papillary layer of the dermis. It has the following characteristics:

- Adnexal structures (e.g., sweat glands, hair follicles) are often involved, but enough of these structures are preserved for function that the epithelium lining them can proliferate and allow for regrowth of skin.
- The burned area characteristically has blisters over it and is very painful.
- If this type of burn is not cared for properly, edema, which accompanies the injury, and decreased blood flow in the tissue can result in conversion to full-thickness burn.
- This depth of burn correlates to Practice Pattern 7C, Impaired Integumentary Integrity Associated with Partial Thickness Skin Involvement and Scar Formation, in the *Guide to Physical Therapist Practice*.[83]

Deep Partial-Thickness Burn

This type of burn involves destruction of the epidermis with damage of the dermis down into the reticular layer. Characteristics include:[1]

- A mixed red or waxy white color (the deeper the injury, the more white it will appear) in appearance.
- Wet surface from broken blisters and alteration of the dermal vascular network, which leaks plasma fluid.
- Marked edema.
- Diminished sensation to light touch or soft pinprick, but retained sense of deep pressure.
- Healing occurs through scar formation and re-epithelialization. However, if left to heal spontaneously, it will result in a thin epithelium that may lack the usual number of sebaceous glands to keep the skin lubricated.
- This depth of burn best matches Practice Pattern 7C, Impaired Integumentary Integrity Associated with Partial Thickness Skin Involvement and Scar Formation, in the *Guide to Physical Therapist Practice*.[83]
- May be associated with the development of hypertrophic and keloid scars.

Full-Thickness Burn

With this type of burn, all the epidermal and dermal layers are completely destroyed. In addition the subcutaneous fat layer may be damaged to some extent. Full-thickness burns have the following characteristics:

- Skin is charred or a translucent white color, with coagulated vessels visible below. Full-thickness burns are often associated with extensive scarring (*eschar*) because epithelial cells from the skin appendages are not present to repopulate the area.
- The area is insensate (without feeling), but patients complain of pain, which is usually a result of surrounding partial-thickness burns.
- As all of the skin tissue and structures are destroyed, there are no sites available for epithelialization of the wound, and skin grafting of tissue over the wound will be necessary.

The following types of grafts can be used:

- *Autogenous, or autograft*: Skin transplanted from one location to another on the same individual. If the entire thickness of the dermis is included, the appropriate term is *full-thickness skin graft*. If less than the entire thickness of the dermis is included, appropriate terms are *partial* or *split-thickness skin graft*. An appropriate donor site is selected, typically the anterior, lateral, or medial part of the thigh; the buttock; or the medial aspect of the arm. For larger defects, a large, flat donor surface is ideal.
- *Xenograft, or heterograft*: Skin taken from a variety of animals, usually a pig. Heterograft skin became popular because of the limited availability and high expense of human skin tissue. In some cases religious, financial, or cultural objections to the use of human cadaver skin may also be factors. Wound coverage using xenograft or heterograft is a temporary covering used until autograft.
- *Allograft*: Cadaver skin, or homograft, is human cadaver skin donated for medical use. Cadaver skin is used as a temporary covering for excised (cleaned) wound surfaces before autograft (permanent) placement. Unmeshed cadaver skin is put over the excised wound and stapled in place. Postoperatively, the cadaver skin may be covered with a dressing. Wound coverage using cadaveric allograft is removed prior to permanent autografting.

This depth of burn is consistent with Practice Pattern 7D, Impaired Integumentary Integrity Associated with Full-Thickness Skin Involvement and Scar Formation, in the *Guide to Physical Therapist Practice*.[83]

Subdermal Burn

This type of burn involves complete destruction of all tissue from the epidermis down to and through the subcutaneous tissue. This depth of injury correlates with Practice Pattern 7E, Impaired Integumentary Integrity Associated with Skin Involvement Extending into the Fascia, Muscle, or Bone and Scar Formation, in the *Guide to Physical Therapist Practice*.[83]

Electrical Burn

Electrical burns result from the passage of an electric current through the body after the skin has made contact with an electrical source.

> ● **Key Point** Electric current follows the course of least resistance offered by various tissue: the nerves, followed by blood vessels, offer the least resistance while the bone offers the most resistance.

Complications associated with electrical burns include cardiac arrhythmias, ventricular fibrillation, renal failure, spinal cord damage, and respiratory arrest.[1]

Burn Extent

The more body surface area (BSA) involved in a burn, the greater the morbidity and mortality rates and the difficulty in management. An individual's palmar surface represents 1% of the BSA. A simple method to estimate burn extent is to use the patient's palmar surface to measure the burned area. Burn extent is calculated only on individuals with second-degree or third-degree burns. Classification by a percentage of body area burned:

- *Critical:* 10% of body with third-degree burns and 30% or more with second-degree burns, along with complications, e.g., respiratory involvement and smoke inhalation.
- *Moderate:* Less than 10% of body with third-degree burns and 15% to 30% with second-degree burns.
- *Minor:* Less than 2% with third-degree burns and 15% with second-degree burns.

Another quick method is to use the Rule of Nines to estimate the extent of burn injury (**Table 8-5**). The Lund–Browder charts are designed specifically for use with children in order to estimate body areas.

● **Key Point** Burns cause an increased metabolic rate and energy metabolism. How the individual responds to the increased energy demands will dictate recovery.

Complications of Burn Injury

Integument trauma often affects the function of the cardiovascular, pulmonary, renal, metabolic, muscular, nervous, and skeletal systems.

TABLE 8-5	Rule of Nines	
Body Area	**Adults (%)**	**Children (%)**
Head—Anterior	4.5	18
Head—Posterior	4.5	
Arm—Anterior	4.5	9
Arm—Posterior	4.5	
Leg—Anterior	9	14
Leg—Posterior	9	
Chest	18	18
Back	18	18
Genitals	1	1

Pain

Superficial skin damage generally results in more pain than deeper injuries because the free endings are not destroyed in the former. However, as the nerve endings regenerate following a full-thickness burn and eschar is removed, intense pain may result. Pain is the major deterrent in preventing burn patients from participating in exercises and positioning following a burn injury.

Infection

In addition to the tissue damage, infection is a major source of mortality and the most significant cause of loss of function and cosmetic appearance. A number of factors play a role:

- Vasoconstriction leading to peripheral hypoperfusion, particularly in the burned areas, creates a major defect in local host defense, enhancing bacterial invasion.
- Dead tissue, warmth, peripheral hypoperfusion, and moisture are ideal for bacterial growth.
- Streptococci and staphylococci usually predominate shortly after a burn, and gram-negative bacteria after 5 to 7 days; mixed flora are always present.

Infection can be reduced or controlled with the following:

- Culturing of wounds and appropriate antibiotic treatment regimen prescribed
- Application of topical antimicrobial agents— for example, silver nitrate, silver sulfadiazine, erythromycin, gentamycin, neomycin, and triple antibiotic
- Use of physician-prescribed anti-inflammatory agents—for example, corticosteroids, hydrocortisone, ibuprofen, and indomethacin
- Standard and transmission-based precautions
- Hand washing by healthcare practitioners
- Sterile technique
- Vacuum assisted closure (VAC)

Cardiac Complications

These include cardiac arrhythmias caused by hypovolemia, hypoxia, acidosis, or hyperkalemia.

Pulmonary Complications

An individual who has been burned in a closed space should be suspected of having an inhalation injury. Signs of an inhalation injury include facial burns, singed nasal hairs, harsh cough, hoarseness, abnormal breath sounds, respiratory distress, and carbonaceous sputum and/or hypoxemia.[1,84] The primary complications associated with this injury are carbon monoxide poisoning, tracheal damage, upper airway obstruction, pulmonary edema, and pneumonia.[1] Thermal damage to the lower respiratory tract can be caused by steam inhalation or by inhalation of hot gases, which produces immediate upper airway obstruction.

- Airway edema can produce upper airway obstruction that develops more slowly.
- Chemical injury to small airway alveolar capillaries can cause delayed progressive respiratory failure.
- Inhaling toxic products (e.g., cyanide, carbon monoxide) generated by burning material (e.g., wood, plastics) may result in thermal injuries to the pharynx and upper airway as well as in ventilation injuries.

● **Key Point** Inhaled carbon monoxide binds to hemoglobin, greatly reducing O_2 transport.

Hypokalemia

Hypokalemia is common during the early resuscitation period because potassium is not generally included in early fluid replacement, because potassium stores in patients taking diuretics may be depleted, and because some potassium is leached into hypotonic 0.5% silver nitrate dressings. Silver nitrate also leaches sodium and chloride into the dressing, sometimes resulting in severe hyponatremia, hypochloremia, and hypochloremic alkalosis.

Hypoalbuminemia

Hypoalbuminemia results from the combination of dilutional effects of sodium-containing replacement fluids and loss of protein into the subeschar edema fluid. Hypocalcemia may result from hypoalbuminemia because most serum calcium is reversibly bound to albumin.

Metabolic Complications

Because thermal injury results in more loss of body mass than any other disease, continued demands are placed on the metabolic system for the significant healing process. Metabolic acidosis may result from poor tissue perfusion due to hypovolemia (monitored through urine output) or to heart failure. The clinician must consider the catabolic state of the patient when designing exercise programs so that the metabolic stress is not increased.

Peripheral Vasoconstriction

Peripheral vasoconstriction causing local hypoperfusion is due to inadequate fluid replacement during resuscitation. Poor focal tissue perfusion can result from a constricting eschar or fascia.

Myoglobinuria

Myoglobinuria, the release of myoglobin into the urine, can result from ischemic constrictions of muscle, crush injuries, or deep thermal or electrical burns of muscle. Initially, osmotic diuresis is needed until the myoglobinuria clears. Without prompt, accurate management, myoglobinuria may result in renal tubular necrosis. Hemoglobinuria may result from erythrocyte destruction after burns.

Hypothermia

Hypothermia, a condition in which the core temperature of the body is too low to maintain normal metabolism, is common in severely burned patients. It can result in fatal arrhythmias if they are rewarmed too quickly.

Heterotopic Ossification

It is unknown why heterotopic ossification, the abnormal formation of bone, occurs in patients with burn injuries. Suspected etiologies include immobilization, microtrauma, high protein intake, and sepsis.[1]

Hypertrophic Scarring and Wound Contracture

Contractures are especially likely to develop if wounds are not closed promptly. If a body part is left immobile for a protracted period of time, capsular contraction and shortening of tendon and muscle groups (which cross the joints) occur. This rapid process can be prevented by a program of passive ROM, anti-deformity positioning, and splinting. The general rule for splinting is to position the affected joint in the opposite direction from which it will contract.

● **Key Point** Types of scars include:
- *Hypertrophic scar:* A raised scar that stays within the boundaries of the burn wound; characteristically red, raised, firm.
- *Keloid scar:* A raised scar that extends beyond the boundaries of the original burn wound; red, raised, firm.

Hypertrophic scarring is also common in burn patients. Techniques to minimize hypertrophic scarring are discussed below.

Burn Healing and Management

Management of burn injuries may be divided into four general phases, the first three of which (initial evaluation and resuscitation, initial wound excision and biologic closure, and definitive wound closure, including grafting) do not involve physical therapy.[85-97] The fourth phase (rehabilitation, reconstruction, and reintegration) typically involves physical therapy.

The development of specific anticipated goals and expected outcomes is based on the following general goals from the *Guide to Physical Therapist Practice*. They include:

- Enhancement of wound and soft tissue healing
- A reduction in the risk of infection and complications
- A reduction in the risk of secondary impairments
- Achievement of maximal range of motion
- Restoration of preinjury level of cardiovascular endurance
- Achievement of good to normal strength
- Achievement of independent ambulation
- Increased independent function in BADL and IADL
- Minimization of scar formation
- Increased patient, family, and caregiver understanding of expectations and goals and outcomes
- Increased aerobic capacity
- Improved self-management of symptoms

The principal components of burn therapy include the following:

- Passive ROM and gentle stretching. Passive ROM is best performed twice daily, with the clinician taking all joints through a full ROM. The clinician must be sensitive to the patient's pain, anxiety, wound status, extremity perfusion, and security of the patient's airway and vascular access devices. These procedures should be performed in coordination with the intensive care unit (ICU) staff. Attention to the security of endotracheal tubes, nasogastric tubes, and arterial and central venous catheters is paramount, as unexpected loss of these devices can contribute to morbidity and mortality. Techniques that can be used to increase the patient's tolerance for passive ROM include the following:
  - ❑ Timing of the ROM session with medication, wound cleansing, or dressing changes
  - ❑ Administration of opiates or benzodiazepines
  - ❑ Gentle conversation, encouragement, and an unhurried approach to therapy sessions

- Increasing active ROM and progressing to strengthening with resistive exercises. Resisted ROM, isometric exercises, active strengthening, and gait training are important objectives.
- Minimizing dependent edema formation and promoting venous return. Burned and grafted extremities commonly have lingering edema that can contribute to joint stiffness. Reducing this edema facilitates rehabilitation efforts.
- Consideration of pressure garments. The use of custom-fitted elastic garments early after injury is expensive, as they frequently need to be downsized as the edema resolves; however, simply wrapping the fingers with self-adherent elastic helps reduce digital edema. Tubular elastic dressings, elastic wrap dressings, elevation, and retrograde massage also help reduce extremity edema.
- ADL training. As definitive wound closure nears and hospital discharge approaches, the focus of rehabilitation efforts becomes practical. Performance of ADL tasks and the impending return to play/school/work are important considerations.
- Initial scar management. Topical silicone may have a favorable influence on selected evolving hypertrophic scars.
- Proprioceptive and sensation training.
- Positioning and splinting. Proper antideformity positioning minimizes shortening of tendons, collateral ligaments, and joint capsules; it reduces extremity and facial edema.

> **● Key Point** All splints should be inspected at least twice daily for evidence of poor fit or pressure injury; improperly used splints can cause injury. A nursing staff in-service training session minimizes splint-related skin injury.

Although splints are used less frequently, there are several predictable contractures that occur in patients with burns that can be prevented by a proper ROM, positioning, and splinting program. These contractures generally are associated with the flexed position of comfort, except in the hands.

> **● Key Point** The most important therapeutic maneuver is elevation of the extremity, especially for patients with a leg or hand burn. Positioning affected extremities just above the level of the heart reduces edema, which is another important aspect of antideformity positioning. The extremity should be placed above heart level at all times except for periods of 20 minutes or less during the day. Because bed rest with elevation is difficult for an outpatient, hospitalization is often required when the legs are burned.

Upper-Extremity Burn Wound Care

Flexion deformities of the neck can be minimized with thermoplastic neck splints, conformers, and split mattresses. In critically ill patients, positioning the neck in slight extension is often all that can be done. The clinician should ensure that the ventilator tubing does not pull the head so that a contracture develops; without proper care, a rotary contracture can develop, generally with the patient turned toward the ventilator.

An axillary contracture can interfere with important upper extremity functions. Axillary adduction contractures can be prevented by positioning the shoulders widely abducted (to approximately 90 degrees) and externally rotated with axillary splints, padded hanging troughs of thermoplastic material, or a variety of support devices mounted to the bed.

Elbow contractures, which restrict extension, are a common volar soft tissue complication. Elbow flexion contractures are minimized by statically splinting the elbow in extension and forearm supination using a gutter splint, conforming splint, or a palmar or dorsal extension splint. Elbow splints can be alternated with flexion splints to help retain full ROM.

Perhaps the most common upper-extremity deformities are dorsal hand and web space contractures:

- Dorsal hand contractures are prevented ideally by attention to proper positioning presurgically and postsurgically using wrist splints, thumb spica, and palmar or dorsal extension splints.
- In the normal web space, the leading edge of the volar aspect of the web is distal to the dorsal aspect, whereas in the typical dorsal web space contracture, this pattern is reversed (the syndactyly is usually a dorsal deformity). Web space contractures can be minimized by proper early surgery and compressive gloves supplemented with web space conformers.

Lower-Extremity Burn Wound Care

Patients who have been supine for extended periods often tolerate immediate upright positioning poorly. Prior to initial efforts at assisted standing, such patients benefit from tilt table training and graduated sitting. Using gentle elastic wraps prior to placing the patient in an upright position helps to prevent lower-extremity edema, which can hinder recovery.

Prevention of contractures is important even in infants, as these contractures can interfere with subsequent ambulation and should be addressed early in recovery. The lower extremities should align in neutral hip extension, 20 degrees of hip abduction, full extension of the knee, and ankle dorsiflexion. Knee immobilizers can minimize knee flexion contractures. The equinus deformity, in which the ankle is plantar flexed and the foot is in a varus position, is a serious problem that can occur even if the ankles are not burned. This position can be prevented, however, with static splinting of the ankles in the neutral position and performing ROM exercises twice daily. Splints designed for this purpose can cause pressure injury over the metatarsal heads or calcaneus if improperly designed. These injuries can be prevented by using padding to distribute pressure evenly across the metatarsal heads and by extending the footplate of the splint beyond the heel and cutting out the area around the calcaneus. A deep dorsal foot burn may result in a contracture of the metatarsophalangeal joints, so that the toes are brought off the ground, causing the patient to have an abnormal gait.

Scar Management

Hypertrophic scarring is a difficult problem for burn patients, and scar management is an essential aspect of burn therapy. Scars can form in an organized manner termed *normatrophic* scarring, or in a disorganized manner such as that seen with hypertrophic or keloid scars.

General intervention guidelines for scar management include:

- Massage of the area using cream twice per day (once the wound is completely healed)
- Use of sunblock and vitamin E cream on the scar
- Use of silicone gel (softens scar)
- Pressure garments
- Ultrasound treatment or electrical stimulation treatment may be considered

1. True or false: The integument or skin is the largest organ system of the body
2. Give five key functions of the skin.
3. Of the five layers of the epidermis, which layer contains melanocytes?
4. Of the five layers of the epidermis, which layer provides the skin its waterproof characteristic and serves the role of protection from infection?
5. Which of the two layers, the epidermis or dermis, contains sebaceous and sweat glands?
6. The body's first line of defense against infection is/are:
   a. Increased capillary permeability to protein
   b. Localized circulatory responses such as vasodilation
   c. The skin and mucous membranes
   d. Phagocytosis
7. What characteristics of the skin can be assessed using palpation?
8. What is the name of the skin or mucous membrane lesion that is flat, circumscribed, and greater than 1 centimeter in its longest diameter?
9. An elevated lesion of skin or mucous membrane that is solid and greater than 1 centimeter in diameter is called what?
10. An elevated lesion that is fluid filled and greater than 1 centimeter in diameter and is located on skin or mucous membrane is called what?
11. What is the function of granulation tissue in wound healing?
12. What is a keloid?
13. You are attending an in-service training on the foot and ankle, and they speaker uses the term *tinea pedis* to describe a common foot condition. What is the common name used for this condition?
14. What common dermatosis appears as a chronic, bilaterally symmetric, erythematous plaquelike lesion with a silvery scale covering?
15. Which areas of the body of the most prone to decubiti?
16. A patient presents with a history of joint disturbances of arthritis and arthralgias that have been symmetrical and migratory. There is a butterfly rash over the nose and molar area. Which condition would you suspect?
    a. Dermatomyositis
    b. Progressive systemic scleroderma
    c. Ankylosing spondylitis
    d. Systemic lupus erythematosus
17. True or false: Seborrheic keratosis is a malignant tumor of the skin.
18. Which form of skin cancer is associated with patients with HIV?
19. What does the pneumonic ABCDE mean when interpreting skin lesions for their potential for cancer?
20. The most painful classification of burns is:
    a. First degree
    b. Second degree
    c. Third degree
    d. Full thickness
21. What are five major complications associated with electrical burns?
22. Which of the following areas produces hormones and the specialized T lymphocytes?
    a. Tonsils
    b. Lymph nodes
    c. Spleen
    d. Thymus
23. All of the following are not considered manifestations of systemic inflammation except:
    a. Vomiting
    b. Myalgia
    c. Anorexia
    d. Fever
24. The classic signs of inflammation include all of the following except:
    a. Increased temperature
    b. Increased redness
    c. Increased swelling
    d. Pallor
25. Characteristics of basal cell carcinoma include:
    a. A sun-induced malignancy
    b. Accounts for over 50% of all skin cancers
    c. Easily treated if detected early
    d. All of the above
26. You are observing a wound on an area that involves full thickness of the dermis and undermining of the deeper tissues, slight involvement of the muscle, but no bone destruction. Given this information, which of the following stages would best describe this ulcer?
27. What types of hip and knee contractures are particularly common in infants and very young children who have suffered a burn to these areas?
28. What type of wound dressing has the ability to transmit moisture, vapor, or gases from the wound bed to the atmosphere?
29. Alginates, semipermeable foam, hydrocolloids, hydrogels, and semipermeable films are all forms of which type of dressing?

30. What is negative-pressure wound therapy?

31. What are the three most common types of selective debridement?

32. What are the three most common types of non-selective debridement?

References

1. Richard RL, Ward RS: Burns, in O'Sullivan SB, Schmitz TJ (eds): Physical Rehabilitation (ed 5). Philadelphia, F. A. Davis, 2007, pp 1091–1115

2. Eckes B, Hunzelmann N, Moinzadeh P, et al: Scleroderma - news to tell. Arch Dermatol Res, 2007

3. Kreuter A, Altmeyer P, Gambichler T: Treatment of localized scleroderma depends on the clinical subtype. Br J Dermatol 156:1363–1365, 2007

4. Chizzolini C: Update on pathophysiology of scleroderma with special reference to immunoinflammatory events. Ann Med 39:42–53, 2007

5. Zivkovic SA, Medsger TA Jr: Myasthenia gravis and scleroderma: Two cases and a review of the literature. Clin Neurol Neurosurg 109:388–391, 2007

6. Verrecchia F, Laboureau J, Verola O, et al: Skin involvement in scleroderma: Where histological and clinical scores meet. Rheumatology (Oxford) 46:833–841, 2007

7. Ashida R, Ihn H, Mimura Y, et al: Clinical features of scleroderma patients with contracture of phalanges. Clin Rheumatol 26:1275–1277, 2007

8. Karnen FP, Kongko HR, Kasjmir YI: Scleroderma in a young man. Acta Med Indones 38:213–216, 2006

9. Jablonska S, Blaszczyk M: New treatments in scleroderma: dermatologic perspective. J Eur Acad Dermatol Venereol 16:433–435, 2002

10. Chen YJ, Wu CY, Shen JL: Predicting factors of interstitial lung disease in dermatomyositis and polymyositis. Acta Derm Venereol 87:33–38, 2007

11. Yoshidome Y, Morimoto S, Tamura N, et al: A case of polymyositis complicated with myasthenic crisis. Clin Rheumatol 26:1569–1570, 2007

12. Pongratz D: Therapeutic options in autoimmune inflammatory myopathies (dermatomyositis, polymyositis, inclusion body myositis). J Neurol 253:v64–v65, 2006

13. Ytterberg SR: Treatment of refractory polymyositis and dermatomyositis. Curr Rheumatol Rep 8:167–173, 2006

14. Zampieri S, Ghirardello A, Iaccarino L, et al: Polymyositis-dermatomyositis and infections. Autoimmunity 39:191–196, 2006

15. Bronner IM, Linssen WH, van der Meulen MF, et al: Polymyositis: An ongoing discussion about a disease entity. Arch Neurol 61:132–135, 2004

16. Ullrich SE: Sunlight and skin cancer: Lessons from the immune system. Mol Carcinog 46:629–633, 2007

17. Ansems TM, van der Pols JC, Hughes MC, et al: Alcohol intake and risk of skin cancer: A prospective study. Eur J Clin Nutr 62:162–170, 2008

18. Rhee JS, Matthews BA, Neuburg M, et al: The skin cancer index: Clinical responsiveness and predictors of quality of life. Laryngoscope 117:399–405, 2007

19. Telfer NR: Skin cancer: Prevalence, prevention and treatment. Clin Med 6:622; author reply 623, 2006

20. Gloster HM Jr, Neal K: Skin cancer in skin of color. J Am Acad Dermatol 55:741–760; quiz 761–764, 2006

21. Honda KS: HIV and skin cancer. Dermatol Clin 24:521–30, vii, 2006

22. Information from your family doctor: Checking yourself for signs of skin cancer. Am Fam Physician 74:819–820, 2006

23. Information from your family doctor. Melanoma: A type of skin cancer. Am Fam Physician 74:813–814, 2006

24. Dixon A: Skin cancer in patients with multiple health problems. Aust Fam Physician 35:717–718, 2006

25. Sharpe G: Skin cancer: prevalence, prevention and treatment. Clin Med 6:333–334, 2006

26. Thomas DR: Prevention and management of pressure ulcers. Mo Med 104:52–57, 2007

27. Evans J, Stephen-Haynes J: Identification of superficial pressure ulcers. J Wound Care 16:54–56, 2007

28. McNees P, Meneses KD: Pressure ulcers and other chronic wounds in patients with and patients without cancer: A retrospective, comparative analysis of healing patterns. Ostomy Wound Manage 53:70–78, 2007

29. Stewart TP, Magnano SJ: Burns or pressure ulcers in the surgical patient? Adv Skin Wound Care 20:74, 77–78, 80 passim, 2007

30. Spilsbury K, Nelson A, Cullum N, et al: Pressure ulcers and their treatment and effects on quality of life: hospital inpatient perspectives. J Adv Nurs 57:494–504, 2007

31. Whitney J, Phillips L, Aslam R, et al: Guidelines for the treatment of pressure ulcers. Wound Repair Regen 14:663–679, 2006

32. Dini V, Bertone M, Romanelli M: Prevention and management of pressure ulcers. Dermatol Ther 19:356–364, 2006

33. Rycroft-Malone J, McInnes L: The prevention of pressure ulcers. Worldviews Evid Based Nurs 1:146–149, 2004

34. Effective methods for preventing pressure ulcers. J Fam Pract 55:942, 2006

35. Benbow M: Guidelines for the prevention and treatment of pressure ulcers. Nurs Stand 20:42–44, 2006

36. Cullum N, Nelson EA, Nixon J: Pressure ulcers. Clin Evid:2592–2606, 2006

37. Reddy M, Gill SS, Rochon PA: Preventing pressure ulcers: A systematic review. JAMA 296:974–984, 2006

38. Baranoski S: Pressure ulcers: a renewed awareness. Nursing 36:36–41; quiz 42, 2006

39. Ratliff CR: Two case studies of Marjolin's ulcers in patients referred for management of chronic pressure ulcers. J Wound Ostomy Continence Nurs 29:266–268, 2002

40. Ozek C, Cankayali R, Bilkay U, et al: Marjolin's ulcers arising in burn scars. J Burn Care Rehabil 22:384–389, 2001

41. Gschwandtner ME, Ambrozy E, Maric S, et al: Microcirculation is similar in ischemic and venous ulcers. Microvasc Res 62:226–235, 2001

42. Jeter KF, Tintle TE: Rethinking ischemic ulcers: From etiology to treatment outcome. Prog Clin Biol Res 365:45–54, 1991

43. Worley CA: Neuropathic ulcers: diabetes and wounds, part II. Differential diagnosis and treatment. Dermatol Nurs 18:163–164, 2006

44. Worley CA: Neuropathic ulcers: Diabetes and wounds, part I. Etiology and assessment. Dermatol Nurs 18:52, 59, 2006

45. Margolis DJ, Allen-Taylor L, Hoffstad O, et al: Diabetic neuropathic foot ulcers and amputation. Wound Repair Regen 13:230–236, 2005

46. Steeper R: A critical review of the aetiology of diabetic neuropathic ulcers. J Wound Care 14:101–103, 2005

47. Aksenov IV: Neuropathic diabetic foot ulcers. N Engl J Med 351:1694–1695; author reply 1694–1695, 2004

48. Chang HR: Neuropathic diabetic foot ulcers. N Engl J Med 351:1694–1695; author reply 1694–1695, 2004

49. Zulkowski K, Ratliff CR: Managing venous and neuropathic ulcers. Nursing 34:68, 2004

50. Boulton AJ, Kirsner RS, Vileikyte L: Clinical practice. Neuropathic diabetic foot ulcers. N Engl J Med 351:48–55, 2004

51. Gul A, Basit A, Ali SM, et al: Role of wound classification in predicting the outcome of diabetic foot ulcer. J Pak Med Assoc 56:444–447, 2006

52. Oyibo SO, Jude EB, Tarawneh I, et al: A comparison of two diabetic foot ulcer classification systems: The Wagner and the University of Texas wound classification systems. Diabetes Care 24:84–88, 2001

53. Cunningham D: Treating venous insufficiency ulcers with soft silicone dressing. Ostomy Wound Manage 51:19–20, 2005

54. Galvan L: Assessing venous ulcers and venous insufficiency. Nursing 35:70, 2005

55. Kelechi TJ, Edlund B: Chronic venous insufficiency: Preventing leg ulcers is primary goal. Adv Nurse Pract 13:31–34, 2005

56. Berliner E, Ozbilgin B, Zarin DA: A systematic review of pneumatic compression for treatment of chronic venous insufficiency and venous ulcers. J Vasc Surg 37:539–544, 2003

57. Ruckley CV: Socioeconomic impact of chronic venous insufficiency and leg ulcers. Angiology 48:67–69, 1997

58. Fonder MA, Mamelak AJ, Lazarus GS, et al: Occlusive wound dressings in emergency medicine and acute care. Emerg Med Clin North Am 25:235–242, 2007

59. Burd A: Evaluating the use of hydrogel sheet dressings in comprehensive burn wound care. Ostomy Wound Manage 53:52–62, 2007

60. Fleck CA: Innovative dressings improve wound care management. Mater Manag Health Care 16:24–26, 28, 2007

61. Ovington LG: Advances in wound dressings. Clin Dermatol 25:33–38, 2007

62. Leaper DJ: Silver dressings: their role in wound management. Int Wound J 3:282–294, 2006

63. O'Donnell TF, Jr., Lau J: A systematic review of randomized controlled trials of wound dressings for chronic venous ulcer. J Vasc Surg 44:1118–1125, 2006

64. Shreenivas S, Magnuson JS, Rosenthal EL: Use of negative-pressure dressings to manage a difficult surgical neck wound. Ear Nose Throat J 85:390–391, 2006

65. Attinger CE, Janis JE, Steinberg J, et al: Clinical approach to wounds: Debridement and wound bed preparation including the use of dressings and wound-healing adjuvants. Plast Reconstr Surg 117:72S–109S, 2006

66. Jones V, Grey JE, Harding KG: Wound dressings. Bmj 332:777–780, 2006

67. Wicker P: Wound dressings. Br J Theatre Nurs 2:22–25, 1992

68. Willey T: Use a decision tree to choose wound dressings. Am J Nurs 92:43–46, 1992

69. McCulloch JM: Wound healing and management, in Placzek JD, Boyce DA (eds): Orthopaedic Physical Therapy Secrets. Philadelphia, Hanley & Belfus, 2001, pp 171–176

70. Morris GS, Brueilly KE, Hanzelka H: Negative pressure wound therapy achieved by vacuum-assisted closure: Evaluating the assumptions. Ostomy Wound Manage. 53:52–57, 2007

71. Vuerstaek JD, Vainas T, Wuite J, et al: State-of-the-art treatment of chronic leg ulcers: A randomized controlled trial comparing vacuum-assisted closure (V.A.C.) with modern wound dressings. J Vasc Surg. 44:1029–1037; discussion 1038, 2006

72. Timmers MS, Le Cessie S, Banwell P, et al: The effects of varying degrees of pressure delivered by negative-pressure wound therapy on skin perfusion. Ann Plast Surg 55:665–671, 2005

73. Eginton MT, Brown KR, Seabrook GR, et al: A prospective randomized evaluation of negative-pressure wound dressings for diabetic foot wounds. Ann Vasc Surg 17:645–649, 2003

74. Wanner MB, Schwarzl F, Strub B, et al: Vacuum-assisted wound closure for cheaper and more comfortable healing of pressure sores: a prospective study. Scand J Plast Reconstr Surg Hand Surg 37:28–33, 2003

75. Horwitz LR, Burke TJ, Carnegie D: Augmentation of wound healing using monochromatic infrared energy: Exploration of a new technology for wound management. Adv Wound Care 12:35–40, 1999

76. Burke TJ: The effect of monochromatic infrared energy on sensation in subjects with diabetic peripheral neuropathy: A double-blind, placebo-controlled study: Response to Clifft et al. Diabetes Care. 29:1186; author reply 1186–1187, 2006

77. Harkless LB, DeLellis S, Carnegie DH, et al: Improved foot sensitivity and pain reduction in patients with peripheral neuropathy after treatment with monochromatic infrared photo energy—MIRE. J Diabetes Complications.20:81–87, 2006

78. Clifft JK, Kasser RJ, Newton TS, et al: The effect of monochromatic infrared energy on sensation in patients with diabetic peripheral neuropathy: A double-blind, placebo-controlled study. Diabetes Care. 28:2896–2900, 2005

79. Londahl M, Katzman P, Nilsson A, et al: A prospective study: hyperbaric oxygen therapy in diabetics with chronic foot ulcers. J Wound Care 15:457–459, 2006

80. Mathieu D: Role of hyperbaric oxygen therapy in the management of lower extremity wounds. Int J Low Extrem Wounds 5:233–235, 2006

81. Koetters KT: Hyperbaric oxygen therapy. J Emerg Nurs 32:417–419, 2006

82. Lin LC, Yau G, Lin TF, et al: The efficacy of hyperbaric oxygen therapy in improving the quality of life in patients with problem wounds. J Nurs Res 14:219–227, 2006

83. Guide to physical therapist practice: Phys Ther 81:S13–S95, 2001

84. Cioffi WG: Inhalation injury, in Carrougher GJ (ed): Burn care and therapy. St. Louis, C. V. Mosby, 1998, p 35

85. Sheridan RL: Burn Rehabilitation, Available at: http://www.emedicine.com/pmr/topic163.htm, 2004

86. Gomez R, Cancio LC: Management of burn wounds in the emergency department. Emerg Med Clin North Am 25:135–146, 2007

87. Prelack K, Dylewski M, Sheridan RL: Practical guidelines for nutritional management of burn injury and recovery. Burns 33:14–24, 2007

88. Khan N, Malik MA: Presentation of burn injuries and their management outcome. J Pak Med Assoc 56:394–397, 2006

89. Abdi S, Zhou Y: Management of pain after burn injury. Curr Opin Anaesthesiol 15:563–567, 2002

90. DeSanti L: Pathophysiology and current management of burn injury. Adv Skin Wound Care 18:323–332; quiz 332–334, 2005

91. Papini R: Management of burn injuries of various depths. BMJ 329:158–160, 2004

92. Hettiaratchy S, Papini R: Initial management of a major burn: II: Assessment and resuscitation. BMJ 329:101–103, 2004

93. Hettiaratchy S, Papini R: Initial management of a major burn: I—overview. BMJ 328:1555–1557, 2004

94. Bishop JF: Burn wound assessment and surgical management. Crit Care Nurs Clin North Am 16:145–177, 2004

95. Montgomery RK: Pain management in burn injury. Crit Care Nurs Clin North Am 16:39–49, 2004

96. Danks RR: Burn management. A comprehensive review of the epidemiology and treatment of burn victims. JEMS 28:118–139; quiz 140–141, 2003

97. Sheridan RL: Airway management and respiratory care of the burn patient. Int Anesthesiol Clin 38:129–145, 2000

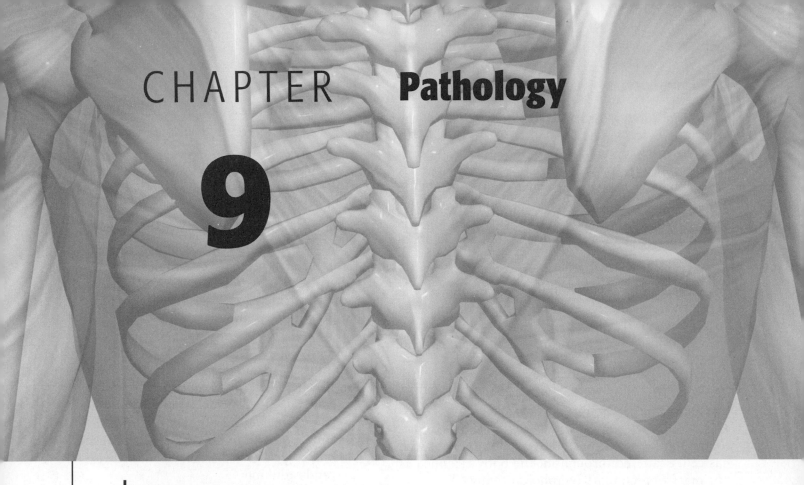

CHAPTER 9 Pathology

The Immune System

Together with a number of physical barriers (the skin, mucous membranes, tears, earwax, mucus, and stomach acid), the immune system defends the body against foreign or hazardous substances that include microorganisms (bacteria, viruses, and fungi), parasites (such as worms), cancer cells, and even transplanted organs and tissues. Antigens are entities that stimulate an immune response in the body. A normal immune response consists of recognizing a foreign antigen, mobilizing forces to defend against it, and attacking it. Disorders of the immune system occur when:

- The body produces an immune response against itself (an autoimmune disorder).
- The body cannot produce suitable immune responses against invading microorganisms (an immunodeficiency disorder).
- A normal immune response to foreign antigens damages normal tissues (an allergic reaction).

To be effective, the immune system must be able to distinguish what is *nonself* (foreign) from what is *self* (auto). Identification molecules on the exterior of all human cells—leukocyte antigens (HLA), or the major histocompatibility complex (MHC)—make this distinction possible. Each individual has unique human leukocyte antigens. Any cell with molecules on its surface that are not identical to those of the body's own cells provokes an attack from the immune system.

T Lymphocytes

T lymphocytes provide the surveillance part of the immune system. They travel through the bloodstream and lymphatic system, looking for antigens in the body. However, unless an antigen undergoes processing into antigen fragments by another white blood cell, called an antigen-presenting cell, a T lymphocyte cannot recognize it. Antigen-presenting cells consist of dendritic cells (which are the most effective), macrophages, and B lymphocytes.

A special molecule called a T-cell receptor, found on the exterior of a T lymphocyte, recognizes the antigen fragment when an HLA molecule presents it. The T-cell receptor then attaches to the part of the HLA molecule presenting the antigen fragment, fitting in it as a key fits in a lock.

Organs of the Immune System

The immune system includes several organs as well as cells scattered throughout the body classified as primary or secondary lymphoid organs.

- *Primary:* Thymus gland and bone marrow—the sites of white blood cell production. Production and preparation of the T lymphocytes (necessary for specific immunity) occur in the thymus gland. The bone marrow produces several types of white blood cells, including neutrophils, monocytes, and B lymphocytes.
- *Secondary:* Spleen, tonsils, liver, appendix, and Peyer's patches in the small intestine. These organs trap microorganisms and other foreign substances and provide a place for mature cells of the immune system to collect, interact with one another and with the foreign substances, and produce a specific immune response.

Autoimmune Diseases

Autoimmune diseases manifest as a self-destructive immune system response directed against normal tissue. Autoimmune diseases can develop according to involvement:

- *Organ specific:* Examples include Hashimoto thyroiditis, Addison disease, Crohn disease, diabetes mellitus, and ulcerative colitis.

- *Nonorgan specific (systemic):* Examples include systemic lupus erythematosus (SLE), fibromyalgia, ankylosing spondylitis, multiple sclerosis, psoriasis, Reiter syndrome, and sarcoidosis.

The etiology of autoimmune diseases is often unknown. The main causes of immunodeficiency can be grouped into primary, secondary, or iatrogenic disorders:

- *Primary disorders:* Involve T cells, B cells, NK (natural killer) cells, phagocytic cells, complement proteins, or lymphoid tissues. Genetically determined immunodeficiency can cause increased susceptibility to infection, autoimmunity, and increased risk of cancer.
- *Secondary disorders:* Result from an underlying disease or cause that depresses or blocks the immune response. These include:
  - ❑ Leukemia or Hodgkin disease
  - ❑ Nonspecific deficiencies in the immune system, which occur because of viral and other infections, malnourishment, alcoholism, cancer, chronic disease, chemotherapy, and radiation
  - ❑ Autoimmune disease, diabetes mellitus, and renal disease
  - ❑ Acquired immunodeficiency syndrome (AIDS)
  - ❑ Organ transplantation—graft versus host disease
- *Iatrogenic disorders:* Induced by immunosuppressive drugs or radiation therapy. Examples of immunosuppressive drugs include corticosteroids, cyclosporine, and cytotoxic drugs.

● **Key Point** Autoimmune disorders share certain clinical features and findings. These include synovitis, pleuritis, myocarditis, vasculitis, myositis, nephritis, and constitutional symptoms (including fatigue, malaise, myalgias, and arthralgias).

Infectious Disease

Types of Organisms

Fungus
Some fungi reproduce by spreading microscopic spores. These spores are often present in the air, where they can be inhaled or come into contact with the body surfaces. Certain types of fungi (such as *Candida*) are commonly present on body surfaces

or in the intestines. Although generally innocuous, these fungi sometimes cause local infections of the skin and nails, vagina, mouth, or sinuses in immunocompromised individuals. In these individuals, fungal infections can be aggressive—spreading quickly to other organs and often proving fatal.

> **● Key Point** Fungal diseases in humans are called *mycoses*.

Even in otherwise healthy people, some fungal infections (for example, blastomycosis and coccidioidomycosis) can have serious outcomes. Several drugs effective against fungal infections are available, but the chemical makeup of fungi makes them difficult to treat. Antifungal drugs may be applied directly to a fungal infection of the skin or other surface, such as the vagina or within the mouth. Antifungal drugs may also be taken by mouth or injected when required to treat more serious infections.

Bacteria

Bacteria are microscopic, single-celled organisms that are encountered in the environment, on the skin, in the airways, in the mouth, and in the digestive and genitourinary tracts of people and animals.

> **● Key Point** Bacteria can be classified according to:
> - Shape—cocci (spherical), bacilli (rodlike), and spirochetes (spiral or helical).
> - Their use of oxygen. Aerobes, bacteria that can live and grow in the presence of oxygen, and anaerobes, bacteria that can tolerate only low levels of oxygen, such as those found in the intestine or in decaying tissue.
> - By color after a particular chemical (Gram) stain is applied. Bacteria that stain blue are called gram positive, whereas those that stain pink are called gram negative.

Gram-positive and gram-negative bacteria differ in the types of infections they produce and in the types of antibiotics that are required to manage them.

> **● Key Point** *Bacteremia* is the presence of viable bacteria in the circulating blood. Most bacteria that enter the bloodstream are rapidly removed by white blood cells. However, if the bacteria become viable, they may establish a focal infection, or the infection may progress to septicemia; the possible sequelae of septicemia include shock, disseminated intravascular coagulation, multiple organ failure, and death.[1]

Mycoplasmas

Mycoplasmas are unusual, self-replicating bacteria that have no cell wall component and very small genomes.[2] For this reason, antibiotics that are active against bacterial cell walls have no effect on mycoplasmas.[2]

Virus

A virus is a subcellular organism made up only of a ribonucleic acid (RNA) or a deoxyribonucleic acid (DNA) nucleus covered with proteins.[2] Viruses are completely dependent on host cells and cannot replicate unless they invade a host cell and stimulate it to participate in the formation of additional virus particles.[2] The virus can either kill the cell it enters or can alter the function of the cell. Some viruses leave their genetic material in the host cell, where it remains dormant for an extended time (*latent infection*)—e.g., herpes viruses. Viruses are not susceptible to antibiotics and cannot be destroyed by pharmacologic means.[2] However, antiviral medications can mitigate the course of the viral illness.[2]

Prions

Prions are newly discovered infectious particles consisting of proteins but lacking nucleic acids.[2] These particles are transmitted from animals to humans and are characterized by a long, latent interval in the host. Examples include Creutzfeldt–Jakob disease and bovine spongiform encephalopathy ("mad cow disease").[2]

Parasites

A parasite[3–5] is an organism that resides on or inside another organism (the host) and causes harm to the host. Parasitic infections are common in rural parts of Africa, Asia, and Latin America and less prevalent in industrialized countries. Parasites enter the body through the mouth or skin. The diagnosis of a parasitic infection can be made from samples of blood, tissue, stool, or urine for laboratory analysis.

Infectious Diseases

Infectious agents are now suspected in the origins of chronic diseases such as sarcoidosis, various forms of inflammatory bowel disease, scleroderma, rheumatoid arthritis, systemic lupus erythematosus, diabetes mellitus, Kawasaki disease, Alzheimer disease, and many forms of cancer. All healthcare professionals need to have an understanding of the infectious process, the sequence of transmission, and approaches, like handwashing, to lessen the spread of infections.

Staphylococcal Infections

Most infections caused by staphylococci are because of *Staphylococcus aureus*.

Staphylococcal Aureus

S. aureus is a gram-positive coccus that occurs with a worldwide distribution. Healthcare workers, anyone with diabetes, and patients on dialysis all have higher rates of colonization. The anterior nares of the nose are the chief site of colonization in adults; other potential sites of colonization include the axilla, rectum, and perineum.[6] Common expressions of staphylococcal infections include skin, wound, and soft tissue infections (burns, surgical wounds, thus pyomyositis, septic bursitis); toxic shock syndrome; endocarditis; osteomyelitis; food poisoning; and infections related to prosthetic devices (prosthetic joints and heart valves and vascular shunts, grafts, and catheters).[6] The clinical manifestations vary enormously according to the site and type of infection.[2] Many antibiotics are effective against *S. aureus*; however, methicillin-resistant *S. aureus* (MRSA) is resistant to most agents.

Streptococcal Infections

Streptococcus pyogenes[7-15] (group A *Streptococcus*) is one of the most common pathogens faced in clinical practice. It causes many diseases in diverse organ systems, ranging from skin infections to infections of the upper respiratory tract. Diagnosis is by culture of group A streptococci from pharyngeal secretions, blood, cerebrospinal fluid, joint aspirate, skin biopsy specimen, sputum, bronchoalveolar lavage fluid, or thoracocentesis fluid. Types include:

- *Group A (pyogenes):* Responsible for pharyngitis, rheumatic fever, scarlet fever, impetigo, necrotizing fasciitis, cellulitis, and myositis
- *Group B (agalactiae):* Responsible for neonatal and adult infections
- *Group C (pneumoniae):* Responsible for pneumonia, otitis media, meningitis, and endocarditis

The interventions for group A streptococcal infections vary depending on the clinical syndrome. In general, penicillin therapy remains the intervention of choice in most situations (except in penicillin-allergic individuals). Remarkably, no penicillin-resistant strains of *S. pyogenes* have yet been encountered in clinical practice.

Osteomyelitis

Osteomyelitis is an infectious process of the bone and its marrow, including infections caused by pyogenic microorganisms, tuberculosis, specific fungal infections (mycotic osteomyelitis), parasitic infections (Hydatid disease), and viral infections or syphilitic infections (Charcot arthropathy).

The proximal tibia is the most common site. Osteomyelitis may or may not produce a fever or an abnormality in white blood cell count.

Hepatitis

Hepatitis[16-22] is defined as an inflammation of the liver. Several different viruses cause viral hepatitis. They are named the hepatitis A, B, C, D, and E viruses. Some cases of viral hepatitis cannot be attributed to the hepatitis A, B, C, D, or E viruses. These types are called non-A-E hepatitis. The hepatitis A, B, C, D, and E viruses cause acute, or short-term, viral hepatitis. The hepatitis B, C, and D viruses can also cause chronic hepatitis, in which the infection is prolonged, sometimes lifelong. Signs and symptoms (some people do not have symptoms) include:

- Low-grade fever—usually an early sign (preicteric phase), with anorexia, nausea, headache, malaise, fatigue, vomiting, abdominal pain, loss of appetite.
- Jaundice (yellowing of the skin and eyes)—usually a sign of the icteric phase, with an enlarged liver with tenderness and abatement of the earlier symptoms.
- Elevated lab values (hepatic transaminases and bilirubin).

Hepatitis A (HAV, Acute Infectious Hepatitis)

Hepatitis A[23-26] spreads mostly through food or water contaminated by feces from an infected person. People at risk include international travelers; people living in areas where hepatitis A outbreaks are common; people who live with or have sex with an infected person; and, during outbreaks, day care children and employees, men who have sex with men, and injection drug users. The best methods of prevention for this type is:

- Getting the hepatitis A vaccine
- Avoiding tap water when traveling internationally

- Practicing good hygiene and sanitation, such as handwashing

Hepatitis A is usually self-limiting, lasting several weeks.

Hepatitis B (HBV, Serum Hepatitis)

Hepatitis B[27–29] is spread through contact with infected blood, sex with an infected person, or from mother to child during childbirth. People at risk are those who have sex with an infected person, gay men, injection drug users, children of immigrants from disease-endemic areas, infants born to infected mothers, people who live with an infected person, healthcare workers, hemodialysis patients, people who received a transfusion of blood or blood products before July 1992 or clotting factors made before 1987, and international travelers. The best prevention for this type is the hepatitis B vaccine. Acute hepatitis B is usually self-limiting. The intervention for chronic hepatitis B includes drug treatment.

Hepatitis C (HCV, Non-A, Non-B)

Hepatitis C[30,31] spreads mostly through contact with infected blood and less commonly, through sexual contact and childbirth. People at risk include injection drug users, people who have sex with an infected person, people who have multiple sex partners, healthcare workers, infants born to infected women, hemodialysis patients, and people who received a transfusion of blood or blood products before July 1992 or clotting factors made before 1987. The best method for prevention is through a reduction in the risk of exposure to the virus (there is no vaccine for hepatitis C) by avoiding behaviors like sharing drug needles or sharing personal items like toothbrushes, razors, and nail clippers with an infected person. The intervention for chronic hepatitis C is pharmacology.

Hepatitis D

Hepatitis D[16,18–20,22] spreads through contact with infected blood. This disease occurs only in people who are already infected with hepatitis B. People at risk include anyone infected with hepatitis B—injection drug users who have hepatitis B have the highest risk. People who have hepatitis B are also at risk if they have sex with a person infected with hepatitis D or if they live with an infected person. Also at risk are people who received a transfusion of blood or blood products before July 1992 or clotting factors made before 1987. The best methods of prevention for this type are:

- Getting immunized against hepatitis B if not already infected
- Avoiding exposure to infected blood, contaminated needles, and an infected person's personal items (e.g., toothbrush, razor, nail clippers)

The intervention for chronic hepatitis D is alpha interferon.

Hepatitis E

Hepatitis E[32] spreads through contaminated food or water (by feces from an infected person). This disease is uncommon in the United States. People at risk include international travelers, people living in areas where hepatitis E outbreaks are common, and people who live or have sex with an infected person. The best way to prevent hepatitis E is to reduce the risk of exposure to the virus (there is no vaccine for hepatitis E) by avoiding tap water when traveling internationally and practicing good hygiene and sanitation. Hepatitis E is usually self-limiting, lasting several weeks to months.

Acquired Immunodeficiency Syndrome

In 1984, three years after the first reports of a disease that was to become known as AIDS, researchers discovered the primary causative viral agent, the human immunodeficiency virus type 1 (HIV-1).[33] In 1986 a second type of HIV, called HIV-2, was isolated from AIDS patients in west Africa, where it may have been present decades earlier.[33] Both HIV-1 and HIV-2 have the same modes of transmission and are associated with similar opportunistic infections as AIDS.[34] The primary cause of AIDS is transmission of the HIV retrovirus by body fluid exchange (in particular blood and semen), which is associated with high-risk behaviors:

- Unprotected sexual contact
- Contaminated needles: sharing, frequent injection of Institute for Applied Biomedicine (IAB) drugs, transfusions (although no longer a major risk)
- Maternal–fetal transmission in utero or at delivery or through contaminated breast milk

Low-risk behaviors for HIV transmission include:

- Occupational transmission: needle sticks
- Casual contact: kissing

The HIV retrovirus chiefly infects human T4 (helper) lymphocytes, the major regulators of the immune response, and destroys or inactivates them.[34] Once

HIV enters the body, cells containing the CD4 antigen, including macrophages and T4 cells, serve as receptors for the HIV retrovirus.[34] After invading a cell, a virus particle (*virion*) injects the core proteins and the two strands of viral RNA into the cell. HIV contains reverse transcriptase, an enzyme that allows for successful replication of the virus in reverse fashion, transcribing the RNA code into DNA.[33]

HIV infection manifests itself in many different ways and differs between adult and pediatric populations. The clinical expressions of HIV infection are classified into three stages:[33,34]

- *Asymptomatic stage:* A patient in the early stages remains asymptomatic, although some individuals can develop an acute, self-limiting infectious mononucleosis-like condition. Laboratory tests are positive despite lack of symptoms.
- *Early symptomatic stage:* As the infection progresses, the immune system becomes increasingly more compromised. This stage, referred to as AIDS-related complex (ARC), may last for weeks or months and is a forerunner to full-blown AIDS. Symptoms and conditions during this stage involve:
  - Generalized adenopathy, deconditioning, anxiety, and depression.
  - Nonspecific symptoms, including weight loss, fatigue, night sweats, swollen lymph glands, loss of appetite, apathy, and fever.
  - Neurological symptoms, including encephalopathy, headache, blurred vision, mild dementia, seizures, and focal neurological signs.
  - Opportunistic infections; the most common are pneumocystis carinii pneumonia (PCP), oral and esophageal candidiasis, cytomegalovirus infection, cryptococcus, herpes simplex, and *Mycobacterium tuberculosis.*
- *HIV advanced disease:* Patients with advanced HIV may experience the following:
  - Neurologic manifestations of central, peripheral, and autonomic nervous systems, including:
    - AIDS encephalopathy (HIV-associated dementia)
    - Peripheral neuropathy: distal, symmetric, and mainly sensory
    - Neuromusculoskeletal diseases: osteomyelitis, bacterial myositis, non-Hodgkin lymphoma, and infectious arthritis

- HIV wasting syndrome, characterized by a disproportionate loss of metabolically active tissue, specifically body cell mass, secondary to weight loss, chronic diarrhea, unexplained weakness, and malnutrition.
- Rheumatologic manifestations.
- HIV-associated myopathy: Progressive painless weakness in the proximal limb muscles.
- Malignancies: The most common are Kaposi sarcoma, non-Hodgkin lymphoma, and primary brain lymphoma.

The diagnosis is by clinical findings and systemic evidence of HIV infection and nonexistence of other known causes of immunodeficiency. Early identification is important so that early and preventive therapies may be introduced. The most commonly performed tests are:

- The enzyme-linked immunosorbent assay (ELISA) test
- Absolute T4 (CD4) cell counts per deciliter of blood; normal CD4 counts are 800 to 1200 per milliliter; symptomatic AIDS CD4 counts are 200 to 500 per milliliter

HIV is now considered as a chronic rather than a terminal illness. Medical management centers on the CD4 cell count and viral load:

- Highly active antiretroviral therapy (HAART); introduced when CD4 cell count drops below 500 cells/mm^3. These drugs do not remove the virus, and lifelong therapy is required.
- Nucleoside analogue reverse-transcriptase inhibitors (NRTIs)—e.g., azidothymidine (AZT).
- Nonnucleoside reverse-transcriptase inhibitors (NNRTIs).
- Protease inhibitors.

Symptomatic treatment includes:

- Education to prevent the spread of infection and disease
- Skin care
- Treatment of opportunistic infections through prophylactic vaccinations
- Maintenance of functional mobility and safety to prevent disability
- Supportive care—e.g., emotional support for patients and family
- Maintenance of good nutritional status
- Fatigue management—e.g., energy conservation techniques, self-care
- Respiratory management as appropriate

- Community management skill training, such as ensuring access to transport station, participating in socialization opportunities, and negotiating healthcare and insurance systems

Intervention

The goals of physical therapy will depend on the presenting signs and symptoms. The clinician must remember to follow universal AIDS/HIV precautions. The following interventions are recommended:[35]

- Exercise. Exercise has clinically significant effects on the immune system. It reduces stress levels and pain, improves appetite, improves cardiovascular endurance and strength, and is an important way to increase the CD4 cells at the early stages of the disease.[34] Exercise should be prescribed using the following guidelines:[34]
  - Moderate aerobic exercise training to improve cardiopulmonary function; this is important in the advanced stages of AIDS
  - Strength training
  - Avoidance of exhausting exercise with symptomatic individuals
  - Mild-level exercises for patients who have opportunistic infections
- Energy conservation techniques, such as balancing rest with activity and scheduling strenuous activities during periods of high energy.
- Stress management and relaxation training.
- Breathing exercises as appropriate.
- Postural education and instruction with body mechanics.
- Neurologic rehabilitation, including balance and proprioceptive training for patients with neurological deficits.
- ADL equipment as appropriate.

Tuberculosis

Tuberculosis (TB) is included in this chapter to reinforce the importance to PTAs of this infectious condition—anyone exposed to TB should have periodic TB testing performed. TB is described in more detail in Chapter 7.

Influenza

Influenza, one of the most contagious airborne communicable diseases, is a common problem in healthcare settings. Its nosocomial transmission is associated with significant morbidity and mortality in acute and long-term healthcare facilities. The mode of transmission is person to person by direct deposition of virus-laden large droplets onto the mucosa of the upper respiratory tract of an immunologically liable person. Once within host cells, cellular dysfunction and deterioration occur, with viral replication and release of viral progeny. Viral shedding occurs at commencement of symptoms or just before the outset of illness (0–24 hours). Shedding continues for 5 to 10 days. Young children may shed the virus longer, placing others at risk for contracting the virus. Influenza results from contamination with one of three key types of virus, A, B, or C. The general appearance among patients who present with influenza varies, with some appearing acutely ill, with some weakness and respiratory findings, while others appearing only mildly sick. On inspection, sufferers may have some or all the following findings:

- Fever; may range from 100 to 104 degrees Fahrenheit
- Tachycardia; most likely results from hypoxia, fever, or both
- Pharyngitis
- Pulmonary findings; active cough, wheezing, rhonchi, or a combination thereof

All healthcare workers must follow the guidelines for isolation precautions (see Chapter 1) to prevent transmission of influenza for both themselves and their patients. This is especially important for the therapist treating aged, immunocompromised, or, chronically ill individuals. As with other diseases, prevention is the most effective strategy. Since the immunization for influenza does not provide immunity for the entire year or for all strains of influenza, recommendations for immunization must be reviewed and acted on individually.

Departmental Infection Control

Sterilization

Sterilization involves removing all microorganisms (such as bacteria, prions, and viruses) from a surface, a piece of equipment, food, or biological culture medium. There are several methods of sterilization.

Heat

A widely used instrument for heat sterilization is the autoclave. Autoclaves commonly use steam heated to 121°C (250°F), at 103 kPa (15 psi) above atmospheric pressure, for 15 minutes. Proper autoclave treatment will inactivate all fungi, bacteria, viruses, and bacterial spores but will not necessarily eliminate prions. Boiling in water for 15 minutes kills non-spore-forming organisms (bacteria and viruses), but it is unsuitable for sterilization because it is ineffective against many bacterial spores and prions. Dry heat can be used to sterilize items. The standard setting for a hot-air oven is at least two hours at 160°C (320°F). A rapid method can heat air to 190°C (374°F) for 6 to 12 hours.

Chemical

Chemicals also are used for sterilization:

- Phenols: general disinfectants
- Halogens, such as chlorine, iodine, and bromine
  - Chlorine bleach is a liquid sterilizing agent. Household bleach, also used in hospitals and biological research laboratories, consists of 5.25% sodium hypochlorite. At this concentration it is most stable for storage, but not most active. Bleach will kill many spores, but it is ineffectual against certain resistant spores. It is also corrosive.
  - Chlorination is used for water disinfection and in filtration systems.
  - Iodines are used in hydrotherapy. They provide full bactericidal activity when organic matter (skin, feces, urine) is present.
- Alcohol
- Quaternary ammonia salts, powerful disinfectants with extra surfactant (detergent) action as well as acting against bacteria, their surfactant action removes excess mucus-containing parasites and bacteria.
  - Glutaraldehyde and formaldehyde solutions are accepted liquid sterilizing agents, provided the immersion time is long enough. It can take up to 12 hours for glutaraldehyde to kill all spores, and even longer for formaldehyde.
  - Ionizing radiation (x-rays, gamma rays) is used to sterilize some medications, plastics, and sutures.
  - Ultraviolet (UV) light can also be used for irradiation, but only on surfaces and some transparent objects (many objects that are transparent to visible light absorb UV), but it is ineffectual in shaded areas, including areas under dirt (which may become polymerized after prolonged irradiation, so it is difficult to remove). It also damages many plastics and is harmful to unprotected skin and eyes.

Filtration

Filtration uses forceful air purification.

Physical Cleaning

Methods of physical cleaning include:

- Ultrasonic—disinfects instruments
- Handwashing with an antimicrobial product

Disinfection

The term *disinfection* applies to the process of reducing the number of viable microorganisms present in a sample (note that *disinfection* is not interchangeable with *sterilization*, which is the killing of *all* microorganisms in a material or on the surface of an object). A disinfectant is a chemical or physical agent that is applied to inanimate objects to kill microbes. Not all disinfectants are capable of sterilizing. An ideal disinfectant should be:

- Fast acting even in the presence of organic substances, such as those in body fluid
- Effective against all types of infectious agents (broadly active) without destroying tissues or acting as a poison if ingested
- Able to easily penetrate material to be disinfected without damaging or discoloring the material
- Easy to prepare and stable even when exposed to light, heat, or other environmental factors
- Inexpensive and easy to obtain and use

Note: An antiseptic is a chemical agent that is applied to living tissue to kill microbes. *Sanitization* is the cleaning of pathogenic microorganisms from public eating utensils and objects, as in the kitchen of a restaurant.

Gastrointestinal System

The gastrointestinal (GI) tract is a long, hollow tube extending from the mouth to the anus. The function of the GI tract is to break down ingested foods and fluids into molecules that can be absorbed and used by the body while simultaneously eliminating waste products.

- *Upper GI tract:* The mouth, esophagus, and stomach
- *Lower GI tract:* The small intestine (duodenum, jejunum, and ileum), and the large intestine (cecum, colon, and rectum)

The function and dysfunction of the various parts of the GI tract are outlined in **Table 9-1.**

TABLE 9-1

Functions and Disorders of the GI Tract

Location	Function/Description	Disorders	Implications for PTA
Mouth	Initiation of chemical and mechanical digestion		
Esophagus	Long tube that transports food from the mouth to the stomach	*Gastroesophageal reflux disease (GERD):* Caused by reflux or backward moving of the gastric contents of the stomach into the esophagus, reducing heartburn. Caused by failure of the lower esophageal sphincter (LES) to regulate flow of food from the esophagus into the stomach and increased gastric pressure. Over time, acidic gastric fluid damages the esophagus, producing reflux esophagitis. Symptoms include heartburn, regurgitation of gastric contents, belching, and chest pain (unrelated to activity). Complications include esophageal strictures, Barrett esophagitis (a precancerous state), and esophageal adenocarcinoma. Medical interventions include acid-suppressing drugs. *Hiatal hernia:* The protrusion of the stomach upward through the diaphragm (rolling hiatal hernia), or displacement of both the stomach and gastroesophageal junction upward into the thorax (sliding hiatal hernia). May be congenital or acquired. Symptoms include heartburn from GERD. Surgery may be indicated.	Positional changes from full supine to a more upright position using pillows or a wedge. Left sidelying is often preferred because right sidelying may promote acid flow into the esophagus. Advise patient to avoid Valsalva maneuver.
Stomach	Secretion of hydrochloric acid and other exocrine functions, including the release of digestive enzymes from the liver, pancreas, and gallbladder to assist with grinding of the food and digestion. GI motility propels food and fluids through the GI system and is provided by rhythmic, intermittent contractions (peristaltic movements) of smooth muscle (except for pharynx and upper one-third of the esophagus).	*Gastritis:* An inflammation of the gastric mucosa or inner layer of the stomach, which can be acute or chronic. *Acute (erosive gastritis):* Caused by severe burns, aspirin or other NSAIDs, corticosteroids, food allergies, or viral or bacterial infections. Symptoms include dyspepsia, nausea, vomiting, and hematemesis. Treatment involves removal of the stimulus of the disease process and pharmacological intervention. *Chronic (nonerosive gastritis):* Usually associated with a *Helicobacter pylori (H. pylori)* bacterial infection. *H. pylori* is a carcinogen and must be treated aggressively. Management is symptomatic and includes avoiding substances like caffeine, nicotine, and alcohol; physician modification and medications, including acid-suppressing proton pump inhibitors, H-2 blockers (medicines that reduce the amount of acid the stomach produces), and antacids. *Peptic ulcer disease:* A disruption or erosion in the gastrointestinal mucosa resulting in ulcerated lesions in areas exposed to acid–pepsin secretions. Can be caused by *H. pylori* infection, chronic NSAID use, excessive secretion of gastric acid, stress, alcohol, smoking, and heredity. Symptoms can include gastric pain, burning or heartburn, nausea, or vomiting that is aggravated by changes in position and the absence of food in the stomach. Symptoms are relieved by food or antacids. Complications include hemorrhage, perforation of the duodenum, and malignancy. Medical management includes use of antibiotics for treatment of *H. pylori* together with acid-suppressing drugs.	Patients taking NSAIDs for a long time should be monitored carefully for pain, bleeding, nausea, or vomiting. Reports of blood in the stool should result in physician referral. Patients should be advised to take medications with food. Pain from peptic ulcers located on the posterior wall of the stomach can present as radiating pain. Pain can also radiate into the right shoulder. Signs of excess bleeding include fatigue, dizziness, pallor, and exercise intolerance.

(continued)

TABLE 9-1	Functions and Disorders of the GI Tract (Continued)		
Location	**Function/Description**	**Disorders**	**Implications for PTA**
Duodenum	Neutralizes acid in food from stomach and mixes pancreatic and biliary secretions with food. Neural control of the GI tract is achieved by the autonomic nervous system, which has both sympathetic and parasympathetic plexuses extending along the length of the GI wall. Major GI hormones include cholecystokinin, gastrin, and secretin.	*Malabsorption syndrome:* A complex of disorders characterized by problems with intestinal absorption of nutrients. Can be caused by gastric or small bowel resection or a number of different factors, including cystic fibrosis, celiac disease, Crohn disease, chronic pancreatitis, and pernicious anemia. Symptoms, based on the root pathology and comorbidities that may exist, include anorexia, weight loss, abdominal bloating, pain and cramps, indigestion, steatorrhea (oil-covered stools), and diarrhea. Treatment includes avoidance of the underlying cause, probiotics, antibiotics, dietary modification, and nutritional support.	PTA must be aware for signs and symptoms of: • Iron-deficiency anemia • Easy bruising and bleeding due to lack of vitamin K • Muscle weakness and fatigue due to lack of protein, iron, folic acid, and vitamin B • Bone loss, pain, and predisposition to develop fractures from lack of calcium, phosphate, and vitamin D • Neuropathy, including tetany and paresthesia due to lack of calcium, vitamin B and D, magnesium, and potassium • Muscle spasms from electrolyte imbalance and lack of calcium • Generalized swelling secondary to protein depletion
		Inflammatory bowel disease (IBD): Refers to two related chronic inflammatory intestinal disorders: Crohn disease and ulcerative colitis. The main difference between Crohn disease and ulcerative colitis is the location and nature of the inflammatory changes: Crohn can affect any part of the GI tract, whereas ulcerative colitis is restricted to the colon and the rectum. Although very different diseases, both may present with any of the following symptoms: abdominal pain, vomiting, diarrhea, rectal bleeding, weight loss, and various associated complaints or diseases, like arthritis. Depending on the level of severity, IBD may require immunosuppression to control the symptoms.	
Jejunum	Absorbs water, electrolytes, and nutrients.	*Irritable bowel syndrome (IBS):* a functional bowel disorder characterized by chronic abdominal pain, discomfort, bloating, and alteration of bowel habits in the absence of any detectable organic cause. In some cases, the symptoms are relieved by bowel movements. Diarrhea or constipation may predominate, or they may alternate. Although there is no cure for IBS, there are treatments that attempt to relieve symptoms, including dietary adjustments, medication, and psychological interventions.	
Ileum	Absorbs bile and intrinsic factors to be recycled.	*Appendicitis:* A medical emergency characterized by inflammation of the vermiform appendix; one of the most common causes of severe acute abdominal pain. Signs and symptoms include localized findings in the right iliac fossa. The abdominal wall becomes very sensitive to gentle palpation (rebound tenderness [Blumberg sign]; pressing a hand on the abdomen elicits less pain than releasing the hand abruptly). Coughing causes point tenderness at McBurney's point (1.5–2 in. above the anterior superior iliac spine in the right lower quadrant).	

| Ileum | Absorbs bile and intrinsic factors to be recycled. |
| Ascending colon, transverse colon, descending colon, sigmoid, rectum, and anus | Water and electrolytes continue to be absorbed. Undigested food is eliminated as feces. |

Peritonitis: An inflammation of the peritoneum, the serous membrane that lines part of the abdominal cavity and viscera. Peritonitis may be localized or generalized, and it may result from infection (often due to rupture of a hollow organ. as may occur in abdominal trauma or appendicitis) or from a noninfectious process. The main manifestations of peritonitis are acute abdominal pain, abdominal tenderness, and abdominal guarding, which are exacerbated by moving the peritoneum—e.g., coughing (forced cough may be used as a test), flexing one's hips, eliciting the Blumberg sign (rebound tenderness). Depending on the severity, the management of peritonitis may include general supportive measures such as vigorous intravenous rehydration and correction of electrolyte disturbances, antibiotics, or surgery (laparotomy).

Diverticulitis: A common digestive disease of the large intestine that develops from diverticulosis (formation of pouches (diverticula) on the outside of the colon). Diverticulitis results if one of these diverticula becomes inflamed. Patients often present with left (more common) or right lower quadrant pain, fever, and leukocytosis (an elevation of the white cell count in blood tests). Patients may also complain of nausea, diarrhea, or constipation. Complications include bowel obstruction, perforation with peritonitis, and hemorrhage.

Colorectal cancer: Includes cancerous growths in the colon, rectum, and appendix. The symptoms of colorectal cancer depend on the location of the tumor in the bowel and can include change in bowel habit (new-onset constipation or diarrhea in the absence of another cause), a feeling of incomplete defecation, a reduction in diameter of stool, or lower gastrointestinal bleeding, including the passage of blood or mucus in the stool. Constitutional symptoms may include fatigue, palpitations, pallor (pale appearance of the skin), unexplained weight loss, and decreased appetite. The treatment depends on the staging of the cancer. When colorectal cancer is caught at early stages (with little spread) it can be curable. However, when it is detected at later stages (when distant metastases are present) it is less likely to be curable.

Hematologic (Blood) Disorders

Hematology is the branch of science that studies the form and structure of blood and blood forming tissues. Blood is a circulating tissue composed of several cells called corpuscles, which constitute about 45% of whole blood. The other 55% is blood plasma, a yellowish fluid that is the blood's liquid medium. The functions of blood cells include:

- To supply nutrients (e.g., oxygen, glucose) and constitutional elements to tissues and to remove waste products (e.g., carbon dioxide, lactic acid)—main function.
- To enable cells (e.g., leukocytes, abnormal tumor cells) and different substances (e.g., amino acids, lipids, hormones) to be transported between tissues and organs.

Blood plasma is essentially an aqueous solution containing 96% water, 4% blood plasma proteins, and trace amounts of other materials, including:

- Albumin (the most abundant constituent)
- Blood clotting factors (fibrinogen)
- Immunoglobulins (antibodies)
- Hormones
- Various other proteins
- Various electrolytes (mainly sodium and chlorine)

● **Key Point** The direct control of erythrocyte production (*erythropoiesis*) is exerted by a hormone called erythropoietin, which is secreted by the kidneys. Erythropoietin acts on the bone marrow to stimulate the maturation and proliferation of erythrocytes by a process called *hematopoiesis*.

Function of the hematological system is integrated with the lymphatic and immune systems. Manifestations of hematological system dysfunction are outlined in **Table 9-2**. Hematologic conditions alter the oxygen-carrying capacity of the blood and the constituents, structure, consistency, and flow of the blood.[35] These changes can contribute to hypo- or hypercoagulopathy, increased work of the heart and breathing, impaired tissue perfusion, and increased risk of thrombus.[35]

Hematologic Dysfunction

Disorders of Iron Absorption

Hemochromatosis

Hemochromatosis[36,37] is an autosomal recessive hereditary disorder characterized by excessive iron absorption by the small intestine.[35] Individuals with this condition lack an effective way to remove iron, and the iron begins to accumulate in the liver, pancreas, skin, heart, and other organs. Hemochromatosis is characterized by:

- Chronic hemolytic anemia. Hemoglobin is released into plasma with resultant reduced oxygen delivery to the tissues.
- Vaso-occlusion, because of the misshapen erythrocytes, which can result in ischemia, occlusion, and infarction of bordering tissue.
- Weakness, fatigue, abdominal pain, arthralgia, or arthritis.
- Enlarged liver and darkened skin.

Diagnosis can be made by a simple genetic test based on family history.[35]

TABLE 9-2	Manifestations of Hematological System Dysfunction	
Manifestation	**Description**
Edema	Buildup of excessive fluid within the interstitial tissues or within body cavities
Infarction	A localized region of necrosis caused by reduction of arterial perfusion below the level required for cell viability
Thrombosis and embolism	*Thrombosis:* Presence of a solid mass of clotted blood within an intact blood vessel or chamber of the heart *Embolism:* A mass of solid, liquid, or gas that moves within a blood vessel to lodge at a site distant from its place of origin
Lymphedema	A chronic swelling of an area due to a buildup of interstitial fluid, especially in the extremities, secondary to obstruction of lymphatic vessels or lymph nodes.
Hypotension and shock	The result of reduced arterial blood circulation and thus decreased perfusion to an organ or tissue

Intervention

Due to the fact that arthropathy occurs in 40% to 60% of individuals with hemochromatosis, a physical therapy intervention is essential in providing flexibility, strength, and proper alignment to promote function; preventing the loss of independence in activities of daily living; and providing assistive devices, orthotics, and splints toward these goals.[35]

Disorders of Erythrocytes
Anemia

Anemia, one of the more common blood disorders, is an abnormality in the quantity or quality (reduction in the oxygen-carrying capacity of erythrocytes) of the blood. Anemia is not a disease but rather a symptom of many other disorders, including:[35]

- Dietary deficiency (nutritional anemia) in iron, vitamin B, and folic acid.
- Decreased production of erythrocytes due to chronic diseases, such as rheumatoid arthritis, tuberculosis, and cancer; bone marrow failure, as in leukemia and aplasia; and inborn or acquired metabolic defect.
- Acute or chronic blood loss causing iron deficiency due to trauma, bleeding peptic ulcer, excessive menstruation, and bleeding hemorrhoids.
- Congenital defects of hemoglobin, as in sickle cell diseases.
- Destruction of erythrocytes in mechanical or autoimmune hemolysis, enzyme defects, and hypersplenism.

> **● Key Point** Exercise intolerance (easy fatigability) can be expected in patients with anemia. Vital signs should be monitored for tachycardia, which is usually accompanied by a sense of generalized weakness, loss of stamina, and exertional dyspnea. Central nervous system symptoms can develop in cases of severe pernicious anemia, whereas neuropathy is observed in the early cases of B_{12} deficiency, allowing for early identification.[35]

Intervention

Treatment of anemia is directed toward alleviating or controlling the causes, relieving the symptoms, and preventing complications.[35] Exercise for any patient with anemia should be approved by the physician. The prevalence of iron-deficiency anemia is likely to be higher in athletic populations and groups, especially in younger female athletes, than in sedentary individuals.[35] A knowledge of the underlying cause of the anemia may be very helpful for the PTA in identifying red flag symptoms, indicating the need for alteration of the program or medical referral.[35] Examples of such symptoms include:[35]

- Evidence of easy bruising in response to the slightest trauma may indicate an alteration in platelet production
- Decreased oxygen delivery to the skin results in impaired healing and loss of elasticity, delaying wound healing and the healing of other musculoskeletal injuries
- Paresthesias, especially numbness mimicking carpal tunnel syndrome, gait disturbances, and extreme weakness, can all indicate anemia caused by vitamin B_{12} deficiency
- Tachycardia and palpitations may occur due to changes in resting cardiac output

Hemostasis Disorders
Sickle Cell Diseases

The sickle cell diseases[38–41] are a group of inherited, autosomal recessive disorders in which the erythrocytes, particularly hemoglobin S, are crescent or sickle shaped instead of being biconcave. The condition is chronic and can be fatal. The two primary pathophysiologic features of sickle cell disorders are chronic hemolytic anemia and vaso-occlusion resulting in ischemic injury.[35]

Sickle cell anemia, a hereditary, chronic form of hemolytic anemia, is merely a result of the disease and not the disease itself.[35] In sickle cell anemia the erythrocytes rupture releasing hemoglobin prematurely into the plasma, thereby reducing oxygen delivery capacity to the tissues. It is important that the PTA be able to recognize the signs and symptoms associated with sickle cell anemia (pain [abdominal, chest, headache], fatigue, weakness, dyspnea on effort, tachycardia, and pallor or yellow skin), and a condition called *sickle cell crisis*, which is an acute episodic condition occurring in children with sickle cell anemia (**Table 9-3**). It also important for the PTA to recognize signs of complications associated with sickle cell anemia, which include cerebrovascular accidents, convulsions, blindness, chronic leg ulcers, avascular necrosis of the femoral head, and bone infarcts.[35]

Hemophilia

Hemophilia is discussed in Chapter 10.

Thrombocytosis

Thrombocytosis[42–45] refers to an increase in the number of circulating platelets (greater than 450,000/mm[3]), which can be primary or secondary. The high platelet count causes an increase in blood viscosity, which can cause intravascular clumping or thrombosis.

Thrombocytopenia

Thrombocytopenia[46–49] refers to a decrease in the number of circulating platelets (less than 150,000/mm³). It is caused by inadequate platelet production from the bone marrow, increased platelet destruction outside the bone marrow, or splenic sequestration. Thrombocytopenia is a common complication of leukemia or metastatic cancer.

The Thalassemias

The thalassemias are a group of inherited, chronic hemolytic anemias commonly affecting people of Mediterranean or southern Chinese ancestry.[50] The thalassemias are characterized by production of extremely thin, fragile erythrocytes, called *target cells*.[35] The onset of thalassemia is usually insidious, and the symptoms resemble those of other hemolytic anemias (jaundice, leg ulcers, splenomegaly), and they lead to bony changes in older children if untreated.[35] The severity depends on whether the infected client is homozygous or heterozygous for the thalassemia trait. Diagnosis is by laboratory testing.

Histiocytosis X

Histiocytosis[51–53] is a generic name for a group of syndromes characterized by an abnormal increase in the number of certain immune cells called *histiocyte cells*, including monocytes, macrophages, and dendritic cells. Most cases of histiocytosis X affect children between ages 1 and 15 years old. The extra immune cells may form tumors, which can affect various parts of the body. In children, histiocytosis X usually involves the bones (80%) and may consist of single or multiple sites. The skull is frequently affected.

Physical Therapy Intervention for Hematologic Disorders

It is important that a physician approve any exercise for the patient with a blood disorder. Physical therapy intervention should be geared toward enhancing flexibility, strength, and appropriate alignment to promote function; preventing contracture formation; preventing falls; and preventing the reduction of independence with ADLs.[35] The PTA can provide methods of pain control, relaxation techniques, emotional support, patient and family education, and assistive devices, orthotics, or splints. In patients with hemostasis disorders, PTAs need to be able to recognize any signs of early (within the first 24 to 48 hours) bleeding episodes (warm, swollen, and painful joints with decreased range of motion,

TABLE 9-3	Signs and Symptoms of Sickle Cell Anemia and Sickle Cell Crisis
Acute and severe pain due to ischemia	
Recurrent joint, extremity, and back pain	
Neurologic manifestations: dizziness, paresthesias, blindness, and cranial nerve palsies	
Renal compensations	

paresthesias, or protective muscle spasm) and sickle cell crisis (**Table 9-3**).[35] The immediate provision of factor replacement by medical personnel to stop the bleeding, and following the PRICE (protection, rest, ice, compression, elevation) principle to promote comfort and healing, are two goals for treating acute joint hemarthrosis or muscle bleed.[35]

● **Key Point** Patients with sickle cell disease must be closely monitored for cardiorespiratory and metabolic responses during exercise.

Genitourinary

The genitourinary system is the organ system of all the reproductive organs and the urinary system. The structures involved in the genitourinary system include the male and female reproductive organs, the kidneys, the bladder, and the ureters. This section will focus on the renal urologic systems.

Water Balance

Fluid found inside the cells, called the *intracellular fluid* (ICF), accounts for two-thirds of the total body fluid. The fluid in the interstitial and intravascular compartment, called the *extracellular fluid* (ECF), makes up the remaining one-third of the body fluid. The ICF and ECF contain electrolytes that are essential to human life. Examples of electrolytes include sodium, calcium, potassium, magnesium, chloride, and bicarbonate. Electrolytes separate into electrically charged particles called *ions* when dissolved in water, allowing them to conduct an electrical charge. This electrical charge is necessary for metabolic activities and essential to the normal function of all cells. The water balance of the body is regulated by the kidneys through a combination of intrinsic and extrinsic mechanisms. The 1 to 2 liters of water normally taken in each day join the body's fluid volume, and nearly the same amount is normally excreted in urine.

The two intrinsic mechanisms that help maintain the water balance are the glomerular tubular balance (GTB) and the countercurrent mechanism:

- *GTB:* The fluid the tubules receive by glomerular filtration determines the amount they reabsorb or excrete
- *Countercurrent mechanism:* A continuous process of concentrating urine as needed

The extrinsic factors for regulating body water include the thirst mechanism and the antidiuretic hormone (ADH), both of which work together. The most common causes and manifestations of fluid and electrolyte imbalances seen in the clinic include burns, surgery, diabetes mellitus, malignancy, acute alcoholism, socioeconomic status, dehydration, edema, fatigue, blood pressure changes, and congestive heart failure. Dehydration can occur because of poor fluid intake or excess output (profuse sweating, vomiting and diarrhea, diuretics) and can lead to uremia and hypovolemic shock. An excess of body fluids can occur because of excessive intake and disturbances of output, including acute renal failure, congestive heart failure, and cirrhosis.

Acid–Base Imbalances

Normal function of body cells depends on the regulation of hydrogen ion concentration so the levels remain within narrow limits to prevent acid–base imbalances.[54] Acid–base imbalances are recognized clinically as abnormalities of serum pH. Normal serum pH is 7.35 to 7.45 (slightly alkaline). Cell function is seriously undermined when the pH falls to 7.2 or lower or rises to 7.55 or higher. Three physiologic systems act interdependently to preserve normal serum pH:

- Blood buffer systems provide immediate buffering of excess acid or base.
- Excretion of acid by the lungs occurs within hours.
- Excretion of acid or reclamation of base by the kidneys occurs within days.

The four general classes of acid–base imbalance are respiratory acidosis, respiratory alkalosis, metabolic acidosis, and metabolic alkalosis (see Chapter 7).

Urinary Tract Disorders[55]

The genitourinary structures involved with urine excretion are:

- *Upper urinary tract:* Kidney and ureter
- *Lower urinary tract:* Bladder and urethra

Urinary Tract Infections

An infection anywhere along the urinary tract is called a *urinary tract infection* (UTI). UTIs are usually classified as upper or lower according to where they occur along the urinary tract. Lower UTIs are infections of the urethra (*urethritis*) or bladder (*cystitis*); upper UTIs are infections of the kidneys (*pyelonephritis*) or ureters (*ureteritis*).[55] Bacteria almost always cause UTIs, although some viruses, fungi, and parasites can infect the urinary tract as well. Bacteria cause more than 85% of UTIs, from the intestine or vagina.[55] Symptoms of urinary tract infections often include:[55]

- A frequent urge to urinate; despite an intense urge to urinate, only a small amount of urine is passed
- Painful, burning feeling around the bladder or urethra during urination (*dysuria*)
- Complaints of pain unrelated to urinating
- Women may feel an uncomfortable pressure above the pubic bone while men may experience fullness in the rectum
- Urine may look milky or cloudy, or reddish if blood (hematuria) is present
- Fever (this may mean the infection has reached the kidneys)
- Pain in the back or side, below the ribs
- Nausea
- Vomiting

Early detection and treatment of this disorder are important to prevent possible permanent structural damage. In the case of insidious onset of back or shoulder pain, especially with the recent history of any infection, a medical screening examination may be warranted.[55]

Interstitial Cystitis

Interstitial cystitis (IC) is a complex, chronic disorder characterized by an inflamed, or irritated, bladder wall. It can lead to scarring and stiffening of the bladder, decreased bladder capacity, glomerulations (pinpoint bleeding), and, rarely, ulcers in the bladder lining. The symptoms of IC vary from person to person but often resemble the symptoms of a urinary tract infection. Symptoms may include:[56,57]

- Decreased bladder capacity.
- An urgent need to urinate often day and night. These include feelings of pressure, pain, and tenderness around the bladder, pelvis, and perineum (the area between the anus and vagina or anus and scrotum), which may

increase as the bladder fills and decrease as it empties.

- Painful sexual intercourse. In men, discomfort or pain occurs in the penis and scrotum. In most women, the symptoms worsen around the menstrual cycle.

Urinary Incontinence

Urinary incontinence may be defined as an involuntary loss of urine that is sufficient to be a problem and occurs most often when bladder pressure exceeds sphincter resistance. The following four categories can be used to classify urinary incontinence:[55]

- *Functional incontinence:* People who suffer from functional incontinence have normal urine control but are unwilling to maintain it (patients with impaired cognition), or they have difficulty reaching a toilet in time because of muscle or joint dysfunction or environmental barriers.
- *Stress incontinence:* Patients with stress incontinence experience loss of urine during activities that increase intraabdominal pressure, such as coughing, lifting, or laughing.
- *Overflow incontinence:* Patients with overflow incontinence have constant leaking of urine from a bladder that is full but unable to empty due to:
  - Anatomic obstruction—e.g., prostate enlargement.
  - Neurogenic bladder—e.g., spinal cord injury.
- *Urge incontinence:* Patients with urge incontinence have the sudden unexpected urge to urinate and the uncontrolled loss of urine; it is often related to reduced bladder capacity, detrusor instability, or hypersensitive bladder.

Medical management of urinary incontinence is aimed at prevention and may include:

- Nutritional counseling to help prevent constipation and to encourage adequate hydration.
- Medications to relieve urge incontinence: estrogen replacement therapy (ERT), anticholinergics, alpha-adrenergic blockers to increase bladder outlet/sphincteric tone, antispasmodics, and combination therapy with tricyclic antidepressant agents and antidiuretic hormone.[58–62]
- Surgical intervention can include catheterization, penile clamps, and surgically implanted artificial sphincters and bladder generators (which send impulses to the nerves that control the bladder function).

Intervention

PTAs can have an important direct role in the intervention of urge and stress urinary incontinence. The PTA is involved in:

- Patient education. The PTA should:
  - Advise the patient to avoid the Valsalva maneuver
  - Advise the patient to avoid activities that strain the pelvic floor and abdominal muscles
  - Provide education on how to preserve an acceptable skin condition through:[63]
    - Adequate protection (e.g., use of adult diapers, underpads)
    - Maintenance of toileting schedule
- Teaching the patient exercises to improve control of pelvic floor and to maintain abdominal function. These exercises include pelvic floor muscle (pubococcygeal muscle) exercises, particularly exercises that address both fast-twitch and slow-twitch muscle fibers that lead to a significant increase in the force of the urethral closure without an appreciable Valsalva effort.[64–66] The Kegel exercises are typically prescribed:
  - Type 1 works on holding contractions, progressing to 10-second holds, resting 10 seconds between contractions.
  - Type 2 works on quick contractions to shut off urine flow. Patients do 10 to 80 repetitions per day, while avoiding squeezing the buttocks or contracting the abdominals.

The PTA should encourage the patient to incorporate Kegel exercises into everyday life, especially with lifting, coughing, laughing, and changing positions.

- Training the patient in progressive strengthening of pelvic floor musculature, using weighted vaginal cones and the pelvic floor exerciser
- Teaching the patient to use biofeedback to reinforce active contractions and relaxation of bladder[67]
- Use of functional electric stimulation for muscle reeducation of bladder and pelvic floor muscles[67]
- Use of noninvasive pulsed magnetic fields (extracorporeal magnetic innervation) for pelvic floor muscle strengthening[63]
- Providing psychological and emotional support

Renal Disorders[55]

Pyelonephritis

Pyelonephritis is an inflammation of the calycis, which is part of the renal pelvis, and the tubules from within one or both kidneys. *Nephritis* is inflammation of the kidney tissue. *Glomerulonephritis* is inflammation of the glomeruli. Pyelonephritis, which is more common in women than in men, is an infectious inflammatory disease involving the kidney parenchyma and renal pelvis.[55] *Escherichia coli,* a bacterium that is normally found in the large intestine, causes about 90% of cases of pyelonephritis.[68,69] Although urine is typically sterile, the distal end of the urethra is commonly colonized by bacterial flora.[55] In a person with a healthy urinary tract, an infection is prevented from moving up the ureters into the kidneys by the flow of urine washing organisms out and by closure of the ureters at their entrance to the bladder.[68,69] Therefore, any physical obstruction to the flow of urine, such as a structural abnormality, kidney stone, pregnancy, an enlarged prostate, or the backflow (reflux) of urine from the bladder into the ureters increases the likelihood of pyelonephritis.

> ● **Key Point** During pregnancy, the enlarging uterus puts pressure on the ureters, which partially obstructs the normal downward flow of urine. Pregnancy also increases the risk of reflux of urine up the ureters by causing the ureters to dilate and reducing the muscle contractions that propel urine down the ureters into the bladder.[68,70]

The signs and symptoms of pyelonephritis often begin suddenly with chills, fever, pain in the lower part of the back (on either side), nausea, and vomiting.[68,69] In a long-standing infection (*chronic pyelonephritis*), the pain may be vague, and fever may come and go or not occur at all. Chronic pyelonephritis occurs only in people who have major underlying abnormalities, such as a urinary tract obstruction or large kidney stones that persist.[71]

Renal Cell Carcinoma[55]

Adult kidney neoplasms account for approximately 2% of all adult cancers. Tobacco smoking and obesity are established risk factors for renal cell carcinomas. Other risk factors include hypertension, reduced consumption of fruits and vegetables, and occupational exposure to substances such as solvents and asbestos. The initial stages of this condition are generally silent with symptoms associated with metastasis. The classic triad associated with renal cancer consists of hematuria, abdominal or flank pain, and a palpable abdominal mass.

Surgical intervention, including radical nephrectomy and regional lymph node dissection, is the intervention of choice for all resectable tumors. PTAs working primarily with the geriatric population need to be aware of the symptoms and signs of this disease. Questions and history related to hematuria, unexplained weight loss, fatigue, fever, and malaise are important, regardless of the reasons for the physical therapy care.

Renal Cystic Disease

A renal cyst is a cavity filled with fluid or renal tubular elements making up a semisolid material.[55] The four types of renal cystic disease are:[55]

- Polycystic kidney disease
- Medullary sponge kidney
- Acquired cystic disease
- Single or multiple cysts

Renal cysts are usually asymptomatic but may include pain, hematuria, fever, and hypertension. PTAs working with a patient with a history of renal cystic disease should be aware of symptoms and signs suggesting that the condition is worsening (gross hematuria, flank pain, renal colic, or a palpable renal mass).[55]

Renal Calculi

Urinary stone disease is the third most common urinary tract disorder, exceeded only by infections and prostate disease.[55] Clinical manifestations include pain associated with urinary tract obstruction (*renal colic*), which usually occurs once the stone has moved out of the kidney into the ureter. The pain is usually acute and unbearable, located on the flank and upper outer abdominal quadrant.[55] Nausea and vomiting; urinary urgency and frequency; blood in the urine; and cool, clammy skin may also be present.[55]

PTAs need to be aware that depending on where the urinary collecting system is obstructed, the condition may be manifested solely by unilateral back pain ranging from the thoracolumbar junction to the iliac crest.[55]

Acute Renal Failure

In acute renal failure, the ability of the kidneys to excrete waste and regulate the homeostasis of blood volume, pH, and electrolytes worsens over a short period of time (hours to days). There is a rise in serum urea and blood creatinine concentration, and a decrease in the renal plasma clearance of creatinine. This compromise in kidney function can be because of a reduced blood flow through the kidneys (atherosclerosis or inflammation of the renal tubules), ischemia, excessive use of nonsteroidal anti-inflammatory drugs or other toxic substances, or trauma.

Chronic Renal Failure

Chronic renal failure (sometimes referred to as renal insufficiency or kidney failure) can be attributed to various conditions that result in permanent loss of nephrons, which in turn results in a progressive decline of glomerular filtration, tubular reabsorption, and endocrine functions of the kidneys.[55] Diabetes mellitus and controlled or poorly controlled high blood pressure are the two leading causes of chronic renal failure.[55] Other causative disorders include urinary tract obstruction and infection, over-the-counter analgesic drug use, hereditary defects of the kidneys, polycystic kidneys, glomerular disorders, increasing age (65 years and older), and systemic lupus erythematosus.[55] *Uremia* is the term used to describe the clinical manifestations of end-stage renal disease. The symptoms of worsening kidney function are unspecific and might include feeling generally unwell and experiencing a reduced appetite. However, chronic kidney disease may also be identified when it leads to one of its recognized complications, such as cardiovascular disease, anemia, or pericarditis.

Dialysis

Dialysis is the process of diffusing blood across a semipermeable membrane for the removal of toxic substances; fluid maintenance, electrolyte, and acid–base balance in the presence of renal failure. The complications of dialysis are multiple and varied:[55]

- Dialysis disequilibrium, the result of drastic changes at the beginning of dialysis; it is manifested by symptoms of nausea, vomiting, drowsiness, headache, and seizures.
- Dialysis dementia, the result of chronic dialysis treatment; it is manifested by signs and symptoms of cerebral dysfunction, including speech difficulties, mental confusion, seizures, and occasionally death.
- Loss of lean body mass, the result of the catabolism and anorexia associated with progressive renal failure. However, weight gain because of fluid retention can mask this loss of body mass.
- Increased susceptibility to infection. Patients on dialysis are immunosuppressed, and the dialysis process requires vascular access for prolonged periods of time.

- Chest and back pain.
- Myopathy.
- Neuropathy.

Physical Therapy Role with Dialysis
Given the multiple and varied complications associated with dialysis, the PTA must record vital signs regularly while the patient is exercising. The PTA must be careful when taking blood pressure to avoid the dialysis shunts (taking blood pressure at the shunt site is contraindicated) and to avoid trauma to the peritoneal catheters.

Endocrine Disorders

The endocrine system is a system of glands, each of which secretes a type of hormone into the bloodstream to regulate the body. Hormones regulate many functions of an organism, including mood, growth and development, tissue function, and metabolism. The field of study that deals with disorders of endocrine glands is endocrinology, a branch of internal medicine. The major glands of the endocrine system are the hypothalamus, pituitary, thyroid, parathyroids, adrenals, pineal body, and the reproductive organs (ovaries and testes). The pancreas is also a part of this system; it has a role in hormone production as well as in digestion.

- The *hypothalamus* secretes hormones that stimulate or suppress the release of hormones in the pituitary gland and is responsible for regulation of the autonomic nervous system.
- The pituitary often is considered the most important part of the endocrine system because it produces hormones that control many functions of other endocrine glands. When the pituitary gland does not produce one or more of its hormones or not enough of them, the condition is called *hypopituitarism*. The pituitary gland is divided into two parts: the anterior lobe and the posterior lobe, each of which release separate hormones.
- The *thyroid* produces hormones that regulate the body's metabolism and also help maintain normal blood pressure, heart rate, digestion, muscle tone, and reproductive functions.
- The *parathyroid* is made up of two pairs of small glands embedded in the surface of the thyroid gland that release parathyroid hormone, which plays a role in regulating calcium levels in the blood and bone metabolism.

- The *adrenal* glands are located on top of each kidney. The adrenal glands are made up of two parts. The outer part is called the *adrenal cortex*, and the inner part is called the *adrenal medulla*. The outer part produces hormones called *corticosteroids*, which regulate the body's metabolism, the balance of salt and water in the body, the immune system, and sexual function. The inner part, or adrenal medulla, produces hormones called *catecholamines* (for example, adrenaline). These hormones help the body cope with physical and emotional stress by increasing the heart rate and blood pressure.

- The *pineal body* secretes a hormone called *melatonin*, which may help regulate the wake–sleep cycle of the body.

- The *ovaries* produce estrogen and progesterone as well as eggs. These hormones control the development of female characteristics (for example, breast growth), and they are also involved in reproductive functions (for example, menstruation and pregnancy).

- The *testes* secrete hormones called *androgens*, the most important of which is testosterone. Androgen hormones affect many male characteristics (for example, sexual development and growth of facial hair) as well as sperm production.

The clinical manifestations of endocrine and metabolic disorders are fatigue, muscle weakness, and occasionally muscle and joint pain. These complaints may be early manifestations of pancreas dysfunction (diabetes mellitus), thyroid (hypothyroidism, hyperthyroidism, and Graves disease), parathyroid disease (hypoparathyroidism, hyperparathyroidism), pituitary dysfunction, and adrenal dysfunction (Addison disease, Cushing syndrome).

Pancreas Dysfunction

Diabetes Mellitus

Diabetes mellitus (DM) is a chronic disorder of carbohydrates, fats, and protein metabolism that is caused by a deficiency or absence of incident secretion by the beta cells of the pancreas, or by defects of the insulin receptors. DM can be associated with devastating complications. The two basic types of diabetes mellitus are type 1 and type 2.

- *Type 1 (insulin-dependent diabetes mellitus)/ IDDM:* Type 1 DM is caused by a decrease in size and number of islet cells resulting in inadequate production of insulin.[72] Type 1 DM can occur at any age, but typically occurs at less than 25 years of age, and is characterized by the marked inability of the pancreas to secrete insulin because of autoimmune destruction of the beta (islet of Langerhans) cells. Treatment includes exogenous insulin (oral or intramuscular injection), exercise, and diet to regulate blood glucose levels.

- *Type 2 (non-insulin-dependent diabetes mellitus/NIDDM):* Formerly called adult-onset diabetes, type 2 diabetes is characterized by a gradual increase in peripheral insulin resistance with an insulin-secretory defect that varies in severity.[73] For type 2 diabetes to develop, both defects must exist. All overweight individuals have insulin resistance, but only those with an inability to increase beta-cell production of insulin develop diabetes.[73] Patients with type 2 diabetes are often asymptomatic, and their disease remains undiagnosed for many years. Early treatment for type 2 diabetes usually involves a trial of medical nutrition therapy (oral insulin, exercise, and diet).

> ● **Key Point** The distinguishing characteristic of a patient with type 1 DM, versus type 2, is that if the patient's insulin is withdrawn, ketosis and eventually ketoacidosis develop.[72] Therefore, type 1 patients are dependent on insulin injections.

Signs and Symptoms of Diabetes Mellitus

The classic signs and symptoms of DM include:

- Hyperglycemia (raised blood sugar)
- Glycosuria (raised sugar in the urine)
- Polyuria (excessive excretion of urine)
- Polydipsia (excessive thirst)
- Excessive hunger (polyphagia) and weight loss
- Fatigue

The morbidity and mortality associated with diabetes are related to the short- and long-term complications. Complications of DM include:

- Hypoglycemia, which:
  - Is characterized by low blood sugar
  - Usually has a rapid onset (within minutes)
  - Results from failure to eat after taking insulin, or excessive insulin
  - Can be precipitated by exercise
  - Leads to CNS changes (e.g., irritability, headache, blurred vision, slurred speech, difficulty concentrating, confusion, incoordination) and sympathetic changes (e.g., diaphoresis, pallor, piloerection, tachycardia, shakiness, hunger)

- Hypoglycemic coma, a loss of consciousness that results from an abnormally low blood sugar level. If the patient is awake, he or she should be given some form of sugar (fruit juice, candy bar); if the patient is unresponsive, medical intervention is necessary.
- Hyperglycemia, characterized by:
  - Abnormally high blood sugar
  - Gradual onset (within days)
  - CNS changes (e.g., confusion, diminished reflexes, paresthesia)
  - Fruity odor to the breath
  - Weakness
  - Complaints of thirst
  - Rapid and weak pulse
  - Rapid and deep respirations
- The patient may lapse into hypoglycemic coma, which can lead to death.
- Increased risk of infections and skin ulcerations. The capacity of the skin to act as a barrier to infection may be compromised when the reduced sensation of diabetic neuropathy results in unnoticed injury. Sensory neuropathy, atherosclerotic vascular disease, and hyperglycemia all predispose diabetic patients to skin and soft tissue infections. These can affect any skin surface but most commonly involve the feet.
- Microvascular disease and complications (e.g., retinopathy, nephropathy). Diabetes increases the risk of myocardial infarction (MI) twofold in men and fourfold in women, and many patients have other risk factors for MI as well.[74,75] The risk of stroke in diabetic patients is double that of nondiabetic people, and the risk of peripheral vascular disease is four times that of people without diabetes.[74,75]
- Neuropathic complications associated with long-term diabetes and poor glucose control. Of the many types of peripheral and autonomic diabetic neuropathy, distal symmetric sensorimotor polyneuropathy (in a glove-and-stocking distribution) is the most frequent. Besides causing pain in its early stages, this neuropathy eventually results in the loss of peripheral sensation. The combination of decreased sensation and peripheral arterial insufficiency often leads to foot ulceration and eventual amputation.
- Blindness. DM is the major cause of blindness in adults aged 20 to 74 years, as well as the leading cause of nontraumatic lower-extremity amputation and end-stage renal disease (ESRD).

A number of tests are used to confirm the diagnosis of DM:

- Fasting plasma glucose test
- Oral glucose tolerance test
- Random plasma glucose test
- Fingerstick blood glucose test

Intervention

Patient Education
Education of the patient/family member should include:

- Emphasis on proper diabetic foot care—e.g., good footwear, hygiene
- Control of risk factors—e.g., obesity, physical inactivity, prolonged stress, smoking
- Injury prevention strategies
- Self-management strategies

Exercise
Exercise[76–82] is another key ingredient in the overall intervention plan, as it has been shown to delay the disease onset, improve blood glucose levels and circulation, reduce cardiovascular risk, and aid in weight control and strength gains. The patient's exercise tolerance is dependent on the adequacy of disease control. As exercise can produce hypoglycemia, the patient's glucose levels should be taken before and following exercise.

The patient should not exercise without eating at least 2 hours before exercise. As a precaution, the PTA or patient should have a carbohydrate snack readily available during exercise. Adequate hydration needs to be maintained both during and after the exercise session. The patient should not exercise:

- When blood glucose levels are high (at or near 250 mg/dL) or if the blood glucose levels are poorly controlled.
- If a urine test is positive for ketones.

> ● **Key Point** If the respiratory rate and pattern suggest Kussmaul respiration (see Chapter 7), diabetic ketoacidosis must be considered immediately and an appropriate referral made.

Thyroid Disorders

The thyroid gland is located at the base of the neck on both sides of the lower part of the larynx and upper part of the trachea. Thyroid diseases can be broadly divided into hyperthyroidism and hypothyroidism.

Hyperthyroidism

Hyperthyroidism[83–85] results from an imbalance of metabolism caused by overproduction of thyroid hormone (*hyperthyroidism*). Hyperthyroidism or thyrotoxicosis occurs when the thyroid releases too many of its hormones over a short (acute) or long (chronic) period of time. Many diseases and conditions can cause this problem, including:

- Graves disease (accounts for 85% of all cases of hyperthyroidism); Graves disease is an autoimmune disease in which the thyroid is overactive, producing an excessive amount of thyroid hormones
- Noncancerous growths of the thyroid gland
- Tumors of the testes or ovaries
- Inflammation (irritation and swelling) of the thyroid because of viral infections or other causes
- Ingestion of excessive amounts of iodine or excessive amounts of thyroid hormone
- Benign (noncancerous) thyroid disease
- Thyroid cancer

The signs and symptoms of Graves disease, and any other condition causing hyperthyroidism, are numerous and include goiter (enlarged thyroid), Graves ophthalmopathy (protrusion of eyes), pretibial myxedema (lumpy, reddish skin of the lower legs), a rapid or irregular heart rate (palpitations), heat intolerance, hyperactivity/increased energy, hyperreflexia, weight loss, and tremor (usually fine shaking or tremor of the outstretched fingers).

Hyperthyroidism is usually treated with anti-thyroid medications, radioactive iodine (which destroys the thyroid and thus stops the excess production of hormones), or surgery to remove the thyroid.

Hypothyroidism

Hypothyroidism[86–89] is the most common pathologic hormone deficiency. It is usually a primary process resulting from failure of the gland to produce adequate amounts of hormone. It may also be caused by a lack of thyroid hormone secretion secondary to the failure of adequate thyrotropin (i.e., thyroid-stimulating hormone)[90] secretion from the pituitary gland or thyrotropin-releasing hormone (TRH) from the hypothalamus (secondary or tertiary hypothyroidism). Cretinism refers to congenital hypothyroidism. The signs and symptoms associated with hypothyroidism include:

- Weight gain
- Increased appetite
- Lethargy and fatigue
- Low blood pressure
- Cold intolerance
- Dry skin and hair
- Possible exercise intolerance and exercise-induced myalgia.
- Reduced cardiac output

Hypothyroidism is usually treated with lifelong thyroid replacement therapy.

Parathyroid Disorders

When treating a patient with a parathyroid disorder, the PTA must be aware of the various signs and symptoms associated with hyperparathyroidism and hypoparathyroidism.

Hyperparathyroidism[91–94]

Primary hyperparathyroidism (HPT) is defined as an abnormal hypersecretion of parathyroid hormone (PTH), producing hypercalcemia (increased serum levels of calcium) and hyperphosphatemia (increased serum levels of phosphate). Primary HPT is the most common cause of elevated PTH and calcium levels. Approximately 85% of cases are found to be caused by an isolated adenoma, 15% by diffuse hyperplasia, and less than 1% by parathyroid carcinoma.

Secondary HPT is a compensatory hyperfunctioning of the parathyroid glands caused by hypocalcemia or peripheral resistance to PTH. Unlike with primary HPT, treating the underlying cause can reverse secondary HPT. Secondary HPT is often associated with a patient with end-organ failure from chronic renal insufficiency. Less commonly, it may be caused by calcium malabsorption, osteomalacia, vitamin D deficiency, or deranged vitamin D metabolism.

Tertiary HPT occurs in a setting of previous secondary HPT in which the glandular hyperfunction and hypersecretion continue despite correction of the underlying abnormality, as in renal transplantation.

Common manifestations of hyperparathyroidism include weakness and fatigue, depression, bone pain, muscle soreness (myalgias), decreased appetite, feelings of nausea and vomiting, constipation, polyuria, polydipsia, cognitive impairment, and osteoporosis. Treatment for the three different types of hyperparathyroidism varies. Generally, treatment is focused at the hypercalcemia; if symptomatic, patients are sent for surgery to remove the parathyroid tumor (parathyroid adenoma) or parathyroid gland.

Hypoparathyroidism

Hypoparathyroidism[95–97] is an uncommon congenital or acquired (parathyroid surgery or total thyroidectomy) condition in which PTH secretion is deficient or absent, resulting in hypocalcemia. Some cases of hypoparathyroidism, categorized as idiopathic, may have an autoimmune basis and other endocrine deficiencies; T-cell dysfunction may also be involved. Signs and symptoms can include tingling lips, fingers, and toes; muscle cramps; abdominal pain; dry hair and brittle nails; muscle spasms (tetany); and seizures. Severe hypocalcemia, a potentially life-threatening condition, is treated as soon as possible with intravenous calcium. Long-term treatment is calcium and vitamin D3 supplementation.

Pituitary Dysfunction

Hyperpituitarism

Hyperpituitarism is the result of excess secretion of adenohypophyseal trophic hormones. Causes include a functional pituitary tumor, hyperplasias and carcinomas of the adenohypophysis, secretion by nonpituitary tumors and certain hypothalamic disorders. Disorders include acromegaly (enlargement of the facial bone structure, enlarged hands and feet, and visceral overgrowth), galactorrhea (abnormal lactation), and amenorrhea. Treatment is via hormone therapy, surgery, or radiation therapy, depending on the cause.

Hypopituitarism

Hypopituitarism, a rare disorder, involves the decreased secretion of one or more of the eight hormones normally produced by the pituitary gland. The signs and symptoms of hypopituitarism vary, depending on which hormones are undersecreted and on the underlying cause of the abnormality. Typical disorders include delayed growth and puberty, sexual and reproductive disorders, and diabetes insipidus. Most hormones controlled by the secretions of the pituitary can be replaced by tablets or injections.

Intervention

Although patients with pituitary dysfunction are treated medically, the PTA must be aware of any signs and symptoms that would indicate an adverse reaction to the medications, including hypoglycemia, bilateral carpal tunnel syndrome, osteophyte formation, bilateral hemianopsia, and postural (orthostatic) hypotension.

Adrenal Disorders

Located on top of both kidneys, the adrenal glands are triangular and measure approximately half an inch in height and 3 inches in length. The inner part is called the *adrenal medulla,* and the outer portion is called the *adrenal cortex.*

> ● **Key Point** The principal hormones produced by the adrenal cortex are cortisol (hydrocortisone), aldosterone, and dehydroepiandrosterone (DHEA). The adrenal cortex also secretes male sex hormones (androgens), glucocorticoids (e.g., cortisol), and mineralocorticoids (e.g., aldosterone).

Dysfunction of the adrenal cortex can be classified according to hypofunction or hyperfunction.

Hypofunction (Addison Disease)

About 70% of cases of Addison disease[98–101] in the United States are due to idiopathic atrophy of the adrenal cortex, probably caused by autoimmune processes. Addison disease occurs when the adrenal glands do not produce enough of the hormone cortisol and, in some cases, the hormone aldosterone. For this reason, the disease is sometimes called *chronic adrenal insufficiency*, or *hypocortisolism*. The disease is characterized by weight loss, muscle weakness, fatigue, low blood pressure (dizziness and syncope), and sometimes darkening of the skin in both exposed and nonexposed parts of the body. Adrenal crisis, a medical emergency, is characterized by profound asthenia; severe pain in the abdomen, lower back, or legs; peripheral vascular collapse; and, finally, renal shutdown. Treatment typically involves long-term pharmacological intervention using synthetic corticosteroids and mineralocorticoids.

Hyperfunction

Hypersecretion of one or more adrenocortical hormones produces distinct clinical syndromes. Excessive production of androgens results in adrenal virilism.[102,103] In adult women, adrenal virilism is caused by adrenal hyperplasia or an adrenal tumor. Depending on whether a male or a female is affected, the symptoms and signs include hirsutism, baldness, acne, deepening of the voice, amenorrhea, atrophy of the uterus, clitoral hypertrophy, decreased breast size, and increased muscularity.

Hypersecretion of glucocorticoids produces Cushing syndrome.[104–110] Hyperfunction of the adrenal cortex resulting from pituitary adrenocorticotropic hormone (ACTH) excess is referred to as Cushing disease, implying a particular physiologic abnormality. Clinical manifestations include rounded "moon" facies with a plethoric appearance. There is truncal obesity with prominent supraclavicular and dorsal cervical fat pads ("buffalo hump"); the distal extremities and fingers are usually quite slender. Muscle wasting and weakness are present. The skin is thin and atrophic, with poor wound healing and easy bruising. Hypertension, renal calculi, osteoporosis, glucose intolerance, reduced resistance to infection, and psychiatric disturbances are common. Cessation of linear growth is characteristic in children. Females usually have menstrual irregularities. In adrenal tumors, an increased production of androgens, in addition to cortisol, may lead to hypertrichosis, temporal region balding, and other signs of virilism in the female.

Excess aldosterone output results in hyperaldosteronism (aldosteronism).[111-115] Aldosterone secretion is regulated by the renin–angiotensin mechanism and to a lesser extent by ACTH.

- Primary aldosteronism (Conn syndrome) is due to an adenoma, usually unilateral, of the glomerulosa cells of the adrenal cortex or, more rarely, to an adrenal carcinoma or hyperplasia. Hypersecretion of aldosterone is manifested by episodic weakness, paresthesias, transient paralysis, and tetany. Diastolic hypertension with polyuria and polydipsia are common.
- Secondary aldosteronism, an increased production of aldosterone by the adrenal cortex caused by stimuli originating outside the adrenal, mimics the primary condition and is related to hypertension and edematous disorders (e.g., cardiac failure, cirrhosis of the liver with ascites).

Intervention

Although these patients are treated medically, the PTA must be aware of any signs and symptoms that would indicate an adverse reaction to the medications, including signs of stress and exhaustion, postural (orthostatic) hypotension, sleep disturbances, degenerative myopathy, increased incidence of osteoporosis, and delayed wound healing.

Metabolic Disorders

Metabolic disorders are a large group of disorders that include carbohydrate disorders, amino acid metabolism disorders, mitochondrial disorders, porphyrin disorders, steroid metabolism disorders, and lysosomal storage disorders.

Metabolic System Pathology

Metabolic system pathologies affect the ability of the cell to perform critical biochemical reactions that involve the processing or transport of proteins (amino acids), carbohydrates (sugars and starches), or lipids (fatty acids).

Tay–Sachs Disease

Tay–Sachs disease (hexosaminidase A deficiency) is an autosomal recessive genetic disorder. Its most common variant, known as infantile Tay–Sachs disease, causes a relentless deterioration of mental and physical abilities that commences around 6 months of age and usually results in death by the age of 4. It is caused by a genetic defect in a single gene, with one defective copy of that gene inherited from each parent. Population studies have shown that the disease is more common in certain groups, including Ashkenazi Jews, Cajun, and French Canadians. As the disease progresses, the child becomes blind, deaf, and unable to swallow. Muscles begin to atrophy and paralysis sets in. There is currently no treatment for this condition.

Wilson Disease

Wilson disease (hepatolenticular degeneration) is an autosomal recessive genetic disorder in which copper accumulates in tissues, manifesting as neurological or psychiatric symptoms and liver disease. Patients with liver problems tend to come to medical attention earlier, generally as children or teenagers, than those with neurological and psychiatric symptoms, who tend to be in their 20s or older. Some are identified only because relatives have been diagnosed with Wilson disease. It is treated with medication that reduces copper absorption or removes the excess copper from the body, but occasionally a liver transplant is required.

Metabolic Bone Disease

Osteoporosis

Osteoporosis is a systemic skeletal disorder characterized by decreased bone mass and deterioration of bony microarchitecture. Osteoporosis results from a combination of genetic and environmental factors that affect both peak bone mass and the rate of bone loss. These factors include medications, diet, race, sex, lifestyle, and physical activity. Osteoporosis may be either primary or secondary. Primary osteoporosis is subdivided into types 1 and 2.

- Type 1, or postmenopausal, osteoporosis is thought to result from gonadal (i.e., estrogen or testosterone) deficiency. Estrogen or testosterone deficiency, regardless of age of occurrence, results in accelerated bone loss. The exact mechanisms of this bone loss are potentially numerous, but, ultimately, an increased recruitment and responsiveness of osteoclast precursors and an increase in bone resorption, which outpaces bone formation, occurs. After menopause, women experience an accelerated bone loss of 1% to 5% per year for the first 5 to 7 years. The end result is a decrease in trabecular bone and an increased risk of Colles and vertebral fractures.

- Type 2, or senile, osteoporosis occurs in women and men because of decreased formation of bone and decreased renal production of 1,25(OH)2 D3 occurring late in life. The consequence is a loss of cortical and trabecular bone and increased risk for fractures of the hip, long bones, and vertebrae.

Secondary osteoporosis, also called type 3, occurs secondary to medications, especially glucocorticoids, or other conditions that cause increased bone loss by various mechanisms.

> ● **Key Point** Osteopenia (low bone density) may be apparent as radiographic lucency but is not always noticeable until 30% of bone mineral is lost.

Osteomalacia

Osteomalacia is characterized by incomplete mineralization of normal osteoid tissue following closure of the growth plates. *Rickets* is defined as the failure of osteoid to calcify in a growing person or animal. Failure of osteoid to calcify in the adult is called *osteomalacia*. Normal bone mineralization depends on interdependent factors that supply adequate calcium and phosphate to the bones. Clinically, osteomalacia is manifested by progressive generalized bone pain, muscle weakness, hypocalcemia, and pseudofractures. In its late stages, osteomalacia is characterized by a waddling gait.[116]

> ● **Key Point** Vitamin D maintains calcium and phosphate homeostasis through its action on bone, the GI tract, kidneys, and parathyroid glands. Vitamin D may be supplied in the diet or produced from a sterol precursor in the skin following exposure to ultraviolet light. Sequential hydroxylation then is required to produce the metabolically active form of vitamin D.

Intervention

Risk factors for skeletal demineralization include those that are modifiable and those that are nonmodifiable. Because anyone can be at risk for developing osteopenia or osteoporosis, every patient should be questioned regarding family history of bone disease and risk factors for low peak bone mass. In addition, the examination of the patient should include:

- Recording of age, sex, and race
- Questions about current and past medication use; cyclosporine, thyroid hormone, glucocorticoids, and some of the chemotherapeutic medications can cause loss of bone density[117,118]
- Questions about reproductive factors, especially with regard to early menopause and estrogen replacement therapy
- Questions about lifestyle factors associated with decreased bone density—e.g., strenuous exercise (such as occurs in marathon runners) that results in amenorrhea
- Questions about dietary factors, especially calcium and vitamin D intake (important because deficiencies of both increase osteoporosis risk), and eating disorders such as anorexia nervosa
- Posture assessment; increased or increasing thoracic kyphosis may be a sign of multiple painless vertebral compression fractures, which may be associated with osteoporosis
- Height measurements
- Assessment of range of motion, which may be decreased as a result of changes in posture
- Assessment of muscle performance; patients with skeletal demineralization also have weak muscles
- Pain assessment
- Assessment of function in terms of gait, locomotion, and balance

Osteoporosis can occur in either a generalized or a regional form. The cardinal feature is a fracture, and the clinical picture depends on the fracture site. Vertebral fracture often manifests as acute back pain after bending, lifting, or coughing or as asymptomatic progressive kyphosis with loss of height. Most fractures occur in the mid- to lower thoracic or upper lumbar spine. The pain is described variably as sharp, nagging, or dull; movement may exacerbate pain; and, sometimes, pain radiates to the abdomen. Acute pain usually resolves after 4 to 6 weeks. In the setting of multiple fractures with severe kyphosis or dowager hump, the pain may become chronic. When kyphosis becomes severe, the patient may develop a restrictive pattern of respiratory impairment. Forearm, hip, and proximal femoral fractures usually occur after falls, with forward falls often resulting in Colles fractures and backward falls resulting in hip fractures. Rib fractures are most often associated with osteoporosis secondary to corticosteroid use or Cushing syndrome, but they can also be observed with other etiologies.

Medical and screening tests of bone mineral density are available:

- Screening tests include finger densitometry and heel (calcaneal) ultrasonography.
- Medical tests include single photon absorptiometry (SPA) and dual energy x-ray absorptiometry (DXA). Radiographs may show fractures or other conditions, such as osteoarthritis, disk disease, or spondylolisthesis. Osteopenia (low bone density) may be apparent as radiographic lucency but is not always noticeable until 30% of bone mineral is lost.
- BMD testing is the best predictor of fracture risk. Although measurement at any site can be used to assess overall fracture risk, measurement at a particular site is the best predictor of fracture risk at that site.

According to guidelines from the National Osteoporosis Foundation, BMD should be measured in the following people:

- Postmenopausal women older than 65 years because, although preventive measures may no longer be effective, these women are at risk and should be treated if they have osteoporosis.
- Postmenopausal women younger than 65 years who have one or more risk factors.
- Postmenopausal women who present with fragility fractures.
- Women who are considering therapy in which BMD will affect that decision.
- Women who have been on hormone replacement therapy (HRT) for prolonged periods.
- Men who experience fractures after minimal trauma.
- People with evidence of osteopenia on radiographs or a disease known to place them at risk for osteoporosis.

BMD is reported as a T-score, which compares the patient's BMD to that of a healthy young adult.

Physical Therapy Intervention
The physical therapy intervention includes:

- Weight-bearing and aerobic exercise, which have been shown to have a positive effect on BMD, although the exact mechanism is not known.[119–121] Regular exercise should be encouraged in all patients, including children and adolescents, in order to strengthen the skeleton during the maturation process. In addition, exercise also improves agility and balance, thereby reducing the risk of falls.
- Postural correction and training, which should address walking, standing, and sitting.

> **● Key Point** Effective medical therapy is available to help prevent and treat osteoporosis, including gonadal hormone replacement, calcitonin, selective estrogen-receptor modulators, and bisphosphonates.[122] However, these agents reduce bone resorption with little, if any, effect on bone formation.[122]

Paget Disease
Paget disease (*osteitis deformans*) of bone is an osteometabolic disorder. The disease is described as a focal disorder of accelerated skeletal remodeling that may affect one or more bones. This produces a slowly progressive enlargement and deformity of multiple bones. Despite intensive studies and widespread interest, its etiology remains obscure. The pathologic process consists of three phases:

- *Phase I:* An osteolytic phase characterized by prominent bone resorption and hypervascularization.
- *Phase II:* A sclerotic phase reflecting previously increased bone formation, but currently decreased cellular activity and vascularity.
- *Phase III:* A mixed phase with both active bone resorption and compensatory bone formation, resulting in a disorganized skeletal architecture. The bones become spongelike, weakened, and deformed. Complications include pathological fractures, delayed union, progressive skeletal deformities, chronic bone pain, neurological compromise of the peripheral and central nervous systems with facial or ocular nerve compression and spinal stenosis, and Pagetic arthritis.

Involvement of the lumbar spine may produce symptoms of clinical spinal stenosis. Involvement of the cervical and thoracic spine may predispose to myelopathy. Although this disorder may be asymptomatic, when symptoms do occur, they occur insidiously. Paget disease is managed either medically or surgically.

Obstetrics and Gynecology

An obstetrician is a physician who has specialized in the management of pregnancy, labor, and postpartum care.[123] Many terms are used in obstetrics to describe the number of pregnancies and deliveries and the stages of pregnancy, labor, and postpartum phase. A number of physiologic changes occur during pregnancy and the postpartum period within the various body systems that can present the PTA with some unique challenges.

Physiologic Changes During Pregnancy

Endocrine System

Changes that occur in the endocrine system during pregnancy include but are not limited to:

- The adrenal, thyroid, parathyroid, and pituitary glands enlarge.
- Hormone levels increase to support the pregnancy and the placenta, and to prepare the mother's body for labor. During pregnancy a female hormone (relaxin) is released that assists in the softening of the pubic symphysis so that during delivery, the female pelvis can stretch enough to allow birth. However, these hormonal changes are also thought to induce a greater laxity in all joints.[124,125] This can result in:
  - ❑ Joint hypermobility, especially throughout the pelvic ring, which relies heavily on ligamentous support[126]
  - ❑ Symphysis pubic dysfunction (SPD)
  - ❑ Sacroiliac joint dysfunction
  - ❑ Increased susceptibility to injury

Symphysis pubic dysfunction and sacroiliac joint dysfunction are discussed in the section "Complications Associated with Pregnancy."

Musculoskeletal System

The average pregnancy weight gain is 20 to 30 pounds.[127] This weight change can produce a number of changes within the musculoskeletal system:

- The abdominal muscles are stretched and weakened as pregnancy develops (see "Complications Associated with Pregnancy").
- Relative ligamentous laxity, both capsular and extracapsular, develops (refer to previous section).
- The rib cage circumference increases, increasing the subcostal angle and the transverse diameter.
- Pelvic floor weakness can develop with advanced pregnancy and childbirth. This can result in stress incontinence (refer to "Urinary Incontinence").

- Postural changes related to the weight of growing breasts, uterus, and fetus, which can cause a shift in the woman's center of gravity in an anterior and superior direction, resulting in problems with balance. In advanced pregnancy, the patient develops a wider base of support and has increased difficulty with walking, stair climbing, and rapid changes in position. Specific postural changes include:[128]
  - ❑ Thoracic kyphosis with scapular retraction
  - ❑ Increased cervical lordosis and forward head
  - ❑ Increased lumbar lordosis

Due to the alterations in ligament extensibility, postural changes become more significant.

● **Key Point** Pregnant females should be taught correct body mechanics and postural exercises to stretch, strengthen, and train postural muscles.

Neurologic

Swelling and increased fluid volume can cause nerve compression of the thoracic outlet, wrists, or groin (brachial plexus, median nerve, and lateral [femoral] cutaneous nerve of the thigh, respectively).[129–131]

Gastrointestinal

Nausea and vomiting may occur in early pregnancy. They are generally confined to the first 16 weeks of pregnancy but occasionally remain throughout the entire 10 lunar months (see "Complications Associated with Pregnancy").[123,132–135] Other changes related to the gastrointestinal system include:[132–135]

- Slowing of intestinal motility
- Development of constipation, abdominal bloating, and hemorrhoids
- Esophageal reflux
- Heartburn (*pyrosis*); fifty percent to 80% of women report heartburn during pregnancy, with its incidence peaking in the third trimester[123]
- An increase in the incidence and symptoms of gallbladder disease

Respiratory System

Adaptive changes that occur in the pulmonary system during pregnancy include:

- The diaphragm elevates with a widening of the thoracic cage. This results in a predominance of costal versus abdominal breathing.

- Mild increases in tidal volume and oxygen consumption, which is caused by increased respiratory center sensitivity and drive due to the increased oxygen requirement of the fetus.[136] With mild exercise, pregnant women have a greater increase in respiratory frequency and oxygen consumption to meet their greater oxygen demand.[136] As exercise increases to moderate and maximal levels, however, pregnant women demonstrate decreased respiratory frequency, lower tidal volume, and maximal oxygen consumption.[136]
- A compensated respiratory alkalosis (see Chapter 7).[137]
- A low expiratory reserve volume (see Chapter 7). The vital capacity and measures of forced expiration are well preserved.[136,138]

Cardiovascular System

The pregnancy-induced changes in the cardiovascular system (see Chapter 6) develop primarily to meet the increased metabolic demands of the mother and fetus. These include:

- Increased blood volume. It increases progressively from 6 to 8 weeks' gestation (pregnancy) and reaches a maximum at approximately 32 to 34 weeks with little change thereafter.[139] The increased blood volume serves two purposes:[140,141]
  - It facilitates maternal and fetal exchanges of respiratory gases, nutrients, and metabolites.
  - It reduces the impact of maternal blood loss at delivery. Typical losses of 300 to 500 milliliters for vaginal births and 750 to 1000 milliliters for Caesarean sections are thus compensated with the so-called autotransfusion of blood from the contracting uterus.
- Increased plasma volume (40% to 50%). It is relatively greater than that of red cell mass (20% to 30%), resulting in hemodilution and a decrease in hemoglobin concentration. Intake of supplemental iron and folic acid is necessary to restore hemoglobin levels to normal (12 g/dl).[140,142,143]
- Increased cardiac output. Cardia output increases to a similar degree as the blood volume.[140,141] During the first trimester, cardiac output is 30% to 40% higher than in the nonpregnant state.[142] During labor, further increases are seen. The heart is enlarged by both chamber dilation and hypertrophy.

Metabolic System

Because of the increased demand for tissue growth, insulin is elevated from plasma expansion, and blood glucose is reduced for a given insulin load. Fats and minerals are stored for maternal use. The metabolic rate increases during both exercise and pregnancy, resulting in greater heat production. Fetoplacental metabolism generates additional heat, which maintains fetal temperature at 0.5° to 1.0°C (0.9° to 1.8°F) above maternal levels.[144–146]

Renal and Urologic Systems

During pregnancy, the renal threshold for glucose drops because of an increase in the glomerular filtration rate, and there is an increase in sodium and water retention.[123] Anatomic and hormonal changes during pregnancy place the pregnant woman at risk for both lower and upper urinary tract infections and for urinary incontinence.[123] As the fetus grows, stress on the mother's bladder can occur. This can result in urinary incontinence (refer to "Urinary Incontinence").

Complications Associated with Pregnancy

Hypertension

Hypertensive disorders complicating pregnancy (**Table 9-4**) are the most common medical risk factors for maternal morbidity and death related to pregnancy.[123]

Symphysis Pubis Dysfunction and Diastasis Symphysis Pubis

The symptoms of symphysis pubis dysfunction (SPD) and diastasis symphysis pubis (DSP)[147–150] vary from person to person. On examination, the patient typically demonstrates an antalgic, waddling gait. Subjectively, the patient reports pain with any activity that involves lifting one leg at a time or parting the legs. Lifting the leg to put on clothes, getting out of a car, bending over, turning over in bed, sitting down or getting up, walking up stairs, standing on one leg, lifting heavy objects, and walking in general

TABLE 9-4	Summary of Types of Hypertension During Pregnancy
Disorder	**Description**
Gestational hypertension	Characterized by epigastric pain, thrombocytopenia, headache.
Preeclampsia	The more severe the hypertension or proteinuria, the more certain is the severity of preeclampsia; symptoms of eclampsia (such as headache, cerebral visual disturbance, and epigastric pain) can occur.
Eclampsia	Mother may develop abruptio placentae, neurological deficits, aspiration pneumonia, pulmonary edema, cardiopulmonary arrest, acute renal failure; maternal death is possible.
Superimposed preeclampsia on chronic hypertension	Risk of abruptio placentae; fetus at risk for growth restriction and death.
Chronic hypertension	Risk of abruptio placentae; fetus at risk for growth restriction and death; pulmonary edema; hypertensive encephalopathy; renal failure.

Data from Boissonnault JS, Stephenson R: The obstetric patient, in Boissonnault WG (ed): Primary Care for the Physical Therapist: Examination and Triage. St. Louis, Elsevier Saunders, 2005, pp 239–270

are all painful. Patients may also report that the hip joint seems stuck in place, or they describe having to wait for it to "pop into place" before being able to walk. Palpation reveals anterior pubic symphyseal tenderness. Occasional clicking can be felt or heard. The range of hip movements will be limited by pain, and there is an inability to stand on one leg. The amount of symphyseal separation does not always correlate with severity of symptoms or the degree of disability. Therefore, the intervention is based on the severity of symptoms rather than the degree of separation as measured by imaging studies.[151]

> **● Key Point** SPD should always be considered when examining patients in the postpartum period who are experiencing suprapubic, sacroiliac, or thigh pain.

Although the symptoms can be dramatically severe in presentation for SPD and DSP, a conservative management approach is often effective in cases of SPD. In more severe cases, the interventions can include bed rest in the lateral decubitus position, pelvic support with a brace or girdle, ambulation with assistance, or devices such as walkers and graded exercise protocols.[151] In all cases, patient education is extremely important in terms of providing advice on how to avoid stress to the area. Many of the suggestions to give include:

- Use a pillow between the legs when sleeping.
- Move slowly and without sudden movements. Keep the legs and hips parallel

and as symmetrical as possible when moving or turning in standing, and in bed. Silk/satin sheets and night garments may make it easier to turn over in bed.
- A waterbed mattress may be helpful.
- When standing, stand symmetrically, with the weight evenly distributed through both legs. Avoid "straddling" movements.
- Sit down to get dressed, especially when putting on underwear or pants.
- An ice pack may feel soothing and help reduce inflammation in the pubic area.

Swimming may help relieve pressure on the joint (the breaststroke may prove aggravating). Deep-water aerobics or deep-water running using flotation devices may also be helpful.

Resolution of symptoms in approximately 6 to 8 weeks with no lasting sequela is the most common outcome in SDP and DSP.[151] Occasionally, patients report residual pain requiring several months of physical therapy, but long-term impairment is unusual. Surgical intervention is rarely required but may be utilized in cases of inadequate reduction, recurrent diastasis, or persistent symptoms.

Low Back Pain
Low back pain[128,152–159] is said to occur in 50% to 90% of pregnant women. However, it is not clear whether the low back pain is the result of the shift in the center of gravity and concomitant changes in the spinal curvature. Because the annulus is a ligamentous

structure, and therefore softens with the release of relaxin, it could be postulated that the low back pain may be related to structural changes in the intervertebral disk. However, frank disk herniations are no more common during pregnancy than at other times. Thus, the pain is likely mechanical in nature.

> ● **Key Point** It is worth noting that complaints of low back pain during pregnancy may be due to a kidney or urinary tract infection.

Coccydynia

Coccydynia,[160–164] pain in and around the region of the coccyx, is relatively common postpartum. Symptoms include pain with sitting. The patient should be provided with seating adaptation (donut cushion) to lessen the weight on the coccyx and to support the lumbar lordosis.

If symptoms persist for more than a few weeks, the displaced coccyx can often be corrected manually by the physical therapist or physician.

Gestational Diabetes

Gestational diabetes is defined as carbohydrate intolerance of variable severity, with onset or first recognition during pregnancy. After the birth, blood sugars usually return to normal levels; however, frank diabetes often develops later in life. Typical causes include:

- Genetic predisposition; high-risk populations include people of Aboriginal, Hispanic, Asian, or African descent
- Family history of diabetes, gestational diabetes, or glucose intolerance
- Increased tissue resistance to insulin during pregnancy, due to increased levels of estrogen and progesterone

Risk factors include:

- Maternal obesity (> 20% above ideal weight)
- Excessive weight gain during pregnancy
- Low level of high-density-lipoprotein (HDL) cholesterol (< 0.9 mmol/L) or elevated fasting level of triglycerides (> 2.8 mmol/L)
- Hypertension or preeclampsia (risk for gestational diabetes is increased to 10% to 15% when hypertension is diagnosed)
- Maternal age greater than 25 years

Most individuals with gestational diabetes are asymptomatic. However, subjectively the patient may complain of:

- Polydipsia
- Polyuria
- Polyphagia
- Weight loss

Diastasis Recti Abdominis

Diastasis recti abdominis is defined as a lateral separation of greater than two fingertip widths of the two bellies of the rectus abdominis at the linea alba (or linea nigra, in pregnancy) that can occur during pregnancy or delivery. If diastasis recti abdominis is confirmed, corrective exercises need to be performed to prevent further muscle trauma. The patient can perform any exercise that does not increase intraabdominal pressure, including partial sit-ups, posterior pelvic tilts while using hands to support the abdominal wall, and transversus abdominis exercises. Traditional abdominal exercises, such as full sit-ups or bilateral straight leg raises, can be resumed when the separation is less than 2 centimeters and when physician clearance is given.

Cesarean Childbirth

Cesarean delivery, also known as cesarean section, is a major abdominal surgery involving two incisions:

- An incision through the abdominal wall
- An incision involving the uterus to deliver the baby

Although not involved in the surgical procedure, the PTA can play an important role postoperatively:

- TENS can be described to decrease incisional pain (electrodes are placed parallel to the incision).
- The PTA can provide patient education:
  - Demonstrate correct breathing and coughing methods to prevent postsurgical pulmonary complications
  - patient on heavy lifting precautions (for 4 to 6 weeks) and use of pillow for incisional support
  - Instruct patient on transverse fictional massage to prevent incisional adhesions
- The PTA can assist the patient with ambulation.
- The PTA can teach the patient helpful exercises:
  - Postural exercises
  - Pelvic floor exercises
  - Gentle abdominal exercises

Hyperemesis Gravidarum

The causes of this condition are largely unknown. Indications that the patient may have this condition include persistent and excessive nausea and vomiting throughout the day and an inability to keep down any solids or liquids. If the condition is prolonged, the patient may also report:[132,135]

- Fatigue, lethargy
- Headache
- Faintness

Various degrees of dehydration may be present: skin may be pale, there may be dark circles under eyes, eyes may appear sunken, mucous membranes may be dry, and skin turgor may be poor.[132,135]

Supine Hypotension

Supine hypotension (also known as inferior vena cava syndrome) may develop in the supine position, especially after the first trimester. The decrease in blood pressure is thought to be caused by the occlusion of the aorta and inferior vena cava by the increased weight and size of the uterus. Spontaneous recovery usually occurs upon change of maternal position. However, patients should be advised not to stand up quickly to decrease the potential for hypotension. Signs and symptoms of this condition include:

- Bradycardia
- Shortness of breath
- Syncope (fainting)
- Dizziness
- Nausea and vomiting
- Sweating or cold, clammy skin
- Headache
- Numbness in extremities
- Weakness
- Restlessness

Psychiatric Changes

Pregnancy-related depression and postpartum depression may occur. Postnatal depression has been documented to occur in 5% to 20% of all postpartum mothers,[165–167] but it can also occur in fathers.[168] Depressive postpartum disorders range from "postpartum blues," which occurs from 1 to 5 days after birth and lasts for only a few days, to postpartum depression and postpartum psychosis, the latter two of which are more serious conditions and require medical or social intervention to avoid serious ramifications of the family unit.[123,169,170]

Intervention

Given the number of changes that occur during pregnancy and the postpartum period within the various body systems, the extent of the physical therapy intervention will depend on the findings of the examination. Therapeutic exercise plays a key role with this patient population. Objective data on the impact of exercise on the mother, the fetus, and the course of pregnancy are limited, and results of the few studies in humans are often equivocal or contradictory.[171] Both exercise and pregnancy are associated with a high demand for energy. Caloric demands with exercise are even higher. The competing energy demands of the exercising mother and the growing fetus raise the theoretic concern that excessive exercise might adversely affect fetal development.[123] Theoretically, because of the physiologic changes associated with pregnancy, as well as the hemodynamic response to exercise, some precautions should be observed during exercise:[171–178]

- Exercise activity should occur at a moderate rate during a low-risk pregnancy. Guidelines permit women to remain at 50% to 60% of their maximal heart rate (monitored intermittently) for approximately 30 minutes per session. Exercise acts in concert with pregnancy to increase heart rate, stroke volume, and cardiac output. However, during exercise, blood is diverted from abdominal viscera, including the uterus, to supply exercising muscle. The decrease in splanchnic blood flow can reach 50% and raises theoretic concerns about fetal hypoxemia.
- Increases in joint laxity due to changes in hormonal levels may lead to a higher risk of strains or sprains, so weight-bearing exercises should be prescribed judiciously. Abdominal and pelvic discomfort from weight-bearing exercise is most likely secondary to tension on the round ligaments, increased uterine mobility, or pelvic instability.
- Women should avoid becoming overtired and should not exercise in the supine position for more than a few minutes after the first trimester (see "Supine Hypotension").
- Positions that involve abdominal compression (flat prone lying) should be avoided in mid- to late pregnancy.
- Adequate hydration and appropriate ventilation are important in preventing the possible teratogenic effects of overheating. Theoretically, when exercise and pregnancy are combined, a rise in maternal core temperature could decrease fetal heat dissipation to the

mother. Some data suggest a teratogenic potential when maternal temperatures rise above 39.2°C (102.6°F), especially in the first trimester.

> **● Key Point** Warning signs associated with exercise during pregnancy include pain, vaginal bleeding, dizziness or feeling faint, tachycardia, dyspnea, chest pain, and uterine contractions.

Complex Disorders

Complex disorders include poorly understood syndromes that do not fit the traditional allopathic model of illness with specific etiology and pathogenesis.

Chronic Fatigue Syndrome

Chronic fatigue syndrome (CFS)[179–184] is an emerging illness characterized by debilitating fatigue, neurological problems, and a variety of flu-like symptoms. The illness is also known as *chronic fatigue immune dysfunction syndrome* (CFIDS), and outside of the United States it is usually known as *myalgic encephalomyelitis* (ME). In the past, CFS has been known as chronic Epstein–Barr virus (CEBV).

> **● Key Point** TThe eight core symptoms of CFS include:
> - Postexertional malaise lasting more than 24 hours
> - Tender lymph nodes
> - Muscle pain
> - Multiple arthralgias without swelling or redness
> - Substantial impairment in short-term memory or concentration
> - Headaches of a new type, pattern, or severity
> - Sore throat
> - Unrefreshing sleep

In addition to the eight core symptoms of CFS, other signs and symptoms include but are not limited to:

- Jaw pain
- Morning stiffness
- Psychological problems, such as depression, irritability, anxiety disorders, and panic attacks
- Tingling sensations

The degree of severity of CFS can differ widely among patients, and it can also vary over time for the same patient. These variations make CFS difficult to diagnose. The etiology of CFS is not yet known, but it can occur after an infection (cold, flu) or shortly after a period of high stress and can sometimes last for years. The diagnosis of CFS is based on exclusion because no single test confirms its presence. Women are diagnosed with chronic fatigue syndrome two to four times as often as men are. According to the International Chronic Fatigue Syndrome Study Group, a person meets the diagnostic criteria of CFS when unexplained persistent fatigue occurs for 6 months or more with at least four of the eight primary signs and symptoms also present.

Fibromyalgia Syndrome

Fibromyalgia syndrome (FMS) is a chronic muscular endurance disorder, with substantial overlap in major depressive disorder, various anxiety disorders, CFS, and multiple regional pain syndromes.[185–188] FMS affects more women than men (9:1) and occurs in people of all ages.[189–191] The exact cause of fibromyalgia is unknown, although it is associated with any condition that diminishes the endurance of the muscles. Pain is the primary symptom of fibromyalgia, often described as aching or burning. The perceived pain in patients with FM derives partly from a generalized decrease in the pain perception threshold, reflecting discrimination of a nociceptive quality from a non-nociceptive quality (e.g., tactile, thermal), and in the threshold for pain tolerance, reflecting an unwillingness to receive more intense stimulation.[192,193] Underlying these threshold changes is altered processing of nociceptive stimuli in the CNS (central sensitization).[192,193] One characteristic of FMS is the presence of multiple tender points. This refers to specific points in the neck, spine, shoulders, and hips that feel tender. Other symptoms include:

- Fatigue and poor sleep
- Depression
- Headaches
- Alternating diarrhea and constipation
- Numbness and tingling in the hands and feet
- Feelings of weakness
- Short-term memory and cognitive difficulties
- Dizziness
- Difficulty breathing; the diaphragm can be so significantly affected in fibromyalgia to the point that it ceases to function as the major breathing muscle, and the accessory muscles of the neck and upper chest take over[34]

The diagnosis of FMS is based on the history and physical exam, which can help to rule out conditions such as myofascial pain syndrome (see next section), rheumatoid arthritis, muscle inflammation, bursitis, or tendonitis.

The multidisciplinary approach with FMS usually involves:

- Empathetic listening and acknowledgment
- Medications
- Psychologic and behavioral approaches; often if stressful situations are resolved, fibromyalgia may improve and medications may not be necessary
- Chronic pain program
- Nutritional consult: higher levels of protein in the diet are recommended
- Physical therapy (see "Physical Therapy Role in Complex Disorders")

Myofascial Pain Syndrome

Myofascial pain syndrome (MPS) is a common, painful disorder that can affect any skeletal muscles in the body. MPS is characterized by the presence of myofascial trigger points (MTrPs).[194–198] An MTrP is a hyperirritable location, approximately 2 to 5 centimeters in diameter,[199] within a taut band of muscle fibers that is painful when compressed and that can give rise to characteristic referred pain, tenderness, and tightness.[200] The patient's reaction to firm palpation of the MTrP (may include withdrawal, wrinkling of the face, or a verbal response) is a distinguishing characteristic of MPS and is termed a *positive jump sign*.[201] This hyperirritability appears to be a result of sensitization of the chemonociceptors and mechanonociceptors located within the muscle, which can be triggered following a microtrauma or macrotrauma, or a sustained muscle contraction from a postural dysfunction.[202] Thus, MTrPs are typically located in areas that are prone to increased mechanical strain or impaired circulation (e.g., upper trapezius, levator scapulae, infraspinatus, quadratus lumborum, gluteus minimus).

Complex Regional Pain Syndrome

Complex regional pain syndrome (CRPS) is an incompletely understood response of the body to an external stimulus, resulting in pain that usually is non-anatomic and disproportionate to the inciting event or expected healing response. A number of terms were previously used to describe CRPS. These included reflex sympathetic dystrophy (RSD), causalgia, neurodystrophy, shoulder hand syndrome, Sudeck atrophy, and sympathalgia. The terms currently in favor are CRPS I (the equivalent of RSD), which has no history of nerve involvement, and CRPS II, also known as causalgia, which does have nerve involvement. Currently, no specific pathologic, histologic, or biochemical markers of this condition exist.

Efferent sympathetic nervous system overactivity and abnormal activity involving spinal internuncial neurons, peripheral nociceptors, and/or mechanoreceptors have been postulated as an etiology for, or at least as a significant component of, CRPS.

CRPS I affects both men and women, but it is more common in women, and while it can occur at any age, it usually affects people between 40 and 60.

Numerous attempts have been made to relate the various stages of disease to signs and symptoms, but because the course of the disease is so unpredictable, and because overlap is common, staging has been difficult. Nevertheless, understanding the stages provides some insight as to the nature and progression of the disease:

- *Stage 1:* Lasts about 1 to 3 months and involves nonfocal pain, burning, swelling with associated joint stiffness, decreased range of motion, and increased skin temperature.
- *Stage 2:* Lasts about 3 to 6 months. Pain continues but decreases over time. Swelling evolves into thickening of the dermis and fascia. Joint stiffness worsens. Early signs of atrophy and osteoporosis become evident, and the extremity becomes cooler. The nails may begin to deteriorate.
- *Stage 3:* The atrophic stage. Pain continues and atrophy is exacerbated by continued decreased range of motion, increased joint stiffness, and joint deterioration. The extremity is cooler with decreased vascularity.

Unfortunately, a diagnosis of CRPS often is delayed because no specific test for CRPS exists. Radionuclide bone imaging (RNBI) is the only generally accepted imaging technique to provide objective and relatively specific evidence of RSD in the upper and lower extremities, predominantly the hands and feet.

If conservative methods fail, a continuum involving sympathetic nerve blocks, sympathectomy, spinal cord stimulation, and morphine pumps are available.

Physical Therapy Role in Complex Disorders

The typical goals for physical therapy with complex disorders[206–210] include:

- To increase function:
  - Relaxation techniques to improve sleep
  - Energy conservation techniques
  - Ergonomic education
  - Methods to decrease pain and fatigue
  - Soft tissue techniques
- Carefully controlled and graded exercises:
  - Cardiovascular fitness training (e.g., low-impact aerobics, walking, water aerobics, stationary bicycling)
  - Flexibility exercises (e.g., stretching tight and sore muscles)
- Lifestyle changes, such as stress reduction and use of relaxation techniques. Anxiety and depression need to be treated to reduce stress.
- Heat, massage, and myofascial release; these provide anecdotal benefit, but they are passive modalities of questionable long-term benefit that do not promote self-efficacy.

Oncology

Oncology is the branch of medicine that deals with tumors, including study of their development, diagnosis, treatment, and prevention. Cancer refers to a large group of diseases characterized by uncontrolled cell growth and the dispersion of abnormal cells. The cause of cancer varies, and it can include lifestyle factors (tobacco use, alcohol use, sexual and reproductive behavior), ethnicity (Black Americans are diagnosed with, and die, more often of cancer than any other racial group in the United States),[211–214] genetic causes (prostate, breast, ovarian, and colon), dietary causes (obesity, high-fat diet, diet low in vitamins A, C, E) and psychological causes (chronic stress). The causative agents are subdivided into two categories:

- Endogenous (genetic)
- Exogenous (environmental or external): viruses (HIV), chemical agents (tar, soot, asphalt, hydrocarbons, nickel, arsenic), physical agents (radiation, asbestos), drugs (cytotoxic drugs, including steroids), tobacco use

Staging and Grading

After a determination as to the type of cancer, the cancer is graded according to the degree of malignancy and differentiation of malignant cells. Staging is the process of describing the extent of disease at the time of diagnosis in order to aid in treatment planning, predict clinical outcome (prognosis), and compare different treatment approaches.

Stage 0 (carcinoma in situ): The abnormal cells are found only in the first layer of cells of the primary site and do not invade the deeper tissues.

Stage I: Cancer involves the primary site, but has not spread to nearby tissues.

Stage IA: A very small amount of cancer, visible under a microscope, is found deeper in the tissues.

Stage IB: A larger amount of cancer is found in the tissues.

Stage II: Cancer has metastasized to nearby areas but is still inside the primary site.

Stage IIA: Cancer has metastasized beyond the primary site.

Stage IIB: Cancer has metastasized to other tissue around the primary site.

Stage III: Cancer has metastasized throughout the nearby area.

Stage IV: Cancer has metastasized to other parts of the body.

Stage IVA: Cancer has metastasized to organs close to the pelvic area.

Stage IVB: Cancer has metastasized to distant organs, such as the lungs.

Clinical manifestations of cancer include but are not limited to:

- Unusual bleeding or discharge
- A lump or thickening of any area (e.g., breast)
- A sore that does not heal
- A change in bladder or bowel habits
- Hoarseness of voice or persistent cough
- Indigestion or difficulty in swallowing
- Unexplained weight loss
- Night pain not related to movement
- Change in the size or appearance of a wart or mole

The common types of cancer are described in **Table 9-5**.

Prevention is the key with cancer. *Primary prevention* includes screening to identify high-risk people and subsequent reduction or elimination of modifiable risk factors (tobacco and alcohol use, diet). It also includes chemoprevention, which is the use of agents to prevent, inhibit, or reverse cancer (aspirin, lycopene, selenium). *Secondary prevention* is aimed at preventing morbidity and mortality by

TABLE 9-5	Common Types of Cancer	
Type	**Description**	**Treatment Options**
Lung	A disease of uncontrolled cell growth in tissues of the lung.	Treatment for lung cancer depends on the cancer's specific cell type, how far it has spread, and the patient's performance status. Common treatments include surgery, chemotherapy, and radiation therapy.
	The main types of lung cancer are small cell lung carcinoma and non-small cell lung carcinoma. This distinction is important, because the treatment varies; non-small cell lung carcinoma (NSCLC) is sometimes treated with surgery, while small cell lung carcinoma (SCLC) usually responds better to chemotherapy and radiation.	
	The most common cause of lung cancer is long-term exposure to tobacco smoke. The occurrence of lung cancer in nonsmokers is often attributed to a combination of genetic factors, radon gas, asbestos, and air pollution including secondhand smoke. The most common symptoms are shortness of breath, coughing (including coughing up blood), and weight loss.	
Pancreatic	A malignant neoplasm of the pancreas. About 95% of exocrine pancreatic cancers are adenocarcinomas. Common symptoms include: pain in the upper abdomen that typically radiates to the back; loss of appetite and/or nausea and vomiting; significant weight loss; painless jaundice (obstruction of the common bile duct as it runs through the pancreas); diabetes mellitus or elevated blood sugar levels.	The prognosis is relatively poor but has improved; the 3-year survival rate is now about 30%, but less than 5% of those diagnosed are still alive 5 years after diagnosis. Complete remission is still rather rare. Surgical treatment of pancreatic cancer depends on the location and stage of the cancer.

TABLE 9-5	Common Types of Cancer (Continued)	
Type	**Description**	**Treatment Options**
Brain	An intracranial solid neoplasm; a tumor (defined as an abnormal growth of cells) within the brain or the central spinal canal. Brain tumors or intracranial neoplasms can be cancerous (malignant) or noncancerous (benign); however, the definitions of malignant or benign neoplasms differ from those commonly used in other types of cancerous or noncancerous neoplasms in the body. Its threat level depends on a combination of factors, like the type of tumor, its location, its size, and its state of development. Primary (true) brain tumors are commonly located in the posterior cranial fossa in children and in the anterior two-thirds of the cerebral hemispheres in adults, although they can affect any part of the brain. Secondary tumors of the brain are metastatic tumors that invaded the intracranial sphere from cancers primarily located in other organs. The most common types of cancers that bring about secondary tumors of the brain are lung cancer, breast cancer, malignant melanoma (skin cancer), kidney cancer, and cancer of the colon (in decreasing order of frequency). The visibility of signs and symptoms of brain tumors mainly depends on two factors: tumor size (volume) and tumor location.	The prognosis of brain cancer varies based on the type of cancer. The types of treatment available include surgery, radiotherapy, chemotherapy, or any combination thereof.
Colorectal	Includes cancerous growths in the colon, rectum, and appendix (refer to Table 9-1).	Invasive cancers that are confined within the wall of the colon (TNM stages I and II) are curable with surgery. If untreated, they spread to regional lymph nodes (stage III), where up to three-quarters are curable by surgery and chemotherapy. Cancer that metastasizes to distant sites (stage IV) is usually not curable, although chemotherapy can extend survival, and in rare cases, surgery and chemotherapy together have seen patients through to a cure. Radiation is used with rectal cancer.
Prostate	A form of cancer that develops in the prostate, a gland in the male reproductive system. The cancer cells may metastasize from the prostate to other parts of the body, particularly the bones and lymph nodes. Prostate cancer may cause pain, difficulty in urinating, problems during sexual intercourse, or erectile dysfunction.	Treatment options for prostate cancer with intent to cure are primarily surgery, radiation therapy, and proton therapy. Other treatments, such as hormonal therapy, chemotherapy, cryosurgery, and high-intensity focused ultrasound (HIFU) also exist. These treatments are used depending on the clinical scenario and desired outcome. The age and underlying health of the man, the extent of metastasis, and response of the cancer to initial treatment are important in determining the outcome of the disease.
Cervical	A malignant neoplasm of the cervix uteri or cervical area. Human papillomavirus (HPV) infection is a factor in the development of nearly 70% of cases of cervical cancer. The early stages of cervical cancer may be completely asymptomatic. Vaginal bleeding or contact bleeding may indicate the presence of malignancy. Also, moderate pain during sexual intercourse and vaginal discharge are symptoms of cervical cancer. In advanced disease, metastases may be present in the abdomen, lungs, or elsewhere.	Annual pap smear screening can identify potentially precancerous changes. Treatment of high-grade changes can prevent the development of cancer. An HPV vaccine effective against the two strains of HPV that cause the most cervical cancer has been licensed in the United States, Canada, Australia, and the European Union.

using drugs, such as tamoxifen for breast cancer. Tertiary prevention aims to manage symptoms, limit complications, and prevent disability.

Curative methods to treat cancer include surgery, radiation, chemotherapy, and biotherapy. Radiation:

- Destroys cancer cells; inhibits cell growth and division
- Is used to treat localized lesions
- Shrinks tumors and prevents spread
- Is used postoperatively to prevent residual cancer cells from metastasizing

Chemotherapy is the use of drugs that destroy cancer cells. It is given orally, subcutaneously, intramuscularly, intravenously, intrathecally (into the subarachnoid space), or intracavitarily (into a body cavity), depending on its action. Chemotherapy is useful in treating widespread or metastatic disease.

Biotherapy strengthens the host's biological response to tumor cells. There are many types of biotherapy, but it is largely experimental. One type of biotherapy is bone marrow (stem cell) transplantation, which is useful for cancers that are responsive to high doses of chemotherapy or radiation. It provides a method of rescuing bone marrow destruction while allowing high doses of chemotherapy.

Palliative methods to treat cancer include:

- Physical therapy (see below)
- Medications (painkillers, narcotics)
- Acupuncture to provide pain relief
- Alternative medicine
- Hospice care, provided for the terminally ill patient and family/friend

Hospice care has the following characteristics:

- It has a multidisciplinary focus.
- Care can be provided at home or in a hospice center.
- Hospice care encompasses provision of supportive services: emotional, physical, social, spiritual, and financial.

Intervention

The physical therapy intervention varies according to the physical condition of the patient, the stage of cancer, and the cancer treatment the patient is undergoing. Functional deficits are often associated with cancer treatments. These deficits can be caused by the medications, the removal of a diseased organ, or a segmental bone, joint, or limb amputation. Consequently, patients undergoing treatment for cancer may have limited motion, soreness, disuse atrophy, pain, fatigue, sensory loss, weakness, sleep disturbance, and lymphedema.[215] If the patient has undergone surgery, the PTA must be alert for any signs and symptoms of deep vein thrombosis and emboli.

> **● Key Point** As a general guideline, people with cancer should not be treated with electric or deep-heating thermal physical agents (ultrasound in particular), even if the site is distant from the neoplasm.

Because many cancer patients have compromised immune systems, healthcare workers must be vigilant in the practice of standard precautions, especially proper handwashing and infection control principles. Some of the procedural interventions that may be used with this population include:

- Patient and family education on the expected goals, the processes involved, and the expected outcomes of the intervention. The patient and family may require assistance with coping mechanisms and working through the grieving process.
- Proper positioning to prevent or correct deformities, preserve integrity, and provide comfort.
- Edema control: elevation of extremities, active range of motion, massage.
- Pain control: TENS, massage.
- Maintaining or improving:
  - ❏ Loss of range of motion: passive, active-assisted, active range of motion exercises
  - ❏ Loss of muscle mass and strength within patient tolerance, weight-bearing limits, and prescribed guidelines
  - ❏ Activity tolerance and cardiovascular endurance
  - ❏ Independence with ADLs

Psychology

Mental health status has been shown to be one of the most important predictors of physical health.[216–218] Psychosocial factors pertain to the psychological development of an individual in relation to his or her social environment. A number of psychosocial factors can influence the direction of physical therapy intervention.

Anxiety

Anxiety disorders are illnesses related to overwhelming anxiety and fear. The following definitions may help the PTA understand the patient's condition:

- *Panic attack:* Repeated episodes of intense fear that strike often and without warning. Physical symptoms include chest pain, heart palpitations, shortness of breath, dizziness, abdominal distress, feelings of unreality, and fear of dying.
- *Obsessive-compulsive disorder:* Repeated, unwanted thoughts or compulsive behaviors that seem impossible to stop or control.
- *Phobias:* Two major types:
  - *Social phobia:* An overwhelming and disabling fear of scrutiny, embarrassment, or humiliation in social situations, which leads to avoidance of many potentially pleasurable and meaningful activities
  - *Specific phobia:* Extreme, disabling, and irrational fear of something that poses little or no actual danger; the fear leads to avoidance of objects or situations
- *Generalized anxiety disorder:* Constant, exaggerated worrisome thoughts and tension about everyday routine life events and activities, lasting at least 6 months. The patient almost always anticipates the worst even though there is little reason to expect it. The patient also experiences physical symptoms, such as fatigue, trembling, muscle tension, headache, or nausea.

Acute Stress Disorder and Post-Traumatic Stress Disorder

Both acute stress disorder (ASD) and post-traumatic stress disorder (PTSD) are specific forms or subsets of anxiety that occur after experiencing or witnessing a traumatic event, such as rape or other criminal assault, war, child abuse, and natural or human-caused disasters. The symptoms of these conditions can include nightmares, flashbacks, numbing of emotions, depression, hostile behavior, and increased irritability. Family members of victims can also develop this disorder. According to the triple vulnerability model, three vulnerabilities need to be present to develop an anxiety disorder:[219,220]

- A biological vulnerability
- A generalized psychological vulnerability (existing experiences of loss of control over unpredictable events)
- A specific psychological vulnerability that links anxiety to specific situations

Chronic pain frequently occurs concurrently with PTSD, and the occurrence of both disorders tend to negatively affect the treatment outcome for each.[220,221] The main design outcome of treatment for PTSD should be engagement in healthy, satisfying, necessary activities.[220]

Coping/Defense Mechanisms

Coping and defense mechanisms are typically unconscious behaviors by which an individual resolves or conceals complex anxieties. The following are some of the more common coping/defense mechanisms:[220]

- *Acting out:* Use of actions, instead of verbal expressions of feelings, to release stress. Acting out occurs because certain feelings, such as anger and hurt, are too difficult to express verbally.
- *Aim inhibition:* Lowering sights to what seems more achievable.
- *Altruism:* Becoming dedicated to helping others in order to manage one's own stress.
- *Attacking:* Trying to beat down that which is threatening.
- *Avoidance:* Mentally or physically avoiding something that causes distress.
- *Compartmentalization:* Separating conflicting thoughts into separated compartments.
- *Compensation:* Making up for a weakness in one area by gaining strength in another.
- *Conversion:* Subconsciously converting stress into physical symptoms.
- *Denial:* Protecting the ego from being overwhelmed by pain through an unrelenting process of disbelief. The patient refuses to acknowledge that an event has occurred.
- *Devaluation:* Being overly critical of others and of oneself; patient may insult therapists and other personnel.
- *Displacement:* Shifting of an intended action or response to an object onto a less threatening object to minimize stress.
- *Dissociation:* Separating oneself from parts of one's life.
- *Humor:* Minimizing of stress by highlighting the ironic or amusing aspects of a stressful situation.
- *Idealization:* Playing up the good points and ignoring limitations of things desired.
- *Identification:* Copying others to take on their characteristics.
- *Intellectualization:* Using intellectual reasoning rather than expressing emotions in order to avoid painful feelings.
- *Omnipotence:* Feeling or acting as if one is better than others to guard against feelings of inadequacy.

- *Passive aggression:* A deliberate and masked way of expressing hidden anger.
- *Projection:* Transferring of one's own unacceptable feelings, thoughts, and beliefs onto another person; patient becomes certain that the other person really feels, thinks, and believes that way.
- *Rationalization:* Using elaborate explanations to reassure oneself that one's actions are driven by sound motives, when the person may truly be unsure.
- *Regression:* Returning to a childlike state to avoid problems.
- *Repression:* Subconsciously hiding uncomfortable thoughts.
- *Somatization:* Turning physical symptoms into psychological problems.
- *Suppression:* Intentionally avoiding thoughts of disturbing feelings, situations, experiences, or problems in order to reduce stress.
- *Trivializing:* Making small of something that is really big.

Depression

Depression is due to inappropriate (i.e., less selective) environmental responsiveness and defective habituation (i.e., a slower return to baseline functioning following a perturbation). The underlying pathophysiology of depression has not been clearly defined, although clinical and preclinical trials suggest a disturbance in CNS serotonin activity as an important factor. The various conditions associated with depression include:

- Learned helplessness. Humans who are exposed to a major stressor are subsequently unable to learn to escape that stressor.
- Desynchronization of circadian rhythms, which manifests in:
  - Decreased total sleep time
  - Increased sleep onset latency
  - Decreased sleep arousal threshold
  - Increased wakefulness
  - More frequent changes between sleep stages, and terminal insomnia
- Behavioral sensitization. Behavior becomes more severe and occurs more rapidly in response to the same dose of a given psychomotor stimulant.

No physical findings have been found to be specific to depression. In more severe cases, an overall decline in grooming and hygiene can be observed,

as well as a change in weight. In addition, depressed patients may show psychomotor retardation, manifested as a slowing or loss of spontaneous movement and reactivity and a flat affect. If untreated, depression can spiral into greater severity and may result in suicide.[222] Fortunately, a number of medical interventions are available, including psychotherapy, medications, electroconvulsive therapy (ECT), light therapy (for seasonal affective disorder), transcranial magnetic stimulation, and vagus nerve stimulation.

From a physical therapy perspective, depression usually affects performance negatively. Depressed patients may not want to make gains in rehabilitation because of decreased motivation and lack of pleasure in life.[220] PTAs can facilitate motivation by providing encouragement, emphasizing strength, offering positive feedback, addressing values, and mobilizing guilt into goal acquisition.[220]

The Grief Process

Grief, itself, is a normal and natural response to a loss of someone or something (loved one, a job, or possibly a role, such as entering retirement). It is important to realize that acknowledging grief promotes the healing process. There are a variety of ways that individuals respond to loss, some healthy and some that may hinder the grieving process.

> **● Key Point** Factors that can hinder the grieving process include avoidance or minimization of one's emotions, use of alcohol or drugs to self-medicate, and use of work (overfunction at workplace) to avoid feelings.
> Healthy responses to grief include allowing sufficient time to experience thoughts and feelings openly to self; acknowledging and accepting all feelings, both positive and negative; using a journal to document the healing process; confiding in a trusted individual; expressing feelings openly (crying offers a release); identifying any unfinished business and attempting to come to a resolution; and attending bereavement groups (which can provide an opportunity to share grief with others who have experienced similar loss).

The grieving process invariably consists of a series of stages unique to each individual. These stages of grief reflect a variety of reactions that may surface as an individual makes sense of how a loss impacts him or her. Experiencing and accepting all feelings remains an important part of the healing process.

Shock, Numbness, Denial, and Disbelief

Shock usually occurs as the initial reaction to a psychological trauma or severe and sudden physical injury.[220] During stressful situations, individuals express themselves through physiological and emotional responses. These reactions serve to protect the individual from an overwhelming experience.

- Numbness is a normal reaction to an immediate loss and should not be confused with "lack of caring."
- Denial often is used as a defense mechanism to alleviate anxiety and pain associated with a disability or illness.[220] Denial, and feelings of disbelief, occur as a specific phase early in the adaptation process and serve to protect the person from having to confront the overwhelming implications of illness or injury at once.[220] Denial and disbelief will diminish as the individual slowly acknowledges the impact of this loss and accompanying feelings.

Bargaining

At times, individuals may ruminate about what could have been done to prevent the loss. Individuals can become preoccupied about ways that things could have been better, imagining all the things that will never be. This reaction can provide insight into the impact of the loss; however, if not properly resolved, intense feelings of remorse or guilt may hinder the healing process. This phase may be marked by externalized hostility toward other people or objects in the environment.

Depression

After recognizing the true extent of the loss, some individuals may experience depressive symptoms. Sleep and appetite disturbance, lack of energy and concentration, and crying spells are some typical symptoms. Feelings of loneliness, emptiness, isolation, and self-pity can also surface during this phase, contributing to this reactive depression. For many, this phase must be experienced in order to begin reorganizing one's life.

Anger

This reaction usually occurs when an individual feels helpless and powerless. Anger may result from feeling abandoned, occurring in cases of loss through death. Feelings of resentment may occur toward one's higher power or toward life in general for the injustice of this loss. After an individual acknowledges anger, guilt may surface due to expressing these negative feelings.

Acknowledgment

Acknowledgment is the first sign that the patient has accepted or recognized the permanency of the condition and its future implications.[220]

Acceptance

Time allows the individual an opportunity to resolve the range of feelings that surface.

Adjustment

Adjustment is the final phase in adaptation and involves the development of new ways of interacting successfully with others and one's environment.[220]

Elisabeth Kübler Ross's Model of Grief Stages[223]

- *Stage 1:* Shock and denial. It is common for people to avoid making decisions or taking action at this point.
- *Stage 2:* Anger. Making decisions at this point is difficult because all one's energy gets put into the emotion rather than problem solving.
- *Stage 3:* Depression and detachment. Because it is hard to make decisions at this stage, one should consider asking a family member, friend, or professional for help if important decisions need to be made.
- *Stage 4:* Dialogue and bargaining. People become more willing to explore alternatives after expressing their feelings.
- *Stage 5:* Acceptance. Decisions are much easier to make because people have found new purpose and meaning as they have begun to accept the loss.

Physical Therapy Approach During the Grieving Process

The PTA plays a role in supporting the patient during the grieving process. The PTA should:

- Discuss quality-of-life issues with patient/family; realize the phases of terminality are being redefined
- Maintain a positive attitude, but avoid excessive cheerfulness
- Focus on the positive: realize and maximize all clinical opportunities
- Learn to deal with the patient's or family's anger during the discharge crisis
- Realize the importance of comfort measures and pain management to patient/family
- Consistently demonstrate warmth and interest
- Try to engage patient's interest in things
- Respect the needs of privacy, independence, and decathexis (the gradual weakening and separating of emotional ties) on the part of the patient

Empathy Versus Sympathy

Empathy is a powerful communication skill that is often misunderstood and underused. Sympathy, on the other hand, is rarely helpful or therapeutic. Appropriate use of empathy as a communication tool facilitates the clinical interview, increases the efficiency of gathering information, and honors the patient's feelings. The key steps to effective empathy include:

- Establishing the boundaries of the professional relationship while recognizing the potential for strong emotions in the clinical setting (i.e., fear, anger, grief, disappointment)
- Providing an environment conducive to the patient's emotional state, learning, and optimal function
- Setting realistic, meaningful goals and involving the patient and family in the goal-setting process
- Legitimizing the patient's feelings by using statements such as "I can imagine that must be..." or "It sounds like you're upset about..."
- Respecting the patient's effort to cope with the predicament, while recognizing secondary gains or unacceptable behavior; unacceptable behaviors should not be reinforced
- Helping the patient to identify feelings, successful coping strategies, and successful conflict resolutions

Psychosocial Pathologies

Affective Disorders

Affective disorders refer to disorders of mood:

- *Psychosis:* A nonspecific cluster of signs and symptoms that may occur in a broad array of medical, neurologic, and surgical disorders, or as a consequence of pharmacologic treatment, substance abuse, or the withdrawal of drugs and alcohol. There are three major categories of this syndrome:
  - ❑ Schizophrenia
  - ❑ Paranoia
  - ❑ Depression
- *Anxiety disorders:* Apprehension of danger and dread accompanied by restlessness, tension, tachycardia, and dyspnea secondary to an unidentifiable reason. Characterized either by an adherence to fixed, false beliefs outside the normal range of a person's subculture or by a hallucinatory experience, and by a formally defined disorder of thought.
- *Behavioral disturbances:* Manifested in a variety of abnormal actions.
- *Neurosis:* A disorder with anxiety as its primary characteristic. Includes depression, obsessive-compulsive states, and hysteria.
- *Delusion:* Commonly defined as a fixed false belief; used in everyday language to describe a belief that is false, fanciful, or derived from deception. In psychiatry, the definition is necessarily more precise and implies that the belief is pathological (the result of an illness or illness process).

Bipolar Disorder

Bipolar disorder, also known as manic-depressive illness, is one of the most common, severe, and persistent mental illnesses. The condition is characterized by periods of deep, prolonged, and profound depression that alternate with periods of excessively elevated and/or irritable mood known as *mania* (characterized by a decreased need for sleep, pressured speech, increased libido, reckless behavior without regard for consequences, grandiosity, and severe thought disturbances, which may or may not include psychosis). Between these highs and lows, patients usually experience periods of higher functionality and can lead a productive life. The etiology and pathophysiology of bipolar disorder have not been determined. However, twin, family, and adoption studies all indicate strongly that bipolar disorder has a genetic component. There are a wide range of medications that are utilized to treat affective disorders.

Neuroses Disorders

The term *neurosis*, also known as *psychoneurosis* or *neurotic disorder*, is a general term that refers to any mental imbalance that causes distress but does not interfere with rational thought or an individual's ability to function in daily life. There are many different specific forms of neuroses: pyromania, obsessive-compulsive disorder, anxiety neurosis, hysteria (in which anxiety may be discharged through a physical symptom), and just as many signs and symptoms: anxiety, sadness or depression, anger, irritability, mental confusion, low sense of self-worth, phobic avoidance, impulsive and compulsive acts, and unpleasant or disturbing thoughts.

Dissociative Disorders

A dissociative disorder occurs when there is a breakdown of one's perception of one's surroundings, memory, identity, or consciousness. There are four main kinds of dissociative disorders:

- *Dissociative amnesia:* An inability to recall important personal information that is more extensive than can be explained by normal forgetfulness. Remembering such information is usually traumatic or produces stress.
- *Dissociative fugue:* Characterized by sudden, unexpected travels from the home or workplace with an inability to recall some or all of one's past. Some of patients with this condition assume a new identity or are confused about their own identity.
- *Dissociative identity disorder:* Formerly referred to as multiple personality disorder; characterized by the existence of two or more identities or personality traits within a single individual. Patients with this disorder demonstrate transfer of behavioral control among alter identities either by state transitions or by inference and overlap of alters who manifest themselves simultaneously. The disorder is observed in 1% to 3% of the general population.
- *Depersonalization disorder:* Also called derealization; characterized by feelings that the objects of the external environment are changing shape and size, or that people are automated and inhuman. The condition features detachment as a major defense. Depersonalization disorder usually begins in adolescence; typically, patients have continuous symptoms. Onset can be sudden or gradual.

Somatoform Disorders

Somatoform disorders represent a group of disorders characterized by physical symptoms that cannot be fully explained by a medical disorder, substance use, or another mental disorder. These somatoform disorders can challenge medical providers who must distinguish between a physical and psychiatric source for the patient's complaints. It is common to find emotional overtones in the presence of pain. These overtones are thought to result from an inhibition of the pain control mechanisms of the central nervous system from such causes as grief, the side effects of medications, or fear of reinjury. Somatosensory amplification refers to the tendency to experience somatic sensation as intense, noxious, and disturbing. Barsky and colleagues[224] introduced the concept of somatosensory amplification as an important feature of hypochondriasis. Somatosensory amplification is

observed in patients whose extreme anxiety leads to an increase in their perception of pain.

Schizophrenia Disorders

Schizophrenia[225–229] is characterized by hallucinations (visual—seeing images, and auditory—hearing voices) and delusions (e.g., altered beliefs, persecutory or grandiose). There are three subtypes of schizophrenia:

- *Paranoid:* The most common type of schizophrenia in most parts of the world. The clinical picture is dominated by relatively stable, often paranoid, delusions, usually accompanied by hallucinations, particularly of the auditory variety, and perceptual disturbances. Disturbances of affect, volition, and speech, and catatonic symptoms, are not prominent.
- *Disorganized:* Characterized by early age of onset and the presence of pronounced thought and speech disorder, altered affect, and strange behavior.
- *Catatonic:* Characterized by auditory and visual hallucinations and most typically the presence of bizarre motor activity. Immobility, bizarre postures, excessive purposeless movements, and mutism characterize the disease. Other symptoms include: prolonged maintenance of a fixed posture (*catalepsy*), grimacing, parrotlike repetition of a word or phrase just spoken by someone else (*echolalia*), repetitive imitation of the movements of another person (*echopraxia*), stupor or excitement.

REVIEW Questions

1. Name four microorganisms that can cause infections in the human.
2. What are rickettsiae?
3. Which of the microorganisms that can cause infections in the human are not susceptible to antibiotics and cannot be destroyed by pharmacologic means?
4. Creutzfeldt–Jakob disease and bovine spongiform encephalopathy ("mad cow disease") are examples of infection by what type of organism?
5. What are nosocomial infections?
6. Which microorganism is one of the most common pathogens faced in clinical practice, causing many diseases at diverse organ systems, ranging from skin infections to infections of the upper respiratory tract?

7. Of the various types of hepatitis, which types are usually self-limiting?

8. Give three examples of high-risk behaviors associated with transmission of the HIV retrovirus.

9. Which is more pathogenic, influenza A or influenza B?

10. Name three chemicals that can be used for sterilization.

11. True or false: The terms *disinfection* and *sterilization* can be used interchangeably.

12. All of the following statements are true about sickle cell disease, except:
    a. This is a group of inherited, autosomal recessive disorders.
    b. The erythrocytes, particularly hemoglobin S, are crescent or sickle shaped instead of being biconcave.
    c. It is contagious.
    d. The condition is chronic and can be fatal.

13. Give four manifestations of cancer.

14. Endocrine pathologies may result in either over-effects or undereffects of the hormone. All of the following could most likely cause the latter type of effect, except:
    a. Faulty target cell receptors
    b. Endocrine tumors
    c. Aberrant hormone synthesis and/or secretion
    d. Altered transport of the hormone in the blood

15. Which of the following, although it is a benign tumor, can have a drastic effect through the destruction of bone in its immediate vicinity?
    a. Osteogenic sarcoma
    b. Chondroma
    c. Osteoma
    d. Giant cell tumor

16. All of the following are thought to have an auto-immune etiology, except:
    a. Dermatomyositis
    b. Rheumatoid arthritis
    c. Osteomalacia
    d. Multiple sclerosis

17. All of the following are examples of malignant glial cell tumors, except:
    a. Retinoblastoma
    b. Astrocytoma
    c. Medullablastoma
    d. Glioblastoma multiform

18. The following are all causes of cancer except:
    a. A localized decrease in mitotic rate, causing aging of the DNA strands
    b. An altered genome due to a mutation of one or more genes

    c. Selective repression of different genetic operons
    d. Increasing age

19. You are treaing a patient with a tumor in the lumbar region that has been staged using the TNM system. With this system, the letters TNM represent which of the following, in the correct order?
    a. Tumor type, number of tumors, tumor metastasis
    b. Tumor location, lymph node involved, mass size of the tumor
    c. Tumor size, lymph node involvement, tumor metastasis
    d. Tumor mass, number of lymph nodes, major organs involved

20. Which of the following neoplasms is malignant?
    a. Fibroma
    b. Osteoma
    c. Chondroma
    d. Neuroblastoma

21. What is fluid in the interstitial and intravascular compartment called?

22. Which organ regulates body water balance?

23. The lymphoid system is composed of all of the following except:
    a. Spleen
    b. Liver
    c. Thymus
    d. Bone marrow

24. The characteristic cell type involved in a chronic inflammatory process is the:
    a. Mast cell
    b. Polymorphonuclear leukocyte
    c. Lymphocyte
    d. Eisinophil

25. Which of the following neoplasms is benign?
    a. Hemangioma
    b. Fibrosarcoma
    c. Microglia
    d. Adenocarcinoma

26. Clinical features of anemia may include:
    a. Tachycardia
    b. Anorexia
    c. Paresthesias
    d. All of the above

27. Which of the following statement is characteristic of hemophilia?
    a. The platelet count is decreased.
    b. There is a delay in coagulation time.
    c. The clot retraction time is decreased.
    d. There is an increase in fibrinolysis.

28. What is the name given to the type of exercises designed to improve control of pelvic floor and to maintain abdominal function that is used to help prevent urinary incontinence?
29. True or false: Diabetes mellitus (DM) is a chronic disorder of carbohydrate, fat, and protein metabolism that is caused by a deficiency or absence of incident secretion by the beta cells of the pancreas or by defects of the insulin receptors.
30. List four classical signs and symptoms of DM.
31. What is Graves disease?
32. What is Addison disease?
33. During pregnancy, which female hormone is released that assists in the softening of the pubic symphysis so that, during delivery, the female pelvis can stretch enough to allow birth?
34. What are the eight core symptoms of chronic fatigue syndrome?
35. You are treating a patient who is oversuspicious and has delusions of persecution. What personality type do you suspect?
    a. Catatonic
    b. Passive-aggressive
    c. Paranoid
    d. None of the above
36. Which of the following is the most serious or severe form of mental disease?
    a. Psychoneurotic disorders
    b. Psychophysiologic disorders
    c. Psychosomatic disorders
    d. Psychotic disorders
37. Which of the following statements does not apply to the defense mechanism of rationalization?
    a. It is one of the most defense mechanisms used by the ego.
    b. The original affect for one object is transferred to another object.
    c. It is used to a certain extent by nearly everyone.
    d. All of the above.
38. The defense mechanism that unconsciously transfers normal body movements to abnormal is called:
    a. Conversion
    b. Rationalization
    c. Regression
    d. Isolation
39. All of the following statements apply to schizophrenia except:
    a. There is a disconnect with reality.
    b. It usually begins at about middle age.

c. The onset may be sudden or it may be gradual.
d. Unconscious material is no longer repressed by the ego.

40. Which of the following is an example of a sensory disturbance developing as a conversion reaction?
    a. A pattern of paresthesia following a dermatome distribution
    b. A pattern of muscle weakness following a myotomal distribution
    c. Stocking-like distribution of anesthesia over an extremity
    d. None of the above
41. A condition of pathological overeating is called:
    a. Polydipsia
    b. Dysphagia
    c. Bulimia
    d. Emesis

References

1. Bass JW, Wittler RR, Weisse ME: Social smile and occult bacteremia. Pediatr Infect Dis J 15:541, 1996
2. Goodman CC, Kelly Snyder TE: Infectious disease, in Goodman CC, Boissonnault WG, Fuller KS (eds): Pathology: Implications for the Physical Therapist (ed 2). Philadelphia, Saunders, 2003, pp 194–235
3. Human nutrition and parasitic infection. Parasitology 107 Suppl:S1–203, 1993
4. Protection and pathology in parasitic infection. Parasite Immunol 22:595, 2000
5. Stear MJ, Wakelin D: Genetic resistance to parasitic infection. Rev Sci Tech 17:143–153, 1998
6. Eady EA, Cove JH: Staphylococcal resistance revisited: Community-acquired methicillin resistant *Staphylococcus aureus*—an emerging problem for the management of skin and soft tissue infections. Curr Opin Infect Dis 16:103–124, 2003
7. Brogan TV, Nizet V, Waldhausen JH: Streptococcal skin infections. N Engl J Med 334:1478, 1996
8. Duggan JM, Georgiadis G, VanGorp C, et al: Group B streptococcal prosthetic joint infections. J South Orthop Assoc 10:209–214; discussion 214, 2001
9. Edwards MS, Baker CJ: Group B streptococcal infections in elderly adults. Clin Infect Dis 41:839–847, 2005
10. Ekelund K, Skinhoj P, Madsen J, et al: Invasive group A, B, C and G streptococcal infections in Denmark 1999–2002: Epidemiological and clinical aspects. Clin Microbiol Infect 11:569–576, 2005
11. Gotoff SP: Group B streptococcal infections. Pediatr Rev 23:381–386, 2002
12. Jaggi P, Shulman ST: Group A streptococcal infections. Pediatr Rev 27:99–105, 2006
13. Lee NY, Yan JJ, Wu JJ, et al: Group B streptococcal soft tissue infections in non-pregnant adults. Clin Microbiol Infect 11:577–579, 2005

14. Mulla ZD: Group A streptococcal infections in long-term care facilities. Am J Infect Control 33:375–376, 2005

15. Weir E, Main C: Invasive group A streptococcal infections. CMAJ 175:32, 2006

16. Amaro R, Schiff ER: Viral hepatitis. Curr Opin Gastroenterol 17:262–267, 2001

17. Gonzalez-Aseguinolaza G, Crettaz J, Ochoa L, et al: Gene therapy for viral hepatitis. Expert Opin Biol Ther 6:1263–1278, 2006

18. Mallat D, Schiff E: Viral hepatitis. Curr Opin Gastroenterol 16:255–261, 2000

19. Marrero R, Schiff E: Viral hepatitis. Curr Opin Gastroenterol 18:330–333, 2002

20. Regev A, Schiff ER: Viral hepatitis. Curr Opin Gastroenterol 15:234–239, 1999

21. Rehermann B, Naoumov NV: Immunological techniques in viral hepatitis. J Hepatol 46:508–520, 2007

22. Trepo C, Zoulim F, Pradat P: Viral hepatitis. Curr Opin Infect Dis 12:481–490, 1999

23. Achord JL: Acute pancreatitis with infectious hepatitis. JAMA 205:837–840, 1968

24. Canosa CA, Gosalvez JA, Abeledo G, et al: Acute infectious hepatitis: Clinical and epidemiological study. Helv Paediatr Acta 32:21–28, 1977

25. Parana R, Codes L, Andrade Z, et al: Clinical, histologic and serologic evaluation of patients with acute non-A-E hepatitis in north-eastern Brazil: Is it an infectious disease? Int J Infect Dis 7:222–230, 2003

26. Tabor E, April M, Seeff LB, et al: Acute non-A, non-B hepatitis: Prolonged presence of the infectious agent in blood. Gastroenterology 76:680–684, 1979

27. Liu CJ, Kao JH: Hepatitis B virus-related hepatocellular carcinoma: Epidemiology and pathogenic role of viral factors. J Chin Med Assoc 70:141–145, 2007

28. Modi AA, Feld JJ: Viral hepatitis and HIV in Africa. AIDS Rev 9:25–39, 2007

29. Wu CA, Lin SY, So SK, et al: Hepatitis B and liver cancer knowledge and preventive practices among Asian Americans in the San Francisco Bay Area, California. Asian Pac J Cancer Prev 8:127–134, 2007

30. Camarero C, Ramos N, Moreno A, et al: Hepatitis C virus infection acquired in childhood. Eur J Pediatr 2007

31. Hahn JA: Sex, drugs, and hepatitis C virus. J Infect Dis 195:1556–1559, 2007

32. Dalton HR, Fellows HJ, Gane EJ, et al: Hepatitis E in New Zealand. J Gastroenterol Hepatol 22:1236–1240, 2007

33. Wong KH, Lee SS, Chan KC: Twenty years of clinical human immunodeficiency virus (HIV) and acquired immunodeficiency syndrome (AIDS) in Hong Kong. Hong Kong Med J 12:133–140, 2006

34. Goodman CC: The immune system, in Goodman CC, Boissonnault WG, Fuller KS (eds): Pathology: Implications for the Physical Therapist (ed 2). Philadelphia, Saunders, 2003, pp 153–193

35. Goodman CC: The hematologic system, in Goodman CC, Boissonnault WG, Fuller KS (eds): Pathology: Implications for the Physical Therapist (ed 2). Philadelphia, Saunders, 2003, pp 509–552

36. Beaton MD, Adams PC: The myths and realities of hemochromatosis. Can J Gastroenterol 21:101–104, 2007

37. Davies MB, Saxby T: Ankle arthropathy of hemochromatosis: A case series and review of the literature. Foot Ankle Int 27:902–906, 2006

38. de Gheldere A, Ndjoko R, Docquier PL, et al: Orthopaedic complications associated with sickle-cell disease. Acta Orthop Belg 72:741–747, 2006

39. Sarrai M, Duroseau H, D'Augustine J, et al: Bone mass density in adults with sickle cell disease. Br J Haematol 11:11, 2007

40. Yoon SL, Black S: Comprehensive, integrative management of pain for patients with sickle-cell disease. J Altern Complement Med 12:995–1001, 2006

41. Sathappan SS, Ginat D, Di Cesare PE: Multidisciplinary management of orthopedic patients with sickle cell disease. Orthopedics 29:1094–1101; quiz 1102–1103, 2006

42. Schafer AI: Thrombocytosis: When is an incidental finding serious? Cleve Clin J Med 73:767–774, 2006

43. Vlacha V, Feketea G: Thrombocytosis in pediatric patients is associated with severe lower respiratory tract inflammation. Arch Med Res 37:755–759, 2006

44. Papageorgiou T, Theodoridou A, Kourti M, et al: Childhood essential thrombocytosis. Pediatr Blood Cancer 47:970–971, 2006

45. Dan K: Thrombocytosis in iron deficiency anemia. Intern Med 44:1025–1026, 2005

46. Salacz ME, Lankiewicz MW, Weissman DE: Management of thrombocytopenia in bone marrow failure: A review. J Palliat Med 10:236–244, 2007

47. Li X, Swisher KK, Vesely SK, et al: Drug-induced thrombocytopenia: an updated systematic review, 2006. Drug Saf 30:185–186, 2007

48. Murphy MF, Bussel JB: Advances in the management of alloimmune thrombocytopenia. Br J Haematol 136:366–378, 2007

49. Girolami B, Girolami A: Heparin-induced thrombocytopenia: A review. Semin Thromb Hemost 32:803–809, 2006

50. Marengo-Rowe AJ: The thalassemias and related disorders. Proc (Bayl Univ Med Cent) 20:27–31, 2007

51. Al-Jahdali H, Al-Shimemeri A, Bamefleh H, et al: Pulmonary histiocytosis X. Ann Saudi Med 18:437–439, 1998

52. de Brito Macedo Ferreira LM, de Carvalho JD, Pereira ST, et al: Histiocytosis X of the temporal bone. Rev Bras Otorrinolaringol (Engl ed) 72:575, 2006

53. Rizvi RM, Nasreen C, Jafri N: Histiocytosis X of the vulva. J Pak Med Assoc 52:430, 2002

54. Goodman CC, Snyder TK: Problems affecting multiple systems, in Goodman CC, Boissonnault WG, Fuller KS (eds): Pathology: Implications for the Physical Therapist (ed 2). Philadelphia, Saunders, 2003, pp 85–119

55. Boissonnault WG, Goodman CC: The renal and urologic systems, in Goodman CC, Boissonnault WG, Fuller KS (eds): Pathology: Implications for the Physical Therapist (ed 2). Philadelphia, Saunders, 2003, pp 704–728

56. Kelada E, Jones A: Interstitial cystitis. Arch Gynecol Obstet 22:22, 2006

57. Sant GR: Etiology, pathogenesis, and diagnosis of interstitial cystitis. Rev Urol 4:S9–S15, 2002

58. Urinary incontinence. Know your drug options. Mayo Clin Health Lett 23:6, 2005

59. Blackwell RE: Estrogen, progestin, and urinary incontinence. JAMA 294:2696–2697; author reply 2697–2698, 2005
60. Bren L: Controlling urinary incontinence. FDA Consum 39:10–15, 2005
61. Castro-Diaz D, Amoros MA: Pharmacotherapy for stress urinary incontinence. Curr Opin Urol 15:227–230, 2005
62. Kelleher C, Cardozo L, Kobashi K, et al: Solifenacin: As effective in mixed urinary incontinence as in urge urinary incontinence. Int Urogynecol J Pelvic Floor Dysfunct 17:382–388, 2006
63. Wilson MM: Urinary incontinence: selected current concepts. Med Clin North Am 90:825–836, 2006
64. Borello-France DF, Zyczynski HM, Downey PA, et al: Effect of pelvic-floor muscle exercise position on continence and quality-of-life outcomes in women with stress urinary incontinence. Phys Ther 86:974–986, 2006
65. Neumann PB, Grimmer KA, Deenadayalan Y: Pelvic floor muscle training and adjunctive therapies for the treatment of stress urinary incontinence in women: A systematic review. BMC Womens Health 6:11, 2006
66. Hay-Smith EJ, Dumoulin C: Pelvic floor muscle training versus no treatment, or inactive control treatments, for urinary incontinence in women. Cochrane Database Syst Rev CD005654, 2006
67. Anders K: Treatments for stress urinary incontinence. Nurs Times 102:55–57, 2006
68. Berger RE: Risk factors associated with acute pyelonephritis in healthy women. J Urol 174:1841, 2005
69. Ramakrishnan K, Scheid DC: Diagnosis and management of acute pyelonephritis in adults. Am Fam Physician 71:933–942, 2005
70. Hill JB, Sheffield JS, McIntire DD, et al: Acute pyelonephritis in pregnancy. Obstet Gynecol 105:18–23, 2005
71. Rollino C, Boero R, Ferro M, et al: Acute pyelonephritis: Analysis of 52 cases. Ren Fail 24:601–608, 2002
72. Toni S, Reali MF, Barni F, et al: Managing insulin therapy during exercise in type 1 diabetes mellitus. Acta Biomed 77 Suppl 1:34–40, 2006
73. Davies MJ: The prevention of type 2 diabetes mellitus. Clin Med 3:470–474, 2003
74. Maier B, Thimme W, Kallischnigg G, et al: Does diabetes mellitus explain the higher hospital mortality of women with acute myocardial infarction? Results from the Berlin Myocardial Infarction Registry. J Investig Med 54:143–151, 2006
75. Toyoda K, Nakano A, Fujibayashi Y, et al: Diabetes mellitus impairs myocardial oxygen metabolism even in non-infarct-related areas in patients with acute myocardial infarction. Int J Cardiol 115:297–304, 2007
76. Cayley WE: The role of exercise in patients with type 2 diabetes. Am Fam Physician 75:335–336, 2007
77. Gaesser GA: Exercise for prevention and treatment of cardiovascular disease, type 2 diabetes, and metabolic syndrome. Curr Diab Rep 7:14–19, 2007
78. Carrier J: Review: Exercise improves glycaemic control and reduces plasma triglycerides and visceral adipose tissue in type 2 diabetes. Evid Based Nurs 10:11, 2007
79. Follow these exercise guidelines to manage type 2 diabetes. Health News 12:12, 2006
80. Feher M: Exercise and sport in diabetes. J Hum Hypertens 20:907, 2006
81. Cauza E, Hanusch-Enserer U, Strasser B, et al: The metabolic effects of long term exercise in Type 2 Diabetes patients. Wien Med Wochenschr 156:515–519, 2006
82. Chipkin SR, Klugh SA, Chasan-Taber L: Exercise and diabetes. Cardiol Clin 19:489–505, 2001
83. Welch TR: Hyperthyroidism: Impact on bone. J Pediatr 150:a3, 2007
84. Maji D: Hyperthyroidism. J Indian Med Assoc 104:563–564, 566–567, 2006
85. Cooper DS: Approach to the patient with subclinical hyperthyroidism. J Clin Endocrinol Metab 92:3–9, 2007
86. Sutandar M, Garcia-Bournissen F, Koren G: Hypothyroidism in pregnancy. J Obstet Gynaecol Can 29:354–356, 2007
87. Lazarus JH: Aspects of treatment of subclinical hypothyroidism. Thyroid 17:313–316, 2007
88. Bungard TJ, Hurlburt M: Management of hypothyroidism during pregnancy. CMAJ 176:1077–1078, 2007
89. Jayakumar RV: Hypothyroidism. J Indian Med Assoc 104:557–560, 562, 2006
90. Zack MB, Fulkerson LL, Hartshorne G, et al: Clinical evaluation of stabilized and nonstabilized PPD-B in patients with group 3 atypical mycobacteria. Chest 63:348–352, 1973
91. Hamidi S, Soltani A, Hedayat A, et al: Primary hyperparathyroidism: A review of 177 cases. Med Sci Monit 12:CR86–89, 2006
92. Mikhail N, Cope D: Evaluation and treatment of primary hyperparathyroidism. JAMA 294:2700, 2005
93. Grey A, Bolland M, Reid IR: Evaluation and treatment of primary hyperparathyroidism. Jama 294:2699–2700, 2005
94. Thaunat M, Gaudin P, Naret C, et al: Role of secondary hyperparathyroidism in spontaneous rupture of the quadriceps tendon complicating chronic renal failure. Rheumatology (Oxford) 45:234–235, 2006
95. Maeda SS, Fortes EM, Oliveira UM, et al: Hypoparathyroidism and pseudohypoparathyroidism. Arq Bras Endocrinol Metabol 50:664–673, 2006
96. Korkmaz C, Yasar S, Binboga A: Hypoparathyroidism simulating ankylosing spondylitis. Joint Bone Spine 72:89–91, 2005
97. De Sanctis C, De Sanctis V, Radetti G, et al: Hypoparathyroidism and pseudohypoparathyroidism. Minerva Pediatr 54:271–278, 2002
98. Nieman LK, Chanco Turner ML: Addison's disease. Clin Dermatol 24:276–280, 2006
99. Lovas K, Husebye ES: Addison's disease. Lancet 365:2058–2061, 2005
100. Marzotti S, Falorni A: Addison's disease. Autoimmunity 37:333–336, 2004
101. Chhangani NP, Sharma P: Addison's disease. Indian Pediatr 40:904–905, 2003
102. Riddick DH, Hammond CB: Adrenal virilism due to 21-hydroxylase deficiency in the postmenarchial female. Obstet Gynecol 45:21–24, 1975
103. David RR: Adrenal virilism in childhood. Ann N Y Acad Sci 142:787–793, 1967
104. Storr HL, Chan LF, Grossman AB, et al: Paediatric Cushing's syndrome: epidemiology, investigation and therapeutic advances. Trends Endocrinol Metab 18:167–174, 2007

105. Makras P, Toloumis G, Papadogias D, et al: The diagnosis and differential diagnosis of endogenous Cushing's syndrome. Hormones (Athens) 5:231–250, 2006

106. Magiakou MA, Smyrnaki P, Chrousos GP: Hypertension in Cushing's syndrome. Best Pract Res Clin Endocrinol Metab 20:467–482, 2006

107. Elte JW: Diagnosis of Cushing's syndrome. Eur J Intern Med 17:311–312, 2006

108. Shibli-Rahhal A, Van Beek M, Schlechte JA: Cushing's syndrome. Clin Dermatol 24:260–265, 2006

109. Newell-Price J, Bertagna X, Grossman AB, et al: Cushing's syndrome. Lancet 367:1605–1617, 2006

110. Miyachi Y: Pathophysiology and diagnosis of Cushing's syndrome. Biomed Pharmacother 54 Suppl 1:113s–117s, 2000

111. Nadar S, Lip GY, Beevers DG: Primary hyperaldosteronism. Ann Clin Biochem 40:439–452, 2003

112. Quinkler M, Lepenies J, Diederich S: Primary hyperaldosteronism. Exp Clin Endocrinol Diabetes 110:263–271, 2002

113. Stowasser M: Hyperaldosteronism: primary versus tertiary. J Hypertens 20:17–19, 2002

114. Stowasser M, Gordon RD: Familial hyperaldosteronism. J Steroid Biochem Mol Biol 78:215–229, 2001

115. Soule S, Davidson JS, Rayner BL: The evaluation of primary hyperaldosteronism. S Afr Med J 90:387–394, 2000

116. Basha B, Rao DS, Han ZH, et al: Osteomalacia due to vitamin D depletion: A neglected consequence of intestinal malabsorption. Am J Med 108:296–300, 2000

117. Briot K: [Non-corticosteroid drug-induced metabolic bone disease]. Presse Med 35:1579–1583, 2006

118. Wolinsky-Friedland M: Drug-induced metabolic bone disease. Endocrinol Metab Clin North Am 24:395–420, 1995

119. Bonaiuti D, Shea B, Iovine R, et al: Exercise for preventing and treating osteoporosis in postmenopausal women. Cochrane Database Syst Rev 3, 2002

120. Marcus R: Role of exercise in preventing and treating osteoporosis. Rheum Dis Clin North Am 27:131–141, vi, 2001

121. Shea B, Bonaiuti D, Iovine R, et al: Cochrane Review on exercise for preventing and treating osteoporosis in postmenopausal women. Eura Medicophys 40:199–209, 2004

122. O'Connell MB: Prescription drug therapies for prevention and treatment of postmenopausal osteoporosis. J Manag Care Pharm 12:S10–19; quiz S26–28, 2006

123. Boissonnault JS, Stephenson R: The obstetric patient, in Boissonnault WG (ed): Primary Care for the Physical Therapist: Examination and Triage. St. Louis, Elsevier Saunders, 2005, pp 239–270

124. Lee HY, Zhao S, Fields PA, et al: Clinical use of relaxin to facilitate birth: Reasons for investigating the premise. Ann N Y Acad Sci 1041:351–366, 2005

125. Lubahn J, Ivance D, Konieczko E, et al: Immunohistochemical detection of relaxin binding to the volar oblique ligament. J Hand Surg [Am] 31:80–84, 2006

126. Goldsmith LT, Weiss G, Steinetz BG: Relaxin and its role in pregnancy. Endocrinol Metab Clin North Am 24:171–186, 1995

127. Wiles R: The views of women of above average weight about appropriate weight gain in pregnancy. Midwifery 14:254–260, 1998

128. Moore K, Dumas GA, Reid JG: Postural changes associated with pregnancy and their relationship with low back pain. Clin Biomech (Bristol, Avon) 5:169–174, 1990

129. Noronha A: Neurologic disorders during pregnancy and the puerperium. Clin Perinatol 12:695–713, 1985

130. Godfrey CM: Carpal tunnel syndrome in pregnancy. Can Med Assoc J 129:928, 1983

131. Graham JG: Neurological complications of pregnancy and anaesthesia. Clin Obstet Gynaecol 9:333–350, 1982

132. Lamondy AM: Managing hyperemesis gravidarum. Nursing 37:66–68, 2007

133. Dodds L, Fell DB, Joseph KS, et al: Outcomes of pregnancies complicated by hyperemesis gravidarum. Obstet Gynecol 107:285–292, 2006

134. Fell DB, Dodds L, Joseph KS, et al: Risk factors for hyperemesis gravidarum requiring hospital admission during pregnancy. Obstet Gynecol 107:277–284, 2006

135. Loh KY, Sivalingam N: Understanding hyperemesis gravidarum. Med J Malaysia 60:394–399; quiz 400, 2005

136. Wise RA, Polito AJ, Krishnan V: Respiratory physiologic changes in pregnancy. Immunol Allergy Clin North Am 26:1–12, 2006

137. Prowse CM, Gaensler EA: Respiratory and acid-base changes during pregnancy. Anesthesiology 26:381–392, 1965

138. Bonica JJ: Maternal respiratory changes during pregnancy and parturition. Clin Anesth 10:1–19, 1974

139. Sadaniantz A, Kocheril AG, Emaus SP, et al: Cardiovascular changes in pregnancy evaluated by two-dimensional and Doppler echocardiography. J Am Soc Echocardiogr 5:253–258, 1992

140. Atkins AF, Watt JM, Milan P, et al: A longitudinal study of cardiovascular dynamic changes throughout pregnancy. Eur J Obstet Gynecol Reprod Biol 12:215–224, 1981

141. Chesley LC: Cardiovascular changes in pregnancy. Obstet Gynecol Annu 4:71–97, 1975

142. Capeless EL, Clapp JF: Cardiovascular changes in early phase of pregnancy. Am J Obstet Gynecol 161:1449–1453, 1989

143. Walters WA, Lim YL: Changes in the materal cardiovascular system during human pregnancy. Surg Gynecol Obstet 131:765–784, 1970

144. Urman BC, McComb PF: A biphasic basal body temperature record during pregnancy. Acta Eur Fertil 20:371–372, 1989

145. Grant A, Mc BW: The 100 day basal body temperature graph in early pregnancy. Med J Aust 46:458–460, 1959

146. Siegler AM: Basal body temperature in pregnancy. Obstet Gynecol 5:830–832, 1955

147. Depledge J, McNair PJ, Keal-Smith C, et al: Management of symphysis pubis dysfunction during pregnancy using exercise and pelvic support belts. Phys Ther 85:1290–1300, 2005

148. Leadbetter RE, Mawer D, Lindow SW: Symphysis pubis dysfunction: A review of the literature. J Matern Fetal Neonatal Med 16:349–354, 2004

149. Owens K, Pearson A, Mason G: Symphysis pubis dysfunction: A cause of significant obstetric morbidity. Eur J Obstet Gynecol Reprod Biol 105:143–146, 2002

150. Allsop JR: Symphysis pubis dysfunction. Br J Gen Pract 47:256, 1997

151. Snow RE, Neubert AG: Peripartum pubic symphysis separation: A case series and review of the literature. Obstet Gynecol Surv 52:438–443, 1997

152. Whitman JM: Pregnancy, low back pain, and manual physical therapy interventions. J Orthop Sports Phys Ther 32:314–317, 2002

153. Mogren IM, Pohjanen AI: Low back pain and pelvic pain during pregnancy: Prevalence and risk factors. Spine 30:983–991, 2005

154. Pool-Goudzwaard AL, Slieker ten Hove MC, Vierhout ME, et al: Relations between pregnancy-related low back pain, pelvic floor activity and pelvic floor dysfunction. Int Urogynecol J Pelvic Floor Dysfunct 16:468–474, 2005

155. Wang SM, Dezinno P, Maranets I, et al: Low back pain during pregnancy: Prevalence, risk factors, and outcomes. Obstet Gynecol 104:65–70, 2004

156. Fast A, Weiss L, Ducommun EJ, et al: Low back pain in pregnancy: Abdominal muscles, sit-up performance and back pain. Spine 15:28–30, 1990

157. Berg G, Hammar M, Moller-Nielsen J, et al: Low back pain during pregnancy. Obstet Gynecol 71:71–75, 1988

158. Bullock JE, Jull GA, Bullock MI: The relationship of low back pain to postural changes during pregnancy. Aust J Physiother 33:10–17, 1987

159. Ostgaard HC, Andersson GBJ, Schultz AB, et al: Influence of some biomechanical factors on low back pain in pregnancy. Spine 18:61–65, 1993

160. Hodges SD, Eck JC, Humphreys SC: A treatment and outcomes analysis of patients with coccydynia. Spine J 4:138–140, 2004

161. Ryder I, Alexander J: Coccydynia: A woman's tail. Midwifery 16:155–160, 2000

162. Maigne JY, Lagauche D, Doursounian L: Instability of the coccyx in coccydynia. J Bone Joint Surg Br 82:1038–1041, 2000

163. Boeglin ER Jr: Coccydynia. J Bone Joint Surg Br 73:1009, 1991

164. Wray CC, Easom S, Hoskinson J: Coccydynia: Aetiology and treatment. J Bone Joint Surg Br 73:335–338, 1991

165. Lee DT, Chung TK: Postnatal depression: An update. Best Pract Res Clin Obstet Gynaecol, 21:183–191, 2007

166. Howard L: Postnatal depression. Clin Evid 1919–1931, 2006

167. Howard L: Postnatal depression. Clin Evid 1764–1775, 2005

168. Cox J: Postnatal depression in fathers. Lancet 366:982, 2005

169. Hanley J: The assessment and treatment of postnatal depression. Nurs Times 102:24–26, 2006

170. Mallikarjun PK, Oyebode F: Prevention of postnatal depression. J R Soc Health 125:221–226, 2005

171. Snyder S, Pendergraph B: Exercise during pregnancy: what do we really know? Am Fam Physician 69:1053, 1056, 2004

172. Parker KM, Smith SA: Aquatic-Aerobic Exercise as a Means of Stress Reduction During Pregnancy. J Perinat Educ 12:6–17, 2003

173. Kramer MS, McDonald SW: Aerobic exercise for women during pregnancy. Cochrane Database Syst Rev 3:CD000180, 2006

174. Morris SN, Johnson NR: Exercise during pregnancy: A critical appraisal of the literature. J Reprod Med 50:181–188, 2005

175. Larsson L, Lindqvist PG: Low-impact exercise during pregnancy: A study of safety. Acta Obstet Gynecol Scand 84:34–38, 2005

176. Fazlani SA: Protocols for exercise during pregnancy. J Pak Med Assoc 54:226–229, 2004

177. Paisley TS, Joy EA, Price RJ Jr.: Exercise during pregnancy: a practical approach. Curr Sports Med Rep 2:325–330, 2003

178. Information from your family doctor: Pregnancy and exercise. Am Fam Physician 68:1168, 2003

179. Centers for Disease Control and Prevention. Inability of retroviral tests to identify persons with chronic fatigue syndrome, 1992. JAMA 269:1779, 1782, 1993

180. Albrecht F: Chronic fatigue syndrome. J Am Acad Child Adolesc Psychiatry 39:808–809, 2000

181. Darbishire L, Ridsdale L, Seed PT: Distinguishing patients with chronic fatigue from those with chronic fatigue syndrome: A diagnostic study in UK primary care. Br J Gen Pract 53:441–445, 2003

182. Lee P: Recent developments in chronic fatigue syndrome. Am J Med 105:1S, 1998

183. Mawle AC: Chronic fatigue syndrome. Immunol Invest 26:269–273, 1997

184. Tan EM, Sugiura K, Gupta S: The case definition of chronic fatigue syndrome. J Clin Immunol 22:8–12, 2002

185. Amital D, Fostick L, Polliack ML, et al: Posttraumatic stress disorder, tenderness, and fibromyalgia syndrome: Are they different entities? J Psychosom Res 61:663–669, 2006

186. Glass JM: Cognitive dysfunction in fibromyalgia and chronic fatigue syndrome: New trends and future directions. Curr Rheumatol Rep 8:425–429, 2006

187. Mehendale AW, Goldman MP: Fibromyalgia syndrome, idiopathic widespread persistent pain or syndrome of myalgic encephalomyelopathy (SME): What is its nature? Pain Pract 2:35–46, 2002

188. Thieme K, Rose U, Pinkpank T, et al: Psychophysiological responses in patients with fibromyalgia syndrome. J Psychosom Res 61:671–679, 2006

189. Cramer CR: Fibromyalgia and chronic fatigue syndrome: An update for athletic trainers. J Athl Train 33:359–361, 1998

190. Goldenberg DL, Burckhardt C, Crofford L: Management of fibromyalgia syndrome. Jama 292:2388–2395, 2004

191. Mease PJ, Clauw DJ, Arnold LM, et al: Fibromyalgia syndrome. J Rheumatol 32:2270–2277, 2005

192. Staud R, Rodriguez ME: Mechanisms of disease: Pain in fibromyalgia syndrome. Nat Clin Pract Rheumatol 2:90–98, 2006

193. Wood PB, Patterson JC 2nd, Sunderland JJ, et al: Reduced presynaptic dopamine activity in fibromyalgia syndrome demonstrated with positron emission tomography: A pilot study. J Pain 8:51–58, 2007

194. McClaflin RR: Myofascial pain syndrome: primary care strategies for early intervention. Postgrad Med 96:56–73, 1994

195. Travell JG, Simons DG: Myofascial Pain and Dysfunction: The Trigger Point Manual. Baltimore, Williams & Wilkins, 1983

196. Fricton JR: Myofascial pain. Baillieres Clin Rheumatol 8:857–880, 1994

197. Vecchiet L, Giamberardino MA, Saggini R: Myofascial pain syndromes: Clinical and pathophysiological aspects. Clin J Pain 7 (Suppl):16–22, 1991

198. Grodin AJ, Cantu RI: Soft tissue mobilization, in Basmajian JV, Nyberg R (eds): Rational Manual Therapies. Baltimore, Maryland, Williams & Wilkins, 1993, pp 199–221

199. Fricton JR: Management of masticatory myofascial pain. Seminars Orthodontics 1:229–243, 1995

200. Esenyel M, Caglar N, Aldemir T: Treatment of myofascial pain. Am J Phys Med Rehab 79:48–52, 2000

201. Fricton JR: Clinical care for myofascial pain. Dental Clin North Am 35:1–29, 1991

202. Dreyer SJ, Boden SD: Nonoperative treatment of neck and arm pain. Spine 23:2746–2754, 1998

203. Wolfe F, Smythe HA, Yunus MB, et al: The American College of Rheumatology 1990 criteria for the classification of fibromyalgia. Arthr Rheum 33:160–172, 1990

204. Fricton JR, Kroening R, Haley D, et al: Myofascial pain syndrome of the head and neck: A review of clinical characteristics of 164 patients. Oral Surg Oral Med Oral Pathol 60:615–623, 1985

205. Fricton JR: Behavioral and psychosocial factors in chronic craniofacial pain. Anesthesia Progress 32:7–12, 1985

206. Cook DB, Nagelkirk PR, Poluri A, et al: The influence of aerobic fitness and fibromyalgia on cardiorespiratory and perceptual responses to exercise in patients with chronic fatigue syndrome. Arthritis Rheum 54:3351–3362, 2006

207. Havermark AM, Langius-Eklof A: Long-term follow up of a physical therapy programme for patients with fibromyalgia syndrome. Scand J Caring Sci 20:315–322, 2006

208. Karper WB, Jannes CR, Hampton JL: Fibromyalgia syndrome: The beneficial effects of exercise. Rehabil Nurs 31:193–198, 2006

209. Kurtais Y, Kutlay S, Ergin S: Exercise and cognitive-behavioural treatment in fibromyalgia syndrome. Curr Pharm Des 12:37–45, 2006

210. Salek AK, Khan MM, Ahmed SM, et al: Effect of aerobic exercise on patients with primary fibromyalgia syndrome. Mymensingh Med J 14:141–144, 2005

211. Flenaugh EL, Henriques-Forsythe MN: Lung cancer disparities in African Americans: health versus health care. Clin Chest Med 27:431–439, vi, 2006

212. Kendall J, Catts ZA, Kendall C, et al: African Americans' knowledge of cancer genetic counseling: An examination of information delivery. Del Med J 78:453–458, 2006

213. O'Keefe SJ, Chung D, Mahmoud N, et al: Why do African Americans get more colon cancer than Native Africans? J Nutr 137:175S–182S, 2007

214. Overmyer M: Search narrows for gene tied to prostate cancer in African-Americans. RN 70:suppl 2, 2007

215. Goodman CC, Snyder TK: Oncology, in Goodman CC, Boissonnault WG, Fuller KS (eds): Pathology: Implications for the Physical Therapist (ed 2). Philadelphia, Saunders, 2003, pp 236–263

216. Extremera N, Fernandez-Berrocal P: Emotional intelligence as predictor of mental, social, and physical health in university students. Span J Psychol 9:45–51, 2006

217. Penedo FJ, Dahn JR: Exercise and well-being: A review of mental and physical health benefits associated with physical activity. Curr Opin Psychiatry 18:189–193, 2005

218. Scott KM, Bruffaerts R, Tsang A, et al: Depression-anxiety relationships with chronic physical conditions: Results from the World Mental Health surveys. J Affect Disord 8:8, 2007

219. Barlow DH: Unraveling the mysteries of anxiety and its disorders from the perspective of emotion theory. Am Psychol 55:1247–1263, 2000

220. Precin P: Influence of psychosocial factors on rehabilitation, in O'Sullivan SB, Schmitz TJ (eds): Physical rehabilitation (ed 5). Philadelphia, F. A. Davis, 2007, pp 27–63

221. Geisser ME, Roth RS, Bachman JE, et al: The relationship between symptoms of post-traumatic stress disorder and pain, affective disturbance and disability among patients with accident and non-accident related pain. Pain 66:207–214, 1996

222. Nemeroff CB: The neurobiology of depression. Sci Am 278:42–49, 1998

223. Kübler-Ross E: On Death and Dying. New York, Macmillan, 1969

224. Barsky AJ, Goodson JD, Lane RS, et al: The amplification of somatic symptoms. Psychosom Med 50:510–19, 1988

225. Eack SM, Newhill CE, Anderson CM, et al: Quality of life for persons living with schizophrenia: More than just symptoms. Psychiatr Rehabil J 30:219–222, 2007

226. Howard L, Kirkwood G, Leese M: Risk of hip fracture in patients with a history of schizophrenia. Br J Psychiatry 190:129–134, 2007

227. Mettner J: Inside schizophrenia. Minn Med 90:14–15, 2007

228. Rabinowitz J, Levine SZ, Haim R, et al: The course of schizophrenia: Progressive deterioration, amelioration or both? Schizophr Res 2007

229. Seeman MV: Symptoms of schizophrenia: Normal adaptations to inability. Med Hypotheses 2007

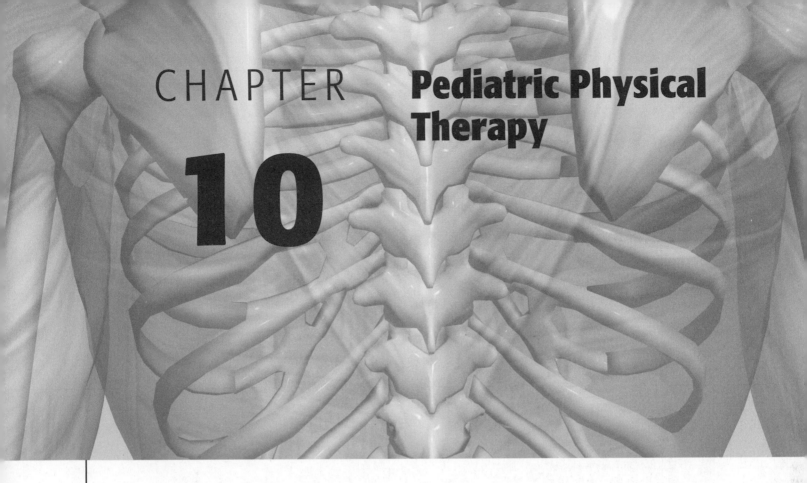

Pediatric Physical Therapy

10

The physical therapy profession focuses on the diagnosis and intervention of dysfunctional human movement throughout the life span. Pediatric physical therapy relates to the period from birth to age 21 years, during which an individual evolves, matures, and ages.

The U.S. federal Individuals with Disabilities Education Act (IDEA) is specific to the pediatric population. IDEA was initially authorized in 1975 as the Education for All Handicapped Children Act. Under the requirements of this federal law, all children who have special needs must be supported in access to free and appropriate public education. This provision is based on an individualized plan. The law has the following provisions:

- Part B provides services at school (usually after age 3 years to 21) and is designed to provide an Individualized Educational Plan (IEP). The IEP identifies the student's specific learning expectations and outlines how the school will address these expectations through appropriate special education programs and services.
- Part C provides services for children less than 3 years old and is designed to provide an Individual Family Service Plan (IFSP). The IFSP is designed to meet the needs of the family as they relate to the child's development, as well as meet the needs of the child.

Developmental Milestones

A milestone is a significant point in development or a significant functional ability achieved during the developmental process. The various developmental milestones for both sensory and motor development are depicted in **Table 10-1** and **Table 10-2**.

TABLE 10-1 Development Milestones According to Position

Age	Prone	Supine	Sitting	Standing	Comments
Newborn (0–1 month)	Displays physiological flexor activity: arms and hands are tucked in close to the body, shoulders are rounded, elbows are flexed, and hands are closed loosely and positioned close to mouth. Lifts head briefly. Moves head to side.	Has no control of neck flexion in supine position, so cannot maintain the head in midline and keeps it rotated to one side.	Lacks trunk muscular control: the back is round and the head flops forward. Can sit in sacral position if supported.	Is capable of primary standing and automatic walking when supported.	Grasp is a reflex in which the hand automatically closes on objects the baby touches due to tactile stimulation of the palm of the hand. The infant: • Has no organized response to postural perturbations • Has poor head control • Is very active when awake • Has random wide-ranging movements, primarily in supine position • Touches and feels, and is soon sucking and learning about the hands • Regards objects in direct line of sight; vision limited to 8 or 9 feet. Follows moving objects midline Skeletal characteristics include coxa valgus, genu varum, tibial varum and torsion, calcaneal varus, and, occasionally, metatarsus adductus.
1 month	Shows improved head lifting in prone position. Has increased cervical rotation mobility. Elbows begin moving forward, arms away from body.	Is able to move head to one side, resulting in lateral vision becoming dominant. Swipes uncontrollably at toys by his or her side. Has wider ranges of movement; heels are able to touch surface.		Displays positive support and primary walking reflexes in supported standing.	The infant: • Has decreasing physiologic flexion (less "recoil") • Shows increasing level of arousal • Engages in neonatal reaching • Is able to visually track a moving object horizontally
2 months	Is able to hold the head steady in all positions and to raise it about 45° due to increased activity of active shoulder abduction. Begins to use arms and hands to support the actions of the head and trunk. Uses hand movements that are more goal directed.	Shows increased asymmetry with more visual interaction.	Has head lag with pull to sit. Begins to develop head and trunk control and has more attempts at sustained extension. Is unable to control head in supported sitting; head bobs.	May not accept weight on lower extremities (astasia–abasia). Ceases neonatal stepping.	The infant has increasing asymmetry/decreased tone. Increased head and trunk control lets the baby use the arms for reaching and playing rather than for support. The baby holds objects placed in the hand.

Age					
3 months	Shows change in the general position of the arms, from a position where the arms are tucked in close to the body with the elbows near the ribs, to one in which the elbows are almost in line with the shoulders, which allows for forearm weight bearing. Can raise face 45° to 90° when prone.	Displays beginning of symmetry; the head is in midline with chin tucking and the hands are in midline on the chest/to mouth.	Attempts pull to sit but falls forward.	Bears minimal weight through extended legs.	This is a period of controlled symmetry. The grasp becomes more controlled and voluntary, and the hands can adjust to the shape of objects. Symmetry is very obvious in the lower extremities as they assume their "frog-legged" position of hip abduction, external rotation and flexion, and knee flexion. The feet come together and the baby is able to take some weight with toes curled in supported standing. Legs are abducted and externally rotated.
4 months	Is able to prop up on the forearms and look around. The head and chest are lifted and maintained in midline. Prone pivots.	Can roll from prone to side and from supine to side, although these are usually accidental occurrences. Is able to bring the hands together in the space above the body due to increased shoulder girdle control. Can move hands to knees. Shows active anterior and posterior pelvic tilt.	Assists in pull to sit by flexing elbows. Very minimal head bobbing, stabilized through shoulder elevation. Tends to sit in a slumped position. Begins to develop protective reactions, first laterally, then forward, and then backward.	Because of the increased head–neck–trunk control, is able to take more weight when placed in standing and can now be held by the hands instead of at the chest. • Legs are extended and the toes are clawed.	Ulnar palmar grasp develops. Baby is able to perform bilateral reaching with the forearm pronated when the trunk is supported. Sidelying activities are performed Baby starts hand-to-mouth activities. Righting and equilibrium reactions are emerging. Findings of concern include poor midline orientation (persistent asymmetric tonic neck reflex), imbalance between flexors and extensors, poor visual attention/tracking, persistent wide base of support in standing, and poor antigravity strength.
5 months	Begins to display equilibrium reactions in prone position. Can roll from prone to supine. Is able to assume and maintain a position of extended arm weight bearing in prone and can weight shift from one forearm to the other end to reach out with one arm.	Has chin tuck, downward gaze. Can touch feet to mouth. Has more active anterior and posterior pelvic tilt. Active roll to sidelying. Manipulates and transfers toys.	Has no head lag when pulled from supine to sit. Assists during pull to sit with chin tuck and head lift. Able to control head in supported sitting, although still leans forward from the hips.	Able to bear almost all weight.	Findings of concern include: • Poor antigravity flexion • Poor tolerance of prone/inability to bear weight to extended arms/poor weight shifting

(continued)

TABLE 10-1 Development Milestones According to Position (Continued)

Age	Prone	Supine	Sitting	Standing	Comments
6 months	Completes turning and can roll from prone to supine. Can lay prone on hands with the elbows extended and is able to weight shift on extended arms from hand to hand and to reach forward due to sufficient shoulder girdle control.	Has active hip extension. Transfers toys. Flexes head independently.	Can sit independently, although initially uses the arms and hands for support.	In standing, is able to bear weight on both legs and bounce. Can independently hold on to the support of a person due to sufficient trunk and hip control.	The baby uses rolling for locomotion. Findings of concern include: • Poor tolerance for prone position • Paucity of movement patterns • Inability to sit independently • Inability to roll or rolling with neck hyperextension
7 months	Has trunk and arms free. Is able to achieve and maintain the quadruped position, although the prone is usually the preferred position. Can pivot on belly, often moving body in a circle.	Tends to avoid except for playing.	Shows more consistent protective reactions. Is able to perform trunk rotation in sitting. Can assume the sitting position from the quadruped position.	Can often pull to stand from the quadruped position. Is able to actively flex and extend both legs simultaneously while standing and supporting independently.	The baby is very active, with a large variety of movements and positions available. The baby may show fear of strangers. Findings of concern include: • Lack of weight shifting in prone • Reliance on more primitive movement patterns as compensations in order to explore • Inability to assume or maintain quadruped • Poor weight bearing in supported stance
8 months	Spends minimal time in prone; able to creep/crawl in the quadruped position by 9 months as the primary means of locomotion.		Shows full equilibrium reactions in sitting, and the beginning of equilibrium reactions in quadruped. Is able to side-sit and is also able to go from sitting to quadruped. May also kneel.	Can stand by leaning on supporting surfaces. Is able to pull to stand. Begins early walking, cruising.	The baby can reach out for objects and reach across the midline of the body without losing balance. The thumb can wrap around objects—now the baby can hold two small objects, such as cubes, in one hand. Findings of concern include: • Poor sitting ability • Inability to use hand for play • Overall reliance on upper extremities

Age			
9 months	Uses a large variety of sitting positions and movement. Is able to pivot and sit for long "periods of time. Often uses sitting as a transitional position.	Uses arms, hands, and body together while pulling up to standing through half-kneel position (9 months). Begins immature stepping. Follows this sequence in rising to standing: kneeling, half kneeling, forward weight shift, squatting, then standing upright.	The index finger starts to move separately from the rest of the hand when poking at objects. This leads to the pincer grasp, with the tips of the thumb and index finer meeting in a precise pattern. The baby's ability to let go of an object smoothly has also improved. Findings of concern include: • Poor standing control • Poor/inadequate sitting • Inability to assume quadruped
10 months	Reaches arms above shoulders. Displays active site sitting. Is rarely stationary.	Begins creeping/climbing; legs are very active. Displays "high guard" (arms held at near shoulder level). Cruises with wide base of support.	
11 months	Is able to play and move hands across midline.	Mostly uses legs. Displays very symmetrical standing with a wide base of support.	
12 to 15 months		Walks unassisted.	
2 years		Runs well. Goes upstairs using reciprocal pattern (reciprocal stair climbing).	The baby is able to self-feed. The baby can build a tower of two cubes.

Data from van Blankenstein M, Welbergen UR, de Haas JH: Le Developpement du Nourrisson: Sa Premiere Annee en 130 Photographies. Paris, Presses Universitaires de France, 1962; and Prechtl HF: New perspectives in early human development. Eur J Obstet Gynecol Reprod Biol 21:347–355, 1986

TABLE 10-2	Gross Motor Checklist for Locomotion Ages 2–5
Age	**Milestone**
2 years	Walks up/down stairs one at the time holding rail
	Walks with heel; displays total gait
	Runs forward well
3 years	Pedals and steers tricycle well
	Jumps forward on both feet
	Alternates feet going upstairs
	Walks backward easily
4 years	Walks downstairs with alternating feet, holding rail
	Gallops
5 years	Is able to walk long distances on toes
	Skips
	Hops forward on one foot
	Displays smooth reciprocal movements in walking and running

Data from Ratliffe KT: Clinical pediatric physical therapy: A guide for the physical therapy team. Philadelphia, Mosby, 1998; and Kahn-D'Angel L: Pediatric Physical Therapy, in O'Sullivan SB, Siegelman RP (eds): National Physical Therapy Examination: Review and Study Guide (ed 9). Evanston, IL, International Educational Resources, 2006

Automatic Postural Responses

Automatic postural responses allow an individual to restore or maintain body equilibrium and remain functionally oriented. These responses are dependent on the organization of the visual, vestibular, and somatosensory systems (see Chapter 5):

- *Righting:* Orientation of the head in space so that the eyes and mouth are in a horizontal plane or the body parts are restored to proper alignment. This response includes vertical righting (orienting head to vertical) and rotational righting (orientation following rotation of a body segment). It operates regardless of the position of the body or where the body is in the environment. Normally, this response develops during the first 6 months of life.
- *Equilibrium:* Complex responses to changes of posture or movement that seek to restore disturbed balance when the body's base of support is subjected to perturbation (push, pull, or tilt).

These responses develop in a position after a child has learned to assume the position (prone, supine, sitting, quadruped, standing) independently. Response is generally in the opposite direction of the force. Examples include:

- ❑ Spinal column concavity on the uphill side on an unstable base of support.
- ❑ Spinal column concavity on the side of the pushing force on a stable base of support.
- ❑ Rotation of the upper trunk and head toward the midline and counter-rotations of the lower trunk.
- ❑ Abduction and extension of the extremities on the downhill side or in the direction of push.
- *Protective (parachute[1] or propping[2]):* Extension movements of the extremities generally in the same direction of the displacing force that shifts the body's center of gravity. Highly context dependent, these movements can be backward, forward, or lateral. These responses develop laterally by 6 to 11 months, then forward, and finally backward by 9 to 12 months.

Primitive Reflexes

Reflexes are involuntary movements or actions that help to identify normal brain and nerve activity. Some reflexes occur only in specific periods of development and are not evident later in development because they become integrated by the CNS (**Table 10-3**). Persistence of these primitive reflexes can interfere with motor milestone attainment.

Motor Control

The term *motor control* refers to processes of the brain and spinal cord that govern posture and movement.[3] It is the ability to regulate or direct the mechanisms essential to movement using perception and cognition. The integral elements of motor control are listed in **Table 10-4**. The field of motor control is directed at studying the nature of movement and how the movement is controlled.

● **Key Point** A *motor plan* is defined as an idea or plan for purposeful movement that is made up of component motor programs.[4] A *motor program* is defined as an abstract representation that, when initiated, results in the production of a coordinated movement sequence.[5]

TABLE 10-3

Primitive Reflexes

Reflex	Description	Normal Age of Response	Potential Negative Consequence if Reflex Persists
Rooting	Stimulus involves light tactile stimulation near the mouth/cheek. Infant moves head in direction of the stimulus and opens the mouth.	Usually occurs around 20 weeks of gestation to 3 months. Usually disappears around 9 months of age.	Interferes with oral motor development, optical righting, visual tracking, midline control of the head, and social interaction.
Sucking	Linked with the rooting reflex stimulus; involves the placing of a nipple or finger in mouth. Can be assessed as to whether it is sustainable and consistent.	Usually fades by around 3 months of age but may persist during sleep until as late as 7 or 8 months.	No major implications.
Moro	One hand supports the infant's head in midline, the other supports the back. The infant is raised to 45 degrees and the head is allowed to fall through 10 degrees. Mature response is abduction with fingers open, then adduction of the limbs and crying.	Normally occurs between 20 weeks of gestation to 5 months.	Interferes with balance and protective reactions in sitting, hand–eye coordination.
Palmar/plantar grasp	Stimulus applied to palm of hand (ulnar side) or soles of feet. The response is a grasping of the digits.	Occurs from birth to 4 months.	Interferes with ability to voluntarily grasp and release objects, and weight bearing on open hand.
Tonic labyrinthine (TLR)	Based on the position of the labyrinth of the inner ear relative to head position. Prone position facilitates flexion. Supine position facilitates extension.	Occurs from birth to 6 months.	Interferes with ability to initiate rolling, ability to prop on elbows with extended hips when prone, and ability to flex trunk and hips to come to sitting position from supine position.
Asymmetric tonic neck reflex (ATNR)	Response is related to position of head turn and extension of extremities on face side or flexion of extremities on skull side.	Occurs around 6 to 8 months.	Interferes with feeding, visual tracking, rolling, development of crawling, and midline use of hands.
Symmetric tonic Neck reflex (STNR)	Infant is positioned in quadruped. Head is positioned in either flexion or extension. The correct response is for the arm and head to do the same thing, and the legs to do the opposite—e.g., if head is extended, arms extend and legs flex.	Occurs around 6 to 8 months.	Interferes with ability to prop on arms in prone position, reciprocal crawling, attaining and maintaining hands and knees position.
Positive supporting	Pressure applied to sole of the foot produces extension of the extremity for weight bearing. Also known as primary standing.	Normally occurs at 35 weeks of gestation to 2 months.	Interferes with standing and walking, balance reactions, and weight shifting.
Neonatal stepping	Walking (reciprocal flexion/extension of legs) motion produced as the infant is moved along a surface while being held under the arms. Also known as automatic walking.	Normally occurs at 38 weeks of gestation to 2 months.	Interferes with standing and walking, balance reactions, reciprocal movements of the lower extremities, and weight shifting
Galant	Skin is touched along the spine from shoulder to hip. Correct response is sidebending of the trunk toward the side of stimulus.	Normally occurs from 30 weeks of gestation to 2 months.	Interferes with sitting balance.
Startle	Infant is exposed to loud, sudden noise. The correct response is similar to the Moro response, but elbows remain flexed and hands closed.	Normally occurs from 28 weeks of gestation to 5 months.	Interferes with sitting balance, protective responses in sitting, and hand–eye coordination.

Data from Capute AJ, Palmer FB, Shapiro BK, et al: Primitive reflex profile: A quantitation of primitive reflexes in infancy. Dev Med Child Neurol 26:375–383, 1984; Damasceno A, Delicio AM, Mazo DF, et al: Primitive reflexes and cognitive function. Arq Neuropsiquiatr 63:577–582, 2005; Schott JM, Rossor MN: The grasp and other primitive reflexes. J Neurol Neurosurg Psychiatr 74:558–560, 2003; Zafeiriou DI: Primitive reflexes and postural reactions in the neurodevelopmental examination. Pediatr Neurol 31:1–8, 2004; and Ratliffe KT: Clinical Pediatric Physical Therapy: A Guide for the Physical Therapy Team. Philadelphia, Mosby, 1998

TABLE 10-4	Integral Elements of Motor Control

The CNS functioning as a fundamentally active agent with the capacity to generate action.

Motor patterns, which are the fundamental units of neuromotor behavior.

The involvement of processes of feedback and comparison of intention and result, which enable the modification of action.

- *Open-loop feedback:* Feedback that is available to the performer but not used to control the action.
- *Closed-loop feedback:* When a decision to move is made in the motor control center (brain). Some of the information is sent to the effector organs (muscles). The rest of the information is sent during the action, and feedback monitors the effectiveness of the movement, allowing for changes to be made during the movement.

A distributed control system that delegates the control of behavior to the most appropriate subsystem.

Memory structures such as schema permit transfer of skills to new situations.

Data from Van Sant AF: Concepts of neural organization and movement, in Connolly BH, Montgomery PC (eds): Therapeutic Exercise in Developmental Disabilities. Thorofare, NJ, SLACK, 2001, pp 1–12

Some of the more common models of motor control are outlined in **Table 10-5**. Factors that govern movement include the task, the environment, and the neuromotor capabilities of the individual. Multiple variables contribute to the initiation and execution of a movement (**Table 10-6**).

● Key Point

- Reflexes are evoked responses and depend on a stimulus to be initiated. They are involuntary, stereotyped, and graded responses to sensory input, and they have no threshold except that the stimulus must be great enough to activate the relevant sensory input pathway.
- Fixed action patterns (sneezing, orgasm) are involuntary and stereotyped, but they typically have a stimulus threshold that must be reached before they are triggered. They are less graded and more complex than reflexes.
- Directed movements (reaching) are voluntary and complex, but they are generally neither stereotyped nor repetitive.
- Rhythmic motor patterns (walking, scratching, breathing) are complex (unlike reflexes), stereotyped (unlike directed movements), and, by definition, repetitive (unlike fixed action patterns), but they are subject to continuous voluntary control. Central pattern generators (CPGs) are neural networks that can endogenously (i.e., without rhythmic sensory or central input) produce rhythmic patterned outputs; these networks underlie the production of most rhythmic motor patterns, such as the gait cycle.[4–7]

Motor Development

Motor development refers to the processes of change in motor behavior that occur over relatively extended time periods.[3]

- Motor development is a complex process that starts in utero and has psychomotor, physiological, biochemical, biomechanical, psychosocial, and even gender considerations.[8]

- Motor development training is the process of producing any change in motor behavior that is related to the age of the individual and includes age-related changes in posture and movement.

● Key Point Recent motor control and development theories include:[3,9,10]

- *Dynamical pattern theory (motor control theory):* General principles of motor coordination include order parameters (variables that incorporate the action of many of a systems subunits and can be used to characterize coordinated behavior) and control parameters (variables that initiate change in order parameters). Some behavioral patterns are more common than others (attractors).
- *Dynamical action theory (motor development theory):* Movement is an emergent property based on multiple factors (e.g., neural maturation, muscle force, biomechanical leverages, emotional state, cognitive awareness, task constraints, and physical environment).

Motor Development Theories

Neural–Maturationist

The neural–maturationist theory is based on the belief that motor patterns emerge in orderly, predetermined genetic sequences that are supported but not fundamentally altered by the environment. This theory depends on the assumption of hierarchic maturation of neural control centers and results in the recognition of general developmental sequences and milestones of development:[11]

- Cephalocaudal
- Central to distal

The neural–maturationist theorists consider the maturational state of the nervous system as the main

TABLE
10-5   Theories of Motor Control

Theory[a]	Description
Maturational-based	**Structure–Function Organization and Reflex Chaining** Sensory inputs are a necessary prerequisite for efferent motor output (stimulus-evoked behavior)—movement occurs in response to a stimulus. Movement is the result of predictable anatomic changes in neural pathways, and complex movement occurs as the result of a compounding of reflex movements. **Hierarchical** The nervous system is organized as a hierarchy, with each successively high level exerting control over the level below it. Separation between voluntary (higher-level) and reflexive (lower-level) movement. Reflexes work together or in sequence to achieve a common purpose, and thus provide the building blocks of complex behavior. Forms the basis of most neurotherapeutic approaches used in physical therapy (Bobath, Brunnstrom). Useful for explaining spontaneous and volitional movement.
Learning-based	**Response Chaining** More emphasis on the role of the environment; action not bound to a specific stimulus (neither spontaneous or volitional movements are dependent on external agents for their initiation). Environment is the controller of the automating process. Linkages exist among muscle groups that allow for movement combinations (synergies). A full complement of motor programs is available and used appropriately in functional contexts prior to birth.[b] Movement dysfunction may be due to motor program centers in the brain and motor program centers at lower levels. **Adams's Closed-Loop Theory[c]** In a closed-loop process, sensory feedback is used for the ongoing production of skilled movement. The closed-loop theory of motor learning also proposes that two distinct types of memory are important in this process: • *Memory trace:* Used in this election and initiation of the movement. • *Perceptual trace:* Built up over a period of practice and becomes the internal reference of correctness. This theory proposes that when learning a new movement skill, an individual gradually develops a perceptual trace for the movement that serves as a guide for later movements, and that the more an individual practices the specific movement, the stronger the perceptual trace becomes. Theoretically, the more time spent in practicing the movement as accurately as possible, the better the learning.
Schmidt's Schema Theory[c,d]	Schmidt's theory emphasizes open-loop control processes and the generalized motor program concept. Three constructs: general motor programs and two types of memory traces, recall schema, and recognition schema. When learning a new motor program, an individual learns a general set of rules that can be applied to a variety of contexts. The generalized motor program is considered to contain the rules for creating the spatial and temporal patterns of muscle activity needed to carry out a given movement.
Dynamical-based systems[e,f]	Seek to address what drives skill acquisition and how an individual moves from one developmental stage of skill to another. The system is composed of a number of identifiable variables (muscle power, body mass, arousal, neural networks, motivation and environmental forces [gravity, friction, etc.]) Movement emerges due to interaction of subsystems, which work together and which change over time. Three key hypotheses: 1. A developing organism is genetically endowed with spontaneously generated behaviors that make up the basic movement repertoire. 2. A sensory system is capable of detecting and recognizing movements having adaptive value. 3. The system has the ability to select movements having adaptive value by varying synaptic strength within and between brain circuits such that successive event selections will progressively modify the movement repertoire.

(continued)

TABLE 10-5	Theories of Motor Control (Continued)

Theory[a]	Description
Central pattern generators (CPGs)[g–k]	These are proposed to account for the basic neural organization and function required to execute coordinated, rhythmic movements, such as locomotion, chewing, grooming (e.g., scratching), and respiration.
	These are commonly defined as *interneural networks,* located in either the spinal court or brainstem, that can order selection and sequencing of motor neurons independent of descending or peripheral afferent neural input.
	They can also modulate the inputs they receive, gating potentially disruptive reflex actions like nociceptive activation of the flexor withdrawal reflex when a limb is fully loaded during the stance phase of locomotion.

Data from (a) Bradley NS, Westcott SL: Motor control: Developmental aspects of motor control in skill acquisition, in Campbell SK, Vander Linden DW, Palisano RJ (eds): Physical Therapy for Children (ed 3). St. Louis, Saunders, 2006, pp 77–130; (b) Comparetti AM: The neurophysiologic and clinical implications of studies on fetal motor behavior. Semin Perinatol 5:183–189, 1981; (c) Shumway-Cook A, Woollacott MH: Motor learning and recovery of function, in Shumway-Cook A, Woollacott MH (eds): Motor Control: Theory and Practical Applications (ed 2). Philadelphia, Lippincott Williams & Wilkins, 2001, pp 26–49; (d) Schmidt RA: Motor schema theory after 27 years: Reflections and implications for a new theory. Res Q Exerc Sport 74:366–375, 2003; (e) Thelen E, Corbetta D: Exploration and selection in the early acquisition of skill. Int Rev Neurobiol 37:75–102, 1994; (f) Thelen E: Motor development: A new synthesis. Am Psychol 50:79–95, 1995; (g) Grillner S, Wallen P: Central pattern generators for locomotion, with special reference to vertebrates. Ann Rev Neurosci 8:233–261, 1985; (h) Hooper SL: Central pattern generators. Curr Biol 10:R176, 2000; (i) Marder E, Bucher D: Central pattern generators and the control of rhythmic movements. Curr Biol 11:R986–996, 2001; (j) Prosiegel M, Holing R, Heintze M, et al: The localization of central pattern generators for swallowing in humans: A clinical-anatomical study on patients with unilateral paresis of the vagal nerve, Avellis' syndrome, Wallenberg's syndrome, posterior fossa tumours and cerebellar hemorrhage. Acta Neurochir Suppl 93:85–88, 2005; and (k) Verdaasdonk BW, Koopman HF, Helm FC: Energy efficient and robust rhythmic limb movement by central pattern generators. Neural Netw 19:388–400, 2006

constraint for developmental progress. Basic motor skills, such as standing and walking, are not learned by experience but are the result of cerebral maturation; the emphasis is on the assessment stages of reflex development and motor milestones as reflections of increasingly higher levels of neural maturation.[12] Based on this theory, the intervention for children with CNS dysfunction is based around methods to inhibit the primitive reflexes and emphasize the facilitation of the righting and equilibrium reactions.[13]

Cognitive Theories
Cognitive-Behavioral
The cognitive-behavioral theory believes that developmental progress occurs through Pavlovian responses to previous stimulation, and by operant processes in

TABLE 10-6	Motor Control Variables

Variable	Description
Sensorimotor	Physiologic mechanisms or processes that reside within the nervous system—e.g., CPGs and the movement synergies and neural mechanisms that alter or regulate them.
Mechanical	The viscoelastic properties of musculoskeletal tissues. Changes in total body mass and relative distribution of mass during development are accompanied by changes in length and center of mass of the body segment, which in turn alter inertial forces due to gravity and during movement.
Cognitive	May include variables that are dependent on conscious and subconscious processes, such as reasoning, memory, or judgment to optimize performance (arousal, motivation, anticipatory or feed-forward strategies, selective use of feedback, practice, and memory).
Task requirements	May include any variable that can contribute to or in some way alter movement, including biomechanical requirements, meaningfulness, predictability, or any other variable associated with a given movement context.

Data from Bradley NS, Westcott SL: Motor control: Developmental aspects of motor control in skill acquisition, in Campbell SK, Vander Linden DW, Palisano RJ (eds): Physical Therapy for Children (ed 3). St. Louis, Saunders, 2006, pp 77–130

which responses are controlled by consequences.[13] Under this theory, behavior is goal oriented and has both direction and purpose: actions are motivated by a desire to achieve a goal or to avoid unpleasant circumstances. Motivation has two purposes:

- To allow internal tension to create a demand for the goal
- To establish the events that an individual will concentrate on

There are two main types of motivators:

- *Deprivation* causes an internal desire to obtain the goal.
- An *incentive* motivates behavior based merely upon the adequacy of the reward.

Cognitive Piagetian

Piaget[14] emphasized an interaction between maturation of cognitive-neural structures and environmental opportunities to promote action. Piaget felt that development proceeds in an ordered series of stages and was largely the result of the individual's experience with the environment. The four stages described by Piaget are:

- *Sensorimotor:* Lasting from birth to approximately 24 months. The child learns about the world primarily through sensory experiences and movement.
- *Preoperational:* From 2 years to approximately 5 or 6 years of age. The child develops the important skill of using symbols, including pictures and spoken words, but is not yet capable of mentally manipulating them in logical order.
- *Concrete operational:* During this stage, from approximately 6 to 11 or 12 years of age, children become capable of what Piaget refers to as mental operations and of applying logical thought to concrete situations.
- *Formal operational:* Beginning at approximately 11 or 12 years of age, this is the period in which the adolescent becomes capable of logical, abstract thinking. During this period, adolescents can imagine all of the *possibilities* in any situation or problem and are capable of analyzing them to determine which are the best approaches.

Piaget describes three processes that are instrumental to adapting to the environment through learning:[14]

- *Assimilation:* The process through which we use our existing mental structures or schemas to take in new information. We need to have an existing schema (idea, concept): prior knowledge to relate to the new information so we can assimilate it. We learn something by connecting new information to something we already know. In order to acquire new ideas or knowledge, we integrate them with and thereby build upon and activate prior knowledge, as in the case of learning to read.
- *Accommodation:* The process through which our existing mental structures or schemas change as we take in new information. We revise these existing schema (ideas, concepts) if new information does not fit with them. That is, if we experience something that is new or different, it modifies our existing knowledge. The mental representations we previously had are changed to accommodate the new experience.
- *Equilibration:* Internal self-efficacy (self-regulation), the balancing that goes on in our minds between assimilation and accommodation. Equilibration is the self-regulatory process through which we balance new experiences with what we already know to achieve a state of equilibrium.

The impact of Piagetian theory on pediatric physical therapy is primarily due to the inclusion of problem-solving activities in therapeutic programs to assist in the cognitive-motivational aspects of facilitating motor development.[13]

Dynamical

The dynamical theory:[15,16]

- Emphasizes process rather than product or hierarchically structured plans
- Places neural maturation on an equal plane with other structures and processes that interact to promote motor development
- Emphasizes that the environment is as important as the organism, and developmental change is seen not as a series of discrete stages, but as a series of states of stability, instability, and phase shifts in which new states become stable aspects of behavior

According to the dynamical theory, cooperating systems, which include musculoskeletal components, sensory systems, central sensorimotor integrated mechanisms, and arousal and motivation, become progressively integrated with the self-organized properties of the system to gradually optimize skilled function.[15,17]

Prenatal Development

The prenatal period of development is also known as the *gestational period*.

> **● Key Point** Note the following definitions:
>
> - *Menstrual age:* The age of a fetus or newborn, in weeks, calculated from the first day of the mother's last normal menstrual period.
> - *Gestational age:* Also known as *fetal age*, the time measured from the first day of the woman's last menstrual cycle to the current date—the time inside of the uterus. A pregnancy of normal gestation is approximately 40 weeks, with a normal range of 38 to 42 weeks.
> - *Preterm (premature):* Born before 37 weeks of gestational age.[18]
> - *Term:* Born within the normal range.
> - *Post term (postmature):* Born after 42 weeks.[18]
> - *Conceptional age:* The age of a fetus or newborn in weeks since conception.
> - *Chronological age:* The time elapsed from date of birth to present day.
> - *Corrected age:* Used for preterm infants; based on the age the child would be if the pregnancy had actually gone to term. The corrected age, generally used for the first 2 years of life, can be calculated as the chronological age minus the number of weeks/months premature.

The prenatal stage of development can be divided into three distinct periods:

- *Germinal:* Begins at the time of fertilization and lasts 2 weeks.
- *Embryonic:* Begins 2 weeks after conception and lasts about 6 weeks.
- *Fetal:* Begins at 7 weeks of gestation and ends at birth. At 14 to 15 weeks, all the preliminary feeding movements, including mouth opening and closing, sustained lip closure, and tongue movements, are present. At 29 weeks audible sucking can be observed.

> **● Key Point** Birth weights:
>
> - Normal (appropriate for gestational age)
> - Large for gestational age: 4000 to 4500 grams (8.8 to 9.9 pounds)
> - Small for gestational age
> - Low birth weight: Less than 2500 grams (5.5 pounds)
> - Very low birth weight: Less than 1500 grams (3.3 pounds)

Infant Screening and Assessment Tools

Developmental screening tests usually are brief, general, play-based tests of skills. Some tests use developmental ages to describe a child's physical, perceptual, social, and emotional maturity. Development tests do not necessarily correlate in any way with intelligence tests.

The Brazelton Neonatal Behavioral Assessment Scale

Population

For infants from birth to the approximate post-term age of 1 month.

Purpose

The Brazelton Neonatal Behavioral Assessment Scale (BNBAS)[19] is based on the assumption that babies communicate through their behavior. It assesses the infant's use of his or her state of consciousness to maintain control of reactions to environmental and internal stimuli, including:

- Regulation of the autonomic nervous systems, including breathing and temperature regulation
- Control of the motor systems
- Control of the states or levels of consciousness
- Social interaction with parents and other caregivers

General Movement Assessment

Population

For preterm and term newborns and young infants.[20]

Purpose

An effective tool for predicting neurologic outcome at 2 years of age, in central patterns (CPs) in particular.[21] The general movement assessment (GMA), which requires examination of the spontaneous movements of preterm and term newborns and young infants, reflects a theoretic view that maturation is not a fixed sequence of differentiation but rather a continuous transformation of behavior in that the developing neural structure must meet the requirements of the organism and its environment.

Dubowitz Neurological Assessment of the Preterm and Full-Term Infant

Population

For preterm and full-term infants soon after birth and during the neonatal period.

Purpose

The Dubowitz Neurological Assessment[18] is screening test based on traditional neuromaturational views of development. It is suitable for use by staff without expertise in neonatal neurology.[22] It is used to detect deviations or resolutions of neurologic problems.[18]

> **● Key Point** A number of studies have shown the Dubowitz assessment to be a valid tool that may be used to develop management protocols in the neonatal intensive care unit (NICU).[23,24]

Movement Assessment of Infants

Population

For infants from birth to 1 year of age.

Purpose

The movement assessment of infants[25] is done to identify motor dysfunction, note changes in the status of motor dysfunction, and help create an appropriate intervention program.

Alberta Infant Motor Scales

Population

For infants from birth to 1 year of age.

Purpose

The Alberta Infant Motor Scales (AIMS), as standardized, discriminative, evaluative, and criterion- and norm-referenced test,[26] is used to identify infants whose motor performance is delayed or aberrant relative to a normal group, to measure change, and to provide parents with information with regard to development.[27] The test highlights what the child can do and notes any deviations from the normal patterns of motor maturation.

> **● Key Point** *Norm-referenced tests* are standardized on the groups of individuals (populations) they are designed to test. They allow the clinician to determine the exact developmental age of a child and to compare the child's performance to the performance typically expected. *Criterion-referenced tests* measure a child's development on particular skills in terms of absolute levels of mastery.[22] These tests have reference points that may not be dependent on a reference group—the child is competing against him- or herself, not a reference group.[22]

Harris Infant Neuromotor Test

Population

For infants from 3 to 12 months of age.

Purpose

The Harris Infant Neuromotor Test (HINT) is designed to identify developmental delay.[28]

Comprehensive Developmental Assessment

Bayley Scales of Infant Development-II

Population

For infants from birth to 15 months.

Purpose

The Bayley scales measure varying stages of growth at each age level, supplemented by extensive longitudinal data on groups of infants.

Motor Assessments

Peabody Development Motor Scales-2

Population

For children from birth to 6 years.

Purpose

The Peabody Development Motor Scales-2 (PDMS-2) is a standardized, descriptive, and norm- and criterion-referenced test used to identify children whose gross or fine motor skills are delayed or aberrant relative to a normal group. The purpose of the PDMS-2 is fivefold:

- To estimate motor competence relative to the child's peers.
- To compare the gross motion motor quotient (GMQ) and fine motor quotient (FMQ) to determine if there is disparity in motor abilities.
- To assess qualitative and quantitative aspects of individual skills.
- To evaluate progress.
- To study the nature of motor development in various populations.

Bruininks Oseretsky Test of Motor Proficiency

Population

For children ages 4.5 to 14.5 years.

Purpose

The Bruininks Oseretsky Test of Motor Proficiency[29] is designed to provide educators, clinicians, and researchers with useful information to assist them in assessing the motor skills of individual students; in developing and evaluating motor training programs; and in assessing serious motor dysfunctions and developmental disabilities in children. The test may also be used as a screening device for differential diagnoses, and it may be easily integrated with other types of educational and psychological measures.

Assessments Designed for Children with Disabilities

Gross Motor Function Measure

Population

The Gross Motor Function Measure (GMFM) test was specifically designed for children with cerebral palsy from 6 months to 18 years of age, but it can be used for any child whose motor function is below age 5 years.

Purpose

The GMFM classification system is a clinical measure designed to evaluate change over time and with intervention in gross motor function in children with cerebral palsy. Assesses motor function (what or how much a child can do) rather than the quality of movement behind motor performance. The test supports functional theory.

Pediatric Evaluation of Disability Inventory

Population
No age limit.

Purpose
The Pediatric Evaluation of Disability Inventory (PEDI) is a norm-referenced test when used with the appropriate age group; it is a criterion-referenced test when used with older children whose function falls in the level of 6 months to 7.5 years. This descriptive and evaluative tool is used to provide a comprehensive clinical assessment of key functional capabilities and performance. The test focuses exclusively on what the child can accomplish and excludes information on how the child accomplishes the task. In addition, it is used for program monitoring, documentation of functional progress, and clinical decision-making. It relies on information gathered from the child's caregiver rather than on direct observation of the child.

Functional Independence Measure for Children

Population
For use with children age 6 months to 7 years.

Purpose
The Functional Independence Measure for Children (WEEFIM) is a minimal data, set-standardized, functional performance measure. This evaluative, discriminative measure uses the actual performance of the child to indicate severity of disability.

Other Tests

School Function Assessment

Population
Used for children in kindergarten through sixth grade.

Purpose
School function assessment reflects the functional and ecological theories based on measurement of a student's performance of tasks that support participation in academic and social aspects of elementary school. The test is norm- or criterion-referenced, and it provides a seminal, comprehensive, and sophisticated method for examining a child within the context of the school environment.

Pediatric Clinical Test of Sensory Interaction for Balance

Population
For children aged 4 to 10 years.

Purpose
The Pediatric Clinical Test of Sensory Interaction for Balance (PCTSIB)[30,31] measures standing balance when sensory input is systematically altered. The PCTSIB assesses a child's standing stability under varying sensory conditions, including standing on stable versus foam surfaces, with and without vision, and with information from body sway relative to the surroundings occluded.

> ● **Key Point** Although the Apgar screening test is not administered by the physical therapist assistant, the results of this test are recorded in the patient's chart. The Apgar test, which is administered to the newborn at 1, 5, and 10 minutes after birth, consists of five tests, which assess heart rate, respiration, reflex irritability, muscle tone, and color. Each test is scored 0, 1, or 2. A score of 7 and above is considered good.

The Role of the Physical Therapist Assistant in the Special Care Nursery

The American Physical Therapy Association's section on pediatrics has published guidelines for physical therapy practice in the newborn intensive care unit (NICU).[32] These guidelines provide the therapist with a structure for clinical training, an algorithm for decision-making, and clinical competencies based on roles, proficiencies, and knowledge areas. The guidelines highlight how the interaction with neonates differs from older populations:

- Conventional methods of manual muscle testing are not appropriate with the neonate, so other strategies must be employed. These include tickling, holding the extremities in positions such as hip and knee flexion, and holding a limb in an antigravity position to stimulate the infant to move or hold the limb.[33,34] The clinician should note whether or not muscles are functioning, which muscles are strong and can move a joint throughout its entire range, and which are weak and can move the joint only partially.

- Normal neonates have physiological flexion of up to 30 degrees at the hips, 10 to 20 degrees at the knees, and ankle dorsiflexion of up to 40 or 50 degrees.[35,36]
- Reflex and behavioral testing is used to evaluate reflex activity such as sucking and swallowing, and the current status of the infant's organization of physiologic response to stress, state control, motor control, and social interaction.
- Although it is difficult to assess pain in a neonate, both physiologic and behavioral responses of the neonate to nociceptive or painful stimuli have been identified.[33] Physiologic manifestations of pain include increased heart rate, increased muscle tone, and dilated pupils.[33] Skin color and character when pain is present include pallor or flushing, diaphoresis, and palmar sweating.[33] Several neonatal pain measures have been developed, including:
  - The Bernese Pain Scale for Neonates[37]
  - The Neonatal Facial Coding System[38]
  - The Pain Assessment in Neonates (PAIN)[39]
  - The face, legs, activity, cry, and consolability (FLACC) measure
- Assessment of pulmonary function in the infant includes observation of and inspection for signs of respiratory distress (retractions, nasal flaring, expiratory granting, inspiratory stridor, use of accessory respiratory muscles, and bulging of intercostal muscles during expiration), chest configuration, color, breathing patterns, and sneezing.

Clinicians who work in special care nurseries should base their intervention strategies on current knowledge of neonatal development and intervention. Common goals of developmental intervention in the NICU include:[40]

- To promote state organization. A neonate's state behaviors reflect both its own internal endogenous processes and exogenous influences from the environment. Newborns who exhibit irregular or "poorly organized" state patterns are more likely to develop conditions ranging from delayed development, aplastic anemia, and hyperactivity to sudden infant death syndrome (SIDS).
- To promote appropriate parent–infant interaction.
- To enhance self-regulatory behavior through environmental modification.

- To promote postural alignment and more normal patterns of movement through therapeutic handling and positioning (**Table 10-7**).
  - To decrease hyperextension of the neck and trunk, reduce elevation of the shoulders, decrease retraction of the scapula, and reduce extension of the lower extremities
  - To enhance ventilation–perfusion ratios and to drain bronchopulmonary segments
  - To increase midline orientation
- To enhance oral motor skills and assist with oral feedings.
- To improve visual and auditory reactions.
- To provide appropriate remediation of orthopedic complications.
- To provide consultation to team members, including the supervising physical therapist, nursing staff, and parents, regarding developmental intervention.

Pediatric Intervention Strategies

Theoretically, early intervention should result in prevention or reduction of secondary impairments, such as contractures and skeletal deformities that are not generally present as primary impairments in early infancy.[15] Rather, they develop later as a result of habitual movement using compensatory patterns or overactive muscles with paretic antagonists or as a result of overall poverty of movement and disuse.[15] When activity limitations persist for long periods and are not remediable or cannot be compensated for, children may fail to succeed in normal life roles, such as participation in school, play, or family activities.[15]

● **Key Point** Therapy planning should start with interdisciplinary assessment of activity and participation in natural environments when a condition that impairs developmental progress and functional capabilities is already well established.[15]

The PTA should focus on a number of important aspects of the therapeutic process of facilitating functional activity and participation, including:[15]

- A search for the constraints in subsystems that limit motor behavior, such as contractures or weakness, leading to treatment goals related to the reduction of impairments.
- The creation of an environment that supports or compensates for weaker or less mature components of the systems that contribute to development of motor control so as to promote activity and participation. Positioning equipment or orthoses (Chapter 14) can be

TABLE 10-7	Ideal Pediatric Positioning			
Region	Sitting	Prone	Supine	Sidelying
Head and neck	Head in neutral position Facing forward Head evenly on shoulders	Head in neutral position Facing to one side Slight cervical flexion	Head in neutral position Facing forward Slight cervical flexion	Head in neutral position Facing forward Slight cervical flexion
Trunk	Straight Shoulders over hips Neutral rotation	Straight Shoulders in line with hips Neutral rotation	Straight Shoulders in line with hips Neutral rotation of trunk	Straight Shoulders in line with hips Slight sidebending okay
Shoulders and arms	Arms fully supported Elbows in flexion Shoulders internally rotated 0° to 45°	Arms fully supported Arms forward of trunk Flexion at shoulders Flexion at elbows	Arms fully supported Arms forward of trunk Forearms rest on trunk or pillow	Both arms supported Lower arm forward, not lying on point of shoulders Lower arm in neutral rotation Upper arm may have 0° to 40° internal rotation
Pelvis and hips	Pelvis in line with the trunk Hips at 90° of flexion Neutral rotation of pelvis Hips symmetrically abducted 10° to 20°	Pelvis in line with trunk Hips in extension Neutral rotation of pelvis Hips symmetrically abducted 10° to 20°	Pelvis in line with trunk Hips in 30 to 90° of flexion Neutral rotation of pelvis Hips symmetrically abducted 10° to 20°	Pelvis in line with trunk Hips in flexion Neutral rotation of pelvis Hips symmetrically abducted 10° to 20°
Legs and feet	Knees at 90° Ankles at 90° Feet and thighs fully supported	Knees extended Feet supported at 90°	Knees supported in flexion Feet held at 90°	Knees in flexion Feet positioned at 90° Pillow between knees

Data from Ratliffe KT: Clinical Pediatric Physical Therapy: A Guide for the Physical Therapy Team. Philadelphia, Mosby, 1998

prescribed to help maintain skeletal alignment, prevent or reduce development of contractures and deformities, and to facilitate functional abilities. A number of design options should be considered when prescribing an orthosis:

- *Passive deformity management:* Used to reverse a flexible deformity and passively position specific joints and segments to maintain current posture and prevent further deformity
- *Active deformity management:* Used to reverse fixed deformity by actively stretching tissues to allow specific joints and segments to be aligned more optimally
- *Passive function:* Used to reverse a flexible deformity and place specific joints and segments in static positions suitable for passive functional activity, such as using a standing frame or sitting in a wheelchair
- *Active function:* Used to enhance stability or mobility of specific joints and segments in a way that facilitates active function, such

as balancing, standing or walking, or motor retraining

- Attention to setting up a therapeutic environment that affords opportunities to practice tasks in a meaningful and functional context.
- The use of activities that promote exploration of a variety of movement patterns that might be appropriate for a task. This may necessitate addressing patient mobility in his or her environment, and the need for adaptive equipment. Goals for using adaptive equipment (**Table 10-8**) include:
  - To gain or reinforce normal movement
  - To achieve normal postural alignment
  - To prevent contractures and deformities
  - To increase opportunity to participate in social or educational programs
  - To provide mobility and encourage exploration
  - To increase independence in activities of daily living and self-help skills

<table>
<tr><td colspan="2">

TABLE 10-8   Pediatric Adaptive Equipment

</td></tr>
</table>

Equipment	Description
Standers	Promote weight bearing and stretching, and, depending on the child's diagnosis, can help with the proper formation of the hip joint and building bone density. Promote bone mineralization and respiratory, bowel, and bladder function. Help teach mobility skills. Allow child to gain important emotional and social support by enabling him or her to interact with the rest of the world from a "normal" position.
Sidelyers	Used in cases when the patient has a tonic labyrinthe reflex (TLR), which can elicit more extensor tone in supine and more flexor tone in prone.
Adaptive seating	Seating can be customized to meet the specific support and posture needs of the individual. As a general rule, seating systems should be customized to maintain head in neutral position, the trunk upright, and the hips, knees, and ankles in correct alignment. For children with cerebral palsy, seating systems can be designed with a sacral pad and knee block to correct pelvic tilt, decrease pelvic rotation, and abduct/de-rotate the hip joint.
Orthoses	Orthoses are frequently required to maintain functional joint position, especially in nonambulatory or hemiplegic patients. Frequent reevaluation of orthotic devices is important because children quickly outgrow them and can undergo skin breakdown from improper use. Ankle-foot-orthoses (AFOs) are commonly used. Submalleolar orthosis for forefoot and midfoot malalignment.

- ❑ To assist in improving physiological functions
- ❑ To increase comfort

> **● Key Point**   It is extremely important that the patient and primary caregivers are involved in the goal-setting and decision-making process to ensure realistic and meaningful solutions. When correctly prescribed and used, assistive technology, especially therapeutic positioning, may address the dimensions of impairment, particularly by helping to prevent secondary impairments such as skin breakdown, cardiopulmonary compromise due to scoliosis or slouched posture, and contractures or deformity due to inadequately supported body segments.

The goal in selecting a mobility device is to provide an appropriate means of getting from one location to another efficiently. It is commonly agreed that positioning needs take precedence over the issuance of a mobility device. Mobility devices include wheelchairs, walkers, and crutches (refer to Chapter 14). The search for control parameters, such as speed of movement or force production, that can be manipulated by intervention to facilitate the attainment of therapeutic goals, especially during sensitive periods of development during which behavior is less stable is important.

The following guidelines are intended to enhance the learning experience for the pediatric patient:[41]

- *Context:* Children learn more rapidly in stimulating and varied physical environments. Effective learning contexts are those that promote initiations by the learner as well as reciprocity and shared control over the interaction between the child and the PTA. This can be accomplished by providing timely and explicit feedback rather than simply corrective feedback.
- *Motivation:* Motivated learning is intentional learning for improvement.
- *Creative behavior:* Encouraging creative behavior is a powerful means of enhancing the child's learning.

> **● Key Point**   A wide variety of methods can be employed when treating children to make the exercises more enjoyable and stimulating. These include the use of:
> - Balls of different sizes to promote strengthening, balance, and coordination
> - Colored wedges to facilitate or increase muscle contraction needed depending on position of wedge
> - Bolsters, which combine the characteristics of ball and wedge
> - Swings to promote sensory integration
> - Scooter boards for prone stability/mobility tasks
> - Toys
> - Music
> - Pets
> - Hippotherapy (horseback-riding therapy),[42–44] which offers many potential cognitive, physical, and emotional benefits and can be used to help improve the child's tone, ROM, strength, coordination, and balance

- *Appropriate instructions:* These provide a method to convey information about the task requirements. Appropriate instructions:
  - ❑ Should include a description of the task based on the learner's competencies as well as on relevant environmental elements—brevity and meaningfulness are important

- ❑ Can be verbally presented and/or demonstrated
- ❑ Help the child to separate task-relevant information from task-irrelevant information
- *Demonstration or modeling:* Children tend to be more visually dependent than adults. Observational motor learning is an effective strategy for developing the perceptual skills necessary for children to selectively attend to environmental cues.
  - ❑ The demonstrations must be task specific and can be enhanced by verbal labeling, rehearsal, and temporal spacing of demonstrations
  - ❑ Peer modeling (the use of another child to demonstrate) also may be used
- *Purposeful tasks:* These should be active, voluntarily regulated, goal directed, and meaningful to the learner. They should promote the practice of relevant, functional, purposeful tasks, use spatial and temporal anticipation strategies to increase the readiness of the child to respond, and use routine rather than random activities to influence reaction time and facilitate anticipation skills.
- *Feedback:* The provision of feedback is essential. The feedback system has an important place in the process of the organizational development. Feedback describes the situation when information about the result of an event in the past can influence an occurrence or occurrences of the same event in the present or future. Feedback differs from reinforcement in that it combines immediately with the input to drive the response, without changing the responsiveness of the system to future signals. In contrast, reinforcement changes the responsiveness of the system to future signals, without combining with the immediate input.

Interventions for Specific Conditions

Conditions Specific to the Infant

Tetralogy of Fallot

Tetralogy of Fallot (TOF) is a congenital heart defect that is classically understood to involve four anatomical abnormalities:

- *Pulmonary stenosis:* A narrowing of the right ventricular outflow tract; can occur at the pulmonary valve, or just below the pulmonary valve.

- *Overriding aorta:* An aortic valve with biventricular connection, situated above the ventricular septal defect and connected to both the right and the left ventricles. The degree to which the aorta is attached to the right ventricle is referred to as its degree of "override."
- *Ventricular septal defect:* A hole between the two ventricles of the heart.
- *Right ventricular hypertrophy:* A secondary anomaly that develops due to the misarrangement of the external ventricular septum and the increased obstruction to the right outflow tract.

TOF is the most common cyanotic heart defect, and the most common cause of "blue baby" syndrome. Cyanosis develops within the first few years of life, or at birth. TOF is initially treated with pharmacological means but may demand surgical repair.

Respiratory Distress Syndrome

Infant respiratory distress syndrome, previously known as *hyaline membrane disease*, is a syndrome caused in premature infants by developmental insufficiency of surfactant production and structural immaturity in the lungs. It can also result from a genetic problem with the production of surfactant-associated proteins. Respiratory distress syndrome begins shortly after birth and manifests by:

- Dyspnea/tachypnea; over a period of hours to days, hypoxemia worsens, and the patient appears dyspneic and more tachypneic
- Cyanosis during breathing efforts
- Flaring of the nostrils
- Tachycardia
- Use of accessory muscles and chest wall retractions (recession)
- Diffuse rales and expiratory grunting

Treatment varies according to severity but can involve:

- Oxygen with a small amount of continuous positive airway pressure (CPAP). If this is insufficient, an endotracheal tube (breathing tube) is inserted into the trachea, and intermittent breaths are given by mechanical ventilation.
- Intravenous fluids to stabilize the blood sugar, blood salts, and blood pressure.
- An exogenous preparation of surfactant, either synthetic or extracted from animal lungs, given through the breathing tube into the lungs.
- Chest physical therapy.

Arthrogryposis

Arthrogryposis,[45–49] or arthrogryposis multiplex congenita, comprises nonprogressive neurological conditions characterized by multiple joint contractures and rigid joints found throughout the body at birth.

Although joint contractures and associated clinical manifestations vary from case to case, there are several common characteristics:

- Involved extremities are fusiform or cylindrical in shape, with thin subcutaneous tissue and absent skin creases.
- Deformities are usually symmetric, and severity increases distally, with hands and feet typically being the most deformed.
- The patient may have joint dislocation, especially the hips and, occasionally, the knees.
- Distal joints are affected more frequently than proximal joints.
- Range of motion in the jaw frequently is limited.

Intervention

The goals of physical therapy are:

- To minimize contractures through range of motion, positioning, splinting, and stretching
- To utilize adaptive equipment
- To provide family education regarding interaction, therapeutic handling, and positioning

Prader–Willi Syndrome

Prader–Willi syndrome (PWS)[50–53] is a chromosomal microdeletion/disomy disorder arising from deletion or disruption of genes in the proximal arm of chromosome 15 or maternal disomy of the proximal arm of chromosome 15 (genomic imprinting).

Intervention

The goals of physical therapy are:

- To enhance postural control
- To emphasize exercise and fitness
- To promote gross and fine motor skills training

Brachial Plexus Injury

Brachial plexus injury occurs most commonly in large babies, frequently with shoulder dystocia or breech delivery. Traumatic lesions associated with brachial plexus injury are fractured clavicle, fractured humerus, subluxation of cervical spine, cervical cord injury, and facial palsy.

- *Erb palsy (Erb–Duchenne palsy):* A paralysis of the arm caused by injury to the upper group of the arm's main nerves; specifically, the upper trunk C5–C6 is severed. These nerves form part of the brachial plexus, comprising the ventral rami of spinal nerves C5–C8, and T1. These injuries arise most commonly, but not exclusively, from shoulder dystocia during a difficult birth. The involved extremity lies adducted, prone, and internally rotated. Moro, biceps, and radial reflexes are absent on the affected side. Grasp reflex is usually present. Five percent of patients have an accompanying (*ipsilateral*) phrenic nerve paresis. The three most common treatments for Erb palsy are: nerve transfers (usually from the opposite leg), subscapularis releases, and latissimus dorsi tendon transfers.
- *Klumpke paralysis:* A rare form of paralysis involving the muscles of the forearm and hand, resulting from a brachial plexus injury in which the eighth cervical (C8) and first thoracic (T1) nerves are injured either before or after they have joined to form the lower trunk. The injury can result from difficulties in childbirth. The most common etiological mechanism is caused by a traumatic vaginal delivery, necessitated by shoulder dystocia. The subsequent paralysis affects, principally, the intrinsic muscles of the hand and the flexors of the wrist and fingers.

Acquired Conditions

Osgood–Schlatter

Osgood–Schlatter (OS)[54] disease (traction apophysis) is a benign, self-limiting knee condition that is one of the most common causes of knee pain in the adolescent. During periods of rapid growth, stress from contraction of the quadriceps is transmitted through the patellar tendon onto a small portion of the partially developed tibial tuberosity. This may result in a partial avulsion fracture through the ossification center.

Intervention

Specific procedural interventions include:

- Bracing (neoprene knee brace). More persistent cases may require cast immobilization for 6 to 8 weeks.
- Quadriceps stretching exercises, including hip extension for a complete stretch of the extensor mechanism, and stretching exercises for the hamstrings.
- The traditional approach of activity limitations is no longer considered necessary.

Idiopathic Scoliosis

Scoliosis[55–68] represents a disturbance of the intercalated series of spinal segments that produces a three-dimensional deformity (lateral curvature and vertebral rotation) of the spine.

● **Key Point** Despite an extensive amount of research devoted to discovering the cause of idiopathic scoliosis, the mechanics and specific etiology are not clearly understood. It is known, however, that there is a familial prevalence of idiopathic scoliosis.

Using the James classification system, scoliosis has three age distinctions. These distinctions, though seemingly arbitrary, have prognostic significance.

- *Infantile idiopathic:* Children are diagnosed when they are younger than 3 years, usually manifesting shortly after birth.
- *Juvenile idiopathic:* Children are diagnosed when they are aged 3 to 9 years.
- *Adolescent idiopathic:* Manifests at or around the onset of puberty and accounts for approximately 80% of all cases of idiopathic scoliosis.

● **Key Point** Scoliosis is generally described as to the location of the curve or curves. One should also describe whether the convexity of the curve points to the right or left. If there is a double curve, each curve must be described and measured. The magnitude of a rib hump is quantified using a scoliometer (an inclinometer) with the forward bending test. If scoliosis is neglected, the curves may progress dramatically, creating significant physical deformity and even cardiopulmonary problems with especially severe curves. Screening is done in schools across the United States. Generally, curvatures less than 30 degrees will not progress after the child is skeletally mature.

Intervention

Physical therapy intervention for scoliosis is based on skeletal maturity of the child, growth potential of the child, and curve magnitude. A patient with scoliosis that is greater than 40 degrees usually requires surgical spinal stabilization. A patient with scoliosis that ranges between 25 and 40 degrees requires a spinal orthosis and physical therapy intervention:

- *Orthoses:* The active theory of orthotics is that curve progression is prevented by muscle contractions responding to the brace wear.

● **Key Point** Patients are often instructed on exercises to be performed while wearing a brace (pelvic tilts, thoracic flexion, and lateral shifts) to improve the active forces, although there is little evidence to support that this works. Electrical muscle stimulation, spinal manipulation, and nutritional therapies have all been shown to be ineffective for managing the spinal deformity associated with idiopathic scoliosis.

- *Exercise:* The primary benefits of exercise are to help with correct alignment following the bracing program; to maintain proper respiration and chest mobility; to maintain muscle strength, particularly in abdominals; to maintain or improve range of motion and spinal flexibility; and to help reduce back pain, to improve overall posture, and to resume prebracing functional skills.

Skeletal Fracture

The mechanical properties and healing qualities of skeletal bone are described in Chapter 4. Fractures of bone in pediatric patients may be due to direct trauma such as a blow, or indirect trauma such as a fall on an outstretched hand (FOOSH) injury, or a twisting injury. The point on a bone at which the metaphysis connects to the physis is an anatomic point of weakness. The various types of fractures are described in Chapter 4. Three types of fractures are worth noting in the pediatric population:

- *Avulsion:* Occurs when a piece of bone attached to a tendon or ligament is torn away. In children, ligaments and tendons are stronger than bone.
- *Growth plate (physeal):* May be defined as a disruption in the cartilaginous physis of long bones that may or may not involve epiphyseal or metaphyseal bone (Figure 10-1). Injuries to the physes are more likely to occur in the pediatric population, in part due to the greater structural strength and integrity of the

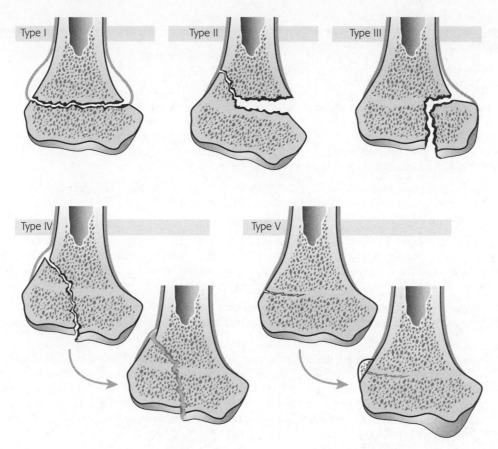

Type I　Type II　Type III

Type IV　Type V

Figure 10-1　Growth plate fractures.

ligaments and joint capsules than of the growth plates, and the fact that the physes of an adult has ossified. Growth plate fractures can have severe consequences because of the potential for growth plate closure, which inhibits future growth, resulting in limb length discrepancies. Conversely, an injury near, but not at, the physis can stimulate increased bone growth.

- *Greenstick:* A type of simple fracture in which only one side of the bone is fractured, while the opposite side is bent (　Figure 10-2　). Because the bones in a pediatric patient have not fully developed, they are less rigid and brittle. This type of fracture tends to heal faster than other types.

The most common clinical presentation with a pediatric fracture is pain, weakness, and functional loss of the involved area. The most common areas for pediatric fracture include the distal radius, the

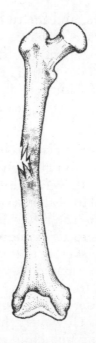

Figure 10-2　Greenstick fracture.

TABLE 10-9	Salter and Harris Classification of Physeal Fractures

Type	Description
I	This fracture typically traverses through the hypertrophic zone of the cartilaginous physis, splitting it longitudinally and separating the epiphysis from the metaphysis. When these fractures are undisplaced, they may not be readily evident on radiographs due to the lack of bony involvement. In many instances, only mild to moderate soft tissue swelling is noted radiographically. In general, the prognosis for this type of fracture is excellent. Usually, only closed reduction is necessary for displaced fractures; however, open reduction and internal fixation may be necessary if a stable satisfactory reduction cannot be maintained.
II	The fracture splits partially through the physis and includes a variably sized triangular bone fragment of metaphysis. This particular fracture pattern occurs in an estimated 75% of all physeal fractures, and it is the most common physeal fracture.
III	This fracture pattern combines physeal injury with an articular discontinuity. This fracture partially involves the physis and then extends through the epiphysis into the joint. It has the potential to disrupt the joint surface. This injury is less common and often requires open reduction and internal fixation to ensure proper anatomical realignment of both the physis and the joint surface.
IV	This fracture runs obliquely through the metaphysis, traverses the physis and epiphysis, and enters the joint. Good treatment results for this fracture are considered to be related to the amount of energy associated with the injury and the adequacy of reduction.
V	These lesions involve compression or crush injuries to the physis and are virtually impossible to diagnose definitively at the time of injury. Knowledge of the injury mechanism simply makes one more or less suspicious of this injury. No fracture lines are evident on initial radiographs, but they may be associated with diaphyseal fractures. SH V fractures are generally very rare; however, family members should be warned of the potential disturbance in growth, and that if growth disturbance occurs, treatment is available (depending upon the child's age and remaining growth potential).
VI	An additional classification of physeal fractures not considered in the original SH classification but now occasionally included is SH VI, which describes an injury to the peripheral portion of the physis and a resultant bony bridge formation that may produce considerable angular deformity.

elbow, the clavicle, and the tibia. The Salter and Harris classification is preferred and is the accepted standard in North America for diagnosing physeal fracture patterns (**Table 10-9**). The most common of the Salter–Harris fractures is II, followed by I, III, IV, and V.

Intervention
In most cases, the medical management of a fracture involves immobilization through casting, splints, or surgical fixation to allow full healing to occur. Pediatric fractures tend to heal faster than an equivalent one in an adult. This can be advantageous: children typically require shorter immobilization times. A disadvantage, however, is that any malpositioned fragments become immovable or fixed much earlier than in adults (3 to 5 days in a young child, 5 to 7 days in an older child, as opposed to 8 to 10 days in an adult). However, the normal process of bone remodeling in a child may correct malalignment, making near-anatomic reductions less

important in children than in adults. Remodeling can be expected if the patient has two or more years of bone growth remaining. Rotational deformity remodels poorly, if at all, and is therefore corrected by surgical reduction. A further complication is that pediatric fractures may stimulate longitudinal growth of the bone, making the bone longer than it would have been had it not been injured. This is particularly true for fractures of the femoral or tibial shaft.

Children tolerate prolonged immobilization much better than adults, and disabling stiffness or loss of range of motion is distinctly unusual after pediatric fractures. Physical therapy, if needed, typically begins after this immobilization period, and depending on the type of fracture, it can involve any or all of the following depending on the location of the fracture:

■ Pain management techniques including the use of non-contraindicated electrotherapeutic modalities (see Chapter 13) and manual techniques, including joint mobilizations by the physical therapist (see Chapter 4)

- Range of motion exercises
- Strengthening exercises, beginning with submaximal isometrics and progressing to multi-angle isometrics, then concentric, eccentric, and plyometrics as appropriate
- Gait and/or crutch training with an appropriate assistive devices and following the prescribed prescription for weight bearing (see Chapter 16)
- Proprioception exercises for balance and coordination (see Chapter 12)
- Functional training, including adaptive, supportive, or protective devices and activities of daily living and self-care
- Patient and family education to decrease the risk of reinjury and to promote healing

Little Leaguer's Elbow

Little Leaguer's elbow is a common term for an avulsion lesion to the medial apophysis. The repetitive motions involved in the various phases of throwing place enormous strains on the elbow, particularly during the late cocking and acceleration phases, which can result in inflammation, scar formation, loose bodies, ligament sprains or ruptures, and the more serious conditions of osteochondritis, or an avulsion fracture. Little League elbow may start insidiously or suddenly. Usually, a sudden onset of pain is secondary to fracture at the site of the lesion.

Clinical findings include a history of pain on the medial side of the elbow, with and without throwing. Physical findings relate to the specific lesion, but they are commonly a persistent elbow discomfort or stiffness due to aggravation by the injury. A locking or "catching" sensation indicates a loose body.

Intervention

Management is conservative, involving rest and elimination of the offending activity for 3 to 6 weeks. If osteochondritis dissecans is present, the joint needs protection for several months. The patient cannot return to pitching until full and normal motion has returned. To prevent elbow disorders, young athletes should adhere to the rules of Little League, which limit the number of pitches per game, per week, and per season, and the number of days of rest between pitching. The pitch count is the most important of these statistics.

Surgical intervention is reserved for patients with symptoms of a loose body or osteochondritis, or who fail to respond to conservative therapy.

Juvenile Rheumatoid Arthritis

Juvenile rheumatoid arthritis (JRA)[69,70] is a group of diseases of unknown etiology that are manifested by chronic joint inflammation. JRA is defined as persistent arthritis, lasting at least 6 weeks, in one or more joints in a child younger than 16 years of age, when all other causes of arthritis have been excluded. JRA can be classified as systemic, oligoarthritis (pauciarticular disease), or polyarticular disease according to onset within the first 6 months.

> ● **Key Point** *Systemic-onset JRA* is characterized by spiking fevers, typically occurring several times each day, with temperature returning to the reference range or below the reference range. May also be accompanied by an evanescent rash, which is typically linear, affecting the trunk and extremities. *Pauciarticular disease* is characterized by arthritis affecting four or fewer joints (typically, larger joints like the knees, ankles, or wrists) while *polyarticular disease* affects at least five joints. Both large and small joints can be involved, often in symmetric bilateral distribution. Severe limitations in motion are usually accompanied by weakness and decreased physical function.

No specific test exists to identify the presence of JRA, and most physicians use a combination of blood tests, x-rays, and the clinical presentation to make an initial diagnosis. The exact etiology of JRA is unclear, but the prevailing theory is that it is an autoimmune inflammatory disorder, activated by an external trigger, in a genetically predisposed host.

Intervention

The treatment of JRA is best undertaken by an experienced team of health professionals, including members from pediatric rheumatology, nursing, and physical and occupational therapy. Pharmacological intervention may include NSAIDs, immunosuppressive medications, tumor necrosis factor (TNF) inhibitors (TNF promotes the inflammatory process), disease-modifying antirheumatic drugs, and corticosteroids. From the physical therapy viewpoint, the supervising PT develops a prioritized problem list and an intervention plan to reduce current impairments, maintain or improve function, prevent or minimize secondary problems, and provide education and support to the child and family.[71] Specific interventions can include any or all of the following:

- Range of motion and stretching exercises
  - *Acute stage:* Passive and active, assisted to avoid joint compression
  - *Subacute/chronic stages:* Active exercises

- Strengthening; avoid substitutions and minimize instability, atrophy, deformity, pain, and injury
  - *Acute and subacute stages:* Isometric exercises progressing cautiously to resistive
  - *Chronic stage:* Judicious use of concentric exercises
- Endurance exercises; provide encouragement to exercise—fun and recreational activities, swimming
- Joint protection strategies and body mechanics education
- Mobility assistive devices as needed
- Rest, as needed; balance rest with activity by using splinting (articular resting)
- Posture and positioning to maintain joint range of motion; patients should spend 20 minutes per day in prone to stretch the hip and knee flexors
- Therapeutic modalities for pain control; paraffin for hands
- Instructions on the wearing of warm pajamas and use of sleeping bag or electric blanket

Slipped Capital Femoral Epiphysis

The hip is the largest joint in the body and is important for postural stability, as well as mobility. Disorders of the developing hip can cause delays or deficiencies in gross motor development with resultant developmental lag in other areas. Slipped capital femoral epiphysis (SCFE)[72–78] is classified as a disorder of epiphyseal growth (**Table 10-10**) and represents a unique type of instability of the proximal femoral growth plate due to a Salter–Harris type 1 fracture through the proximal femoral physis. The cause of SCFE is unclear. Stress around the hip causes a shear force to be applied at the growth plate and causes the epiphysis to move posteriorly and medially. In addition, the position of the proximal physis normally changes from horizontal to oblique during preadolescence and adolescence, redirecting hip forces from compression forces to shear forces. The severity of SCFE is measured in grades of slippage.

The patient usually presents with an antalgic limp and pain in the groin. The leg is usually held in external rotation, both when supine and when standing. With attempts to flex the hip, the legs move into external rotation.

> ● **Key Point** Knowledge of SCFE and its manifestations will facilitate prompt referral by the PTA to the supervising physical therapist and ultimately to an orthopedic surgeon.

Intervention

The PTA may be involved in the hospital on an inpatient or outpatient basis, work in home care, or work at school. Functions of the PTA with the pediatric population include ordering equipment, providing mobility training, teaching and monitoring range of motion and strengthening exercises, or consulting about environmental adaptations. The goals of treatment are:[76]

- To avoid further damage or remodeling of the affected hip joint to keep the displacement to a minimum
- To maintain motion
- To delay or prevent premature degenerative arthritis

TABLE 10-10	Epiphyseal Disorders: Slipped Capital Femoral Epiphysis	
Epiphyseal Disorder	**Incidence**	**Clinical Features and Diagnosis**
Slipped capital femoral epiphysis (SCFE) (adolescent coxa vara)	Males (13–16 years of age) are two to five times more likely to be affected than females (11–14 years of age). 25% to 33% bilateral, especially with boys younger than 12 years. More common in blacks.	Obesity (75% of cases). Mild hip pain referred to the medial aspect of the knee. Slight limp that increases with fatigue; positive Trendelenburg sign. Posture: lower extremity unloaded into flexion, external rotation, and abduction to avoid impingement of metaphysis on the anterior lip of acetabulum. Reduced hip flexion, internal rotation, abduction. Diagnosis is confirmed with x-ray; AP and lateral views helpful, but frog view with positive Kline's line is definitive.

Data from Hallisy KM: The adolescent population, in Boissonnault WG (ed): Primary Care for the Physical Therapist: Examination and Triage. St. Louis, Elsevier Saunders, 2005, pp 175–237

Following surgical fixation, using one or two pins or screws, usually in situ, the PT completes a careful and thorough examination of the motion of the hip joint. Subsequent measurements should be taken after every operation and removal of the cast. The weight-bearing status can vary but is usually non-weight bearing or touch-down weight bearing. Full weight bearing is permitted when the growth plate has fused (within approximately 3 to 4 months).

> ● **Key Point** Complications from surgery include chondrolysis and/or necrosis of the femoral head, both of which increase the likelihood of significant joint degeneration in later years.

Range of motion exercises for the hip should be done in all planes, with particular emphasis on hip flexion, internal rotation, and abduction. Strengthening of the involved extremity is introduced when sufficient healing has occurred. Gait training post-surgery is initiated once lower-extremity strength and range of motion are adequate for ambulation skills.

Legg–Calvé–Perthes Disease

Legg–Calvé–Perthes disease (LCPD) is the name given to idiopathic osteonecrosis of the capital femoral epiphysis of the femoral head. LCPD has an unconfirmed etiology, but it may involve an interruption of the blood supply to the capital femoral epiphysis known as *osteochondroses* (avascular necrosis of the epiphysis).[79-85] As with those patients with an SCFE, knowledge of this disease and its manifestations will facilitate early recognition and referral by the PTA to the supervising physical therapist. Patients tend to have a limp and frequently have a positive Trendelenburg sign resulting from pain or hip abduction weakness.[76] Limited hip range of motion is noted, especially in hip abduction and internal rotation. The child complains of pain in the groin, hip, or knee (referred pain).[76] The disease process takes from 2 to 4 years to complete.[82] Controversy exists regarding the appropriate treatment, or whether treatment is even necessary.[76] The goal of treatment is to relieve pain, as well as to maintain the spherical shape of the femoral head and to prevent extrusion of the enlarged femoral head from the joint. Physical therapy may be provided at home, at school, or in the clinic. Treatment methods include:

- Observation only
- Range of motion exercises in all planes of hip motion (especially internal rotation and abduction)
- Bracing
- Casting
- Surgery

Intervention

Specific procedural interventions can be used to relieve the forces incurred during weight bearing (crutch training, aquatic therapy). Gait training may be initiated with an orthosis or with bracing. The specific gait pattern and assistive devices depend on the type of orthosis. Patient and family education is necessary to teach hip protection strategies, which will minimize degenerative changes as the child ages.

Scheuermann Disease

Scheuermann disease, which is found in approximately 10% of the population and in males and females equally, typically is seen in pubescent athletes.[86] The disease involves a defect to the ring apophysis of the vertebral body and anterior wedging of the affected vertebrae, as a result of a flexion overload of the anterior vertebral body (Figure 10-3).[87] The end

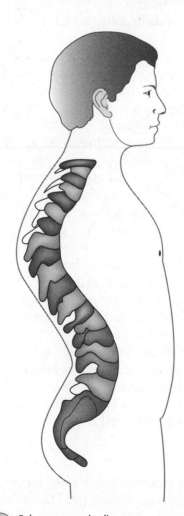

Figure 10-3   Scheuermann's disease.

plate can crack, thus making it possible for disk material to bulge into the vertebral body (Schmorl node). The initial onset is typically asymptomatic, but as the condition progresses, the patient may complain of an aching sensation in the upper spine. In addition, there may be observational evidence of an increased thoracic kyphosis and pain with thoracic extension and rotation, usually detected during a school physical or noted by the parents.

Intervention

The intervention depends on the severity but typically involves postural education, a modification of the aggravating activity, exercise, or bracing. The exercise program involves the stretching of the pectoralis major and minor muscles, and muscle-strengthening exercises for the thoracic spine extensors (seated rotation, and extension in lying exercises) and the scapular adductors.[88]

Osteochondritis Dissecans

Osteochondritis dissecans (OCD) is a rare cause of anterior knee or elbow pain in the young athlete. OCD is a joint disorder in which cracks form in the articular cartilage and the underlying subchondral bone due to vascular deprivation (*avascular necrosis*). The result is fragmentation (*dissection*) of both cartilage and bone, and the free movement of these osteochondral fragments within the joint space, causing pain and further damage. If it occurs in the knee, it involves the weight-bearing portions of the medial and lateral femoral condyles. Occasionally, pain may not be the most prominent symptom, but a catching sensation with joint motion may be the primary complaint if there is a loose body within the joint space. If the lesion is small, a painful arc is present during active and passive movement. Nonsurgical treatment is rarely an option because the capacity for articular cartilage to heal is limited. As a result, even moderate cases require some form of surgery. When possible, nonoperative forms of management such as protected weight bearing (partial or non-weight bearing) and immobilization are used. Surgical treatment varies widely and includes arthroscopic drilling of intact lesions, securing of cartilage flap lesions with pins or screws, drilling and replacement of cartilage plugs, stem cell transplantation, and joint replacement.

Intervention

Postoperative rehabilitation usually involves immobilization then physical therapy. During the immobilization period, isometric exercises are commonly used to restore muscle lost to atrophy without disturbing the cartilage of the affected joint. Once the immobilization period has ended, physical therapy involves protection of the joint's cartilage surface and underlying subchondral bone with maintenance of muscle strength and range of motion and low-impact activities, such as walking or swimming.

Osteogenesis Imperfecta

Osteogenesis imperfecta (OI) is an inherited condition resulting from abnormality in the type I collagen (found in bones, organ capsules, fascia, cornea, sclera, tendons, meninges, and dermis), which causes the bones to be brittle. In the most severe forms, the infant is born with multiple fractures sustained in utero or during the birth process.

Intervention

Typical participation restrictions for an infant with OI depend on the severity of the case and the types of immobilizations employed.[89–92]

> **● Key Point** When handling an infant, it is important not to put forces across the long bones; instead, support the head and trunk with the arms and legs gently draped across the supporting arm. It is also important to change the carrying position of the infant periodically because he or she develops strength by accommodating to postural changes. The caregiver and clinician must be aware of the signs of a fracture, which include inflammation (warmth of the site, edema, and pain), bruising, irritability, and deformity.

Possible interventions include:

- An aquatic exercise program
- Braces and splints; usually required in moderate to severe OI to begin standing activities on solid surfaces
- Gait training, which is progressed in the usual fashion (parallel bars and moving to various assistive devices); commonly initiated when the child has achieved strength with a rating of at least 3/5 (Fair) and when range of motion has reached a plateau

> **● Key Point** Remember that when children use walkers or crutches, a large percentage of the body weight is borne by the upper extremities, necessitating precautions against bowing deformities of the radius and ulna.

- Wheelchair, which is often required for mobility by children with severe types of OI because of the shortened extremities. Wheelchairs are often specially ordered and may require adaptations

Asthma (Hyperreactive Airway Disease)

Asthma is a chronic inflammatory disorder of the airways, characterized by (particularly at night, or in the early morning) recurrent episodes of wheezing, breathlessness, chest tightness, and coughing. In extreme cases, asthma can lead to respiratory failure. Asthma is typically caused by environmental and genetic factors, but other factors, such as food allergens, stress, fatigue, and viral infections, have also been implicated. The medical treatment for asthma includes the use of bronchodilators.

> ● **Key Point** Exercise-induced asthma (EIA), or exercise-induced bronchospasm, is an asthma variant defined as a condition in which exercise or vigorous physical activity triggers acute bronchospasm in persons with heightened airway reactivity to numerous exogenous and endogenous stimuli.

Intervention

Physical therapy intervention for asthma[93] may include any or all of the following:

- Patient education on how to self-monitor asthma symptoms, patterns, and response to medications, and to perform and record peak flow readings (where appropriate).[94,95]
- Patient education on breathing exercises (specific diaphragmatic training from recumbent to upright positions, and eventually to sporting conditions), postural education, relaxation techniques, and endurance and strength training.[96–99]
- Home exercise program incorporating lengthening of neck accessory muscles through active stretching, mid trunk stabilization exercises, and controlled breathing techniques.

Traumatic Brain Injury

The various causes of traumatic brain injury (TBI) are described in Chapter 5.

Intervention

The intervention will depend on the impairments and functional limitations found in the examination and listed in the POC. Common impairments include:[100]

- Abnormal muscle tone
- Postural asymmetry
- Decreased muscle strength
- Loss of range of motion
- Ataxia

- Poor balance
- Behavior state changes
- Poor motor planning
- Poor visual perceptual skills
- Impaired cognition

Activity limitations may include:[100]

- Decreased age-appropriate mobility
- Delayed gross motor skills
- Poor school performances
- Decreased attention to environment

Specific goals for the intervention may include:

- To maintain or improve joint ROM (positioning, casting, and passive ROM)
- To maximize functional mobility; intervention is directed at assisting the child in the achievement of the highest possible levels of independent functioning in his or her home, school, and residential community
- To maximize strength and postural control
- To stimulate/arouse level of consciousness
- To facilitate gross and fine motor development through appropriate positioning, postures, and movements
- To maximize patient/caregiver competence with therapeutic positioning and handling
- To provide a home program

Congenital Conditions

Congenital Muscular Torticollis

Congenital muscular torticollis (CMT)[101–108] (from the Latin *torti*, meaning "twisted," and *collis*, meaning "neck") refers to presentation of the neck in a twisted or bent position due to a unilateral shortening of the sternocleidomastoid (SCM) muscle. The position adopted by the head and neck is one of:

- Side bending of the neck to the same side as the contracture
- Rotation of the neck to the opposite side as the contracture

> ● **Key Point** CMT is named for the side of the involved SCM muscle—e.g., a left CMT involves the left SCM and results in sidebending of the head and neck to the left and rotation to the right. There is little agreement as to the etiology of CMT. Theories include direct injury to the SCM muscle (due to birth trauma or intrauterine malpositioning), abnormal vascular patterns, rupture of the muscle, infective myositis, fibrosis of the SCM, neurogenic injury, and hereditary factors.

In addition, the infant may exhibit asymmetric neck extension and forward head posture due to upper cervical extension.

> ● **Key Point** In infants with CMT, neck range of motion is decreased for ipsilateral rotation, contralateral lateral flexion, and contralateral asymmetric flexion and extension. The infant is not able to maintain a midline alignment of the head with the torso in static postures or during movement because of the neck muscle imbalance and muscle contracture.

Complications associated with CMT include:

- Worsening of any scoliosis or skull and facial asymmetry
- Having a detrimental influence on compensatory movement patterns affecting motor control development
- Persistent asymmetry of early reflexes and reinforcement of an asymmetric postural preference
- Neglect of the ipsilateral hand, through decreased visual awareness of the ipsilateral visual field
- Interference of symmetric development of head and neck righting reactions
- Delayed propping and rolling over the involved side and limited vestibular, proprioceptive, and sensorimotor development. In the older child this may result in asymmetric weight bearing in sitting, crawling, walking, and transitional movement skills as well as incomplete development of automatic postural reactions

Intervention

Intervention[106] is directed toward resolving each impairment or activity limitation identified by the physical therapy examination. The goals of physical therapy typically include:

- To increase range of motion using passive neck ROM exercises (ipsilateral rotation, contralateral lateral flexion, and contralateral asymmetric extension from a starting point of neutral cervical spine alignment), active assistive ROM, strengthening, and postural control exercises.
- To provide family and caregiver education on how to carry and position the infant to promote elongation of the involved SCM and how to promote active contraction of the contralateral SCM.
- Developmental exercises. For example, with a left CMT:[106]
  - *Supported sitting:* The infant's head is prevented from tilting to the left. Toy

placement is used to promote head rotation to the left. Manual guidance is given to the left upper extremity for forward flexion, external rotation, and forearm supination during reach and grasp.
  - *Supine:* Toys are placed slightly to the left to promote rotation of the head to the left, while the central axis alignment of head to body is maintained with sustained light traction on the occiput or base of the skull. Reaching and grasping activities allow the infant to exercise in an open kinetic chain to activate left upper extremity flexion, external rotation, elbow extension, horizontal abduction, and adduction.
  - *Sidelying (on the left):* Soft supports are placed anterior and posterior to the infant's trunk to allow the infant to be positioned in a three-quarters sidelying position
- Assistive devices may be used to help obtain, maintain, or restrain motion in infants or children who are 4 months of age or older. These devices include a fabricated-to-fit, soft neck collar, or a *tubular orthosis for torticollis* (TOT).

Cystic Fibrosis

Cystic fibrosis (CF) is an autosomal recessive disorder of exocrine gland function, involving multiple organ systems (lungs, liver, intestine, pancreas) and chiefly resulting in chronic respiratory infections, pancreatic enzyme insufficiency, and associated complications in untreated patients. The failure of epithelial cells to transport chloride and the associated water results in a buildup of viscous secretions in the respiratory tract, pancreas, liver, gastrointestinal tract, and sweat glands. The increased viscosity of these secretions makes them difficult to clear. Although CF is a terminal disease, the median age of death has increased to 35 years of age due to early detection and comprehensive management.

> ● **Key Point** Sweat chloride analysis is used to distinguish CF from other causes of severe pulmonary and pancreatic insufficiencies and to define patients requiring further analysis.[109]

The clinical characteristics of CF include:[110]

- Postural abnormalities; comparative dimensions of the chest in the anterior–posterior and transverse planes may reveal the barrel chest deformity common to obstructive lung diseases[111]

- Poor weight gain
- Modifications of breathing pattern, or signs of respiratory distress
- Chronic productive cough
- Recurrent infections
- Salty-tasting skin

Patients with cystic fibrosis often require management by a multidisciplinary team including physicians, nurses, nutritionists, physical therapists, respiratory therapists, counselors, and social workers. The goals of the intervention are:

- To maintain adequate nutritional status
- To prevent pulmonary and other complications
- To encourage physical activity
- To provide adequate psychosocial support

Specific chest physical therapy techniques for the infant include but are not limited to:[110,112]

- Postural draining, percussion, and vibrations. Timing the physical therapy around feeding schedules may be necessary to reduce the risk of gastroesophageal reflux. Postural drainage positions are easily achieved by arranging the infant in the required manner on the caregiver's lap. The applied force of percussion should vary with the size and condition of the infant, and conscientious monitoring of the infant's response to treatment should guide the amount of vigor used.
- Education for the family in the application of prescribed physical therapy modalities should be ongoing. The patient may also be trained to use autogenic drainage, a positive expiratory pressure (PEP) device, or flutter valve therapy. Mechanical percussors ease the work involved with manual percussion and provide the child with an aid to self-treatment.

The intervention for the preschool and school-age period depends on the severity of illness. The goals should encompass an improvement in exercise tolerance with continued attention to secretion clearance techniques (postural drainage, percussion, and vibration), correction and maintenance of proper postural alignment, and continued education of the caregivers. Exercise has also been shown to be a useful therapeutic modality for secretion clearance, increases in peak oxygen consumption, increased maximal work capacity, and improved expiratory flow rates.[113,114]

Developmental Dysplasia of the Hip

Developmental dysplasia of the hip (DDH), formerly referred to as congenital hip dysplasia (CHD), involves an abnormal growth/development of the hip including the osseous structures, such as the acetabulum and the proximal femur, and the labrum, capsule, and other soft tissues, which results in a failure of the femoral head to rest in the acetabulum of the pelvis. The condition may occur at any time, from conception to skeletal maturity, but it usually develops in the last trimester of pregnancy. The various types of developmental dysplasia of the hip in infancy include:

- *Dysplasia:* Acetabular may be shallow or small with diminished lateral borders. It may occur alone or with any level of femoral deformity or displacement.
- *Subluxation:* The femoral head is displaced to the rim of the acetabulum, sliding laterally.
- *Dislocated:* The femoral head is displaced completely outside the acetabulum, but it can be reduced with manual pressure.
- *Tetraologic:* The femoral head lies completely outside the hip socket and cannot be reduced with manual pressure.

Intervention

The treatment of this condition depends on the child's age and the severity of the condition. Although surgical intervention is an option in severe cases, the conservative approach is discussed here. Conservative treatment will be most effective for infants whose subluxation or dislocation have been discovered and treated early, within the first 6 months of life. The conservative approach involves maintaining the hip in flexion and abduction through bracing, splinting, or diapering until it is adequately remodeled.

- *Diapering:* The child is placed in two or three diapers to hold the legs in abduction, and parents are instructed to position the infant in hip flexion as well.
- *Pavlik harness*: A Pavlik harness is used if symptoms persist after several weeks (Figure 10-4). The harness, which is initially worn 24 hours a day for 6 to 12 weeks, restricts hip extension and adduction and allows the hip to be maintained in flexion and abduction, the "protective position."[76] The position of flexion and abduction enhances normal acetabular development, and the kicking motion allowed in this position stretches the contracted hip adductors and promotes spontaneous reduction of the dislocated hip.[76] After the initial period, the harness is worn 12 hours per day for 3 to 6 additional months, or until both clinical and radiographic signs are normal. In infants older than 9 months of age who are beginning to walk independently, an abduction orthosis can be used as an alternative to the Pavlik harness.[76] If the Pavlik harness is used, it is important to teach the parents to place the hips in the correct position—too much flexion or abduction can cause excessive pressure through the femoral heads, resulting in possible avascular necrosis.

The PTA may provide strengthening and range of motion activities, progressive gait training, caregiver training for transfers, or mobility and exercise, or the PTA may consult for adaptive equipment and functional access for the child.

Equinovarus

Clubfoot, or talipes equinovarus, is a congenital deformity consisting of hindfoot equinus (i.e., plantarflexion), hindfoot varus, and forefoot varus (the forefoot is curved inward in relation to the heel, the heel is bent inward in relation to the leg, and the ankle is fixed in plantarflexion with toes pointed down). Clubfoot can be classified as:

- Postural or positional (not true clubfoot)
- Fixed or rigid; either flexible (i.e., correctable without surgery) or resistant (i.e., requires surgical release)

Intervention

Treatment consists of manipulation (reducing the talonavicular joint by moving the navicular laterally and the head of the talus medially) by the PT, taping, stretching, bracing, and serial casting, which is most effective if started immediately after birth. The role of the PTA involves monitoring of the casts, providing developmental intervention to promote typical functional skills, and to assist in stretching and splinting.

Congenital Limb Deficiencies

Children with limb deficiencies (CLD) or amputations need to make substantial adaptations to achieve effective function as growth and maturation occur. A variety of genetic syndromes have been implicated in patterns of skeletal abnormalities in children, but the cause is unknown in approximately 60% to 70% of cases. Congenital limb deficiencies can be classified into two major groups:

- *Transverse deficiencies:* A limb that has developed normally to a certain point, with structures beyond that point absent. For example, a child's lower extremity has a fully developed femur but no tibia, fibula, tarsal, metatarsals or phalanges.

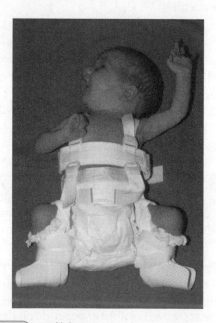

Figure 10-4 Pavlik harness.

- *Longitudinal deficiencies:* A limb that has elements in the long axis of the limb that are absent. For example, a child who is missing the radius and thumb in one upper extremity, with the ulna, carpals, and other digits present.

The clinical presentation varies according to the type of CLD, the level of the deficiency, and the number of deficiencies or limbs involved.

Intervention

The intervention for this population is directed toward helping the child develop appropriate functional and developmental skills while reducing any secondary impairments, such as soft tissue contractures. The PTA may be involved in problem solving, checking prosthetic fit, and communicating with team members.

Cerebral Palsy

Cerebral palsy (CP)[21,42,43,116–159] is considered to be a nonprogressive defect or lesion in single or multiple locations in the immature brain resulting in disorders of posture and controlled movement. Clinical presentation is highly variable. CP is diagnosed when a child does not reach motor milestones and exhibits abnormal muscle tone or quanlitative differences in movement patterns such as asymmetry.

> **● Key Point** In most cases of CP the exact cause is unknown but is most likely multifactorial (intracranial hemorrhage; intrauterine infection; birth asphyxia; Rh incompatibility; multiple births; early prenatal, perinatal, or postnatal injury due to vascular insufficiency; or CNS malformation).

CP has been classified in a number of ways. A classification based on the area of the body exhibiting motor impairment yields the designations of *monoplegia* (one limb), *diplegia* (primarily lower limbs, although upper limbs can be involved), *hemiplegia* (upper and lower limbs on one side of the body), and *quadriplegia* (all limbs). Another classification is based on the most obvious movement abnormality resulting from common brain lesions: spastic, athetoid, ataxic, low tone, or a combination.

- *Spastic:* Constitutes 75% of patients with cerebral palsy. Patients have signs of upper motor neuron involvement, including hyperreflexia, clonus, extensor Babinski response, persistent primitive reflexes, and overflow reflexes (i.e., crossed adductor).
- *Athetoid:* Low muscle stiffness with fluctuating muscle tone and poor functional stability,

especially in the proximal joint. Patient tends to exhibit slow, involuntary, continuous writhing movements of the upper and lower extremities.
- *Ataxic:* Low postural tone with poor balance.
- *Low tone:* Diminished resting muscle tone and decreased ability to generate voluntary muscle force.

Impairments in CP are problems of the neuromuscular and skeletal systems that are either an immediate result of the existing pathophysiologic process or an indirect consequence that has developed over time:

- *Primary impairments of the muscular system:* Insufficient force generation, spasticity, abnormal extensibility, and exaggerated or hyperactive reflexes.
- *Primary impairments of the neuromuscular system:* Poor selected control of muscle activity, poor regulation of activity in muscle groups in anticipation of postural changes and body movement (anticipatory regulation), and decreased ability to learn unique movements.
- *Secondary impairments of the skeletal system:* Malalignment such as torsion or hip deformities.

> **● Key Point** The clinical term *tone* is used to describe the impairments of spasticity and abnormal extensibility. Supraspinal and interneuronal mechanisms appear to be responsible for spasticity.

Intervention

The physical therapy intervention should include:

- Family and caregiver education and support
- Maximization of gross motor activity using a variety of movement and postures to promote sensory variety (reaching, rolling, sitting, crawling, transitional movements, standing, and prewalking skills)
- Promoting normalization of tone using positioning that promotes the full lengthening of spastic or hypoextensible muscles
- Promoting functional voluntary movement of limbs by incorporating active movements such as the handling of toys that require two hands and that encourage the infant to develop flexor control and symmetry while promoting anterior, posterior, and lateral control
- Helping the child compensate for activity limitations when necessary

- Tasks that are purposeful, relevant, developmentally appropriate, active, goal-directed, and meaningful to the child[160]

> ● **Key Point** The focus of treatment in the preschool years is to include activities such as transitional movements against gravity, ball gymnastics, treadmill use, and practice of functional skills such as ascending and descending stairs. These activities can help to improve force generation of muscles and prevent atrophy.[155]
>
> During the school age and adolescent years, the focus is to maintain muscle extensibility (casting, stretching, daily ROM exercises) and force generation, joint integrity (joint mobilizations), and fitness while considering the stresses of growth, maturation, and increasing demand in life skills and participation in community activities (horseback riding, swimming, skiing, sailing, canoeing, camping, fishing, yoga, and tai chi).

Down Syndrome (Trisomy 21)

Down syndrome is a chromosomal abnormality characterized by the presence of an extra copy of genetic material on the 21st chromosome, either in whole (trisomy 21) or in part (such as due to translocations). Translocation occurs when part of a chromosome breaks off during cell division and attaches to another chromosome.

> ● **Key Point** When some of the cells in the body are normal and other cells have trisomy 21, it is referred to as *mosaic Down syndrome.*

The extra chromosome 21 that occurs in Down syndrome affects almost every organ system and results in a wide spectrum of phenotypic consequences. Impairments associated with this condition include hypotonia, ligamentous laxity, and associated joint hypermobility (especially craniovertebral), scoliosis, decreased force generation of muscles, feeding impairments, congenital heart defects, visual and hearing losses, and cognitive deficits (mental retardation). The exact etiology of Down syndrome is currently unknown. During pregnancy, a female can be tested for alpha-fetoprotein (a fetal liver protein), estriol (a pregnancy hormone), human chorionic gonadotropin (hCG, a pregnancy hormone), and inhibin-alpha (INHA). Invasive screening tests include amniocentesis, chorionic villus sampling (CVS), or percutaneous umbilical cord blood sampling (PUBS).

Intervention

The role of physical therapy depends on the particular manifestations of the disorder but can include:

- Minimizing gross motor delay; although physical therapy will not accelerate developmental milestones, it can help the patient avoid compensatory patterns.
- Techniques to counteract hypotonia (see
- Chapter 5)
- Strengthening exercises
- Encouraging verbal–motor function
- Emphasis on exercise and fitness for the management of obesity
- Balance and coordination exercises
- Maximizing respiratory function
- Nutritional consult
- Learning strategies based on level of mental retardation
- Family and caregiver education

Duchenne Muscular Dystrophy

The muscular dystrophies (MD) associated with defects in dystrophin[161–170] (dystrophin is integral to the structural stability of the myofiber) range greatly.

> ● **Key Point** Duchenne muscular dystrophy (DMD), the best-known form of muscular dystrophy, is characterized by rapid progression of muscle degeneration that affects boys and, very rarely, girls. The etiology of DMD is inheritance as an X-linked recessive trait, with the mother being the silent carrier. DMD typically manifests with weakness in the pelvis and upper limbs, resulting in clumsiness, frequent falling, inability to keep up with peers while playing, and an unusual gait (lateral trunk sway—waddling). One of the characteristic signs is that the individual needs to push on his or her legs with the hands in order to attain an upright position (Gower sign). The posterior calf is usually enlarged as a result of fatty and connective tissue infiltration, or by compensatory hypertrophy of the calves secondary to weak tibialis anterior muscles. As DMD progresses, a wheelchair may be needed during adolescence. Most patients with Duchenne MD die in their early 20s because of muscle-based breathing and heart problems.

Intervention

Medical management focuses on maintaining function of the unaffected musculature for as long as possible through the use of glucocorticoids and immunosuppressant medications in an effort to maximize the quality of life. The focus of physical therapy is to:

- Maintain available strength. Mild, non-jarring physical activity such as swimming is encouraged. Manual muscle testing should be evaluated on a consistent basis.
- Retard the development of contractures. This can be achieved through ROM exercises, stretching of the iliotibial band/tensor fascia latae, iliopsoas, hamstrings, and Achilles tendon, and the use of night splints. Range of motion testing should be

evaluated on a consistent basis to determine the pattern and rate of disability.

- Encourage mobility. Braces, such as ankle–foot orthoses and knee–ankle–foot orthoses, are important adjuncts in prolonging the period of ambulation/mobility and delaying wheelchair dependency. However, the use of orthoses for a standing program or continuation of supported walking should be considered a personal rather than therapeutic decision.[171]
- Promote family involvement in a home program.

> ● **Key Point** The role of exercise in the treatment of muscular dystrophy is controversial.

Once wheelchair dependency becomes inevitable (usually at the 9- to 14-year age range), attention should shift to prophylaxis against the deleterious consequences of immobility:

- The chair should be customized to the patient's needs. Eventually, a power wheelchair is necessary because upper-extremity and truncal weakness will typically not allow use of a motorized scooter.[171]
- The fit of the wheelchair must be closely monitored to provide adequate support. Strategic cushioning and supports can help maintain alignment of the spine and pelvis, and reduces the incidence of pressure sores with attendant skin breakdown, which often occur in the sacral and coccygeal regions. The footrests should be modified to support the ankle in a neutral position. A reclining back will allow a position change while sitting in a wheelchair and will help deter flexion contracture formation at the hip.[171]
- Adaptive devices, such as specially designed wheelchair tables and ball-bearing splints, maximize upper-extremity mobility in muscles that cannot resist gravity.
- Emphasis should shift toward an exercise program of active assistive and active exercises of the upper extremities. Key muscle groups for maintenance of strength for transfers include the shoulder depressors and triceps.[171] The shoulder flexor and abductor and elbow flexor muscle groups are key areas for exercises to maintain routine ADLs such as self-feeding and hygiene.[171]
- Breathing exercises, postural drainage, or intermittent pressure breathing treatments should be included in the management program based on results of pulmonary evaluation.

Spina Bifida

Myelodysplasia, of which spina bifida is a subclassification, refers to a defective development of any part (especially the lower segments) of the spinal cord.[35,36,172–176] Spina bifida includes a continuum of congenital anomalies of the spine due to insufficient closure of the neural tube and failure of the vertebral arches to fuse. Spina bifida is classified into *aperta* (visible or open) and *occulta* (not visible, or hidden). The three main types of spina bifida are:

- *Spina bifida occulta:* "Occulta" means hidden, and the defect is not visible. This type is rarely linked with complications or symptoms, and it is usually discovered accidentally during an x-ray or MRI for some other reason.
- *Meningocele (spina bifida aperta):* The membrane that surrounds the spinal cord may enlarge, creating a lump or "cyst." This is often invisible through the skin and causes no problems. If the spinal canal is cleft, or "bifid," the cyst may expand and come to the surface. In such cases, since the cyst does not enclose the spinal cord, the cord is not exposed. The cyst varies in size, but it can almost always be removed surgically if necessary, leaving no permanent disability.
- *Myelomeningocele (spina bifida cystica):* The most complex and severe form of spina bifida, myelomeningocele usually involves neurological problems that can be very serious or even fatal. A section of the spinal cord and the nerves that stem from the cord are exposed and visible on the outside of the body; or, if there is a cyst, it encloses part of the cord and the nerves. This condition accounts for 94% of cases of true spina bifida. The most severe form of spina bifida cystica is myelocele, or myeloschisis, in which the open neural plate is covered secondarily by epithelium and the neural plate has spread out onto the surface.

Intervention[177]
Function
The type of impairment and functional prognosis according to neurosegmental level is outlined in **Table 10-11**.

TABLE 10-11 Impairment and Functional Prognosis According to Neurosegmental Level

Neurosegmental Level	Muscles Innervated	Preambulation Orthoses	Ambulation Orthoses	Assistive Devices	Functional Prognosis	Musculoskeletal Problems
Thoracic	Abdominal	Standing frame	Reciprocating gait orthosis	Parallel bars Walker Forearm crutches	Wheelchair	Spinal deformity Decubiti
Upper lumbar	All of the above muscles innervated, and hip flexors	Standing frame	Reciprocating gait orthosis	Parallel bars Walker Forearm crutches	Wheelchair Possible household or therapeutic ambulation Standing transfers	Hip flexion contractures
Mid lumbar	All of the above muscles innervated, and knee extensors, hip adductors	None	HKAFO KAFO AFO (depending on quad strength)	Parallel bars Walker Forearm crutches	Wheelchair for community, orthoses for household ambulation	Hip dislocation, subluxation
Low lumbar	All of the above muscles innervated, and hip abductors, knee flexors, ankle and foot dorsiflexors, evertors, inverters, toe flexors	None	KAFO AFO	Parallel bars Walker Forearm crutches None	Household or community ambulators	Foot deformities
Lumbosacral	All of the above muscles innervated, and ankle plantar flexors, foot intrinsic muscles	None	AFO or none AFO recommended to maintain gait quality and decrease compensatory overactivity of muscles	Walker None	Community ambulators	Foot pressure sores

Data from Kahn-D'Angel L: Pediatric Physical Therapy, in O'Sullivan SB, Siegelman RP (eds): National Physical Therapy Examination: Review and Study Guide (ed 9). Evanston, IL, International Educational Resources, 2006, pp 232; and Ryan K, Eman J, Ploski C: Goal attainment and habilitation of infants and children with spina bifida. APTA, National Conference, 1991

Positioning

Postural stability is essential to effectively perform functional tasks. Symmetric alignment is important to minimize joint stress and deforming forces and to permit muscles to function at the optimal length. Typical postural problems include forward head, rounded shoulders, kyphosis, scoliosis, excessive lordosis, anterior pelvic tilt, rotational deformities of the hip or tibia, flexed hips and knees, and pronated feet. Static and dynamic balance should be observed in sitting, four-point positioning, kneeling, half-kneeling, and standing, as well as during transitions between these positions. Adaptive equipment is recommended based on age. For example:

- A standing frame may be used in children aged 1 to 2 years to diminish the degree of osteoporosis and to limit the contracture of the hip, knee, and ankle.
- A parapodium may be helpful for children aged 3 to 12 years, allowing patients in an erect posture greater experience standing and manipulating work with their upper extremities at a table or desk.

Bracing

The goal of bracing is to prevent contractures and to allow patients to function at the maximum level possible with their neurological lesion and their intelligence. Bracing also ensures a normal developmental progression, allowing for appropriate age-related activities, with the goal of ambulation.

Exercise

Passive ROM exercises should be brief and should be performed only two to three times each day. Passive ROM exercises must continue throughout the child's life. Exercises, including stretching, can also be used for the correction of muscle imbalances.

Gait Training

Independent ambulation generally is a function of having an intact quadriceps muscle with good or excellent plus strength levels. Patients who do not have adequate quadriceps function may require bilateral Lofstrand crutches or may be primarily restricted to a wheelchair. Functional ambulation generally is described according to the following levels, developed by Hoffer:[178]

- *Community ambulator:* Indoors or outdoors, crutches with or without braces.
- *Household ambulator:* Only indoors, crutches with or without braces.
- *Nonfunctional ambulator:* Wheelchair, crutches, and braces in therapy.
- *Nonambulator:* Wheelchair bound. Focus is on wheelchair mobility, transfers, transitions, and decubiti prevention.

Spinal Muscular Atrophy

The spinal muscular atrophies (SMAs) are characterized by primary degeneration of the anterior horn cells of the spinal cord.

> ● **Key Point** SMA is typically inherited as autosomal recessive. No cure or treatment is currently available for SMA, but physical therapy is commonly advocated.[171]

The primary impairment in all forms of SMA is muscle weakness. Secondary impairments include postural compensations resulting from muscle weakness, contractures, and occasionally scoliosis. Respiratory distress is present early in acute childhood SMA.

Intervention

The primary focus of physical therapy is to improve the quality of life and to minimize disability through access to play, functional use of orthoses and adaptive equipment, and strategies to minimize disabilities secondary to the impairments (positioning, vestibular, and visual stimulation).[171]

Hemophilia

Hemophilia is a bleeding disorder inherited as a sex-linked autosomal recessive trait. Because the genes involved are located on the X chromosome, males are affected (females are carriers) because they have only one X chromosome.[179–183] The condition is caused by an abnormality of plasma clotting proteins (clotting factor VIII in hemophilia A; clotting factor IX in hemophilia B, or Christmas disease) necessary for blood coagulation. The condition is characterized by prolonged bleeding, although the blood flow is not any faster than what occurs in a normal person with the same injury. There are two primary types:

- Hemophilia A (classic hemophilia—Factor VIII deficiency); 80% of all cases
- Hemophilia B (Christmas disease—Factor IX deficiency)

The hallmark of hemophilia is hemorrhage into the joints. This bleeding is painful and leads to long-term inflammation and deterioration of the joint. Complications include:

- Joint contracture(s) and deformities (especially at the hip, knee, elbow, and ankle joints).
- Hemophiliac arthropathy, which may occur in severe forms. The articular cartilage softens, turns brown (due to hemosiderin), and becomes pitted and fragmented.[184] This can result in permanent deformities, misalignment, loss of mobility, and extremities of unequal lengths.
- Muscle weakness and atrophy around affected joints.
- Peripheral nerve compression by hematoma.
- Postural (nonstructural) scoliosis.
- Decreased aerobic fitness.
- Difficulties with ADLs.

Currently, no known cure or prenatal treatment for hemophilia exists.[184]

Intervention

Specific goals include:

- To prevent contractures
- To maintain manual traction and mobilization
- To implement progressive/dynamic splinting
- To implement serial casting/dropout casts
- To teach active ROM exercises (passive ROM is generally contraindicated)
- To maintain strength. Isometric strengthening exercises initially, then the patient moves to graded progressive exercises
- To prevent or diminish disability
- To improve gait through training
- To implement proprioceptive training
- To provide bracing/splints to provide stabilization and protection

Pediatric Oncology

Cancer is the chief cause of death by disease and the second-leading cause of death overall, following trauma, in children ages 1 to 14 years.

> ● **Key Point**   Common signs and symptoms of cancer in children can include fever, pain, a mass or swelling, bruising, pallor, headaches, neurologic changes, and visual disturbances.

Leukemia

Acute lymphoblastic leukemia (ALL) is a malignant disease of the bone marrow in which early lymphoid precursors proliferate and replace the normal hematopoietic cells of the marrow, resulting in a marked decrease in the production of normal blood cells.

Neuroblastoma

Neuroblastoma, an embryonal malignancy of the sympathetic nervous system, is the most common extracranial childhood cancer and the most common tumor occurring during infancy.[185]

Lymphomas

Hodgkin Lymphoma

Hodgkin lymphoma (HL),[186–188] formerly known as Hodgkin disease, is a malignant disorder that arises primarily in peripheral lymph nodes and is most common in young adults in the 20- and 30-year age range. The etiology of HL is unknown.

Non-Hodgkin Lymphoma

The non-Hodgkin lymphomas (NHLs)[189–193] constitute a heterogeneous group of lymphoid system neoplasms with varying presentation, natural history, and response to therapy.

Wilms Tumor

Wilms tumor (WT) is the fifth most common pediatric malignancy and the most common renal tumor in children.[185,194–199] The etiology essentially remains unknown.

Bone Tumors

Osteogenic Sarcoma

Technically, any sarcoma that arises from bone is called an osteogenic sarcoma. Therefore, this term includes fibrosarcoma, chondrosarcoma, and osteosarcoma, all named for their cell of origin.[200–206] Osteogenic sarcoma (osteosarcoma) is the most common form of bone cancer in children and the third most common cancer in adolescence. It is thought to arise from a primitive mesenchymal bone-forming cell and is characterized by production of osteoid. Although an osteosarcoma can occur in any bone, it most commonly occurs in the long bones of the extremities near metaphyseal growth plates (distal femur, tibia, and humerus).

Ewing Sarcoma

Ewing sarcoma, a highly malignant primary medullary bone tumor, is derived from red bone marrow and is most frequently observed in the bone shaft of children and adolescents aged 4 to 15 years.[207–211]

Physical Therapy Role in Oncology Cases

The physical therapy intervention varies according to the physical condition of the patient, the stage of cancer, and the treatment the patient is undergoing. It involves:

- Educating patient and family on the expected goals, processes involved, and the expected outcomes of the intervention
- Assisting patient and family in coping mechanisms and through the grieving process
- Teaching proper positioning to prevent or correct deformities, preserve integrity, and provide comfort
- Controlling edema through elevation of extremities, active range of motion, and massage
- Controlling pain through such modalities as TENS or massage
- Preserving or correcting loss of range of motion through passive, active-assisted, and active range of motion exercises
- Preserving or correcting loss of muscle mass and strength within patient tolerance, weight-bearing limits, and prescribed guidelines
- Preserving or increasing activity tolerance and cardiovascular endurance
- Preserving or increasing independence

REVIEW Questions

1. Describe the purpose of the the Individuals with Disabilities Education Act (IDEA).
2. Describe the purpose of the Individual Family Service Plan (IFSP).
3. Define the term *motor control*.
4. Define the term motor development.
5. How many weeks old is a preterm (premature) infant?
6. At approximately what age (in months) would you expect a normally developing child to be able to perform rolling?
7. At approximately what age (in months) would you expect a normally developing child to be able to perform independent sitting?
8. At approximately what age (in months) would you expect a normally developing child to be able to perform creeping (quadruped)?
9. At approximately what age (in months) would you expect a normally developing child to be able to walk?
10. Developmentally, tonic stability is most evident when a child can do what?
    a. Lift the head while in prone
    b. Hold the head in neutral while sitting upright

c. Maintain pivot prone posture
    d. None of the above
11. Define *knowledge of results* when used in relation to extrinsic feedback.
12. Describe how you would test for the Moro reflex.
13. Describe how you would test for the symmetric tonic neck reflex (STNR).
14. What would be the correct response to the stimulus of turning the head to one side with the asymmetric tonic neck reflex (ATNR).
15. If a child is being held and the dorsum of his or her foot is rubbed against the table, which provokes the foot to be placed on the table, what is this reflex called?
16. According to Brunnstrom, what is the flexor synergy pattern of the lower extremity at the hip, knee and ankle?
17. According to Rood, what is the effect in terms of the agonists and antagonists of stretching an extensor muscle such as the soleus?
    a. The agonists and antagonists are inhibited.
    b. The agonists and antagonists are facilitated.
    c. The agonist is inhibited and the antagonist is facilitated.
    d. The antagonist is inhibited and the agonist is facilitated.
18. Give six characteristics that you would see in a child with cystic fibrosis.
19. All of the following are pathologies of the skeletal system that are present at birth in the neonate, except:
    a. Talipes equinovarus
    b. Scoliosis
    c. Syndactyly
    d. Osteogenesis imperfecta
20. While observing a patient's foot, you notice the following deformity: foot inversion, forefoot adduction, and plantar flexion. What is the name of this deformity?
    a. Talipes equinovarus
    b. Talipes calcaneovalgus
    c. Talipes valgus
    d. Talipes calcaneus
21. Which of the following statements does not apply to osteogenesis imperfecta?
    a. It is a rare congenital skeletal disease.
    b. The bones are extremely fragile.
    c. It is of unknown etiology.
    d. The tendency for fractures is more severe following puberty.

22. The most common and serious deformities as far as congenital dislocations are concerned affect the:
  a. Spine
  b. Hip
  c. Shoulder
  d. Knee

23. Which of the following statements best describes lower-extremity positioning in standing during the first 2 years of life of a child with no dysfunction?
  a. Femoral retroversion, femoral internal rotation, foot supination
  b. Femoral anteversion, femoral external rotation, foot pronation
  c. Femoral retroversion, femoral external rotation, foot pronation
  d. Femoral anteversion, femoral internal rotation, foot supination

24. The clinical picture of scoliosis includes:
  a. Inequality of leg length
  b. Lateral curvature of the spine
  c. Rotation of the spine
  d. All of the above

25. Ewing sarcoma:
  a. Is a malignant tumor.
  b. Can simulate a low-grade osteomyelitis.
  c. Typically has an onset characterized by pain.
  d. All of the above.

26. You are treating an overweight teenage male who has symptoms of moderate or groin and knee pain. His leg abducts and externally rotates during hip flexion. The most likely diagnosis is:
  a. Congenital dislocated hip
  b. Legg–Calvé–Perthes disease
  c. Slipped capital femoral epiphysis
  d. None of the above

27. You are beginning a treatment of a 6-year-old boy with his mother. The mother reports that earlier this morning she pulled the child from a seated position by grasping the boy's right wrist. The child then experienced immediate pain at the right elbow. Which of the following is the most likely diagnosis?
  a. Pulled elbow
  b. Little Leaguer's elbow
  c. Radial head fracture
  d. Muscle strain

28. While treating an infant, you observed that there is limitation of abduction of the flexed right hip and an asymmetry of the gluteal folds. What deformity would you suspect?
  a. Osgood–Schlatter's disease
  b. Osteogenesis imperfecta
  c. Acetabular dysplasia
  d. Osteochondritis dissecans

29. You are treating a patient with Sever disease. What joint should be the focus of your treatment?
  a. Shoulder
  b. Knee
  c. Ankle
  d. Hip

30. Which of the spina bifida types is the most severe form?

31. In which of the spina bifida types may neurologic manifestations be absent?

32. Which spina bifida type is associated with a herniated sac that contains the spinal cord in which the central canal is dilated and greatly distended with cerebrospinal fluid?

33. You are reassessing a 10-year-old boy diagnosed with Duchenne muscular dystrophy. Which of the following do you feel is the most important information to determine?
  a. The boy's most serious physical problems from the perspective of his parents/caretakers.
  b. The results of the motor examination.
  c. The child's developmental milestones, according to the parents.
  d. The results from the WeeFim.

34. A patient presents with neck pain and a deformity of the neck that causes rotation and tilting of the head in the opposite direction. Which diagnosis best describes this patient's condition?

35. You are treating a 15-year-old female distance runner for foot pain of unknown etiology. As you palpate along the medial aspect of the foot and ankle you palpate the head of the first metatarsal bone and the metatarsophalangeal joint. Immediately proximal to this you identify the first cuneiform. What large bony prominence would you expect to find next if you continue to move in and a proximal direction?
  a. Talar head
  b. Navicular
  c. Cuboid
  d. None of the above

36. You are treating a 14-year-old girl who has a body mass index (BMI) of 18. The girl reports extreme difficulty with eating, induced vomiting, and severe constipation. Which of the following would you most likely suspect?

   a. Multiple sclerosis

   b. Anorexia nervosa

   c. Bulemia

   d. Juvenile arthritis

37. The most appropriate school physical therapy intervention to use during class for a child with decreased sitting balance but normal tone would be to:

   a. Use a therapeutic ball to promote sitting balance.

   b. Adapt a desk and wheelchair to provide adequate sitting balance.

   c. Use a prone stander.

   d. Use a sidelyer.

38. Which of the following is characterized by tendinitis of the patella tendon and osteochondroses of its tibial attachment?

   a. Legg–Perthes disease

   b. Rickets

   c. Paget disease

   d. Osgood–Schlatter disease

References

1. Milani-Comparetti A, Gidoni EA: Routine developmental examination in normal and retarded children. Dev Med Child Neurol 9:631–638, 1967

2. Dargassies SS: Neurodevelopmental symptoms during the first year of life. I. Essential landmarks for each key-age. Dev Med Child Neurol 14:235–246, 1972

3. Van Sant AF: Concepts of neural organization and movement, in Connolly BH, Montgomery PC (eds): Therapeutic Exercise in Developmental Disabilities (ed 2). Thorofare, NJ, SLACK, 2001, pp 1–12

4. O'Sullivan SB: Strategies to improve motor function, in O'Sullivan SB, Schmitz TJ (eds): Physical Rehabilitation (ed 5). Philadelphia, F. A. Davis, 2007, pp 471–522

5. Schmidt R, Lee T: Motor control and learning (ed 4). Champaign, IL, Human Kinetics, 2005

6. Thompson S, Watson WH 3rd: Central pattern generator for swimming in Melibe. J Exp Biol 208:1347–1361, 2005

7. Yamaguchi T: The central pattern generator for forelimb locomotion in the cat. Prog Brain Res 143:115–122, 2004

8. Lewis C: Physiological response to exercise in the child: Considerations for the typically and atypically developing youngster, Proceedings from the American Physical Therapy Association combined sections meeting. San Antonio, TX, 2001

9. Schöner G, Kelso JAS: Dynamic pattern generation in behavioral and neural systems. Science 239:1513–1520, 1988

10. Kelso JAS: A dynamical basis for action systems, in Gazzaniga MS (ed): Handbook of cognitive neuroscience. New York, Plenum Press, 1984, pp 321–356

11. Gesell A: The Embryology of Behavior. New York, Harper & Row, 1945

12. Horak FB: Assumptions underlying motor control for neurologic rehabilitation, in Lister MJ (ed): Contemporary Management of Motor Control Problems: Proceedings of the II STEP Conference. Alexandria, VA, Foundation for Physical Therapy, 1991, pp 11–27

13. Campbell SK: The child's development of functional movement, in Campbell SK, Vander Linden DW, Palisano RJ (eds): Physical Therapy for Children. St. Louis, Saunders, 2006, pp 33–76

14. Piaget J: The Origins of Intelligence in Children. New York, International Universities Press, 1952

15. Palisano RJ, Campbell SK, Harris SR: Evidence-based decision-making in pediatric physical therapy, in Campbell SK, Vander Linden DW, Palisano RJ (eds): Physical Therapy for Children. St. Louis, Saunders, 2006, pp 3–32

16. Thelen E: Motor development: A new synthesis. Am Psychol 50:79–95, 1995

17. Shumway-Cook A, Woollacott MH: The growth of stability: Postural control from a development perspective. J Mot Behav 17:131–147, 1985

18. Dubowitz L, Dubowitz V: The Neurological Examination of the Full-Term Newborn Infant. Philadelphia, J. B. Lippincott, 1981

19. Brazelton TB: Neonatal Behavioral Assessment Scale. Philadelphia, J. B. Lippincott, 1973

20. Einspieler C, Prechtl HF, Ferrari F, et al: The qualitative assessment of general movements in preterm, term and young infants: review of the methodology. Early Hum Dev 50:47–60, 1997

21. Prechtl HF: State of the art of a new functional assessment of the young nervous system: An early predictor of cerebral palsy. Early Hum Dev 50:1–11, 1997

22. Connolly BH: Tests and assessment, in Connolly BH, Montgomery PC (eds): Therapeutic Exercise in Developmental Disabilities. Thorofare, NJ, SLACK, 2001, pp 15–33

23. Campbell SK: Test-retest reliability of the Test of Infant Motor Performance. Pediatric physical therapy 11:60–66, 1999

24. Mercuri E, Guzzetta A, Laroche S, et al: Neurologic examination of preterm infants at term age: comparison with term infants. J Pediatr 142:647–655, 2003

25. Chandler LS, Andrews MS, Swanson MW: Movement Assessment of Infants. Rolling Bay, WA, Chandler, Andrews, and Swanson, 1980

26. Blanchard Y, Neilan E, Busanich J, et al: Interrater reliability of early intervention providers scoring the alberta infant motor scale. Pediatr Phys Ther 16:13–18, 2004

27. Piper MC, Pinnell LE, Darrah J, et al: Construction and validation of the Alberta Infant Motor Scale (AIMS). Can J Public Health 83 Suppl 2:S46–S50, 1992

28. Harris SR, Daniels LE: Content validity of the Harris Infant Neuromotor Test. Phys Ther 76:727–37, 1996

29. Bruininks RH: Bruininks Oseretsky Test of Motor Proficiency: Examiner's Manual. Circle Pines, MN, American Guidance Service, 1978

30. Richardson PK, Atwater SW, Crowe TK, et al: Performance of preschoolers on the Pediatric Clinical Test of Sensory

Interaction for Balance. Am J Occup Ther 46:793–800, 1992

31. Deitz JC, Richardson PK, Westcott SL, et al: Performance of children with learning disabilities on the Clinical Test of Sensory Interaction for Balance. Phys Occup Ther Pediatr 16:1–21, 1996

32. Sweeney JK, Heriza CB, Reilly MA, et al: Practice guidelines for the physical therapist in the neonatal intensive care unit (NICU). Pediatric Physical Therapy 11:119–132, 1999

33. Kahn-D'Angel L, Unanue-Rose RA: The Special Care Nursery, in Campbell SK, Vander Linden DW, Palisano RJ (eds): Physical Therapy for Children (ed 3). St. Louis, Saunders, 2006, pp 1053–1097

34. Schneider JW, Krosschell K, Gabriel KL: Congenital spinal cord injury, in Umphred DA (ed): Neurological Rehabilitation (ed 3). St. Louis, Mosby, 1995, pp 454–483

35. Mitchell LE, Adzick NS, Melchionne J, et al: Spina bifida. Lancet 364:1885–1895, 2004

36. Dias L: Orthopaedic care in spina bifida: past, present, and future. Dev Med Child Neurol 46:579, 2004

37. Cignacco E, Mueller R, Hamers JP, et al: Pain assessment in the neonate using the Bernese Pain Scale for Neonates. Early Hum Dev 78:125–131, 2004

38. Grunau RE, Holsti L, Whitfield MF, et al: Are twitches, startles, and body movements pain indicators in extremely low birth weight infants? Clin J Pain 16:37–45, 2000

39. Hudson-Barr D, Capper-Michel B, Lambert S, et al: Validation of the Pain Assessment in Neonates (PAIN) scale with the Neonatal Infant Pain Scale (NIPS). Neonatal Netw 21:15–21, 2002

40. Sheahan MS, Farmer-Brockway N: The high-risk infant, in Tecklin JS (ed): Pediatric physical therapy (ed 2). Philadelphia, JB Lippincott, 1994, pp 56–88

41. Larin HM: Motor learning, in Campbell SK (ed): Physical Therapy for Children. Philadelphia, W. B. Saunders, 1995, pp 157–181

42. Sterba JA: Does horseback riding therapy or therapist-directed hippotherapy rehabilitate children with cerebral palsy? Dev Med Child Neurol 49:68–73, 2007

43. Casady RL, Nichols-Larsen DS: The effect of hippotherapy on ten children with cerebral palsy. Pediatr Phys Ther 16:165–172, 2004

44. Meregillano G: Hippotherapy. Phys Med Rehabil Clin N Am 15:843–54, vii, 2004

45. Mallia Milanes G, Napolitano R, Quaglia F, et al: Prenatal diagnosis of arthrogryposis. Minerva Ginecol 59:201–202, 2007

46. Mennen U, van Heest A, Ezaki MB, et al: Arthrogryposis multiplex congenita. J Hand Surg [Br] 30:468–474, 2005

47. Bernstein RM: Arthrogryposis and amyoplasia. J Am Acad Orthop Surg 10:417–424, 2002

48. Hardwick JC, Irvine GA: Obstetric care in arthrogryposis multiplex congenita. BJOG 109:1303–1304, 2002

49. O'Flaherty P: Arthrogryposis multiplex congenita. Neonatal Netw 20:13–20, 2001

50. Cassidy SB, Dykens E, Williams CA: Prader-Willi and Angelman syndromes: Sister imprinted disorders. Am J Med Genet 97:136–146, 2000

51. Martin A, State M, Koenig K, et al: Prader-Willi syndrome. Am J Psychiatr 155:1265–1273, 1998

52. Cassidy SB, Schwartz S: Prader-Willi and Angelman syndromes: Disorders of genomic imprinting. Medicine (Baltimore) 77:140–151, 1998

53. Cassidy SB: Prader-Willi syndrome. J Med Genet 34:917–923, 1997

54. Mital MA, Matza RA: Osgood-Schlatter's disease: the painful puzzler. Physician Sports Med 5:60, 1977

55. Patrick C: Spinal conditions, in Campbell SK, Vander Linden DW, Palisano RJ (eds): Physical Therapy for Children. St. Louis, Saunders, 2006, pp 337–358

56. McKenzie RA: Manual correction of sciatic scoliosis. N Z Med J 76:194–199, 1972

57. Blum CL: Chiropractic and pilates therapy for the treatment of adult scoliosis. J Manip Physiol Ther 25:E3, 2002

58. Miller NH: Genetics of familial idiopathic scoliosis. Clin Orthop Rel Res 401:60–64, 2002

59. Kane WJ: Scoliosis prevalence: A call for a statement of terms. Clin Orthop 126:43–46, 1977

60. Miller NH: Cause and natural history of adolescent idiopathic scoliosis. Orthop Clin North Am 30:343–352, vii, 1999

61. Dobbs MB, Weinstein SL: Infantile and juvenile scoliosis. Orthop Clin North Am 30:331–341, vii, 1999

62. Greiner KA: Adolescent idiopathic scoliosis: radiologic decision-making. Am Fam Physician 65:1817–1822, 2002

63. Lonstein JE, Winter RB: Adolescent idiopathic scoliosis. Nonoperative treatment. Orthop Clin North Am 19:239–246, 1988

64. Lenke LG: Lenke classification system of adolescent idiopathic scoliosis: Treatment recommendations. Instr Course Lect 54:537–542, 2005

65. Lenke LG, Edwards CC, 2nd, Bridwell KH: The Lenke classification of adolescent idiopathic scoliosis: How it organizes curve patterns as a template to perform selective fusions of the spine. Spine 28:S199–S207, 2003

66. Weinstein SL, Ponseti IV: Curve progression in idiopathic scoliosis. J Bone Joint Surg Am 65:447–455, 1983

67. Ponseti IV, Pedrini V, Wynne-Davies R, et al: Pathogenesis of scoliosis. Clin Orthop Relat Res 268–280, 1976

68. Ponseti IV, Friedman B: Prognosis in idiopathic scoliosis. J Bone Joint Surg Am 32A:381–395, 1950

69. Duffy CM, Arsenault L, Duffy KN, et al: The Juvenile Arthritis Quality of Life Questionnaire: Development of a new responsive index for juvenile rheumatoid arthritis and juvenile spondyloarthritides. J Rheumatol 24:738–746, 1997

70. Brewer EJ, Jr., Bass J, Baum J, et al: Current proposed revision of JRA Criteria. JRA Criteria Subcommittee of the Diagnostic and Therapeutic Criteria Committee of the American Rheumatism Section of the Arthritis Foundation. Arthritis Rheum 20:195–199, 1977

71. Klepper SE: Juvenile Rheumatoid Arthritis, in Campbell SK, Vander Linden DW, Palisano RJ (eds): Physical Therapy for Children. St. Louis, Saunders, 2006, pp 291–323

72. Kalogrianitis S, Tan CK, Kemp GJ, et al: Does unstable slipped capital femoral epiphysis require urgent stabilization? J Pediatr Orthop B 16:6–9, 2007

73. Kamarulzaman MA, Abdul Halim AR, Ibrahim S: Slipped capital femoral epiphysis (SCFE): A 12-year review. Med J Malaysia 61 (Suppl A):71–78, 2006

74. Flores M, Satish SG, Key T: Slipped capital femoral epiphysis in identical twins: is there an HLA predisposition?

Report of a case and review of the literature. Bull Hosp Joint Dis 63:158–160, 2006

75. Aronsson DD, Loder RT, Breur GJ, et al: Slipped capital femoral epiphysis: Current concepts. J Am Acad Orthop Surg 14:666–679, 2006

76. Leach J: Orthopedic conditions, in Campbell SK, Vander Linden DW, Palisano RJ (eds): Physical Therapy for Children (ed 3). St. Louis, Saunders, 2006, pp 481–515

77. Umans H, Liebling MS, Moy L, et al: Slipped capital femoral epiphysis: A physeal lesion diagnosed by MRI, with radiographic and CT correlation. Skeletal Radiol 27:139–144, 1998

78. Busch MT, Morrissy RT: Slipped capital femoral epiphysis. Orthop Clin North Am 18:637–647, 1987

79. Herring JA, Kim HT, Browne R: Legg-Calve-Perthes disease. Part II: Prospective multicenter study of the effect of treatment on outcome. J Bone Joint Surg Am 86-A:2121–2134, 2004

80. Herring JA, Kim HT, Browne R: Legg-Calve-Perthes disease. Part I: Classification of radiographs with use of the modified lateral pillar and Stulberg classifications. J Bone Joint Surg Am 86-A:2103–2120, 2004

81. Moens P, Fabry G: Legg-Calve-Perthes disease: One century later. Acta Orthop Belg 69:97–103, 2003

82. Thompson GH, Price CT, Roy D, et al: Legg-Calve-Perthes disease: Current concepts. Instr Course Lect 51:367–84, 2002

83. Gross GW, Articolo GA, Bowen JR: Legg-Calve-Perthes Disease: Imaging Evaluation and Management. Semin Musculoskelet Radiol 3:379–391, 1999

84. Roy DR: Current concepts in Legg-Calve-Perthes disease. Pediatr Ann 28:748–752, 1999

85. Townsend DJ: Legg-Calve-Perthes disease. Orthopedics 22:381, 1999

86. Bradford DS, Loustein JE, Moe JH, et al: Moe's Textbook of Skoliosis and other Spinal Deformities (ed 2). Philadelphia, WB Saunders, 1987

87. Benson MK, Byrnes DP: The clinical syndromes and surgical treatment of thoracic intervertebral disc prolapse. J Bone Joint Surg 57B:471–477, 1975

88. Winkel D, Matthijs O, Phelps V: Thoracic Spine, in Winkel D, Matthijs O, Phelps V (eds): Diagnosis and Treatment of the Spine. Maryland, Aspen, 1997, pp 389–541

89. Bleakney DA, Donohoe M: Osteogenesis imperfecta, in Campbell SK, Vander Linden DW, Palisano RJ (eds): Physical Therapy for Children (ed 3). St. Louis, Saunders, 2006, pp 401–419

90. Binder H: Rehabilitation of infants with osteogenesis imperfecta. Connect Tissue Res 31:S37–S39, 1995

91. Gerber LH, Binder H, Weintrob J, et al: Rehabilitation of children and infants with osteogenesis imperfecta: A program for ambulation. Clin Orthop Relat Res 254–262, 1990

92. Binder H, Hawks L, Graybill G, et al: Osteogenesis imperfecta: Rehabilitation approach with infants and young children. Arch Phys Med Rehabil 65:537–541, 1984

93. Massery M, Magee CL: Asthma: Multisystem Implications, in Campbell SK, Vander Linden DW, Palisano RJ (eds): Physical Therapy for Children (ed 3). St. Louis, Saunders, 2006, pp 851–879

94. Calfee CS, Katz PP, Yelin EH, et al: The influence of perceived control of asthma on health outcomes. Chest 130:1312–1318, 2006

95. Manning P, Greally P, Shanahan E: Asthma control and management: A patient's perspective. Ir Med J 98:231–232, 234–235, 2005

96. Lucas SR, Platts-Mills TA: Physical activity and exercise in asthma: Relevance to etiology and treatment. J Allergy Clin Immunol 115:928–934, 2005

97. Mintz M: Asthma update: part I. Diagnosis, monitoring, and prevention of disease progression. Am Fam Physician 70:893–898, 2004

98. Ram FS, Robinson SM, Black PN, et al: Physical training for asthma. Cochrane Database Syst Rev: CD001116, 2005

99. Welsh L, Kemp JG, Roberts RG: Effects of physical conditioning on children and adolescents with asthma. Sports Med 35:127–141, 2005

100. Kerkering GA: Brain injuries: Traumatic brain injuries, near drowning, and brain tumors, in Campbell SK, Vander Linden DW, Palisano RJ (eds): Physical Therapy for Children (ed 3). St. Louis, Saunders, 2006, pp 709–734

101. Britton TC: Torticollis: What is straight ahead? Lancet 351:1223–1224, 1998

102. Kiesewetter WB, Nelson PK, Pallandino VS, et al: Neonatal torticollis. JAMA 157:1281–1285, 1955

103. Morrison DL, MacEwen GD: Congenital muscular torticollis: Observations regarding clinical findings, associated conditions, and results of treatment. J Pediatr Orthop 2:500–505, 1982

104. Anastasopoulos D, Nasios G, Psilas K, et al: What is straight ahead to a patient with torticollis? Brain 121:91–101, 1998

105. Kiwak KJ: Establishing an etiology for torticollis. Postgrad Med 75:126–134, 1984

106. Karmel-Ross K: Congenital Muscular Torticollis, in Campbell SK, Vander Linden DW, Palisano RJ (eds): Physical Therapy for Children (ed 3). St. Louis, Saunders, 2006, pp 359–380

107. Bredenkamp JK, Hoover LA, Berke GS, et al: Congenital muscular torticollis: A spectrum of disease. Arch Otolaryngol Head Neck Surg 116:212–216, 1990

108. Whyte AM, Lufkin RB, Bredenkamp J, et al: Sternocleidomastoid fibrosis in congenital muscular torticollis: MR appearance. J Comput Assist Tomogr 13:163–164, 1989

109. Shah U, Moatter T: Screening for cystic fibrosis: the importance of using the correct tools. J Ayub Med Coll Abbottabad 18:7–10, 2006

110. Agnew JL, Ashwell JA, Renaud SL: Cystic Fibrosis, in Campbell SK, Vander Linden DW, Palisano RJ (eds): Physical Therapy for Children (ed 3). St. Louis, Saunders, 2006, pp 819–850

111. Humberstone N: Respiratory assessment and treatment, in Irwin S, Tecklin JS (eds): Cardiopulmonary physical therapy. St. Louis, Mosby, 1990, pp 283–322

112. Thomas J, Cook DJ, Brooks D: Chest physical therapy management of patients with cystic fibrosis: A meta-analysis. Am J Respir Crit Care Med 151:846–850, 1995

113. Zach MS, Purrer B, Oberwaldner B: Effect of swimming on forced expiration and sputum clearance in cystic fibrosis. Lancet 2:1201–1203, 1981

114. Orenstein DM, Franklin BA, Doershuk CF, et al: Exercise conditioning and cardiopulmonary fitness in cystic

fibrosis: The effects of a three-month supervised running program. Chest 80:392–398, 1981

115. Graf R: Hip sonography: Diagnosis and management of infant hip dysplasia (ed 2). New York, Springer, 2006

116. Witt P, Parr C: Effectiveness of Trager psychophysical integration in promoting trunk mobility in a child with cerebral palsy: A case report. Phys Occup Ther Pediatr 8:75–94, 1988

117. Gage JR, Deluca PA, Renshaw TS: Gait analysis: Principles and applications with emphasis on its use with cerebral palsy. Inst Course Lect 45:491–507, 1996

118. Abel MH, Damiano DL, Pannunzio M, et al: Muscle-tendon surgery in diplegic cerebral palsy: Functional and mechanical changes. J Pediatr Orthop 19:366–375, 1999

119. Blair E, Stanley F: Issues in the classification and epidemiology of cerebral palsy. Mental Retard Devel Disab Res Rev 3:184–193, 1997

120. Davids JR, Foti T, Dabelstein J, et al: Voluntary (normal) versus obligatory (cerebral palsy) toe-walking in children: A kinematic, kinetic, and electromyographic analysis. J Pediatr Orthop 19:461–469, 1999

121. Gage JR: Gait Analysis in Cerebral Palsy. London, MacKeith Press, 1991

122. Mayston M: Evidence-based physical therapy for the management of children with cerebral palsy. Dev Med Child Neurol 47:795, 2005

123. Harris SR, Roxborough L: Efficacy and effectiveness of physical therapy in enhancing postural control in children with cerebral palsy. Neural Plast 12:229–243, 2005

124. Palisano RJ, Snider LM, Orlin MN: Recent advances in physical and occupational therapy for children with cerebral palsy. Semin Pediatr Neurol 11:66–77, 2004

125. Wilton J: Casting, splinting, and physical and occupational therapy of hand deformity and dysfunction in cerebral palsy. Hand Clin 19:573–84, 2003

126. Engsberg JR, Ross SA, Wagner JM, et al: Changes in hip spasticity and strength following selective dorsal rhizotomy and physical therapy for spastic cerebral palsy. Dev Med Child Neurol 44:220–226, 2002

127. Engsberg JR, Ross SA, Park TS: Changes in ankle spasticity and strength following selective dorsal rhizotomy and physical therapy for spastic cerebral palsy. J Neurosurg 91:727–732, 1999

128. Barry MJ: Physical therapy interventions for patients with movement disorders due to cerebral palsy. J Child Neurol 11 (Suppl 1):S51–S60, 1996

129. Campbell SK, Gardner HG, Ramakrishnan V: Correlates of physicians' decisions to refer children with cerebral palsy for physical therapy. Dev Med Child Neurol 37:1062–1074, 1995

130. Harryman SE: Lower-extremity surgery for children with cerebral palsy: Physical therapy management. Phys Ther 72:16–24, 1992

131. Mayo NE: The effect of physical therapy for children with motor delay and cerebral palsy: A randomized clinical trial. Am J Phys Med Rehabil: 70:258–267, 1991

132. Stine SB: Therapy—physical or otherwise—in cerebral palsy. Am J Dis Child 144:519–520, 1990

133. Campbell SK, Anderson JC, Gardner HG: Use of survey research methods to study clinical decision making: refer-

ral to physical therapy of children with cerebral palsy. Phys Ther 69:610–615, 1989

134. Bower E: The effects of physical therapy on cerebral palsy. Dev Med Child Neurol 31:266, 1989

135. Harris SR: Commentary on "The effects of physical therapy on cerebral palsy: A controlled trial in infants with spastic diplegia." Phys Occup Ther Pediatr 9:1–4, 1989

136. Horton SV, Taylor DC: The use of behavior therapy and physical therapy to promote independent ambulation in a preschooler with mental retardation and cerebral palsy. Res Dev Disabil 10:363–375, 1989

137. Physical therapy for cerebral palsy. N Engl J Med 319:796–797, 1988

138. Palmer FB, Shapiro BK, Wachtel RC, et al: The effects of physical therapy on cerebral palsy: A controlled trial in infants with spastic diplegia. N Engl J Med 318:803–808, 1988

139. Sommerfeld D, Fraser BA, Hensinger RN, et al: Evaluation of physical therapy service for severely mentally impaired students with cerebral palsy. Phys Ther 61:338–344, 1981

140. Sussman MD, Cusick B: Preliminary report: The role of short-leg, tone-reducing casts as an adjunct to physical therapy of patients with cerebral palsy. Johns Hopkins Med J 145:112–114, 1979

141. Abdel-Salam E, Maraghi S, Tawfik M: Evaluation of physical therapy techniques in the management of cerebral palsy. J Egypt Med Assoc 61:531–541, 1978

142. Marx M: Integrating physical therapy into a cerebral palsy early education program. Phys Ther 53:512–514, 1973

143. Mathias A: Management of cerebral palsy: Physical therapy in relation to orthopedic surgery. Phys Ther 47:473–482, 1967

144. Stroumbou-Alamani S: Current concepts in the medical treatment of cerebral palsy. Physical therapy. Arch Ital Pediatr Pueric 25:113–120, 1967

145. D'Wolf N, Donnelly E: Physical therapy and cerebral palsy. Clin Pediatr (Phila) 5:351–355, 1966

146. Footh WK, Kogan KL: Measuring the effectiveness of physical therapy in the treatment of cerebral palsy. J Appl Toxicol 43:867–873, 1963

147. Paine RS: Physical therapy in the management of cerebral palsy. Dev Med Child Neurol 5:193, 1963

148. Gelperin A, Payton O: Evaluation of equanil as adjunct to physical therapy for children with severe cerebral palsy. Phys Ther Rev 39:383–388, 1959

149. Schwartz FF: Physical therapy for children with cerebral palsy. J Int Coll Surg 21:84–87, 1954

150. Brooks W, Callahan M, Schleich-Korn J: Physical therapy and the adult with cerebral palsy; report of a conference on vocational guidance. Phys Ther Rev 33:426–428, 1953

151. Bailey LA: Physical therapy in the treatment of cerebral palsy. Phys Ther Rev 30:230–231, 1950

152. Grogan DP, Lundy MS, Ogden JA: A method for early postoperative mobilization of the cerebral palsy patient using a removable abduction bar. J Pediatr Orthop 7:338–340, 1987

153. Katz K, Arbel N, Apter N, et al: Early mobilization after sliding achilles tendon lengthening in children with spastic cerebral palsy. Foot Ankle Int 21:1011–1014, 2000

154. Palisano R, Rosenbaum P, Walter S, et al: Development and reliability of a system to classify gross motor function

in children with cerebral palsy. Dev Med Child Neurol 39:214–223, 1997

155. Olney SJ, Wright MJ: Cerebral Palsy, in Campbell SK, Vander Linden DW, Palisano RJ (eds): Physical Therapy for Children. St. Louis, Saunders, 2006, pp 625–664

156. Rosenbaum P: Cerebral palsy: What parents and doctors want to know. BMJ 326:970–974, 2003

157. Lepage C, Noreau L, Bernard PM: Association between characteristics of locomotion and accomplishment of life habits in children with cerebral palsy. Phys Ther 78:458–469, 1998

158. Westberry DE, Davids JR, Jacobs JM, et al: Effectiveness of serial stretch casting for resistant or recurrent knee flexion contractures following hamstring lengthening in children with cerebral palsy. J Pediatr Orthop 26:109–114, 2006

159. Hoare B, Wasiak J, Imms C, et al: Constraint-induced movement therapy in the treatment of the upper limb in children with hemiplegic cerebral palsy. Cochrane Database Syst Rev CD004149, 2007

160. Clayton-Krasinski D, Klepper S: Impaired neuromotor development, in Cameron MH, Monroe LG (eds): Physical Rehabilitation: Evidence-Based Examination, Evaluation, and Intervention. St Louis, MO, Saunders/Elsevier, 2007, pp 333–366

161. Eagle M, Bourke J, Bullock R, et al: Managing Duchenne muscular dystrophy: The additive effect of spinal surgery and home nocturnal ventilation in improving survival. Neuromuscul Disord 17:470–475, 2007

162. King WM, Ruttencutter R, Nagaraja HN, et al: Orthopedic outcomes of long-term daily corticosteroid treatment in Duchenne muscular dystrophy. Neurology 68:1607–1613, 2007

163. Freund AA, Scola RH, Arndt RC, et al: Duchenne and Becker muscular dystrophy: A molecular and immunohistochemical approach. Arq Neuropsiquiatr 65:73–76, 2007

164. Zhang S, Xie H, Zhou G, et al: Development of therapy for Duchenne muscular dystrophy. Zhongguo Xiu Fu Chong Jian Wai Ke Za Zhi 21:194–203, 2007

165. Velasco MV, Colin AA, Zurakowski D, et al: Posterior spinal fusion for scoliosis in duchenne muscular dystrophy diminishes the rate of respiratory decline. Spine 32:459–465, 2007

166. Main M, Mercuri E, Haliloglu G, et al: Serial casting of the ankles in Duchenne muscular dystrophy: can it be an alternative to surgery? Neuromuscul Disord 17:227–230, 2007

167. Karol LA: Scoliosis in patients with Duchenne muscular dystrophy. J Bone Joint Surg Am 89 (Suppl 1):155–162, 2007

168. Grange RW, Call JA: Recommendations to define exercise prescription for Duchenne muscular dystrophy. Exerc Sport Sci Rev 35:12–17, 2007

169. Deconinck N, Dan B: Pathophysiology of duchenne muscular dystrophy: current hypotheses. Pediatr Neurol 36:1–7, 2007

170. Wagner KR, Lechtzin N, Judge DP: Current treatment of adult Duchenne muscular dystrophy. Biochim Biophys Acta 1772:229–237, 2007

171. Stuberg WA: Muscular dystrophy and spinal muscular atrophy, in Campbell SK, Vander Linden DW, Palisano RJ (eds): Physical Therapy for Children. St. Louis, Saunders, 2006, pp 421–451

172. Shaer CM, Chescheir N, Erickson K, et al: Obstetrician-gynecologists' practice and knowledge regarding spina bifida. Am J Perinatol 23:355–362, 2006

173. Woodhouse CR: Progress in the management of children born with spina bifida. Eur Urol 49:777–778, 2006

174. Verhoef M, Barf HA, Post MW, et al: Functional independence among young adults with spina bifida, in relation to hydrocephalus and level of lesion. Dev Med Child Neurol 48:114–119, 2006

175. Ali L, Stocks GM: Spina bifida, tethered cord and regional anaesthesia. Anaesthesia 60:1149–1150, 2005

176. Spina bifida. Nurs Times 101:31, 2005

177. Hinderer KA, Hinderer SR, Shurtleff DB: Myelodysplasia, in Campbell SK, Vander Linden DW, Palisano RJ (eds): Physical Therapy for Children (ed 3). St. Louis, Saunders, 2006, pp 735–799

178. Hoffer MM, Feiwell E, Perry R, et al: Functional ambulation in patients with myelomeningocele. J Bone Joint Surg Am 55:137–148, 1973

179. Williams V, Griffiths A, Tapp H, et al: A hemophilic son of a hemophiliac: Did my son inherit my hemophilia? J Thromb Haemost 5:210–211, 2007

180. Lusher JM, Brownstein AP: Hemophilia and HIV. J Thromb Haemost 12:12, 2007

181. Hoots WK, Nugent DJ: Evidence for the benefits of prophylaxis in the management of hemophilia A. Thromb Haemost 96:433–440, 2006

182. Evatt BL: The tragic history of AIDS in the hemophilia population, 1982–1984. J Thromb Haemost 4:2295–301, 2006

183. Hilliard P, Funk S, Zourikian N, et al: Hemophilia joint health score reliability study. Haemophilia 12:518–525, 2006

184. Goodman CC: The hematologic system, in Goodman CC, Boissonnault WG, Fuller KS (eds): Pathology: Implications for the Physical Therapist (ed 2). Philadelphia, Saunders, 2003, pp 509–552

185. Kim S, Chung DH: Pediatric solid malignancies: neuroblastoma and Wilms' tumor. Surg Clin North Am 86:469–87, xi, 2006

186. Roman E, Ansell P, Bull D: Leukaemia and non-Hodgkin's lymphoma in children and young adults: Are prenatal and neonatal factors important determinants of disease? Br J Cancer 76:406–415, 1997

187. Fiorillo A, Migliorati R, Fiore M, et al: Non-Hodgkin's lymphoma in childhood presenting as thyroid enlargement. Clin Pediatr (Phila) 26:152–154, 1987

188. Brecher ML, Sinks LF, Thomas RR, et al: Non-Hodgkin's lymphoma in children. Cancer 41:1997–2001, 1978

189. Medina-Sanson A, Chico-Ponce de Leon F, Cabrera-Munoz Mde L, et al: Primary central nervous system non-Hodgkin lymphoma in childhood presenting as bilateral optic neuritis. Childs Nerv Syst 22:1364–1368, 2006

190. Cairo MS, Raetz E, Lim MS, et al: Childhood and adolescent non-Hodgkin lymphoma: New insights in biology and critical challenges for the future. Pediatr Blood Cancer 45:753–769, 2005

191. Sandlund JT, Santana V, Abromowitch M, et al: Large cell non-Hodgkin lymphoma of childhood: clinical characteristics and outcome. Leukemia 8:30–34, 1994

192. Traggis D, Jaffe N, Vawter G, et al: Non-Hodgkin lymphoma of the head and neck in childhood. J Pediatr 87:933–936, 1975

193. Crist WM, Mahmoud H, Pickert CB, et al: Biology and staging of childhood non-Hodgkin lymphoma. An Esp Pediatr 29 (Suppl 34):104–109, 1988

194. Nathan PC, Ness KK, Greenberg ML, et al: Health-related quality of life in adult survivors of childhood wilms tumor or neuroblastoma: A report from the childhood cancer survivor study. Pediatr Blood Cancer 49: 704–15, 2006

195. Kutluk T, Varan A, Buyukpamukcu N, et al: Improved survival of children with wilms tumor. J Pediatr Hematol Oncol 28:423–426, 2006

196. Breslow NE, Beckwith JB, Perlman EJ, et al: Age distributions, birth weights, nephrogenic rests, and heterogeneity in the pathogenesis of Wilms tumor. Pediatr Blood Cancer 47:260–267, 2006

197. Seyed-Ahadi MM, Khaleghnejad-Tabari A, Mirshemirani A, et al: Wilms' tumor: A 10 year retrospective study. Arch Iran Med 10:65–69, 2007

198. Abd El-Aal HH, Habib EE, Mishrif MM: Wilms' Tumor: The experience of the pediatric unit of Kasr El-Aini Center of Radiation Oncology and Nuclear Medicine (NEM-ROCK). J Egypt Natl Canc Inst 17:308–311, 2005

199. Cook A, Farhat W, Khoury A: Update on Wilms' tumor in children. J Med Liban 53:85–90, 2005

200. Dahlin DC, Coventry MB: Osteogenic sarcoma: A study of six hundred cases. J Bone Joint Surg Am 49A:101–110, 1967

201. Wilson AW, Davies HM, Edwards GA, et al: Can some physical therapy and manual techniques generate potentially osteogenic levels of strain within mammalian bone? Phys Ther 79:931–938, 1999

202. Picci P: Osteosarcoma (Osteogenic sarcoma). Orphanet J Rare Dis 2:6, 2007

203. Berg EE: Osteogenic sarcoma. Orthop Nurs 25:348–349; quiz 350–351, 2006

204. Lin SY, Chen WM, Wu HH, et al: Extraosseous osteogenic sarcoma. J Chin Med Assoc 68:542–545, 2005

205. Wang LL: Biology of osteogenic sarcoma. Cancer J 11:294–305, 2005

206. Deitch J, Crawford AH, Choudhury S: Osteogenic sarcoma of the rib: A case presentation and literature review. Spine 28:E74–E77, 2003

207. Iwamoto Y: Diagnosis and Treatment of Ewing's Sarcoma. Jpn J Clin Oncol 37:79–89, 2007

208. Scotlandi K: Targeted therapies in Ewing's sarcoma. Adv Exp Med Biol 587:13–22, 2006

209. Chun JM, Kim SY, Kim JH: Ewing's sarcoma of the rotator cuff tendon: A case report. J Shoulder Elbow Surg 15:e41–43, 2006

210. Bernstein M, Kovar H, Paulussen M, et al: Ewing's sarcoma family of tumors: Current management. Oncologist 11:503–519, 2006

211. Hajdu SI: The enigma of Ewing's sarcoma. Ann Clin Lab Sci 36:108–110, 2006

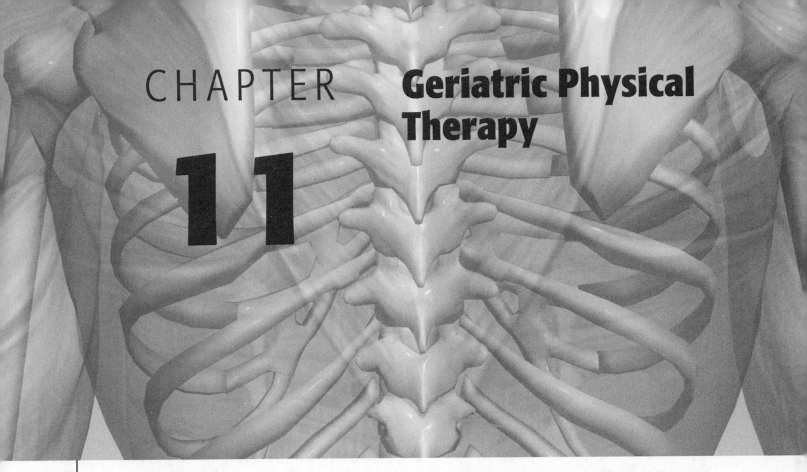

CHAPTER 11
Geriatric Physical Therapy

Aging is the accumulation of diverse adverse changes that increase the risk of death.[1] The rate of aging—that is, the rate at which aging changes occur—normally varies from individual to individual, resulting in differences in the age of death, the onset of various diseases, and the impact of aging on function.[1]

The Aging Process

Aging changes can be attributed to a combination of development, genetic defects, the environment, disease, and an inborn factor, the aging process. These aging changes are responsible for both the commonly recognized sequential alterations that accompany advancing age beyond the early period of life, and the progressive increases in the probability of experiencing a chronic debilitating disease.[1] The incidence of chronic conditions has been shown to increase with advancing age and, because aging is often accompanied by a deterioration of general health, the geriatric population is especially vulnerable to loss of function and independence. In addition, because elderly individuals often suffer from several diseases at the same time (comorbidities), such as cardiovascular disorders, osteoporosis, arthritis, and diabetes, the interaction of these diseases produces a cumulative effect.

> **● Key Point** Note the following definitions:
> - *Geriatrics:* The branch of medicine that focuses on health promotion and the prevention and treatment of disease and disability in later life.
> - *Gerontology:* The study of the aging process and the science related to the care of the elderly.
> - *Ageism:* Defined by Webster as "any attitude, action, or institutional structure that subordinates a person, group or perception purely on the basis of age." When that bias is the primary motivation behind acts of discrimination against that person or group, then those acts constitute age discrimination.
> - *Senescence:* The combination of processes of deterioration that follow the period of development of an organism.

Musculoskeletal impairments are among the most prevalent and symptomatic health problems of middle and old age.[2] The subsequent loss of strength, motion, and increasing pain prevents elderly individuals from making full use of their abilities and from participating in the regular physical activity necessary to maintain optimum mobility, general health, and, in some cases, independence.[3]

Theories of Aging

A wide array of theories exist as to why aging occurs, why species have the life spans they do, and what kinds of factors are likely to influence the aging process.

- *Genetic theories* focus on the mechanisms for aging located in the nucleus of the cell, implicating mutations and chromosomal anomalies that accumulate with age.
- *Neuroendocrine-immuno theories* focus on the gradual decline in the system's ability to produce necessary antibodies to fight disease and decrease in its ability to distinguish between antibodies and proteins. In essence, the immune system itself becomes self-destructive and reacts against itself. Examples of such autoimmune diseases are lupus, scleroderma, and adult-onset diabetes.
- *Environmental theories* focus on the accumulative damage caused by free-radical (any molecule that has a free electron) reactions.[4] Theoretically, a free radical reacts with healthy molecules in a destructive way. It is known that diet, lifestyle, drugs (e.g., tobacco, alcohol), radiation, and so on are all accelerators of free radical production within the body. However, there is also natural production of free radicals within the body as a by-product of energy production, particularly from the mitochondria.
- *Planned obsolescence theories* focus on the genetic programming of senescence genes in the DNA.[1] According to this theory, individuals are born with a unique code and a preprogrammed life span of physical and mental functioning, and certain genes regulate the rate of aging.
- *Telomere-shortening theories* focus on scientific findings that telomeres (DNA-protein complexes that cap the ends of chromosomes and promote genetic stability) play a critical role in determining the number of times a cell divides, its health, and its life span.

Aging is a heterogeneous process and therefore differs greatly among individuals, producing a great variability in health and functional status in the older population. Many changes are associated with aging throughout adulthood and into old age. **Table 11-1** summarizes these system changes. While some elderly adults succumb to the functional limitations and disability associated with aging, disease, or injury, many elderly adults retain high levels of activity and functional abilities well into advanced age.

> ● **Key Point** Normal aging can be defined as age-related changes that are the result of the passage of time rather than the result of pathologic conditions. Chronologic age should not be used to determine potential for recovery or the appropriateness of referral for rehabilitation.

Coexisting pathologic processes can exacerbate the effects of other conditions and result in greater functional limitations and disability. Throughout youth and early adulthood, the body has reserve physiologic capacities and system redundancies that enable the body to adapt to the physical challenges and injury without a loss of functional abilities. The gradual decline of health and increased incidence of injury and disease experienced by older individuals can be partially attributed to the gradual loss of this physiologic reserve.[3] Without this physiologic reserve, an older individual is more susceptible to functional limitations and disability, resulting in frailty. Frailty is viewed as usual aging, and it is on the opposite end of the spectrum from successful aging.[3] It is important to remember that frailty is not a natural consequence of aging and that the performance of physical activity throughout the aging years can produce a number of physiologic benefits:

- Substantial improvements can be made in almost all aspects of cardiovascular functioning.
- Individuals of all ages can benefit from muscle strengthening exercises. In particular, resistance training can have a significant impact on the maintenance of independence in old age.
- Regular activity helps prevent and/or postpone the age-associated declines in flexibility, balance, and coordination.

Conversely, disuse exacerbates the aging process and negatively impacts the physiologic reserve in the face of disease and injury.

TABLE 11-1	Summary of Multisystem Changes in the Elderly

System	Changes
Musculoskeletal	Muscle mass and strength decrease at a rate of about 30% between the ages of 60 and 90
	Change in muscle fiber type, white and red; type II fibers (fast twitch) decrease by about 50%
	Decrease in recruitment of motor units
	Decreased tensile strength of bone (more than 30% of women over the age of 65 have osteoporosis)
	Joint flexibility reduced by 25% to 30% over the age of 70
Neuromuscular	Atrophy of neurons; nerve fibers decrease and change in structure
	Myoneural junction decreases in transmission speed
	Decrease in nerve conduction velocity by about 0.4% a year after age 70
	Slowing of motor neuron conduction, which contributes to alterations in the autonomic system
	Decreasing reflexes result from decrease in nerve conduction; ankle jerk is absent in about 70%, and knee and biceps jerk are absent in about 15%
	Overall slow and decreased responsiveness in reaction time (simple reflexes less than complex)
	Increased postural sway (less in women than in men, with linear increase with age)
Neurosensory	Decrease in sweating (implications for modalities and exercise)
	10% to 20% decrease in brain weight by age 90
	Decrease in mechanoreceptors
	Decrease in visual acuity and ability to accommodate to lighting changes resulting from increased density of lens
	Decrease in hearing capabilities
Cardiovascular and pulmonary	Decrease in cardiac output by about 0.7% a year after 20 years of age
	Increased vascular resistance
	Decreased arterial elasticity
	Decreased cardiac reserve; decreased physical and psychological response to stress
	Increased irritation of myocardium contributes to increased risk of atrial fibrillation and arrhythmias
	Decrease in lung function (from age 25 to age 85, as much as 50% decrease in maximal voluntary ventilation due to an increase in air resistance; about 40% decrease in vital capacity)
	Respiratory gas exchange surface decreases at a rate of about 0.27 m² a year (maximum oxygen consumption for sedentary individuals of any age is 0.62 to 0.7 mL per minute)
	Decrease in elastin in the lungs (increased rigidity) and chest wall soft tissues results in decrease in chest wall compliance
	Decrease in vital capacity and decrease in pulmonary blood flow contribute to lower oxygen saturation levels
	Decreased cough reflex
Urogenital and renal	Gradual overall structure changes in all renal components
	Decreased glomerular filtration rate and creatinine clearance
	Change in response to sodium intake
	Muscle hypertrophy in the urethra and bladder
Gastrointestinal	Decreased peristalsis
	Diminished secretions of pepsin and acid in the stomach
	Decreasing hepatic and pancreatic enzymes
Immunologic	Decrease in overall function with respect to infection
	Decreased temperature regulation
	Decrease in T cells

Data from Bottomley JM: The geriatric population, in Boissonnault WG (ed): Primary Care for the Physical Therapist: Examination and Triage. St. Louis, Elsevier Saunders, 2005, pp 288–306; and Bottomley JM: Summary of system changes: Comparing and contrasting age-related changes, in Bottomley JM, Lewis CB (eds): Geriatric rehabilitation: A clinical approach (ed 2). Upper Saddle River, NJ, Prentice-Hall, 2003, pp 50–75

Definitions

Ageism

Ageism is defined by Webster as "any attitude, action, or institutional structure which subordinates a person, group or perception purely on the basis of age." When that bias is the primary motivation behind acts of discrimination against that person or group, then those acts constitute age discrimination.

Life Span

There are two kinds of life span:

- *Maximum life span:* The greatest age reached by any member of a species.
- *Average life span:* The average age reached by members of a population. This figure has shown changes over time, largely due to medical advances. The average life span was 47 years in 1900 and 75 years in 1990. As of the year 2000, in the United States the life expectancy for females is 80 years. For males, the comparable figure is 74 years.

Life Expectancy

Life expectancy, the number of years an individual can expect to live, is based on average life spans. Men generally have higher death rates than women at every age. Thus, the health, social, and economic problems of the oldest old are likely to remain primarily the problems of women.

Senescence

Senescence can be defined as the combination of processes of deterioration that follow the period of development of an organism.

Mortality

Mortality refers to the number of deaths (from a disease or at general) per 1000 people and is typically reported on an annual basis. Reductions in mortality have resulted in impressive increases in life expectancy that have contributed to the growth of the older population, especially at the oldest ages.

Morbidity

Morbidity refers to the number of people who have a disease (prevalence) compared with the total number of people in a population at a particular point in time. The term *morbidity* can also refer to:

- The state of being diseased (from Latin *morbidus*, meaning sick, unhealthy)
- The degree or severity of a disease

- The incidence of a disease; the number of new cases in a particular population during a particular time interval

Physiological Changes and Adaptations in the Old Adult

Some of the changes associated with aging throughout adulthood are discussed below.

Impaired Strength

The decline in strength in elderly individuals has been associated with increases in falls, functional decline, and impaired mobility. However, much of the atrophy that occurs reflects the effects of disuse, not mere age-related changes.[5] The decrease in muscle performance with advancing age affects men and women differently—women experience a less steep absolute decline in strength than men.

> ● **Key Point** Resistive exercise in this age group should be directed toward the muscles most susceptible to atrophic changes.[6,7] Additionally, exercises should be geared toward increasing power, not just strength.

Impaired Balance

Age-related balance dysfunctions can occur through a loss of sensory elements (degenerative changes in the otoconia of the utricle and saccule; loss of vestibular hair cell receptors), the ability to integrate information and issue motor commands (decreased number of vestibular neurons), and muscle weakness. Diseases common in aging populations lead to further deterioration in balance function in some patients (e.g., Ménière disease, benign paroxysmal positional vertigo [BPPV], cerebrovascular disease, vertebrobasilar artery insufficiency, cerebellar dysfunction, cardiac disease).

In addition to vestibular dysfunction, dizziness can also cause a loss of balance. Dizziness can have a multitude of different causes, including cardiac abnormalities and medications. Classes of medications that may predispose a person to vestibular dysfunction include:

- Tricyclic antidepressants (may cause hypotension)
- Antihypertensives
- Anticonvulsants
- Anti-anxiety drugs (may cause confusion)
- Antipsychotics (may cause hypotension)
- Sedatives
- Postural hypotension

The clinical implications of impaired balance include:

- Diminished acuity
- Delayed reaction times by the patient
- Longer response times from the patient
- Reduced function of vestibular ocular reflex (VOR), leading to diminished retinal image stability with head movements
- Altered sensory organization, leading to higher dependence upon somatosensory inputs
- Disorganized postural response patterns, leading to diminished ankle torque, increased hip torque, and increased postural sway

Intervention Strategies for Impaired Balance

To help a patient improve balance, the PTA should:

- Determine the presence of any disease states that can contribute to balance disorders
- Assess static and dynamic balance in elderly patients
- Use fall-risk questionnaires to help identify fall risk
- Assess need for appropriate and safe assistive devices/adaptive equipment

- Train patient to perform the following exercises:
  - Strengthening and flexibility exercises
  - Weight-bearing exercises to help prevent osteoporosis
  - Balance and gait exercises
- Assist patient with transfer training (sit-to-stand transitions)
- Assist patient in functional training (turning, walking, negotiating stairs)
- Perform pharmacological reevaluation as appropriate
- Modify living environment (**Table 11-2**)
- Provide safety education

Impaired Coordination

The most salient age-related changes impacting coordinated movement include:

- Decreased strength
- Slowed reaction time
- Decreased range of motion
- Postural changes
- Impaired balance

These changes may be accentuated further by alterations in sensation, perceptual impairments, and diminished vision and hearing acuity.

TABLE 11-2	Home Safety Checklist		

All Living Spaces	Bathrooms	Outdoors
_____ Remove throw rugs	_____ Install grab bars in the bathtub or shower and by the toilet	_____ Repair cracked sidewalks
_____ Secure carpet edges	_____ Use rubber mats in the bathtub or shower	_____ Install handrails on stairs and steps
_____ Remove low furniture and objects on the floor	_____ Take up floor mats when the bathtub or shower is not in use	_____ Trim shrubbery along the pathway to the home
_____ Reduce clutter	_____ Install a raised toilet seat	_____ Install adequate lighting by doorways and along walkways leading to doors
_____ Remove cords and wires on the floor		
_____ Check lighting for adequate illumination at night (especially in the pathway to the bathroom)		
_____ Secure carpet or treads on stairs		
_____ Install handrails on staircases		
_____ Eliminate chairs that are too low to sit in and get out of easily		
_____ Avoid floor wax (or use nonskid wax)		
_____ Ensure that the telephone can be reached from the floor		

Data from Rubenstein LZ: Falls. In Yoshikawa TT, Cobbs EL, Brummel-Smith K (eds): Ambulatory Geriatric Care. St. Louis: Mosby, 1993, pp 296–304; and Dutton M: McGraw-Hill's NPTE (National Physical Therapy Examination). New York, McGraw-Hill, 2009

Impaired Cognition

Age-related changes in the brain start at around age 60. Normal, nonprogressive, and negligible declines among the aged do not dramatically impact daily functioning until the early 80s, but the more serious disorders/diseases can significantly affect cognitive function in old age. Not all cognitive disorders are irreversible, but many require timely identification and intercession to offset permanent dysfunction.

Dementia

Primarily a disease of the elderly, *dementia*[8-16] is a generic term most often applied to geropsychological problems (see "Delirium, Dementia"), applying broadly to a progressive, persistent loss of cognitive and intellectual functions, including:

- Memory, especially with short-term memory; long-term memory is usually retained (impairments tend to be task dependent, under novel conditions)
- Language; reduction in, or inappropriate use of, vocabulary
- Visuospatial skill (see "Impaired Balance")
- Emotion; can be emotionally labile

In addition, personality changes may occur without impairment in perception or consciousness. Dementia is often confused with delirium (also known as *acute confusional state*). Delirium presents with:

- A rapid onset and fluctuating course, which is potentially reversible
- Attention and focal cognitive deficits

In contrast, dementia progresses slowly, is irreversible, causes profound memory deficits, and is associated with global cognitive deficits.

Intervention Strategies for Impaired Cognition

There are a variety of intervention strategies:

- Overall approach may focus either on a patient's current cognitive functioning or on decline in functioning from a previous level. An advantage of addressing cognitive decline, rather than current functioning, is that the influences of education, premorbid intelligence, and cultural differences are discounted in the intervention. With cognitive tests, the measurement of decline strictly requires two or more measurement points, which is often difficult to attain.
- Correction of medical problems associated with cognitive deficits (cardiovascular disease, hypertension, diabetes, or hypothyroidism).

- Pharmacological reevaluation if drug toxicity suspected.
- Nutritional assessment as appropriate.
- Cognitive training activities (e.g., chess, crossword puzzles).
- Provision of a stimulating and enriching environment.
- Use of context-based tasks versus memorization.

Pathological Conditions Associated with the Elderly

Musculoskeletal Disorders and Diseases

Osteoarthritis

Osteoarthritis (OA), also known as *degenerative joint disease*, is a clinical condition of synovial joints. OA is characterized by:

- Development of fissures
- Cracks and general thinning of joint cartilage
- Bone damage
- Hypertrophy of the cartilage
- Synovial inflammation

The degenerative changes are most pronounced on the articular cartilage in weight-bearing areas of the large joints. Two types of OA are commonly recognized: primary and secondary OA.[17-19]

Primary OA

Primary OA is the most common form. Primary OA has no known cause, although it appears to be related to aging and heredity. It most often affects:

- The distal interphalangeal (DIP) joints and, less often, the proximal interphalangeal (PIP) joints of the hands
- The hip
- The knee
- The metatarsophalangeal and tarsometatarsal joints of the feet
- Possibly the cervical and lumbar spine

Secondary OA

Secondary OA may occur in any joint due to articular injury. These injuries include fracture, repetitive joint use, obesity, or metabolic disease (e.g., osteoporosis, osteomalacia). Secondary OA may occur at any age. OA of the hip and knee represent two of the most significant causes of adult pain and physical disability. Estimates of people older than 55 years who are afflicted with OA range from 70%

to 85%, and OA is listed eighth as a worldwide cause of disability. The characteristics of secondary OA include:

- Pain
- Muscle spasm
- Muscle atrophy
- Stiffness
- Crepitus, swelling, inflammation, and joint effusion
- Loss of range of motion
- Deformity
- Impaired function

The medical intervention for OA includes:

- Nonsteroidal anti-inflammatory drugs (NSAIDs)
- Corticosteroid injections
- Topical analgesics
- Surgical joint replacement

The goals of physical therapy intervention include:

- To reduce pain and muscle spasm through the use of modalities and relaxation training
- To maintain or improve range of motion and correct muscle imbalances through therapeutic exercises:
  - ❏ Strengthening exercises
  - ❏ Flexibility exercises
- To improve balance and ambulation
- To provide assistive devices as needed (e.g., canes, walkers, orthotics, reachers)
- To promote aerobic conditioning using low- to non-impact exercises (e.g., walking program, pool exercises)
- To provide patient education and empowerment:
  - ❏ Joint protection strategies
  - ❏ Energy conservation techniques
  - ❏ Activities to avoid
- To promote a healthy lifestyle—e.g., losing weight

Osteoporosis

Osteoporosis is a systemic skeletal disorder characterized by decreased bone mass and deterioration of bony microarchitecture (see Chapter 9).

Fractures

Fractures commonly occur among seniors and can have a significant impact on the morbidity, mortality, and functional dependence of this population.

Fractures in the elderly have their own set of problems. The fractures heal more slowly. Furthermore, older adults are prone to complications, such as:

- Pneumonia
- Changes in mental status
- Decubiti
- Comorbidity
- Decreased vision
- Poor balance

The following are deemed to be the most common fractures to occur in the elderly population.

Pathological Fractures

Pathological fractures occur from low-energy injuries to an area of bone weakness with a preexisting abnormality or disease. The differential diagnosis for low-energy injuries to the bone is based on the determination as to why the fracture occurred.

Stress Fractures

Stress fractures,[20] including fatigue and insufficiency fractures, are fractures that occur in the absence of a specific acute precipitating traumatic event. Multiple clinical reports have described stress fractures in persons with rheumatoid arthritis, lupus erythematosis, osteoarthritis, pyrophosphate arthropathy, renal disease, osteoporosis, and joint replacements, and in older patients who have no apparent musculoskeletal disease.

Proximal Humerus Fractures

Proximal humerus fractures have been conservatively estimated to account for 5% of all fractures. These fractures occur in older patients who primarily are osteoporotic. Like hip fractures, proximal humerus fractures represent a major morbidity in the elderly population. The most common mechanism for these fractures is a fall on an outstretched hand (FOOSH) from a standing height. The majority of fractures are nondisplaced, and nonoperative treatment is often selected. When fracture displacement occurs, operative intervention is selected. Operative treatment includes closed reduction with percutaneous fixation, open reduction and internal fixation, and proximal humeral head replacement. The following describes the common findings with this type of fracture:

- Complaints of pain and loss of function of the involved extremity. In general, unstable fractures are much more painful and often may require surgical stabilization to allow for adequate pain relief.

- Swelling and ecchymoses about the shoulder and upper arm. The presence of extensive ecchymosis may become visible 24 to 48 hours following injury.

A neurovascular examination by the PT to determine concurrent neurovascular injury is essential. The axillary nerve is the most common nerve injured.

The intervention goals in proximal humerus fractures are to allow bone and soft tissue healing to maximize function of the upper extremity while minimizing risk. Displaced fractures are those that if left untreated have the greatest likelihood of producing limited function. The physical therapy intervention includes:

- Gentle ROM exercises, which may begin after 7 to 10 days if the fracture is stable.
- More aggressive-passive and active-assisted range of motion can begin once bony union has occurred.

Distal Radius Fracture

The distal radial fracture[21] is the most common forearm fracture. It is usually caused by a FOOSH. It can also result from direct impact or axial forces. The classification of these fractures is based on distal radial angulation and displacement, intra-articular or extra-articular involvement, and associated anomalies of the ulnar or carpal bones. The most common complication of associated soft-tissue injury is peripheral nerve dysfunction. The median nerve is most commonly affected, but the ulnar nerve may also be injured.

- *Median nerve:* Usually affected as the result of direct trauma by fracture or displacement, or injury through a proximal radial fragment or displacement of a volar fragment.
- *Ulnar nerve:* Usually affected as the result of medial displacement of the radial fragment or by the ulnar head being anteriorly displaced.

Other complications include:

- Injury to arteries occurs with open and closed fractures; it can also occur with markedly displaced fractures and dislocations of the radius and ulna.
- Tendon lacerations occur from high-energy injuries and should be suspected with open fractures and high-velocity injuries. The extensor pollicis longus tendon is most frequently ruptured.

- Intercarpal injuries, including ligament sprains and scaphoid fractures, may accompany fracture dislocations of the distal forearm. Fractures through the radial styloid can disrupt both the radioscapholunate and scapholunate interosseus ligament, causing a disruption between the two bones.

Most distal radial fractures are diagnosed by conventional radiography. CT and MRI are used to evaluate complex distal radial fractures for the evaluation of associated injuries and for surgical planning.

Proximal Femur/Hip Fracture

Fracture of the hip can have devastating consequences: the mortality rate is 20%. About 50% of patients will not resume their premorbid level of function following a hip fracture. This is particularly true in older persons, where the hip fracture most often results from a simple fall; in a small percentage, the fracture occurs spontaneously in the absence of a fall. The typical signs and symptoms of a proximal femur/hip fracture include:

- Patient complains of pain and inability to move the hip. With stress fractures in young athletes and nondisplaced fractures, the patient may complain of pain in hip or knee and may be ambulatory.
- Patient may have a history of other osteoporotic fractures, such as Colles or vertebral fractures.

The various types of proximal femur/hip fracture include:

- *Femoral head fracture:* Most often, these fractures occur as a result of hip dislocation; therefore, the position of the extremity is abduction, external rotation, and flexion or extension for anterior dislocation. With posterior dislocation (the most common type), the extremity is held in an adducted and internally rotated position.
- *Femoral neck fracture:* Together with intertrochanteric fractures, these fractures constitute the vast majority of all hip fractures. The extremity is held in a slightly shortened, abducted, and externally rotated position, unless the fracture is only a stress fracture or severely impacted. In this case, the hip is held in a natural position.
- *Intertrochanteric fracture:* Extremity is held in a markedly shortened and externally rotated position.

- *Subtrochanteric fracture:* Proximal femur usually is held in a flexed and externally rotated position.

The majority of hip fractures are treated surgically. Treatment protocols are based on the type of fracture and surgical procedure used (internal fixation versus prosthetic replacement). The goals are to restore the pre-injured levels of function, mobility, and self-care.

Fractures of the Spine
Compression fracture of the vertebral body is common and ranges from mild to severe. More severe fractures can cause significant pain, leading to inability to perform activities of daily living and life-threatening decline in the elderly patient who already has decreased reserves. While the diagnosis can be suspected from history and physical examination, plain radiographs, as well as occasional computed tomography or magnetic resonance imaging, are often helpful in accurate diagnosis and prognosis. Traditional conservative treatment includes bed rest and pain control. Procedures such as vertebroplasty can be considered in those patients who do not respond to initial treatment. PTAs can help patients prevent compression fractures by addressing predisposing factors, identifying high-risk patients, and educating patients and the public about measures to prevent falls.

Neurologic Disorders and Diseases
Cerebrovascular Accident (Stroke)
A cerebrovascular accident or stroke syndrome encompasses a heterogeneous group of pathophysiologic causes, including thrombosis, embolism, and hemorrhage that results in a sudden loss of circulation to an area of the brain, resulting in a corresponding loss of neurologic function.

● Key Point Any process that disrupts blood flow to a portion of the brain unleashes an ischemic cascade, leading to the death of neurons and cerebral infarction.

Strokes are currently classified as either hemorrhagic or ischemic, although the two can coexist.

- *Hemorrhagic:* Accounts for only 10% to 15% of all strokes, but it is associated with higher mortality rates than the ischemic variety.[22] It results from abnormal bleeding into the extravascular areas of the brain. Causes include, but are not limited to, intracranial aneurysm, hypertension, arteriovenous malformation (AVM), and anticoagulant therapy.

- *Ischemic:*[23–27] The most common type, affecting about 80% of individuals with stroke. Results when a clot blocks or impairs blood flow. Risk factors for ischemic stroke include advanced age (the risk doubles every decade), hypertension, smoking, heart disease (e.g., coronary artery disease, left ventricular hypertrophy, chronic atrial fibrillation), and hypercholesterolemia. Ischemic strokes are most often caused by extracranial embolism or intracranial thrombosis.
  - Emboli may arise from the heart, the extracranial arteries or, rarely, the right-sided circulation (*paradoxical emboli*). The sources of cardiogenic emboli include valvular thrombi (e.g., in mitral stenosis, endocarditis, prosthetic valves); mural thrombi (e.g., in myocardial infarction [MI], atrial fibrillation, dilated cardiomyopathy); and atrial myxomas.
  - Lacunar infarcts, which are cystic cavities that form after an infarct, commonly occur in patients with small vessel disease, such as diabetes and hypertension.
  - The most common sites of thrombotic occlusion are cerebral artery branch points, especially in the distribution of the internal carotid artery. Arterial stenosis, atherosclerosis, and platelet adherence cause the formation of blood clots that either embolize or occlude the artery. Less common causes of thrombosis include polycythemia and sickle cell anemia.

● Key Point Any process that causes dissection of the cerebral arteries also can cause thrombotic stroke (e.g., trauma, thoracic aortic dissection, arteritis).

Common symptoms of stroke include abrupt onset of hemiparesis, monoparesis, or quadriparesis; monocular or binocular visual loss; visual field deficits; diplopia; dysarthria; ataxia; vertigo; aphasia; or sudden decrease in the level of consciousness.

● Key Point Stroke should be considered in any patient presenting with an acute neurologic deficit (focal or global) or altered level of consciousness.

Stroke is largely preventable. Potentially modifiable risk factors include smoking, obesity, lack of exercise, diet, and excess alcohol consumption.

The major neuroanatomic stroke syndromes are caused by disruption of their respective cerebrovascular distributions. Correlating the patient's neurologic deficits with the expected sites of arterial compromise may assist in determining the intervention:[28-34]

- *Anterior cerebral artery (ACA) occlusion:* Primarily affects frontal and parietal lobe function, producing altered mental status, impaired judgment, neglect, contralateral hemiplegia/hemiparesis and hypesthesia, bowel and bladder incontinence, behavioral changes, apraxia (if located in the nondominant hemisphere), or aphasia (if located in the dominant hemisphere).
- *Middle cerebral artery (MCA):* The most common stroke syndrome. Occlusions commonly produce contralateral hemiparesis, contralateral hypesthesia, ipsilateral hemianopsia (blindness in one half of the visual field), and gaze preference toward the side of the lesion. Agnosia is common, and receptive or expressive aphasia may result if the lesion occurs in the dominant hemisphere. Since the MCA supplies the upper extremity motor strip, weakness of the arm and face is usually worse than that of the lower limb.
- *Posterior cerebral artery occlusions:* These affect vision and thought, producing homonymous hemianopsia, pain and temperature sensory loss, contralateral hemiplegia (central area), cortical blindness, visual agnosia, altered mental status, and impaired memory.

> **● Key Point** Vertebrobasilar artery occlusions are notoriously difficult to detect because they cause a wide variety of cranial nerve, cerebellar, and brainstem deficits. These include vertigo, nystagmus, diplopia, visual field deficits, dysphagia, dysarthria, facial hypesthesia, syncope, and ataxia. Loss of pain and temperature sensation occurs on the ipsilateral face and contralateral body. In contrast, anterior strokes produce findings on one side of the body only.

The neuroanatomic stroke syndrome subtypes include:

- *Anterior communicating artery:* Produces incontinence, impairment of intellect, loss of innovative abilities, and paraparesis.
- *Anterior inferior cerebellar artery:* Produces ipsilateral ataxia, loss of contralateral pain and temperature, ipsilateral deafness, ipsilateral facial paralysis, and ipsilateral sensory loss to the face.
- *Posterior inferior cerebellar artery (PICA):* The largest branch of the vertebral artery, and one of the three main arterial blood supplies for the cerebellum.

- *Paramedian area: Produces paralysis of one or more cranial nerves on the same side of the body as the lesion, and varying degrees of impairment of sensation and loss of motor function of the arm and leg on the contralateral side.*
- *Lateral area:* Produces symptoms of dysfunction of the cerebellum and of the nuclei and tracks in the lateral portion of the brainstem, in particular the motor nuclei of the fifth, seventh, and tenth cranial nerves; the sensory nuclei of the fifth and eighth cranial nerves; the descending sympathetic pathways; and the spinothalamic tract.
- *Internal carotid artery:* Produces aphasia (when in the dominant hemisphere), contralateral hemiplegia, hemianesthesia, hemianopia, and unilateral loss of vision.
- *Posterior inferior cerebral artery:* Produces ataxia, contralateral hemianalgesia, difficulty swallowing, ipsilateral weakness of the tongue and vocal cords, and nystagmus.
- *Superior cerebral artery:* Produces contralateral hemianesthesia/hemianalgesia, contralateral facial weakness, and ipsilateral ataxia.

The medical examination for stroke also includes a number of routine laboratory and diagnostic tests, including:[35]

- Urinalysis
- Blood analysis
- Fasting blood glucose levels
- Blood chemistry profile, including creatinine phosphokinase isoenzyme (CPK-MB), which is elevated with cardiac infarction
- Thyroid function tests
- Full cardiac workup (radiograph of chest, ECG, and echocardiography; see Chapter 6)
- Pertinent imaging studies, including CT scan, MRI, PET scan, transcranial and carotid Doppler, and cerebral angiography

Physical Therapy Intervention
The primary impairments associated with stroke include:[35]

- Loss of or impaired sensation
- Pain—headache, neck and face pain
- Visual changes, including neglect and visual field deficits
- Alterations in motor function, including weakness, alterations in tone, abnormal synergy patterns, abnormal reflexes, altered coordination, bowel and bladder changes, and altered motor programming

- Impairments in postural control and balance
- Impairments of speech, language, and swallowing
- Impairments of perception and cognition
- Changes in emotional status

Patients may recover following a stroke in two different, but related, ways:

- A reduction in the extent of neurologic impairment as the result of spontaneous natural neurologic recovery that limits the extent of the stroke, or from other interventions that enhance neurologic functioning. A patient demonstrating this form of recovery presents with improvements in motor control, language ability, or other primary neurologic functions.
- The improved ability to perform daily functions within the limitations of the physical impairments. A patient who has sensorimotor, cognitive, or behavioral deficits resulting from stroke may regain the capacity to carry out ADLs such as feeding, dressing, bathing, and toileting, even if some degree of residual physical impairment remains. The ability to perform these tasks can improve through adaptation and training in the presence or absence of natural neurologic recovery, thought to be the element of recovery on which rehabilitation exerts the greatest effect.

In many instances, the recovery from a stroke occurs in the sequential manner described by Brunnstrom (see Chapter 5) or by Fugl-Meyer and colleagues:[37]

1. Reflexes recur after a period of initial flaccidity with no voluntary movement.
2. Voluntary movement is possible only within the dynamic flexion and extension synergies.
3. Voluntary control in isolated joint movements emerges with a mixing of synergies.
4. Increasing voluntary control is out of synergy; coordination deficits are present.
5. The patient has maximum scores in stages 1 through 4—control and coordination of movement near normal.

The goals for the physical therapy intervention should include:

- To maintain or improve range of motion:
  - Positioning techniques
  - Passive ROM/Self ROM
  - Soft tissue/joint mobilizations
- To maintain or improve strength:
  - Graded strength training combined with careful monitoring of blood pressure, heart rate, and ratings of perceived exertion (RPE)
- Improve postural control and functional mobility:[35]
  - Rolling activities
  - Transfer training (supine to sit; sit to supine; sit to stand; sit down transfers)
  - Sitting exercises focusing on correct alignment, control, weight shifts, and reaching
  - Bridging
  - Standing activities (modified plantigrade, upright standing, and weight shifts)
  - Locomotor and gait training as appropriate
- Improve manipulation and dexterity skills
- Assess the need for environmental modifications and/or assistive devices (orthotics, foot and ankle controls [AFO], knee controls, and wheelchairs)
- Minimize secondary complications:
  - Spasticity (refer to Chapter 5)
  - Contracture and deformity prevention
  - Decubiti
  - Confusion
  - Decreased sensorimotor function
- Improve feeding and swallowing deficits using a multidisciplinary approach

Refer to Chapter 5 for details about motor learning strategies.

Degenerative Diseases

Degenerative diseases generally are characterized by the loss of neurons and secondary gliosis (scarring) without evidence of major inflammation or necrosis of tissue.

Parkinson Disease

Parkinson disease[38-50] (PD) is a progressive neurodegenerative disorder associated with a loss of pigmented dopaminergic nigrostriatal neurons in the substantia nigra and the presence of Lewy bodies. The term *parkinsonism* is used to refer to a group of disorders that produce abnormalities of basal ganglia function. PD, or idiopathic parkinsonism, is the most common form. Most cases of idiopathic PD are believed to be due to a combination of genetic and environmental factors (e.g., use of pesticides, living in a rural environment, exposure to herbicides, proximity to industrial plants or quarries).

The onset of PD is typically asymmetric, with the most common initial finding being an asymmetric resting tremor in an upper extremity. As with most tremors, the amplitude increases with stress and resolves during sleep. After several months (or as much as a few years) the tremor may affect the extremities on the other side, but asymmetry often is maintained. PD tremor also may involve the tongue, lips, or chin. Other signs and symptoms include:

- The axial posture becomes progressively flexed and strides become shorter.
- Decreased swallowing may lead to excess saliva and ultimately drooling.
- Sleep disturbances may occur.

Symptoms of autonomic dysfunction are common and include constipation, sweating abnormalities, sexual dysfunction, and seborrheic dermatitis.

The three cardinal signs of PD are resting tremor, rigidity, and bradykinesia. Of these cardinal features, two of three are required to make the clinical diagnosis. Postural instability is the fourth cardinal sign, but it emerges later in the disease, usually after 8 years or more.

- *Tremor:* The characteristic PD tremor is present and most prominent with the limb at rest.
  - ❑ The usual frequency of the tremor is 3 to 5 Hz.
  - ❑ The tremor may appear as a pill-rolling motion of the hand or a simple oscillation of the hand or arm.
  - ❑ The same tremor may be observed with the arms outstretched (position of postural maintenance), and a less prominent, higher frequency kinetic tremor is also common.
- *Rigidity:* Refers to an increase in resistance to passive movement about a joint.
  - ❑ The resistance can be either smooth (lead pipe) or oscillating (cogwheeling).
  - ❑ Rigidity usually is tested by flexing and extending the patient's relaxed wrist. The rigidity can be made more obvious with voluntary movement in the contralateral limb.
- *Bradykinesia:* Refers to slowness of movement but also includes a lack of spontaneous movements and decreased amplitude of movement. Bradykinesia may be expressed as micrographia (small handwriting), hypomimia (decreased facial expression), decreased blink rate, cogwheeling eye pursuit, decreased pupillary reflexes, dysarthria, and hypophonia (soft speech).

- *Postural instability:* Refers to imbalance and loss of righting reflexes. Its emergence is an important milestone, because it is poorly amenable to treatment and a common source of disability in late disease. The clinician should check for the ability to maintain both static and dynamic balance, reactive adjustments and anticipatory adjustments. Patients may experience freezing when starting to walk (start-hesitation), during turning, or while crossing a threshold, such as going through a doorway.

Other impairments associated with PD include:

- Dementia, which generally occurs late in PD and affects 15% to 30% of patients. Short-term memory and visuospatial function may be impaired, but aphasia is not present.
- Poor oromotor control/dysphagia, which can affect nutritional status.
- Impaired respiratory status and cardiovascular deconditioning leading to decreased chest expansion and vital capacity.
- Contractures, especially in flexors and adductors.
- Autonomic dysfunction, leading to increased sweating.
- Muscle weakness associated with disuse atrophy.
- Gait dysfunction; festination common, generalized lack of extension.

Parkinson disease can be staged for examination and intervention purposes using the Hoehn and Yahr classification:[51]

I. Minimal or absent disability, unilateral symptoms.
II. Minimal bilateral or midline involvement, no balance involvement.
III. Impaired balance, some restrictions in activity.
IV. All symptoms present and severe. Patient stands and walks only with assistance.
V. Confinement to bed or wheelchair.

The medical management for PD is largely pharmacologic:

- *Early neuroprotective therapy:* Monoamine oxidase inhibitors (MAOs) to improve metabolism of intracerebral dopamine.
- *Symptomatic therapy:* Levadopa, anticholinergic agents, and dopamine agonists.

Medications usually provide good symptomatic control for 4 to 6 years, after which the disability progresses despite best medical management, and many patients develop long-term motor complications, including fluctuations and dyskinesia.

Surgical intervention may include ablative surgery (pallidotomy or thalamotomy), deep brain stimulation to block nerve signals that cause the symptoms, and neural transplantation of cells capable of surviving and delivering dopamine into the striatum of patients with advanced PD.

Physical Therapy Intervention

The goal of the physical therapy intervention of PD is to provide control of signs and symptoms for as long as possible while attempting to prevent or minimize the secondary impairments associated with disuse and inactivity. It is important that the clinician monitor changes associated with the disease progression and any side effects that may be caused by the pharmacological interventions. The following strategies are recommended:

- Patient education:
  - Compensatory strategies to initiate movement
  - Flexibility exercises
  - Postural and balance training
  - Mobility training
  - Energy conservation techniques
  - Safety in the home and community
  - Relaxation techniques, including gentle rocking and slow rhythmic, rotational movements of the extremities
- Strengthening exercises emphasizing overall improvement with mobility, postural control, and balance (PNF techniques)
- Cardiovascular endurance exercises
- Assessment for adaptive and supportive equipment
- Gait training
- Family/caregiver education

Alzheimer Disease

Alzheimer disease (AD), the most common cause of dementia, is an acquired cognitive and behavioral impairment of sufficient severity to markedly interfere with social and occupational functioning. The anatomic pathology of AD includes neurofibrillary tangles (NFTs), senile plaques (SPs) at the microscopic level, and cerebrocortical atrophy, which predominantly involves the association regions and particularly the medial aspect of the temporal lobe. The cause of AD is unknown.

Patients with AD most commonly present with insidiously progressive memory loss, to which other aspects of cognitive impairment are added over several years. After memory loss occurs, patients may also have language disorders (e.g., anomia, progressive aphasia) and impairment in their visuospatial skills and decision-making functions. The earliest evidence of AD is the onset of chronic, insidious memory loss that is slowly progressive over several years. This loss can be associated with slowly progressive behavioral changes. Although other neurologic systems (e.g., extrapyramidal cerebellar systems) can also be affected, the most prominent finding as the disease progresses to its moderate and severe stages is progressive memory impairment. Other common neurologic presentations include changes in language ability (e.g., anomia, progressive aphasia), impaired visuospatial skills, and impaired executive function.

Medical Intervention

Therapeutic approaches to AD are based on developing theories of its pathogenesis and on the need to alleviate its cognitive and behavioral manifestations. To date, no interventions have been shown to convincingly prevent AD or slow its progression. Medical treatments for AD include psychotropic medications and behavioral interventions.

Physical Therapy Intervention

Both physical and mental activities are recommended for patients with AD. Many experts recommend mentally challenging activities, such as doing crossword puzzles and brainteasers, both to prevent deterioration and to slow its rate. The mental activities should be kept within a reasonable level of difficulty for the patient, they should preferably be interactive, and they should be designed to allow the patient to recognize and correct mistakes. Most important, these activities should be administered in a manner that does not cause excessive frustration and that ideally motivates the patient to engage in them frequently.

Cognitive Disorders

Delirium, Dementia

Delirium, dementia, and certain other alterations in cognition are often referred to as mental status change (MSC), acute confusional state (ACS), or organic brain syndrome (OBS). Acute alterations in brain function are commonly referred to as MSC or ACS, while chronic alterations and any

MSC specifically due to nonpsychiatric causes are generally referred to as OBS.

- Delirium presents with acute onset of impaired awareness, easy distraction, confusion, and disturbances of perception (e.g., illusions, misinterpretations, visual hallucinations). Recent memory is usually deficient, and the patient often is disoriented to time and place. The patient may be agitated or obtunded, and the level of awareness may fluctuate over brief periods. Speech may be incoherent, pressured, nonsensical, perseverating, or rambling, which may make the taking of subjective complaints from the patient impossible.
- Dementia presents with a history of chronic, steady decline in short- and long-term memory and is associated with difficulties in social relationships, work, and activities of daily life. In contrast to delirium, processing is normal. However, delirium can be superimposed on an underlying dementing process. Earlier stages of dementia may present subtly, and patients may minimize or attempt to hide their impairments. Patients at this stage often have an associated depression.

The end result of these dysfunctions is impairment of cognition that affects some or all of the following: alertness, orientation, emotion, behavior, memory, perception, language, praxis, problem solving, judgment, and psychomotor activity.

> **● Key Point** Any serious infection can lead to mental status changes. A rapid pulse rate is seen in patients with fever, sepsis, dehydration, and various cardiac dysrhythmias and in overdoses of stimulants, anticholinergics, quinidine, theophylline, tricyclic antidepressants, or aspirin.

> **● Key Point** In the elderly, the combined effects of visual and auditory impairments; dementia or other chronic brain dysfunction; medication side effects, particularly polypharmacy; and/or unfamiliar environment or nighttime darkness can lead to acute confusion or psychosis, which is known as sundowning. As the name implies, this condition usually occurs in the evening hours.

Physical Therapy Intervention
The physical therapy intervention will depend on the extent of the disease. The goals typically include:

- To improve self-care abilities to carry out ADLs (e.g., grooming, hygiene, continence)
- To provide a safe environment to prevent falls, injury, or further dysfunction
- To provide a soothing environment by reducing environmental distractions to help decrease agitation and to increase attention
- To improve motor function
- To improve gait and balance, while providing regular physical activity
- To provide reorienting information: calendars, memory aids

Depression
The many possible causes of depression (refer to Chapter 9) in the elderly have many different sources. Causes may be:

- Psychological
- Environmental
- Physical
- Related to personality traits

Psychological factors include:

- Unresolved, repressed traumatic experiences from childhood or later life that may surface when a senior slows down
- Previous history of depression
- Damage to body image (from amputation, cancer surgery, or heart attack)
- Fear of death or dying
- Frustration with memory loss
- Difficulty adjusting to stressful or changing conditions (i.e., housing and living conditions, loss of loved ones or friends, loss of capabilities)
- Substance abuse (alcohol)

Environmental factors include:

- Loneliness, isolation
- Impact of retirement (whether the individual has chosen to stop working, been laid off, or been forced to stop because of chronic health problems or a disability)
- Being unmarried (especially if widowed), or recent bereavement
- Lack of a supportive social network
- Decreased mobility due to illness or loss of driving privileges

Physical factors include:

- Genetics—inherited tendencies toward depression
- Comorbidities (such as Parkinson, Alzheimer, cancer, diabetes, or stroke)
- Vascular changes in the brain
- Vitamin B_{12} deficiency
- Chronic or severe pain

Personality characteristics (may also be symptomatic of unresolved trauma) include:

- Low self-esteem
- Extreme dependency
- Pessimism

Cardiovascular Disorders and Diseases

Hypertension

Hypertension is one of the most common worldwide diseases afflicting humans and is an important public health challenge. Regulation of normal blood pressure is a complex process. Although this regulation is a function of cardiac output and peripheral vascular resistance, both of these variables are influenced by multiple factors (see Chapter 6). The classification of hypertension based on age (expressed in mm Hg) is outlined in Chapter 6. Hypertension may be either essential or secondary.

Essential Hypertension

A possible pathogenesis of essential hypertension[52–61] has been proposed in which multiple factors, including genetic predisposition, excess dietary salt intake, and adrenergic tone, may interact to produce hypertension. Although genetics appears to contribute to essential hypertension, the exact mechanism has not been established. After a long consistent asymptomatic period, persistent hypertension develops into complicated hypertension, in which target organ damage to the aorta and small arteries, heart, kidneys, retina, and central nervous system is evident. The progression begins with prehypertension in persons aged 10 to 30 years (by increased cardiac output), to early hypertension in persons aged 20 to 40 years (in which increased peripheral resistance is prominent), to established hypertension in persons aged 30 to 50 years, and, finally, to complicated hypertension in persons aged 40 to 60 years.

Secondary Hypertension

The historical and physical findings that suggest the possibility of secondary hypertension are a history of known renal disease, abdominal masses, anemia, and urochrome pigmentation.

Hypertension can be associated with the following:

- Cardiac involvement manifested as left ventricular hypertrophy (LVH), left atrial enlargement, aortic root dilatation, atrial and ventricular arrhythmias, systolic and diastolic heart failure, and ischemic heart disease. A history of cardiovascular risk factors includes hypercholesterolemia, diabetes mellitus, and tobacco use (including chewing tobacco).
- Central nervous system involvement manifested as hemorrhagic and atheroembolic stroke or encephalopathy.
- Renal involvement. A reduction in renal blood flow in conjunction with elevated afferent glomerular arteriolar resistance increases glomerular hydrostatic pressure secondary to efferent glomerular arteriolar constriction.

An accurate measurement of blood pressure is the key to diagnosis (see Chapter 6). Palpation of all peripheral pulses should be performed.

Intervention

No consensus exists regarding optimal drug therapy for treatment of hypertension. Most intervention approaches address lifestyle modifications:

- Lose weight if overweight.
- Limit alcohol intake to no more than 1 oz. (30 mL) of ethanol (i.e., 24 oz. [720 mL] of beer, 10 oz. [300 mL] of wine, 2 oz. [60 mL] of 100-proof whiskey) per day or 0.5 (15 mL) ethanol per day for women and people of lighter weight.
- Increase aerobic activity (30 to 45 minutes most days of the week).
- Reduce sodium intake to no more than 100 mmol/d (2.4 g sodium or 6 g sodium chloride).
- Maintain adequate intake of dietary potassium (approximately 90 mmol/d).
- Maintain adequate intake of dietary calcium and magnesium for general health.
- Stop smoking and reduce intake of dietary saturated fat and cholesterol for overall cardiovascular health.

Coronary Artery Disease

See Chapter 6.

Pulmonary Disorders and Diseases

Chronic Bronchitis/Chronic Obstructive Pulmonary Disease

For discussions of chronic bronchitis/chronic obstructive pulmonary disease, asthma, pneumonia, and lung cancer, see Chapter 7.

Integumentary Disorders and Diseases

Decubitus Ulcers

See Chapter 8.

Metabolic Pathologies

Diabetes Mellitus

See Chapter 9.

Common Functional Problem Areas in the Geriatric Population

Immobility–Disability

Immobility is a common occurence by which a host of diseases and problems in the elderly produce further disability. Persons who are chronically ill, aged, or disabled are particularly susceptible to the adverse effects of prolonged bed rest, immobilization, and inactivity. Common causes of immobility in the elderly include:

- *Musculoskeletal system:* Arthritis, osteoporosis, fractures (especially hip and femur), and podiatric problems.
- *Cardiopulmonary system:* Chronic coronary heart disease, chronic obstructive lung disease, severe heart failure, and peripheral vascular disease.
- *Neurologic system:* Cerebrovascular accident, Parkinson disease, cerebellar dysfunction, neuropathies, cognitive, psychological and sensory problems (dementia, depression, fear and anxiety), pain, and impaired vision.
- *Environmental causes:* Forced immobilization (restraint use) and inadequate aids for mobility.
- *Malnutrition.*
- *Deconditioning.*

Physical Therapy Intervention

Intervention strategies should include the following, while monitoring vital signs:

- Minimize duration of bed rest. Avoid strict bed rest unless absolutely necessary.
- Be aware of possible adverse effects of medications.
- Encourage the continuation of daily activities that the patient is able to perform as tolerated but avoid overexertion.
- Implement bathroom privileges or bedside commode.
- Let patient stand 30 to 60 seconds during transfers (bed to chair).
- Encourage taking meals at a table.
- Encourage the wearing of street clothes.
- Encourage daily exercises as a basis of good care. Exercises should emphasize:
  - Balance and proprioception
  - Strength and endurance
  - Coordination and equilibrium
  - Aerobic capacity
  - Posture
  - Gait
  - Cadence
  - Base of support
  - Gait deviations
  - Assistive device; design possible ways to enhance mobility through the use of assistive devices (e.g. walking aids, wheelchairs) and making the home accessible
- Ensure that a sufficient fluid intake (1.5 to 2 liters of fluid intake per day as possible) and adequate nutritional levels are being maintained.
- Encourage socialization with family, friends, or caregivers.
- If the patient is bed-bound, maintain proper body alignment and change positions every few hours. Pressure padding and heel protectors may be used to provide comfort and prevent pressure sores.
  - Skin integrity; protecting the integrity of the skin is important in providing effective treatment to prevent skin breakdown
  - Protective sensations; a loss of protective sensations prevents the patient from feeling pain, pressure and other sensations
  - Discriminatory sensations; this is the ability to sense the intensity, location, quality and duration of symptoms

Falls and Instability

Falls can be markers of poor health and declining function, and they are often associated with significant morbidity.[62] More than 90% of hip fractures occur as a result of falls, with most of these fractures occurring in persons over 70 years of age. One-third of community-dwelling elderly persons and 60% of nursing home residents fall each year. Risk factors for falls in the elderly include increasing age, medication use, cognitive impairment, and sensory deficits. Common causes of falls in the elderly include:[63]

- Accident, environmental hazard, fall from bed
- Gait disturbance, balance disorders or weakness, pain related to arthritis
- Vertigo
- Medications or alcohol
- Confusion and cognitive impairment
- Postural (orthostatic) hypotension
- Visual disorder
- Central nervous system disorder, syncope, drop attacks, epilepsy

Elderly persons who survive a fall experience significant morbidity. Hospital stays are almost twice as long in elderly patients who are hospitalized after a fall than in elderly patients who are admitted for another reason.

Balance and Gait Testing

Several simple tests have exhibited a strong correlation with a history of falling (see Chapter 3). These functional balance measures are quantifiable and correlate well with the ability of older adults to ambulate safely in their environment.

Overall physical function also should be assessed. This is accomplished by evaluating the patient's ADLs and instrumental activities of daily living (IADLs).

Physical Therapy Intervention

With patients who have a history of falling, the intervention is directed at the underlying cause of the fall and in preventing recurrence. Functional training should include:

- Sit-to-stand transitions
- Turning
- Provision of appropriate assistive devices/adaptive equipment
- Patient and family/caregiver education:
  - Identification of risks
  - Safety issues
  - Adequate lighting at home
  - Contrasting colors
  - Reduction of clutter

Nutritional Deficiency

Nutritional status is an important aspect of health. Nutrition takes on greater importance in the context of chronic illness.[64–69] With increase in age, there is an increased risk of developing nutritional deficiencies that can lead to such debilitating consequences as functional dependency, morbidity, and mortality. Some older persons are at increased risk for nutritional deficiency because of multiple drug therapies, dental problems, economic hardship, and reduced social contacts. These problems arise from many varied environmental, social, and economic factors that are compounded by physiological changes of aging. A statement on nutrition screening is needed in order to:

- Incorporate nutritional screening in the clinical care of older persons
- Heighten awareness of the multiple risk factors having an impact upon nutritional status of older persons

The Food and Nutritional Board of the Institute of Medicine no longer uses the term Recommended Daily Allowances. Rather, they use Dietary Reference Intakes (DRI). DRIs are reference values to estimate the nutrient intakes to be used for planning and assessing diets for healthy people. Many of the DRIs for older adults are not based on large studies of older people; rather, they are derived by extrapolation from data obtained for younger persons. The DRI adjustments for older adults have been made based on the reduction in physiologic function, changes in body composition, and metabolic adaptation in adults over 51 years of age and then again over 71 years of age.

Physical Therapy Role

A proper and continuous nutritional assessment of a patient's nutritional status is important to identify patients that are at risk. Although not directly involved with the patient's nutritional status, the PTA should attempt to:

- Maintain or improve the patient's physical function
- Assist in the monitoring of the patient's nutritional intake by observing any physical or mental changes that could be nutritionally related
- Request nutritional consults as necessary
- Communicate with social worker for elderly food programs (Meals on Wheels, federal food stamp programs)
- Make recommendations for home health aides:
  - Assistance in grocery shopping
  - Meal preparation

General Principles of Geriatric Rehabilitation

The following areas should be emphasized in the intervention of the elderly population:

- Safety:
  - Level of cognition, vision, hearing, proprioception
  - Appropriate and safe use of assistive devices
- Home/living environment.
- Level of activity/exercise. The absolute contraindications for exercising older adults include but are not limited to:
  - Severe cardiac disease with unstable angina pectoris
  - Acute myocardial infarction (<2 days after infarction)
  - Severe valvular heart disease
  - Rapid or prolonged atrial or ventricular arrhythmias/tachycardias

- ❑ Uncontrolled hypertension
- ❑ Profound orthostatic hypotension
- ❑ Acute thrombophlebitis
- ❑ Acute pulmonary embolism (<2 days after event)
- ❑ Known or suspected dissecting aneurysm
- ■ Health promotion:
  - ❑ Determine effects of normal aging versus disease pathologies
  - ❑ Provide education on healthy lifestyle and prevention of disability
  - ❑ Maximize independence
  - ❑ Enhance coping skills
- ■ Support systems:
  - ❑ Help prevent social isolation
  - ❑ Educate caregivers, friends, and family
  - ❑ Provide empowerment
  - ❑ Involve patient in decision-making
  - ❑ Be the patient's advocate for needed services

Ethical and Legal Issues

The Living Will (Advanced Care and Medical Directive)

Through advances in medical technology, some patients who formerly would have died can now be kept alive by artificial means. Sometimes a patient may desire such treatment because it is a temporary measure potentially leading to an improvement in health. At other times, such treatment may be undesirable because it may only prolong the process of dying rather than restore the patient to an acceptable quality of life. The Advanced Care Medical Directive (ACMD), established by the federal Patient Self-Determination Act of 1990, was designed to address such issues. Advance directives are documents signed by a competent person giving direction to healthcare providers about treatment choices in certain circumstances. There are two types of advance directives:

- ■ A durable power of attorney for health care ("durable power") allows a patient to name a "patient advocate" to act on behalf of the patient and carry out his or her wishes (see "Healthcare Proxy" below).
- ■ A living will allows a patient to state his or her wishes in writing but does not name a patient advocate.

The regulations for ACMD vary by state. However, in order to be deemed a legal document the ACMD must be signed by the principal and witnessed by two adults. There are generally two broad types of situations in which the directive may apply:

- ■ Terminal illness, in which death is expected in a relatively short time.
- ■ Permanent disability in an intolerable situation. This is a highly individualized decision.

Many standard health care declarations instruct physicians to withhold "extraordinary care" or "life-sustaining or life-prolonging" treatments.

Refusal of Treatment

If deemed mentally competent (the patient understands his or her condition and the consequences any decision may have), every adult has the right to decide to accept or refuse any medical treatment. There are basically two broad reasons to refuse a certain treatment:

- ■ The benefit of the treatment is not great enough to justify its risk or discomfort. This is the basis for most treatment decisions, and it involves the individual attitudes each patient will bring to the decision. Some people will endure unpleasant and risky treatments for a chance to live longer; others prefer a more comfortable, shorter life, using the least possible medical intervention.
- ■ The treatment will prolong life under intolerable conditions. Even an easily tolerated treatment with minimal discomfort might be unacceptable if it prolongs life in the face of unwanted circumstances. A feeding tube may be simple, safe, comfortable, and highly effective in preventing death from starvation and dehydration. Nevertheless, some may not want it used if another irreversible condition exists (for example, a persistent vegetative state).

"Do Not Resuscitate" Orders

"Do Not Resuscitate" (DNR) orders apply only to cardiopulmonary resuscitation, and there are specific rules concerning how they are to be written and who may authorize them.

Healthcare Proxy

A healthcare proxy is an agent who makes healthcare decisions for the patient when he or she has been determined to be incapable of making such decisions.

Informed Consent

Informed consent is the process by which a competent and fully informed patient can participate in choices about his or her health care. It is generally accepted that complete informed consent includes a discussion of the following elements:

- The nature and purpose of the decision/procedure.
- Reasonable alternatives to the proposed intervention.
- The relevant risks, benefits, consequences, and uncertainties related to each alternative.
- The likelihood of success or failure of the intervention.
- An assessment of patient understanding. In order for the patient's consent to be valid, he or she must be considered competent to make the decision at hand and the consent must be voluntary. If the patient is not deemed competent, consent must be obtained from a legal guardian or healthcare proxy.
- The acceptance of the intervention by the patient.

REVIEW Questions

1. What is the name given to the study of the aging process and the science related to the care of the elderly?

2. The degenerative changes associated with osteoarthritis are most pronounced on the articular cartilage of which type of joints?

3. When assessing the risk of falling in an elderly patient, all the following factors are known to increase risk, except:
   a. Using a walker
   b. Taking three prescription medications
   c. Fear of falling
   d. History of falls

4. A 67-year-old woman says she has fallen twice in the past year. All the following should be considered, except:
   a. Asking about her use of alcohol
   b. Reviewing her use of over-the-counter medications
   c. Measuring serum 25-hydroxyvitamin D concentration
   d. Performing aauditory examination

5. Which of these interventions would *not* help reduce risk of falling in a 70-year-old man who lives in a nursing home?
   a. Gait training
   b. An exercise program

   c. Educating the staff about ways to prevent falls
   d. Evaluating whether assistive devices are being used appropriately

6. An 80-year-old man who lives at home says he has never fallen but would like to reduce his risk of falling. All these interventions would be appropriate, except:
   a. A multifactorial program that includes exercise with balance training
   b. A multifactorial program that includes a review of medications
   c. A single intervention that consists of education on risk factor modification
   d. A single intervention that consists of vitamin D supplementation

7. You are advising a 72-year-old individual who wants to take part in a graduated conditioning program. Which of the following would be appropriate advice for the healthy elderly?
   a. Intensity prescribed using maximal age-related HR.
   b. An initial conservative approach to reduce characteristic muscle fatigability.
   c. An emphasis on low intensity and increased duration of exercise to avoid injury.
   d. All of the above.

8. You find a patient on the floor who complains of pain in the right groin and gluteal area. The right hip is flexed, abducted, and internally rotated. The most likely diagnosis is:
   a. Dislocated tibia
   b. Fractured femoral head
   c. Dislocated hip
   d. Fractured acetabulum

9. You are treating a patient with a recent arterial occlusion in the brain, specifically in the dominant left hemisphere. The patient demonstrates contralateral hemiplegia and loss of sensation. Which artery has most likely been occluded?
   a. Middle cerebral artery
   b. Anterior cerebral artery
   c. Posterior cerebral artery
   d. None of the above

10. Give four potentially modifiable risk factors for stroke.

11. The most appropriate positioning strategy for a patient recovering from acute stroke who is in bed and demonstrates a flaccid upper extremity is:
    a. Sidelying on the sound side with the affected upper extremity supported on a pillow with

the shoulder protracted and elbow extended
   b. Sidelying on the affected side with the affected upper extremity flexed overhead
   c. Supine with the affected hand positioned on stomach
   d. None of the above

12. A 72-year-old patient recovering from stroke reports to you that he has been prescribed "blood thinners." During his rehabilitation, it would be important to advise the patient to watch for:
   a. Hematuria and ecchymosis
   b. Edema and dermatitis
   c. Headaches and nausea
   d. None of the above

13. Which of the following is not a typical change associated with aging?
   a. Reduction in blood flow
   b. Reduction in muscle mass
   c. Increase in ventricular size
   d. Reduction of nerve conduction velocity

14. The most common stroke syndrome involves which artery of the brain?

15. A lesion of which artery in the brain affects vision and thought, producing homonymous hemianopsia, pain and temperature sensory loss, contralateral hemiplegia (central area), cortical blindness, visual agnosia, altered mental status, and impaired memory?

16. What disease involves a progressive neurodegenerative disorder associated with a loss of pigmented dopaminergic nigrostriatal neurons in the substantia nigra and the presence of Lewy bodies?

17. What are considered the three cardinal signs of Parkinson disease?

18. What is the earliest clinical symptom associated with Alzheimer disease?

19. What are the two types of advance direc-tives?

20. The process by which a competent and fully informed patient can participate in choices about his or her health care is called what?

References

1. Harman D: Aging: phenomena and theories. Ann N Y Acad Sci 854:1–7, 1998
2. Jette AM, Branch LG, Berlin J: Musculoskeletal impairments and physical disablement among the aged. J Gerontol 45:M203–M208, 1990
3. Voight C: Rehabilitation considerations with the geriatric patient, in Prentice WE Jr, Voight ML (eds): Techniques in Musculoskeletal Rehabilitation. New York, McGraw-Hill, 2001, pp 679–696
4. Harman D: Free radical involvement in aging. Pathophysiology and therapeutic implications. Drugs Aging 3:60–80, 1993
5. Hall C, Thein-Brody L: Impairment in Muscle Performance, in Hall C, Thein-Brody L (eds): Therapeutic Exercise: Moving Toward Function. Baltimore, MD, Lippincott Williams & Wilkins, 2005, pp 57–86
6. Evans WJ: High-velocity resistance training for increasing peak muscle power in elderly women. Clin J Sport Med 13:66, 2003
7. Fielding RA, LeBrasseur NK, Cuoco A, et al: High-velocity resistance training increases skeletal muscle peak power in older women. J Am Geriatr Soc 50:655–662, 2002
8. Treatment of dementia and agitation: a guide for families and caregivers. J Psychiatr Pract 13:207–216, 2007
9. Elble RJ: Gait and dementia: Moving beyond the notion of gait apraxia. J Neural Transm 114:1253–1258, 2007
10. Holthe T, Thorsen K, Josephsson S: Occupational patterns of people with dementia in residential care: An ethnographic study. Scand J Occup Ther 14:96–107, 2007
11. Man-Son-Hing M, Marshall SC, Molnar FJ, et al: Systematic review of driving risk and the efficacy of compensatory strategies in persons with dementia. J Am Geriatr Soc 55:878–884, 2007
12. Missotten P, Ylieff M, Di Notte D, et al: Quality of life in dementia: A 2-year follow-up study. Int J Geriatr Psychiatry, 2007
13. Mitchell SL, Kiely DK, Miller SC, et al: Hospice Care for Patients with Dementia. J Pain Symptom Manage, 2007
14. Newton JP: Dementia, oral health and the failing dentition. Gerodontology 24:65–66, 2007
15. Pedraza O, Smith GE, Ivnik RJ, et al: Reliable change on the Dementia Rating Scale. J Int Neuropsychol Soc:1–5, 2007
16. Solfrizzi V, D'Introno A, Colacicco AM, et al: Alcohol consumption, mild cognitive impairment, and progression to dementia. Neurology 68:1790–1799, 2007
17. Lawrence RC, Hochberg MC, Kelsey JL, et al: Estimates of the prevalence of selected arthritic and musculoskeletal diseases in the United States. J Rheumatol 16:427–441, 1989
18. Birchfield PC: Osteoarthritis overview. Geriatric Nursing 22:124–130; quiz 130–131, 2001
19. Kee CK: Osteoarthritis: manageable scourge of aging. Rheumatology 35:199–208, 2000
20. Buckwalter JA, Brandser EA: Stress and insufficiency fractures. Am Fam Physician 56:175–182, 1997
21. Richards B, Riego de Dios R: Radius, distal fractures, Available at: http://www.emedicine.com/radio/topic822.htm, 2004
22. Locksley HB: Hemorrhagic strokes. Principal causes, natural history, and treatment. Med Clin North Am 52:1193–1212, 1968
23. Khealani BA, Syed NA, Maken S, et al: Predictors of ischemic versus hemorrhagic strokes in hypertensive patients. J Coll Physicians Surg Pak 15:22–25, 2005
24. Leys D, Lamy C, Lucas C, et al: Arterial ischemic strokes associated with pregnancy and puerperium. Acta Neurol Belg 97:5–16, 1997
25. Ryglewicz D, Hier DB, Wiszniewska M, et al: Ischemic strokes are more severe in Poland than in the United States. Neurology 54:513–515, 2000

26. Sagui E, M'Baye PS, Dubecq C, et al: Ischemic and hemorrhagic strokes in Dakar, Senegal: a hospital-based study. Stroke 36:1844–1847, 2005

27. Yahia AM, Kirmani JF, Xavier AR, et al: Characteristics and predictors of aortic plaques in patients with transient ischemic attacks and strokes. J Neuroimaging 14:16–22, 2004

28. Baker AB: Common Stroke Syndromes and Their Management. Postgrad Med 37:268–272, 1965

29. Brown MM: Identification and management of difficult stroke and TIA syndromes. J Neurol Neurosurg Psychiatry 70 Suppl 1:I17–I22, 2001

30. Chambers BR, Bladin PF, McGrath K, et al: Stroke syndromes in young people. Clin Exp Neurol 18:132–144, 1981

31. Golden GS: Stroke syndromes in childhood. Neurol Clin 3:59–75, 1985

32. Jordan LC, Hillis AE: Aphasia and right hemisphere syndromes in stroke. Curr Neurol Neurosci Rep 5:458–464, 2005

33. Stone WM: Ischemic stroke syndromes: classification, pathophysiology and clinical features. Med Health R I 81:197–203, 1998

34. Vroom FQ: Stroke: malignant and benign syndromes. South Med J 66:898–904, 1973

35. O'Sullivan SB: Stroke, in O'Sullivan SB, Schmitz TJ (eds): Physical Rehabilitation (ed 5). Philadelphia, F. A. Davis, 2007, pp 705–776

36. Wityk RJ, Pessin MS, Kaplan RF, et al: Serial assessment of acute stroke using the NIH Stroke Scale. Stroke 25:362–365, 1994

37. Fugl-Meyer AR, Jaasko L, Leyman I, et al: The post-stroke hemiplegic patient: A method for evaluation of physical performance. Scand J Rehabil Med 7:13–31, 1975

38. Afifi M: Clinical spectrum of Parkinson's disease. Singapore Med J 48:484–485; author reply 486, 2007

39. Playfer JR: Ageing and Parkinson's disease. Pract Neurol 7:4–5, 2007

40. Clarke CE, Moore AP: Parkinson's disease. Am Fam Physician 75:1045–1048, 2007

41. Konczak J, Krawczewski K, Tuite P, et al: The perception of passive motion in Parkinson's disease. J Neurol 254:655–663, 2007

42. Bertucci Filho D, Teive HA, Werneck LC: Early-onset Parkinson's disease and depression. Arq Neuropsiquiatr 65:5–10, 2007

43. Schrag A, Dodel R, Spottke A, et al: Rate of clinical progression in Parkinson's disease: A prospective study. Mov Disord 22:938–945, 2007

44. Hermanowicz N: Drug therapy for Parkinson's disease. Semin Neurol 27:97–105, 2007

45. Idiaquez J, Benarroch EE, Rosales H, et al: Autonomic and cognitive dysfunction in Parkinson's disease. Clin Auton Res 17:93–98, 2007

46. Ross OA, Farrer MJ, Wu RM: Common variants in Parkinson's disease. Mov Disord 22:899–900, 2007

47. Vaugoyeau M, Viel S, Assaiante C, et al: Impaired vertical postural control and proprioceptive integration deficits in Parkinson's disease. Neuroscience 146:852–863, 2007

48. Haehner A, Hummel T, Hummel C, et al: Olfactory loss may be a first sign of idiopathic Parkinson's disease. Mov Disord 22:839–842, 2007

49. Ziemssen T, Reichmann H: Non-motor dysfunction in Parkinson's disease. Parkinsonism Relat Disord 13:323–332, 2007

50. Whitton PS: Inflammation as a causative factor in the aetiology of Parkinson's disease. Br J Pharmacol 150:963–976, 2007

51. Hoehn MM, Yahr MD: Parkinsonism: Onset, progression and mortality. Neurology 17:427–442, 1967

52. Avdic S, Mujcinovic Z, Asceric M, et al: Left ventricular diastolic dysfunction in essential hypertension. Bosn J Basic Med Sci 7:15–20, 2007

53. Binder A: A review of the genetics of essential hypertension. Curr Opin Cardiol 22:176–184, 2007

54. Cuspidi C, Meani S, Valerio C, et al: Age and target organ damage in essential hypertension: Role of the metabolic syndrome. Am J Hypertens 20:296–303, 2007

55. El-Shafei SA, Bassili A, Hassanien NM, et al: Genetic determinants of essential hypertension. J Egypt Public Health Assoc 77:231–246, 2002

56. Hollenberg NK, Williams GH: Nonmodulation and essential hypertension. Curr Hypertens Rep 8:127–131, 2006

57. Kennedy S: Essential hypertension 2: Treatment and monitoring update. Community Pract 79:64–66, 2006

58. Kennedy S: Essential hypertension: recent changes in management. Community Pract 79:23–24, 2006

59. Krzych LJ: Blood pressure variability in children with essential hypertension. J Hum Hypertens 21:494–500, 2007

60. Parrilli G, Manguso F, Orsini L, et al: Essential hypertension and chronic viral hepatitis. Dig Liver Dis 39:466–472, 2007

61. Pierdomenico SD: Blood pressure variability and cardiovascular outcome in essential hypertension. Am J Hypertens 20:162–163, 2007

62. Fuller GF: Falls in the elderly. Am Fam Physician 61:2159–2168, 2173–2174, 2000

63. Rubenstein LZ: Falls, in Yoshikawa TT, Cobbs EL, Brummel-Smith K (eds): Ambulatory geriatric care. St. Louis, Mosby, 1993, pp 296–304

64. Baxter J: Screening and treating those at risk of nutritional deficiency. Community Nurse 6:S1–S2, S5, 2000

65. Callen BL, Wells TJ: Screening for nutritional risk in community-dwelling old-old. Public Health Nurs 22:138–146, 2005

66. Corish CA, Flood P, Kennedy NP: Comparison of nutritional risk screening tools in patients on admission to hospital. J Hum Nutr Diet 17:133–139; quiz 141–143, 2004

67. Hedberg AM, Garcia N, Trejus IJ, et al: Nutritional risk screening: Development of a standardized protocol using dietetic technicians. J Am Diet Assoc 88:1553–1556, 1988

68. Melnik TA, Helferd SJ, Firmery LA, et al: Screening elderly in the community: The relationship between dietary adequacy and nutritional risk. J Am Diet Assoc 94:1425–1427, 1994

69. Reilly HM: Screening for nutritional risk. Proc Nutr Soc 55:841–853, 1996

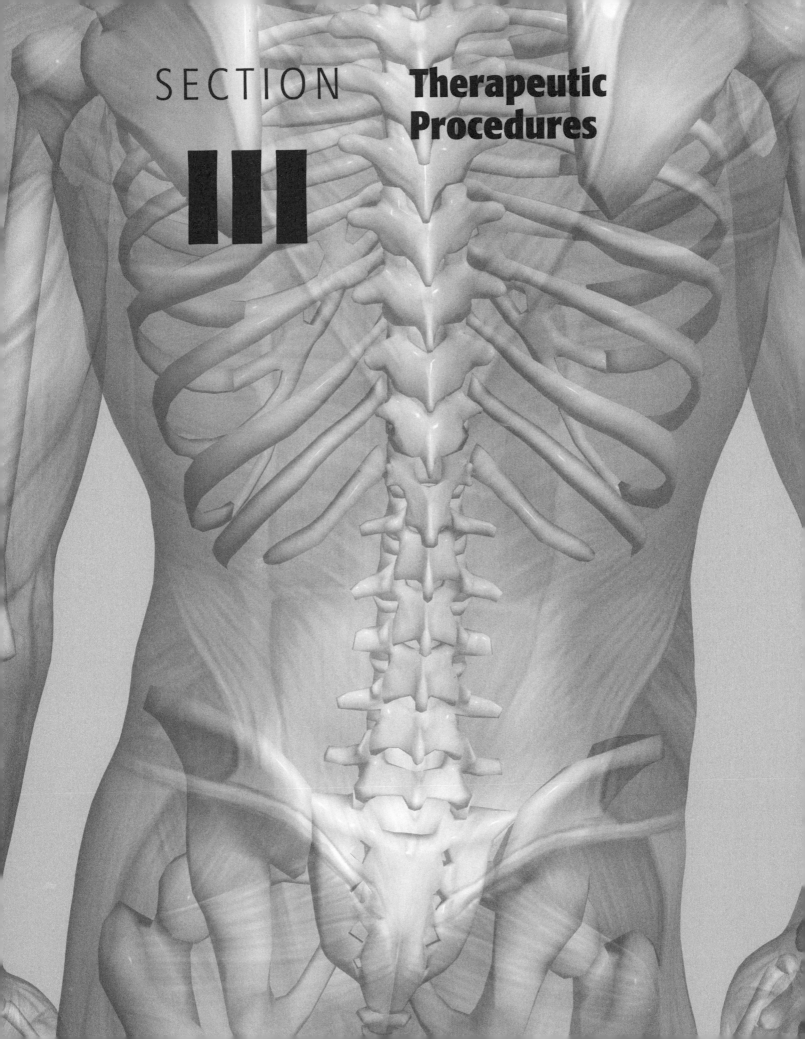

SECTION

III

Therapeutic Procedures

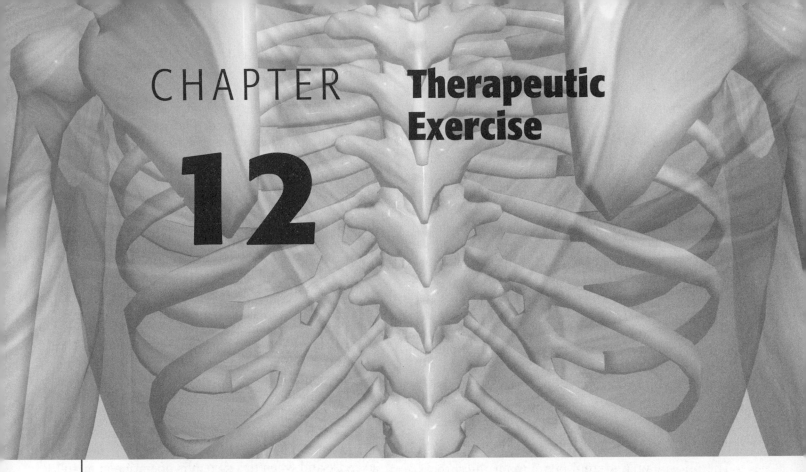

CHAPTER 12

Therapeutic Exercise

Therapeutic exercise is fundamental to physical therapy, and an important component of the vast majority of interventions. Performed accurately, therapeutic exercise can restore, maintain, and improve a patient's functional status by increasing strength, endurance, and flexibility. Therapeutic exercise enables the patient/client to:

- Reduce or minimize impairments
- Enhance function
- Optimize overall health
- Improve fitness and well-being

When prescribing a therapeutic exercise program it is important to consider the functional loss and disability of the patient.

Physiology of Exercise

Muscles are metabolically active and must generate energy to move. The creation of energy occurs initially from the breakdown of certain nutrients from foodstuffs. The energy required for exercise is stored in a compound called *adenosine triphosphate* (ATP). ATP is produced in the muscle tissue from blood glucose or glycogen. Fats and proteins can also be metabolized to generate ATP. Glucose not needed immediately is stored as glycogen in the resting muscle and liver. Stored glycogen can later be converted back to glucose and transferred to the blood to meet the body's energy needs. If the duration or intensity of the exercise increases, the body relies more heavily on fat stored in adipose tissue to meet its energy needs. During rest and submaximal exertion, both fat and carbohydrates are used to provide energy in approximately a 60% to 40% ratio.

During physical exercise, energy turnover in skeletal muscle can increase by 400 times compared with muscle at rest, and muscle oxygen consumption can increase by more than 100 times.[1] The energy required to power muscular activity is derived from the hydrolysis of ATP to ADP (adenosine diphosphate) and inorganic phosphate (P_i). Despite the large fluctuations in energy demand just mentioned, muscle ATP remains practically constant and demonstrates a remarkable precision of the system in adjusting the rate of the ATP-generating processes to the demand.[2] There are three energy systems that contribute to the resynthesis of ATP via ADP rephosphorylation. The relative contribution of these energy systems to ATP resynthesis has been shown to depend upon the intensity and duration of exercise.[3] It is worth noting that at no time during either rest or exercise does any single energy system provide the complete supply of energy. The three energy systems are the phosphagen system, the glycolysis system, and the oxidative system.

Phosphagen System

The phosphagen system is an anaerobic process, meaning it can proceed without oxygen (O_2). Within the skeletal muscle cell at the onset of muscular contraction, phosphocreatine (PCr) represents the most immediate reserve for the rephosphorylation of ATP. The phosphagen system provides ATP primarily for short-term, high-intensity activities (i.e., sprinting) and is active at the start of all exercises regardless of intensity.[4] One disadvantage of the phosphagen system is that because of its significant contribution to the energy yield at the onset of near maximal exercise, the concentration of PCr can be reduced to less than 40% of resting levels within 10 seconds of the start of intense exercise.[5]

Glycolysis System

The glycolysis system is an anaerobic process that involves the breakdown of carbohydrates—either glycogen stored in the muscle or glucose delivered in the blood—to produce ATP. Because this system relies upon a series of nine different chemical reactions, it is slower to become fully active. However, glycogenolysis has a greater capacity to provide energy than does PCr, and therefore it supplements PCr during maximal exercise and continues to rephosphorylate ADP during maximal exercise after PCr reserves have become essentially depleted.[4] The process of glycolysis can go one of two ways, termed *fast glycolysis* and *slow glycolysis*, depending

on the energy demands within the cell. If energy must be supplied at a high rate, fast glycolysis is used primarily. If the energy demand is not as high, slow glycolysis is activated. The main disadvantage of the fast glycolysis system is that during very high intensity exercise, hydrogen ions dissociate from the glycogenolytic end product of lactic acid.[2] An increase in hydrogen ion concentration is believed to inhibit glycotic reactions and directly interfere with muscle excitation–contraction and coupling, which can potentially impair contractile force during exercise.[4]

Oxidative System

As its name suggests, the oxidative system requires O_2 and is consequently termed the "aerobic" system. The oxidative system is the primary source of ATP at rest and during low-intensity activities. While being unable to produce ATP at an equivalent rate to that produced by PCr breakdown and glycogenolysis, the oxidative system is capable of sustaining low-intensity exercise for several hours.[4] However, because of an increased complexity, the time between the onset of exercise and when this system is operating at its full potential is around 45 seconds.[6]

> **● Key Point** In most activities, both aerobic and anaerobic systems function simultaneously with the ratio being determined by the intensity and duration of the activity. In general, high-intensity activities of short duration rely more heavily on the anaerobic system, whereas low-intensity activities of longer duration rely more on the aerobic system.

Measures of Energy Expenditure

The energy value of the food eaten can be quantified in terms of the calorie. A kilocalorie (kcal) is the amount of heat necessary to raise 1.0 kilogram of water by 1.0 degrees Celsius. A metabolic equivalent unit, or MET, is defined as the energy expenditure for sitting quietly, talking on the phone, or reading a book, which, for the average adult, approximates 3.5 milliliters of oxygen uptake per kilogram of body weight per minute (3.5 mL O_2/kg/min—1.2 kcal/min for a 70-kg individual). METs are defined as multiples of resting energy metabolism. For example, a 2-MET activity requires two times the metabolic energy expenditure of sitting quietly. The harder the body works during the activity, the higher the MET (**Table 12-1**). Any activity that burns 3 to 6 METs is considered moderate-intensity physical activity. Any activity that burns more than 6 METs is considered vigorous-intensity physical activity.

TABLE 12-1

General Physical Activities Defined by Level of Intensity in Accordance with CDC and ACSM Guidelines

Moderate Activity, 3.0 to 6.0 METs (3.5 to 7 kcal/min)	Vigorous Activity, Greater than 6.0 METs (more than 7 kcal/min)
Walking at a moderate or brisk pace of 3 to 4.5 mph on a level surface inside or outside, such as	Racewalking and aerobic walking (5 mph or faster)
• Walking to class, work, or the store	Jogging or running
• Walking for pleasure	Wheeling your wheelchair
• Walking the dog	Walking and climbing briskly up a hill
• Walking as a break from work	Backpacking
Walking downstairs or down a hill	Mountain climbing, rock climbing, rapelling
Racewalking—less than 5 mph	Roller skating or in-line skating at a brisk pace
Using crutches	
Hiking	
Roller skating or in-line skating at a leisurely pace	
Bicycling 5 to 9 mph, level terrain, or with few hills	Bicycling more than 10 mph or bicycling on steep uphill terrain
Stationary bicycling—using moderate effort	Stationary bicycling—using vigorous effort
Aerobic dancing—high impact	Aerobic dancing—high impact
Water aerobics	Step aerobics
	Water jogging
	Teaching an aerobic dance class
Calisthenics—light	Calisthenics—push-ups, pull-ups, vigorous effort
Yoga	Karate, judo, tae kwon do, jujitsu
Gymnastics	Jumping rope
General home exercises, light or moderate effort, getting up and down from the floor	Performing jumping jacks
Jumping on a trampoline	Using a stair climber machine at a fast pace
Using a stair climber machine at a light to moderate pace	Using a rowing machine—with vigorous effort
Using a rowing machine—with moderate effort	Using an arm cycling machine—with vigorous effort
Weight training and bodybuilding using free weights or Nautilus- or Universal-type weights	Circuit weight training
Boxing—punching bag	Boxing—in the ring, sparring
	Wrestling—competitive
Ballroom dancing	Professional ballroom dancing—energetically
Line dancing	Square dancing—energetically
Square dancing	Folk dancing—energetically
Folk dancing	Clogging
Modern dancing, disco	
Ballet	
Table tennis—competitive	Tennis—singles
Tennis—doubles	Wheelchair tennis
Golf, wheeling or carrying clubs	—
Softball—fast pitch or slow pitch	Most competitive sports
Basketball—shooting baskets	Football
Coaching children's or adults' sports	Basketball
	Wheelchair basketball
	Soccer
	Rugby
	Kickball
	Field or rollerblade hockey
	Lacrosse

The Basal Metabolic Rate

The basal metabolic rate (BMR), the sum total of cellular activity in all metabolically active tissues while under basal conditions, is the minimal amount of oxygen needed in order to support life.

- A person's BMR varies according to overall body size, gender, age, fat-free mass, and endocrine function.
- In general, the BMR tends to be 5% to 10% lower in women than men. There is a decline in BMR of 2% to 3% per decade of life, which is most likely due to the reduction in physical activity associated with aging.

Measures of Body Composition

Hydrostatic Weighing

Hydrostatic weighing (i.e., underwater weighing) is a method for measuring the mass density of a body, based on the Archimedes principle. The individual is fully immersed in water. Calculations are then made using the following three measurable values: the weight of the body outside the water, the weight of the immersed body, and the density of the water. The residual volume in the lungs can add error if not measured directly (the standard error for this method is estimated at 2% to 2.5%).

Plethysmography

A plethysmograph is an instrument for measuring changes in volume within an organ or whole body (usually resulting from fluctuations in the amount of blood or air it contains). A displacement plethysmography is similar in principle to hydrostatic weighing, except that air is used, which is more convenient and comfortable than water. From the subject's body density, relative proportions of body fat and lean body mass are calculated based on the density of fat and lean tissue. Because lean tissue is denser than fat tissue, a higher density reflects a higher proportion of lean tissue.

Skinfold Measurements

Taking skinfold measurements at three to nine standardized sites is a common method for determining body fat composition. Usually only the right side is measured (for consistency). The nine standard skinfold sites include: abdomen, triceps, biceps, chest, medial calf, mid axillary, subscapular, suprailiac, and the thigh. The tester pinches the skin at the appropriate site to raise a double layer of skin and the underlying adipose tissue, but not the muscle. The calipers are then applied 1 centimeter below and at right angles to the pinch, and a reading in millimeters (mm) is taken two seconds later. The mean of two measurements is taken. If the two measurements differ greatly, a third is done, and the median value taken.

Body Mass Index

Body mass index (BMI) is a measure of body fat based on height and weight. Body fat can be divided into two types:

- *Essential fat:* Necessary for normal physiological function, serving as a source of energy and a storage site for some vitamins.
- *Storage fat:* Stored in adipose tissue.

● **Key Point** Fat-free mass (FFM) includes muscle, skin, bone, and viscera.

Separate calculations are used for boys and girls aged 2 to 20 and for adult men and women. Further subdivisions can be made according to gender for adults. The limitations of relying on the BMI include:

- It may overestimate body fat in athletes and others who have a muscular build.
- It may underestimate body fat in older persons and others who have lost muscle mass.

Two methods can be used to calculate BMI:

- BMI (kg/m²) = weight in kilograms/height in meters²
- BMI (lbs/inches²) = (weight in pounds × 703)/ height in inches²

● **Key Point** The standard error with estimating fat percentage with the BMI is approximately 5%.

Bioelectrical Impedance Analysis

Bioelectrical impedance analysis (BIA) measures body composition by sending a low, safe electrical current through the body fluids contained mainly in the lean and fat tissue. BIA measures the impedance or opposition to the flow of this electric current.

- Impedance is low in lean tissue, where intracellular fluid and electrolytes are primarily contained.
- Impedance is high in fat tissue.

Impedance is thus proportional to body water volume (TBW). Prediction equations, previously generated by correlating impedance measures against an independent estimate of TBW, can be used subsequently to convert the measured impedance to a corresponding estimate of TBW. Lean body mass is then calculated from this estimate using an assumed hydration fraction for lean tissue. Fat mass is calculated as the difference between body weight and lean body mass.

● **Key Point** BIA values are affected by numerous variables, including body position, hydration status, consumption of food and beverages, ambient air and skin temperature, recent physical activity, and conductance of the examining table. Reliable BIA requires standardization and control of these variables.

Muscle Fiber Types

The basic function of a muscle is to contract. On the basis of their contractile properties, different types of muscle fibers have been recognized within skeletal muscle: type I (slow-twitch red oxidative), and type II (fast-twitch white glycolytic). Type II fibers can be broken down further into three distinct subsets:[9] type II, A; type II, AB; and type II, B (**Table 12-2**).

- Slow-twitch fibers have a high capacity for oxygen uptake. They are, therefore, suitable for activities of long duration or endurance, including the maintenance of posture.
- Fast-twitch fibers have a low capacity for oxygen uptake and are therefore suited to quick, explosive actions, including such activities as sprinting.

● **Key Point** In fast-twitch fibers, the sarcoplasmic reticulum embraces every individual myofibril. In slow-twitch fibers, it may contain multiple myofibrils.[10]

Theory dictates that a muscle with a large percentage of the total cross-sectional area occupied by slow-twitch type I fibers should be more fatigue resistant than one in which the fast-twitch type II fibers predominate.

Recruitment of Motor Units

The force and speed of a muscle contraction are based on the requirement of an activity and are dependent on the ability of the central nervous system to control the recruitment of motor units.[11] Slow-twitch fiber motor units have low thresholds and are relatively more easily activated than the motor units of the fast-twitch fibers. Consequently, the slow-twitch fibers are the first to be recruited, even when the resulting limb movement is rapid.[12]

TABLE 12-2 Comparison of Muscle Fiber Types

Characteristics	Type I	Type II A	Type II AB	Type II B
Diameter	Small	Intermediate	Large	Very large
Capillaries	Many	Many	Few	Few
Resistance to fatigue	High	Fairly high	Intermediate	Low
Glycogen content	Low	Intermediate	High	High
Respiration	Aerobic	Aerobic	Anaerobic	Anaerobic
Twitch rate	Slow	Fast	Fast	Fast
Major storage fuel	Triglycerides	Creatine phosphate Glycogen	Creatine phosphate Glycogen	Creatine phosphate Glycogen

Muscle Function

Muscle groups are classified as follows:

- *Agonist muscle:* Contracts to produce the desired movement.
- *Antagonist muscle:* Typically opposes the desired movement and is responsible for returning a limb to its initial position. Antagonists ensure that the desired motion occurs in a coordinated and controlled fashion by relaxing and lengthening in a gradual manner.
- *Synergist muscle (supporters):* Muscle groups that perform, or assist in performing, joint motions. Although synergists can work with the agonists, they can also oppose the agonists as occurs in force couples.

- *Neutralizers:* These muscles help cancel out, or neutralize, extra motion from the agonists to make sure that the force generated works within the desired plane of motion—for example, when the flexor carpi ulnaris and extensor carpi ulnaris neutralize the flexion/extension forces at the wrist to produce ulnar deviation.
- *Stabilizers (fixators):* Provide the necessary support to help stabilize an area so that another area can be moved—for example, the trunk core stabilizers become active when the upper extremities are being used.

Stable posture results from a balance of competing forces, whereas movement occurs when competing forces are unbalanced.[14]

Types of Muscle Contraction

The word *contraction*, used to describe the generation of tension within muscle fibers, conjures up an image of a shortening of muscle fibers. However, a contraction can produce a shortening or a lengthening of the muscle, or no change in the muscle length. In addition, a muscle contraction produces compression at the joint surfaces of neighboring joints.

There are three basic types of muscle contraction:

- *Isometric contraction:* Provides a static contraction with a variable and accommodating resistance without producing a change in muscle length. Examples of isometric exercise include muscle setting exercises, stabilization exercises, and multiple angle isometrics.
- *Concentric contraction:* Provides a dynamic contraction whereby tension is produced and shortening of the muscle takes place, approximating the origin and insertion of the contracting muscle.
- *Eccentric contraction:* Provides a dynamic contraction whereby tension is produced as lengthening of the muscle occurs. The net action is opposite that produced by concentric contraction in that the origin and insertion of the contracting muscle move further apart during the contraction. In reality, the muscle does not actually lengthen; it merely returns from its shortened position to its normal resting length.

Active Length–Tension Relationship

Muscles are elastic in nature and are therefore constantly being lengthened or shortened. This change in length of a muscle is known as its excursion. Typically, a muscle can only shorten or elongate about half its resting length. In its most basic form, the length–tension relationship states that isometric tension generated in skeletal muscle is a function of the magnitude of overlap between actin and myosin filaments (see Chapter 4). For each muscle cell, there is an optimum length, or range of lengths, at which the contractile force is strongest. At the optimum length of the muscle, there is near-optimal overlap of actin and myosin, allowing for the generation of maximum tension at this length.

- If the muscle is in a shortened position relative to the optimum length, the overlap of actin and myosin reduces the number of sites available for cross-bridge formation. *Active insufficiency* of a muscle occurs when the muscle is incapable of shortening to the extent required to produce full range of motion at all joints crossed simultaneously.[11,16–18] For example, the finger flexors cannot produce a tight fist when the wrist is fully flexed, as they can when it is in neutral position.
- If the muscle is in a lengthened position relative to the optimum length, the actin filaments are pulled away from the myosin heads such that they cannot create as many cross-bridges.[19] *Passive insufficiency* of the muscle occurs when the two-joint muscle cannot stretch to the extent required for full range of motion in the opposite direction at all joints crossed.[11,16–18] For example, a larger range of hyperextension is possible at the wrist when the fingers are not fully extended.

The length–tension relationship is often represented graphically (Figure 12-1). At short muscle lengths, an increase in length brings an increase in force, giving a positive slope to the length–tension function. At medium lengths, filament overlap allows the largest number of cross-bridges to form, and thus the force is maximum, and the slope is zero. At longer lengths, the slope becomes negative in that the force decreases with increasing length because available cross-bridge sites decrease.

Passive Length–Tension Relationship

A muscle generates greater internal elastic force when it is stretched, as demonstrated by a muscle's

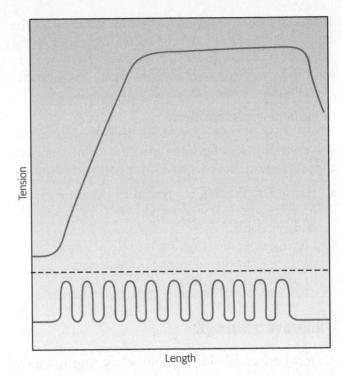

Figure 12-1   Length-tension curve.

passive length tension curve (refer to Figure 12-1). As a muscle is progressively stretched, the tissue is slack until it reaches a critical length where it begins to generate tension. Beyond this critical length, the tension builds exponentially. It is not uncommon for muscles to use active contractions with passive lengthening. For example, consider the bicep when pulling an object toward the body, a movement that combines simultaneous and rapid elbow flexion with shoulder extension. As the biceps contracts to perform elbow flexion, it is simultaneously elongated or stretched across the extending shoulder. Such an activity helps maintain a near constant (and optimal) overall length of the biceps during the activity and allows the biceps to produce a more constant force throughout the range of motion.[20]

Force–Velocity Relationship

The rate of muscle shortening or lengthening substantially affects the force that a muscle can develop during contraction.

Shortening Contractions

As the speed of a muscle shortening increases, the force it is capable of producing decreases.[21,22] The slower rate of shortening is thought to produce greater forces than can be produced by increasing the number of cross-bridges formed. This relationship can be viewed as a continuum, with the optimum velocity for the muscle somewhere between the slowest and fastest rates. At very slow speeds, the force that a muscle can resist or overcome rises rapidly, up to 50% greater than the maximum isometric contraction.[21,22]

Lengthening Contractions

When a muscle contracts while lengthening (*eccentric contraction*), the force production differs from that of a shortening (*concentric*) contraction:

- Rapid lengthening contractions generate more force than do slow ones (slower lengthening contractions).
- During slow lengthening muscle actions, the work produced approximates that of an isometric contraction.[21,22]

Improving Strength

To most effectively increase muscle strength, a muscle must work with increasing effort against progressively increasing resistance.[23,24] If a resistance is applied to a muscle as it contracts so that the metabolic capabilities of the muscle are progressively overloaded, adaptive changes occur within the muscle, which make it stronger over time.[21,25] These adaptive changes include:[22,24,26–30]

- An increase in the efficiency of the neuromuscular system. This increased efficiency results in:
  - An increase in the number of motor units recruited
  - An increase in the firing rate of each motor unit
  - An increase in the synchronization of motor unit firing
- The endurance of the muscle improves.
- Stimulation of slow-twitch (Type I) fibers (when performing workloads of low intensity), and stimulation of fast-twitch (Type IIa) fibers (when performing workloads of high intensity and short duration).
- Remodeling (*hypertrophy*). The muscle hypertrophies due to an increase in the number and size of the myofilaments (actin and myosin).
- An increase in blood flow to exercising muscles via contraction and relaxation.
- The power of the muscle improves.
- Improved bone mass (Wolfe's Law).
- Increase in metabolism, calorie burning, and weight control.

- Increased intramuscular pressure results from a muscle contraction of about 60% of its force-generating capacity.
- Cardiovascular benefits when using large muscle groups. Strength training of specific muscles has a brief activation period and uses a relatively small muscle mass, thereby producing less cardiovascular metabolic demand than vigorous walking, swimming, and other such activities.

Conversely, a muscle can become weak or atrophied through:

- Disease
- Neurologic compromise
- Immobilization
- Disuse

Contraindications of Strength Training

Absolute contraindications to strength training include unstable angina, uncontrolled hypertension, uncontrolled dysrhythmias, hypertrophic cardiomyopathy, and certain stages of retinopathy. Patients with congestive heart failure, myocardial ischemia, poor left ventricular function, or autonomic neuropathies must be carefully evaluated before initiating a strength-training program.

Exercise Principles

There are three exercise principles worth mentioning:

- *SAID principle:* The specific adaptation to imposed demand (SAID) principle acknowledges that the human body responds to explicit demands placed upon it with a specific and predictable adaptation. Therefore, the focus of the exercise prescription should be to improve the strength and coordination of functional or sports-specific movements with strengthening and flexibility exercises that approximate the desired activity in terms of its frequency, intensity, and duration.
- *Overload principle:* The principle of overload states that a greater than normal stress or load on the body is required for training adaptation to take place. To increase strength, the muscle must be challenged at a greater level than it is accustomed to. High levels of tension will produce adaptations in the form of hypertrophy and recruitment of more muscle fibers.

- *Reversibility principle:* Any adaptive changes in the body systems, such as increased strength or endurance, in response to a resistance exercise program, are temporary unless training-induced improvements are regularly used through functional activities or resistance exercises.[31] These changes can begin within a week or two after the cessation of resistance exercises and will continue until the training effects are lost.[15,32]

Types of Exercise

Isometric Exercises

Isometric exercises provide a static contraction with a variable and accommodating resistance without producing a change in muscle length. This type of exercise has an obvious role where joint movement is restricted, either by pain, or by bracing/casting. Their primary role in this regard is to prevent atrophy and prevent a decrease of ligament, bone, and muscle strength. A 6-second hold of 75% of maximal resistance is sufficient to increase strength when performed repetitively. The disadvantages of isometric exercises are:

- The strength gains are developed at a specific point in the range of motion and not throughout the range (unless performed at multi-angles).
- Not all of a muscle's fibers are activated. There is predominantly an activation of slow-twitch (Type I) fibers.
- There are no flexibility or cardiovascular fitness benefits.
- Peak effort can be injurious to the tissues due to vasoconstriction and joint compression forces.
- There is limited functional carryover.[33]
- Considerable internal pressure can be generated, especially if the breath is held during contraction, which can result in:
  □ Further injury to patients with weakness in the abdominal wall (hernia)
  □ Cardiovascular impairment (by increasing blood pressure through the Valsalva maneuver, even if the exercise is performed correctly)

Concentric/Isotonic Exercises

Concentric/isotonic contractions are commonly used in the rehabilitation process and occur frequently in activities of daily living—the biceps curl and the lifting of a cup to the mouth are respective examples.

Concentric exercises are dynamic and allow the clinician to vary the load from constant, using free weights, to variable, using an exercise machine. The speed of contraction can also be manipulated depending on the goal of the intervention.

Eccentric Exercises

Maximum eccentric exercises produce more force than maximal concentric contraction. Eccentric strength is important for many functional activities and can provide a source of shock absorption during closed-chain functional activities. The clinical indications for the use of eccentric exercise are numerous.[34]

Functional Exercises

Functional strength is the ability of the neuromuscular system to perform the various types of contractions involved with multi-joint functional activities in an efficient manner and in a multi-planar environment.[35] Functional exercises use combinations of concentric and eccentric contractions in the performance of activities that relate to a patient's needs and requirements. Effective rehabilitation targets specific muscles with regard to functional muscle activity patterns and overall conditioning, and it utilizes a progression of increased activity, while preventing further trauma.[36] Incremental gains in function should be seen as strength increases.

Isokinetic Exercise

Isokinetic exercise requires the use of special equipment that produces an accommodating and variable resistance. The main principle behind isokinetic exercise is that peak torque (the maximum force generated through the range of motion) is inversely related to angular velocity, the speed that a body segment moves through its range of motion. Thus, an increase in angular velocity decreases peak torque production. Advantages of this type of exercise include:

- Both high speed/low resistance and low speed/high resistance regimens result in excellent strength gains.[37–40]
- Both concentric or eccentric resistance exercises can be performed on isokinetic machines.
- The machines provide maximum resistance at all points in the range of motion as a muscle contracts.
- The gravity-produced torque created by the machine adds to the force generated by the muscle when it contracts, resulting in a higher torque output than is actually created by the muscle.

The disadvantages of this type of exercise include:

- Expense
- The potential for impact loading and incorrect joint axis alignment[41]
- Questionable functional carryover[33]
- Open-chain exercise
- Single muscle/motion

Types of Resistance

Resistance can be applied to a muscle by any external force or mass, including any of the following.

Gravity

Gravity alone can supply sufficient resistance with a weakened muscle. With respect to gravity, muscle actions may occur:

- In the same direction of gravity (downward)
- In the opposite direction to gravity (upward)
- In a direction perpendicular to gravity (horizontal)
- In the same or opposite direction to gravity but at an angle

Body Weight

A wide variety of exercises have been developed using no equipment, relying only on the patient's body weight for the resistance (e.g., push-ups).

Small Weights/Surgical Tubing/Theraband

These are economical ways of applying resistance and are typically used to strengthen the smaller muscles or to increase the endurance of larger muscles by increasing the number of reps. Free weights also provide more versatility than exercise machines, especially for three-dimensional exercises. The disadvantage of free weights is that they offer no variable resistance throughout the range of motion, so the weakest point along the length–tension curve of each muscle limits the amount of weight lifted.

Exercise Machines

In situations where the larger muscle groups require strengthening, a multitude of specific indoor exercise machines can be used. These machines are often used in the more advanced stages of a rehabilitation program when more resistance can be tolerated, but they also can be used in the earlier stages depending on the size of the muscle undergoing rehabilitation. Examples of these machines include the multi-hip, the lat pull-down, the leg extension, and the leg curl machines. Exercise machines are often fitted with an oval-shaped cam or wheel that mimics the length of tension curve of the muscle (Nautilus, Cybex).

Although these machines are a more expensive alternative to dumbbell or elastic resistance, they do offer some advantages:

- They provide more adequate resistance for large muscle groups than can be achieved with free weights/cuff weights or manual resistance.
- They are typically safer than free weights because control throughout the range is provided.
- They provide the clinician with the ability to quantify and measure the amount of resistance that the patient can tolerate over time.

The disadvantages of exercise machines include:

- The inability to modify the exercise to be more functional or three-dimensional
- The inability to modify the amount of resistance at particular points of the range

Manual Resistance

Manual resistance is a type of active exercise in which another person provides resistance manually. An example of manual resistance is proprioceptive neuromuscular facilitation (PNF).

The advantages of manual resistance, when applied by a skilled clinician, are:[42]

- Control of the extremity position and force applied. This is especially useful in the early stages of an exercise program when the muscle is weak.
- More effective reeducation of the muscle or extremity, through the use of diagonal or functional patterns of movement.
- Critical sensory input to the patient through tactile stimulation and appropriate facilitation techniques (e.g., quick PNF stretch).
- Accurate accommodation and alterations in the resistance applied throughout the range. For example, an exercise can be modified to avoid a painful arc in the range.
- Ability to limit the range. This is particularly important when the amount of range of motion needs to be carefully controlled (postsurgical restrictions or pain).

The disadvantages of manual resistance include:

- The amount of resistance applied cannot be measured quantitatively.
- The amount of resistance is limited by the strength of the clinician/caregiver or family member.

There can be difficulty with consistency of the applied force throughout the range and with each repetition.

> ● **Key Point** Water can be used as a form of resistance (see Chapter 13). Water provides resistance proportional to the relative speed of movement of the patient and the water and the cross-sectional area of the patient in contact with the water.[43]

Correct Progression

For exercises to be effective, the patient must be compliant and be able to train without exacerbating the condition.[44] The therapeutic exercise program always begins with an exercise the patient can perform, before progressing in difficulty toward a functional outcome. The early goals of exercise are concerned with increasing circulation, preventing atrophy, increasing protein synthesis, and reducing the level of metabolites.[44] Each progression is made more challenging by altering one of the parameters of exercise (type/mode of exercise, intensity, duration, and frequency), which are modified according to patient response.

- *Type of exercise:* Type of exercise relates to the specific activity being performed, including the mode of resistance (see "Types of Resistance") and type of activity being performed (see "Types of Exercise").
- *Intensity:* Intensity refers to how much effort is required to perform the exercise. For aerobic activities, the exercise intensity should be at a level that is 40% to 85% maximal aerobic power (Vo_2 max) or 55% to 90% of maximal heart rate.[45]
- *Related Perceived Exertion (RPE):* It is now recognized that an individual's perception of effort (relative perceived exertion) is closely related to the level of physiological effort (refer to Table 6-5).[7,8] It is important, therefore, to closely monitor the patient's response to exercise. Any discomfort or reproduction of symptoms that lasts more than 1 to 2 hours after the intervention is unacceptable. Patient responses that can modify the intensity include increases in pain level, muscle fatigue, time taken to recover from fatigue, cardiovascular response, compensatory movements, insufficient balance, level of motivation, and degree of comprehension.
- *Duration:* Duration refers to the length of the exercise session. In most functional exercises, fatigue must be considered so that the patient's

tolerance is not exceeded. The exercise should be performed in a pain-free range until fatigue occurs. Fatigue may also occur as a lack of coordination observed by the clinician but not perceived by the patient. Physical conditioning occurs over a period of 15 to 60 minutes depending on the level of intensity. Average conditioning time is 20 to 30 minutes for moderate-intensity exercise. However, individuals who are severely compromised are more likely to benefit from a series of short exercise sessions (3 to 10 minutes) spaced throughout the day.

- *Frequency:* Frequency refers to how often the exercise is performed. Frequency of activity is dependent upon intensity and duration; the lower the intensity, the shorter the duration, the greater the frequency. The recommended frequency is 3 to 5 sessions per week at moderate intensities and duration (>5 METs).

> ● **Key Point** If pain is reported by the patient *before* a resistive activity or before the end feel during passive range of motion, the patient's symptoms are considered irritable. The intervention in the presence of irritability should not be aggressive.[46] If pain occurs *after* resistance, then the patient's symptoms are not considered irritable, and exercise, particularly stretching, can be more aggressive.

Delayed-Onset Muscle Soreness

Muscular soreness may result from all forms of exercise. Acute muscle soreness develops during or directly after strenuous and aerobic exercise performed to the point of fatigue. The soreness is theoretically related to the decreased blood flow and reduced oxygen that creates a temporary buildup of lactic acid and potassium. Using a cool-down period of low-intensity exercise that facilitates the return of oxygen to the muscle can minimize the adverse effects of this type of soreness. A type of soreness that is related to eccentric exercise is delayed-onset muscle soreness (DOMS).[34] This type of soreness, which occurs between 48 and 72 hours after exercise, may last for up to 10 days. Prevention of this type of muscle soreness involves careful design of the eccentric program, including prepatory techniques, accurate training variables, and appropriate aftercare.[34] The intervention for DOMS includes aerobic submaximal exercise with no eccentric component (swimming, biking, or stepper machines), pain-free flexibility exercises, and high speed (300 degrees/second) concentric only isokinetic training.[34,47]

Exercise Hierarchy

A hierarchy exists for ROM and resistive exercises during the subacute (neovascularization) stage of healing, to ensure that any progression is done in a safe and controlled fashion. The hierarchy for the ROM exercises is *passive ROM → active-assisted ROM → active ROM*.

- Passive range of motion does not prevent muscle atrophy, increase strength or endurance, or assist circulation to the same extent that active, volunteer muscle contraction does.
- Active range of motion does not maintain or increase strength, or develop skill or coordination, except in the movement patterns used.

● Key Point It is important to remember when making the transition from passive ROM to active ROM that gravity has a significant impact, especially in individuals with weak musculature. These individuals may require assistance when the segment moves up against gravity or moves downward with gravity.

The mobility activities chosen can be performed in cardinal planes or in multiple planes using functional movement patterns. Once these are tolerated well by the patient, a resistive exercise progression is initiated. Gentle resistance exercises in the form of isometrics can be introduced very early in the rehabilitative process. The typical progression for isometric exercises is:

- Single angle submaximal isometrics performed in the neutral position
- Multiple angle submaximal isometrics performed at various angles of the range
- Multiple angle maximal isometrics

Although some soreness can be expected, sharp pain should not be provoked.

Optimal strength-specific programs include the use of both eccentric and concentric muscle actions and the performance of both single-joint and multijoint exercises. The hierarchy for the resistive exercise progression is based on patient tolerance and response to ensure that any progress made is done in a safe and controlled fashion. The typical sequence occurs in the following order:[48]

- Small arc submaximal concentric/eccentric
- Full ROM submaximal concentric/eccentric
- Full ROM submaximal eccentric
- Functional ROM submaximal concentric
- Functional ROM submaximal eccentric
- Full ROM submaximal eccentric isokinetic
- Functional ROM submaximal eccentric isokinetic

At regular intervals, the clinician should ensure that:

- The patient is adherent with the exercise program at home.
- The patient understands the rationale behind the exercise program.
- The patient is performing the exercise program correctly and at the appropriate intensity.
- The patient's exercise program is being updated appropriately based on clinical findings and patient response.

● Key Point Neuromuscular electrical stimulation (NMES) can be an effective component of a rehabilitation program for muscle weakness (see Chapter 13).

A number of precautions must be observed with patients who are performing strength training:

- Muscles that are weak or fatigued rely on other muscles to produce the movement if the resistance is too high. This results in incorrect stabilization and poor form.
- Overworking of the muscles can occur if the exercise parameters (frequency, intensity, duration) are advanced too quickly.
- Adequate rest must be provided (3 to 4 minutes are needed to return the muscle to 90% to 95% of pre-exercise capacity, with the most rapid recovery occurring in the first minute) after each vigorous exercise.
- The rest period between sets can be determined by the time the breathing rate, or pulse, of the patient returns to the steady state.

Warm-Up and Cool-Down Periods

Each exercise session should include a 5- to 15-minute warm-up and a 5- to 15-minute cool-down period.

- Warm-up:
  - Includes low-intensity cardiorespiratory activities
  - Serves to prepare the heart and circulatory system from being suddenly overloaded
- Cool-down:
  - Includes low-intensity cardiorespiratory activities and flexibility exercises
  - Helps prevent abrupt physiological alterations that can occur with sudden cessation of strenuous exercise, such as adaptive shortening, and lactic acid buildup

The length of the warm-up and cool-down sessions may need to be longer for deconditioned or older individuals.

Circuit Training

The term *circuit* refers to a number of carefully selected exercises arranged consecutively. In the original format, 9 to 12 stations composed the circuit, but this number may vary according to the circuit's design. Each circuit training participant moves from one station to the next with little (15–30 seconds) or no rest, performing a 15- to 45-second work bout of 8 to 20 repetitions at each station. The circuit training workout program may be performed with exercise machines, handheld weights, elastic resistance, calisthenics, or any combination of these. Commonly prescribed exercises for circuit training include bench press, seated row, leg press, seated press, lat pulldown, upright row, leg extension, leg curl, triceps push-down, arm curl, and an abdominal exercise (crunch).

Interval Training

Interval training includes an exercise period followed by a prescribed rest interval. It is perceived to be less demanding than continuous training and tends to improve strength and power more than endurance. With appropriate spacing of work and rest intervals, a significant amount of high-intensity work can be achieved and is greater than the amount of work accomplished with continuous training. The longer the work interval, the more the anaerobic system is stressed and the less important is the duration of the rest period. In a short work interval, a work recovery ratio of 1:1 or 1:5 is appropriate to stress the aerobic system.

Open and Closed Kinetic Chain Exercises

The expression *kinetic chain* is used to describe the function or activity of an extremity and/or trunk in terms of a series of linked chains. According to kinetic chain theory, each of the joint segments of the body involved in a particular movement constitutes a link along one of these kinetic chains. As each motion of a joint is often a function of other joint motions, the efficiency of an activity can be dependent on how well these chain-links work together.[49]

Closed Kinetic Chain

Examples of a closed kinetic chain exercise (CKCE) involving the lower extremities include the squat and the leg press. The activities of walking, running, jumping, climbing, and rising from the floor all incorporate closed kinetic chain components.

An example of a CKCE for the upper extremities is the push-up, or using the arms to rise out of a chair.

Open Kinetic Chain

Open kinetic chain exercises (OKCE) involving the lower extremity include the seated knee extension and prone knee flexion. Upper-extremity examples of OKCE include the biceps curl and the military press.

Improving Muscular Endurance

To increase muscle endurance, exercises are performed against light resistance for many repetitions, so that the amount of energy expended is equal to the amount of energy supplied. This phenomenon, called *steady state*, occurs after some 5 to 6 minutes of exercise at a constant intensity level. Working at a level to which the muscle is accustomed improves the endurance of that muscle but does not increase its strength. However, exercise programs that increase strength also increase muscular endurance. Muscular endurance programs are typically indicated early in a strengthening program as the high-repetition and low-load exercises are more comfortable, enhance the vascular supply to muscle, cause less muscle soreness, cause less joint irritation, and reduce the risk of muscle injury.

Aerobic Capacity and Cardiorespiratory Endurance

By definition, cardiorespiratory endurance is the ability to perform whole-body activities (e.g., walking, jogging, biking, swimming) for extended periods of time without undue fatigue. A number of adaptations occur within the circulatory system in response to exercise:

- *Heart rate:* Monitoring heart rate is an indirect method of estimating oxygen consumption as, in general, these two factors have a linear relationship. If a physical therapy intervention requires an increase in systemic oxygen consumption expressed as either an increase in MET levels, kcal, L/O_2, or ml O_2 per kg of body weight per minute, then HR should also increase.[50]

> ● **Key Point** The magnitude at which the HR increases with increasing workloads is influenced by many factors, including age, fitness level, type of activity being performed, presence of disease, medications, blood volume, and environmental factors such as temperature, humidity, and altitude. Failure of the heart rate to increase with increasing workloads (*chronotropic incompetence*) should be of concern for the PTA, even if the patient is taking beta blockers. Beta blockers slow the HR, which can prevent the increase in heart rate that typically occurs with exercise.[50]

- *Stroke volume:* The volume of blood being pumped out with each beat increases with exercise, but only to the point when there is enough time between beats for the heart to fill up (approximately 110 to 120 beats per minute). In the normal heart, as workload increases, stroke volume (SV) increases linearly up to 50% of aerobic capacity, after which it increases only slightly. Factors that influence the magnitude of change in SV include ventricular function, body position, and exercise intensity.

> **● Key Point** Stroke volume (SV) is the amount of blood pumped out by the left ventricle of the heart with each beat. The heart does not pump all the blood out of the ventricle—normally, only about two-thirds.

- *Cardiac output:* Cardiac output (CO), the product of HR and SV, increases linearly with workload because of the increases in HR and SV in response to increasing exercise intensity.

> **● Key Point** Cardiac output (CO) is the amount of blood discharged by each ventricle (not both ventricles combined) per minute, usually expressed as liters per minute. Factors that influence the magnitude of change in CO include age, posture, body size, presence of disease, and level of physical conditioning. A long-term beneficial training effect that occurs with regard to cardiac output of the heart is that the stroke volume increases while the exercise heart rate is reduced at a given standard exercise load.

- *Blood pressure:* Blood pressure, a product of cardiac output and peripheral vascular resistance, is defined as the pressure exerted by the blood on the walls of the blood vessels, specifically *arterial blood pressure* (the pressure in the large arteries). Systolic pressure increases in proportion to oxygen consumption and cardiac output, while diastolic pressure shows little or no increase. Long-term aerobic training can result in reduced systolic and diastolic pressure.

> **● Key Point** The normal blood pressure response is a progressive increase in systolic blood pressure with no change or even a slight decrease in diastolic blood pressure. A failure of the systolic blood pressure to rise with an increase in intensity (called *exertional hypotension*) is considered abnormal and may occur in patients with a number of cardiovascular problems. The slight decrease in diastolic blood pressure is due primarily to the vasodilation of the arteries from the exercise bout. Thus, the expansion in artery size may lower blood pressure during the diastolic phase.[50]

- *Mitochondria:* Exercise leads to an increase in the size and number of mitochondria. Every physical action requires energy. ATP molecules are produced in the mitochondria by the process of oxidative phosphorylation. Mitochondria are found in high concentrations in the muscle cells that require more energy. Though the primary function of mitochondria is to produce energy, they also play an important role in the metabolism and synthesis of certain other substances in the body.
- *Hemoglobin concentration:* The concentration of hemoglobin in circulating blood does not change with training; it may actually decrease slightly.
- *Myoglobin:* Increased myoglobin content is another result of training. Myoglobin, an iron- and oxygen-binding protein found in the muscle tissue, is related to hemoglobin, which is the iron- and oxygen-binding protein in blood, specifically in the red blood cells.
- *Use of fat and carbohydrates:* Exercise leads to improved mobilization and use of fat and carbohydrates.
- *Lung changes:* The following lung changes occur due to exercise:
  - An increase in the volume of air that can be inspired in a single maximal ventilation. Ventilation is the process of air exchange in the lungs.
  - An increase in the diffusing capacity of the lungs.
  - Rapid rise in oxygen consumption during the first minutes of exercise. It levels off as the aerobic metabolism supplies the energy required by the working muscles.

Techniques for Improving or Maintaining Cardiorespiratory Endurance

The detraining effects of cardiorespiratory endurance occur rapidly, after only 2 weeks, when a person stops exercising. Several different training factors must be considered when attempting to maintain or improve cardiorespiratory endurance.

Continuous Training

The FITT principle refers to frequency, intensity, type, and time of exercise.

- *Frequency:* To see at least minimal improvement in cardiorespiratory endurance, it is necessary for the average person to engage in no fewer than three sessions per week. If the intensity is kept constant, there appears to be no additional benefit from twice a week versus four times or three times a week versus five times per week. If the goal is weight loss, 5 to 7 days per week increases the caloric expenditure more than 2 days per week.

- *Intensity:* Recommendations regarding training intensity (overload) vary. Relative intensity for an individual is calculated as a percentage of the maximum function, using V_{O_2} max or maximum heart rate (HR_{max}). To see minimal improvement in cardiorespiratory endurance, the average person must train with a heart rate elevated to at least 60% of its maximal rate. Three common methods of monitoring intensity are employed:
  - ❏ Monitoring heart rate. Two formulas are commonly used:
    Karvonen equation:
    - Target training HR = resting HR + (0.6 [Maximum HR – Resting HR])
    - Maximum heart rate: 220 – age
  - ❏ Rating of perceived exertion (RPE) (refer to Table 6-5). A cardiorespiratory training effect can be achieved at a rating of "somewhat hard" or "hard" (13 to 16).
  - ❏ Calculating the V_{O_2} max or HR directly or indirectly: 3-minute step test, 12-minute run, or 1-mile walk test
- *Type of exercise:* The type of activity chosen in continuous training must be aerobic, involving large muscle groups activated in a rhythmic manner.
- *Time (duration):* Duration is increased when intensity is limited—e.g., by initial fitness level. For minimal improvement to occur, the patient must participate in continuous activity with a heart rate elevated to its working level. Three to 5 minutes per day produces a training effect in poorly conditioned individuals, whereas 20 to 30 minutes, three to five times a week, is optimal for conditioned people.

Continuous training at a submaximal energy requirement can be prolonged for 20 to 60 minutes without exhausting the oxygen transport system. A number of pieces of exercise equipment can be used to improve aerobic capacity and endurance:

- *Treadmill walking:* Progressing from slow to fast and short distances to longer distances with or without an incline.
- *Ergometers:* These come in a variety of forms for both the upper extremities and the lower extremities. The pace progression is from slow to fast, and the goal is to increase the time spent exercising.
- *Free weights and elastic resistance:* The use of low resistance and high repetitions can produce an aerobic effect.

Obese individuals should exercise at longer durations and lower intensities. They should be able to exercise while maintaining a conversation (talk test).

Improving Muscle Power

It has been demonstrated that when a concentric contraction is preceded by a phase of active or passive stretching, elastic energy is stored in the muscle. This stored energy is then used in the following contractile phase. For example, during functional activities, the muscles operate with a strong concentric action, which is usually preceded by a *passive* eccentric loading, as part of a stretch-shortening cycle.[29] The stretch-shortening cycle includes the ability of the muscle to absorb or dissipate shock, while also preparing the stretched muscle for response.[51] Plyometric exercises, described next, are used to improve the ability of the muscles to perform these actions, by enhancing their power, speed, and agility. Having a muscle work dynamically against resistance within a specified period increases power. In the context of rehabilitation, plyometric training is the bridge between strength and power exercises.[52]

Plyometrics

The traditional definition of plyometrics was associated with quick, rapid movement involving a pre-stretch of the contracting muscle, which stores elastic energy in the muscle and activates the myotatic reflex.[53–56] The muscle's ability to use the stored elastic energy is affected by time, the magnitude of the stretch, and the velocity of the stretch.[57]

● **Key Point** The nerve receptors involved in plyometrics are the muscle spindle, the Golgi tendon organ, and the joint capsule/ ligamentous receptors (see Chapter 5).

Movement patterns in both athletics and activities of daily living (ADL) involve repeated stretch-shortening cycles, where a downward eccentric movement must be stopped and converted into an upward concentric movement in a desired direction. The degree of enhanced muscle performance is dependent upon the time frame between the eccentric and concentric contractions.[56]

Acceleration and deceleration are the most important components of all task-specific activities.[44]

These activities utilize variable speed and resistance throughout the range of contraction, stimulating neurological receptors, and increasing their excitability. These neurological receptors play an important role in fiber recruitment and physiologic coordination. Plyometrics serve to improve the reactivity of these receptors by involving muscle stretch-shortening exercises, which consist of three distinct phases:

- A *setting or eccentric* phase in which the muscle is eccentrically stretched and slowly loaded. This phase begins when the athlete mentally prepares for the activity and lasts until the stretch stimulus is initiated.[57]
- A rapid *amortization (reversal)* phase, which is the amount of time between undergoing the yielding eccentric contraction and the initiation of a concentric force.[57] If the amortization phase is slow, elastic energy is wasted as heat, and the stretch reflex is not activated.[57]
- A *concentric response* contraction to develop a large amount of momentum and force.

By reproducing these stretch-shortening cycles at positions of predicted performance, plyometric activities stimulate proprioceptive feedback to fine-tune muscle activity patterns. Stretch-shortening exercise trains the neuromuscular system by exposing it to increased strength loads and improving the stretch reflex.[57]

The goal of plyometric training is to minimize the amount of time required between the yielding eccentric contraction and the initiation of the overcoming concentric contraction. This is particularly useful in activities that require a maximum amount of muscular force in a minimum amount of time. These parameters are difficult to imitate using traditional exercise tools, but they are nonetheless a very important component of the rehabilitative process in order for the patient to make a safe return to sport.

As plyometrics involves ballistic, high-velocity movement patterns, before initiating plyometric exercises, the clinician must ensure that the patient has an adequate strength and physical condition base.[57] Minimal performance criteria for safe plyometrics include the ability to perform one repetition of a parallel squat with a load of body weight on the subject's back (for jumps over 12 inches) for the lower extremity, and a bench press with one-third body weight for the upper extremity.[52] In addition, success in the static stability tests[52] and dynamic stability tests (vertical jump for the lower extremities and medicine ball throw for the upper extremities) may be used as a measure of preparation.[34]

Many different activities and devices can be utilized in plyometric exercises. Plyometric exercises may include diagonal and multiplanar motions with tubing or isokinetic machines. These exercises may be used to mimic any of the needed motions and can be performed in the standing, sitting, or supine positions.

Lower-Extremity Plyometric Exercises
Lower-extremity plyometric exercises involve the manipulation of the role of gravity to vary the intensity of the exercise. Thus, plyometric exercises can be performed horizontally or vertically.

Horizontal plyometrics are performed perpendicular to the line of gravity. These exercises are preferable for most initial clinical rehabilitation plans because the concentric force is reduced and the eccentric phase is not facilitated.[34] Examples of these types of exercises include pushing a sled against resistance and a modified leg press that allows the subject to push off and land on the footplate.

Vertical plyometric exercises (against or with gravitational forces) are more advanced. These exercises require a greater level of control.[34] The drop jump is an example: the subject steps off a box, lands, and immediately executes a vertical jump.

The footwear and landing surfaces used in plyometric drills must have shock-absorbing qualities, and the protocol should allow sufficient recovery time between sets to prevent fatigue of the muscle groups being trained.[58]

Upper-Extremity Plyometric Exercises
Plyometric exercises for the upper extremity involve relatively rapid movements in planes that approximate normal joint function. For example, at the shoulder this would include 90° abduction, trunk rotation, and diagonal arm motions, and rapid external/internal rotation exercises. Plyometrics should be done for all body segments involved in the activity. Hip rotation, knee flexion/extension, and trunk rotation are power activities that require plyometric activation. Plyometric exercises for the upper extremity include wall push-offs, corner push-ups, box push-offs, the rebounder, and weighted ball throws using medicine and other weighted balls (the weight of the ball creates a pre-stretch and an eccentric load when it is caught, creating resistance and demanding a powerful agonist contraction to propel it forward again). The exercises can be performed using one arm or both arms at the same time. The former emphasizes trunk rotation, and the latter emphasizes trunk extension and flexion,

as well as shoulder motion. While force-dependent motor firing patterns should be reestablished, special care must be taken to completely integrate all of the components of the kinetic chain to generate and funnel the proper forces to the appropriate joint.

Improving Flexibility

Flexibility training must involve techniques that stretch both the contractile and inert tissues (see Chapter 4).

Methods of Stretching

Four broad categories of stretching techniques can be used to increase the extensibility of the soft tissues: static, cyclic, ballistic, and proprioceptive neuromuscular facilitation stretching.

Static Stretching

Static stretching involves the application of a steady force for a constant period at a point in the range just past tissue resistance. The duration of static stretch is based on the patient's tolerance and response during the stretching procedure. Static stretches can be applied using a manually applied force, weighted traction, specific low-load braces, or pulley systems that have been modified accordingly to provide this type of stretching (**Table 12-3**).[60]

The advantages of static stretching include the decreased chance of exceeding strain limits of the tissue being stretched, and reduced potential for muscle soreness.[62,63] Research has shown that the tension created in muscle during static stretching is approximately half that created during ballistic stretching.[64] In the early phase, effective stretching should be performed every hour, but with each session lasting only a few minutes. In healthy young and/or middle aged adults, stretch durations of 15, 30, 45, or 60 seconds or 2 minutes to lower-extremity musculature has been shown to produce significant gains in ROM.[65-69] Longer durations are recommended in older patients due to decreased extensibility in the connective tissues (minimum of 30 seconds for younger patients, and 60 seconds in older patients).[65,68] The frequency of stretching needs to occur a minimum of two times per week.[70]

TABLE 12-3	Guidelines for Applying a Low-Load, Prolonged Stretch	
Sequence	Description	Rationale
I	The involved structure is preheated using either moist heat or ultrasound.	To increase extensibility of connective tissue
II	The involved structure is placed in a gravity-assisted position of slight but not maximum stretch.	To promote relaxation
III	A moist heat application is applied for the entire course of treatment.	To increase extensibility of connective tissue To promote relaxation To increase blood flow
IV	A low-load stress/weight is applied gradually. The patient should be allowed to rest or recover for a few minutes during the course of treatment if the sensation of stretch becomes too uncomfortable.	To enhance a long-lasting change in motion
V	The low-load stress/weight is removed but the moist heat application is continued for another 5 minutes.	To increase extensibility of connective tissue To promote relaxation To increase blood flow
VI	Isometric contractions and passive stretching are performed.	To enhance strength gains at the new end of range of motion

Approximately 6 weeks of stretching are necessary to demonstrate significant increases in muscular flexibility.[62,63]

> **● Key Point** Heat should be applied to increase intramuscular temperature prior to, and during, stretching.[71,72] This heat can be achieved either through low-intensity warm-up exercise or through the use of thermal modalities.[72]

The question of whether muscle flexibility or stretching before activity results in a decrease in muscle injuries has yet to be proven.[37,73–77] In addition, there is limited scientific literature to determine the appropriate place for stretching in an exercise program. In one study, static stretching was done before, after, and both before and after each workout. All produced significant increases in range of motion.[78]

Cyclic Stretching

Intermittent cyclic stretching involves a relatively short duration stretch that is repeatedly but gradually applied, released, and then reapplied.[79] The end-range stretch force is applied at a slow velocity, at relatively low intensity, and in a controlled manner. There appears to be no consensus as to the duration of the stretch (5 to 30 seconds) or the optimal number of repetitions (typically based on patient tolerance) during a treatment session.

Ballistic Stretching

This technique uses high-velocity bouncing movements at the end range to stretch a particular muscle. The bouncing movements at the end of range are slight initially but are progressively increased over several repetitions. Due to the increased potential for injury using this technique, it is not appropriate for all patient populations.

In comparisons of the ballistic and static methods, two studies[80,81] have found that both produce similar improvements in flexibility. However, the ballistic method appears to cause more residual muscle soreness or muscle strain than those techniques that incorporate relaxation into the technique.[82–84]

Proprioceptive Muscular Facilitation Stretching

Proprioceptive muscular facilitation (PNF) stretching is one of the most effective forms of flexibility training for increasing range of motion.[85] PNF techniques (see Chapter 5) can be both passive (no associated muscular contraction) or active (performed with a voluntary muscle contraction). However, PNF stretching techniques are not appropriate in

patients with paralysis or spasticity resulting from neuromuscular diseases or injury.

> **● Key Point** The majority of studies have shown the PNF technique to be the most effective stretching technique for increasing ROM through muscle lengthening when compared with the static or slow sustained, and the ballistic or bounce techniques.[86–90]

The different techniques of PNF stretching all facilitate muscular inhibition through autogenic inhibition and are therefore more appropriate where muscle spasm limits motion and less appropriate for stretching fibrotic contractures.[85]

> **● Key Point** Note the following definitions:
> - *Reciprocal inhibition:* Reciprocal inhibition describes the process by which muscles on one side of a joint relax (are inhibited) to accommodate contraction on the other side of the joint.
> - *Autogenic inhibition:* Autogenic inhibition of a muscle is controlled by the Golgi tendon organ (see Chapter 5), the role of which is to monitor tension within a muscle. The stimulation of the Golgi tendon organ by a muscle contraction causes the inhibition or relaxation of the muscle in which it is located.[91]

Often the isometric contraction is referred to as "hold" and the concentric muscle contraction is referred to as "contract." A similar technique involves concentrically contracting the anatagonist muscle group to that being stretched in order to achieve reciprocal inhibition—a reflex muscular relaxation that occurs in the muscle that is opposite the muscle where the Golgi tendon organ is stimulated.

Postisometric Relaxation
A commonly used technique in PNF and other manual techniques is postisometric relaxation (PIR). PIR refers to the effect of the subsequent reduction in tone experienced by a muscle, or group of muscles, after brief periods during which an isometric contraction has been performed.[92] The basis for PIR is related to the theory behind contract–relax in that light, brief isometric contractions of a hypertonic muscle externally stretch the nuclear bag fibers of the muscle spindles. This stretching, in turn, allows a lengthening of muscle during the postisometric phase, without stimulating myostatic reflexes.[93] Phasic muscles that have become adaptively shortened are treated using more forceful isometric contractions.

> **● Key Point** PIR techniques are ideal as an initial technique to gain the patient's trust, especially in cases of reflex contraction or trigger point hypertonicity.[94] These techniques can also be used for joint mobilizations when a manipulation is not desirable.[95]

The most common PNF stretching techniques use a combination of "contracting," "holding," and passive stretching (often referred to as "relaxing"). There appears to be no consensus as to whether to use the relaxation of the agonist or the antagonist to gain motion.[59,96-99] Each technique, although slightly different, involves starting with a passive stretch held for about 10 seconds. A hamstring stretch can be used to illustrate the different variations. The patient is positioned in supine for each example. The patient places one leg extended, flat on the floor, and the other is extended, resting on the clinician's shoulder.

Hold–Relax

The clinician moves the patient's extended leg to a point of mild discomfort. This passive stretch (pre-stretch) is held for 10 seconds. The patient is then asked to isometrically contract the hamstrings by pushing the extended leg against the clinician's shoulder. The clinician applies just enough force so that the leg remains static. This is the "hold" phase and lasts for 6 seconds. The patient is then asked to "relax," and the clinician moves the leg into the new range and completes a second passive stretch, which is held for 30 seconds. The patient's extended leg is then moved further into the range (greater hip flexion) due to the autogenic inhibition of the hamstrings.

> ● **Key Point** The terms *contract-relax* and *hold-relax* are often used interchangeably, but they are not identical. With the contract relax technique the rotators of the limb are allowed to contract concentrically, whereas all of the muscle groups contract isometrically during the pre-stretch contraction of the restricting muscles. For the hold-relax technique, the pre-stretch contraction is isometric in all muscles of the diagonal pattern.

Contract–Relax

The clinician moves the patient's extended leg to a point of mild discomfort. This passive stretch is held for 10 seconds. The patient is then asked to concentrically contract the hamstrings by pushing the extended leg against the clinician's shoulder. The clinician applies just enough force so there is resistance while allowing the patient to push the leg to the floor (i.e., through the full range of motion). This is the "contract" phase. The patient is then instructed to "relax," and the clinician completes a second passive stretch, which is held for 30 seconds. The patient's extended leg should move further into the range (greater hip flexion) due to the autogenic inhibition of the hamstrings.

Hold–Relax with Agonist Contraction

The clinician moves the patient's extended leg to a point of mild discomfort. This passive stretch is held for 10 seconds. The patient is then asked to isometrically contract the hamstrings by pushing the extended leg against the clinician's shoulder. The clinician applies just enough force so that the leg remains static. This is the "hold" phase and lasts for 6 seconds. This initiates autogenic inhibition. The clinician completes a second passive stretch held for 30 seconds, and the patient is asked to flex the hip (i.e., move the leg in the same direction as it is being stretched). This initiates the reciprocal inhibition.

Improving Balance

Balance is a complex motor control task involving the detection and integration of sensory information to assess the position and motion of the body in space and the performance of appropriate musculoskeletal responses to control body position within the context of the environment and task.[100] Balance, or postural equilibrium, is the single most important factor dictating movement strategies, especially in the closed kinetic chain environment. Postural equilibrium involves synchronization between the neurologic system and the musculoskeletal system in order to maintain a stable weight-bearing and antigravity position for a prolonged period of time. Functional tasks require different types of balance control, including:[100]

- *Static balance:* Involves maintaining a stable antigravity position while at rest, such as when standing and sitting.
- *Dynamic balance:* The ability to stabilize the body when the support surface is moving or when the body is moving on a stable surface, such as during sit-to-stand transfers or walking.
- *Automatic postural reactions:* The ability to maintain balance in response to unexpected external perturbations, such as standing on a bus that suddenly decelerates.

To maintain balance, the body must continually adjust its position in space to keep the center of gravity (COG) of an individual over the base of support or to bring the center of gravity back to that position after perturbation. A certain amount of anteroposterior and lateral sway normally occurs while maintaining balance. For example, normal anteroposterior sway in adults is 12 degrees from the most posterior to the most anterior position.[101] If the sway exceeds the limits of stability, some strategy must be employed to regain balance. There are a number of reflex mechanisms that produce quick, relatively invariant movements to ensure that the response matches the postural challenge.

- *Ankle strategy (AP plane):* Movements of the ankle that are activated during quiet stance and during small perturbations to restore a person's COG to a stable position.
- *Weight-shift strategy (lateral plane):* Involves shifting the body weight laterally from one leg to the other.
- *Suspension strategy:* Occurs during balance tasks when a person quickly lowers the body's COG by flexing the knees, causing associated flexion of the ankles and hips.
- *Hip strategy:* Used for rapid and/or large external perturbations or for movement executed with the COG near the limits of stability.

- *Stepping strategy:* A forward or backward step that is used when a large force displaces the COG beyond the limits of stability.

● **Key Point** Since afferent input is altered after joint injury, the training must focus on the restoration of proprioceptive sensibility to retrain these altered afferent pathways and enhance the sensation of joint movement.[102]

Because balance training often involves activities that challenge the patient's limits of stability, it is important that the PTA take steps to ensure the patient's safety. This includes the use of a gait belt, performing the exercises near a railing, and closely guarding the patient. Balance training to promote static balance control involves changing the base of support of the patient while performing various tasks. The usual progression employed involves narrowing of the base of support, raising the center of gravity (COG), and changing the weight-bearing surface from hard to soft, or from flat to uneven, while increasing the perturbation. Challenges to the patient's position can be added in a variety of ways (**Table 12-4**).

TABLE 12-4 **Progressive Challenges for Balance Training**

Position (in order of increasing difficulty)	Target Muscle Groups	Activities	Progressions and Rationale
Supine/prone	Trunk (all muscles) Neck muscles	Rolling to increase segmentation (a hook-lying position is used). Reaching from side lying.	Varying speeds can be used to increase the challenge.
Quadruped	Trunk (extensor Upper extremities Proximal lower extremities	Static holding with applied challenges (e.g., alternating isometrics, rhythmic stabilization). Creeping on all fours.	Alternating isometrics applied in a variety of directions—uniplanar (anterior–posterior, medial–lateral) initially, and then three dimensionally.
Sitting	Trunk Lower extremities (hips)	Decreasing upper extremity support. Reaching activities. Static holding with applied challenges (e.g., alternating isometrics, rhythmic stabilization).	Rhythmic stabilization produces co-contractions of opposing muscle groups. Reaching activities enhance dynamic control of trunk.
Kneeling (including half-kneeling and tall-kneeling)	Trunk Lower extremities (except the foot and ankle)	Static holding with applied challenges (e.g., alternating isometrics, rhythmic stabilization).	
Standing	Trunk Lower extremities	Static standing. Gait: Bilateral support:parallel bars > walker Single-hand support: quad cane > straight cane.	Varying the base of support widths (wide to narrow).

Restoring Postural Equilibrium

When restoring postural equilibrium, it is important to follow a structured sequence:

1. Static control of trunk without extremity movement; stable base provided by proximal segments and trunk to allow functional movements:
   a. Manual perturbation to stable trunk
   b. Weight shifting while maintaining postural equilibrium
2. Dynamic control of trunk without extremity movement:
   a. Fixation of distal segments while proximal segments are moved
   b. Gradual increase of range of motion from small range to large
   c. Reverse applies to those patients who have hyperkinetic movement disorders (ataxia) where the goal is to work from large ranges to small
3. Static control of trunk with extremity movement.
4. Maintenance of trunk stability with increasingly ballistic extremity movements.
5. Exercises to increase strength, endurance, flexibility, and coordination prescribed in conjunction with equilibrium exercises:
   a. Exercises that challenge the endurance capabilities of the core muscles
   b. Progress from extremity exercises with the spine in neutral to extremity exercises with the spine in a variety of functional positions
   c. Education of the patient about how normal alignment of the spine feels in a variety of positions, and how muscles can be used to control those positions:
      i. The clinician should provide verbal, visual, tactile, and proprioceptive cues to enhance learning.
      ii. The clinician should emphasize exercises that involve maintaining functional positions to work the correct muscle groups.

Improving Joint Stabilization

Instability implies that a person has increased joint range of motion but does not have the ability to stabilize and control movement of that joint. Stabilization exercises are dynamic activities that attempt to limit and control any excessive movement. Stabilization activities include patient education, mobility exercises for stiff or hypomobile joints, strengthening exercises in the shortened range for hypermobile segments, and neuromuscular reeducation (NMR).

NMR has been defined as a method of training the enhancement of unconscious motor responses by stimulating both afferent signals and central mechanisms responsible for dynamic joint control.[103] The objective in NMR is to restore proximal stability, muscle control, and flexibility through a balance of proprioceptive retraining and strengthening. NMR attempts to improve the nervous system's ability to generate a fast and optimal muscle-firing pattern, to increase joint stability, to decrease joint forces, and to relearn movement patterns and skills.[103]

NMR is initiated with simple activities and progresses to more complex activities requiring proprioceptive and kinesthetic awareness, once the neuromuscular deficits are minimized.[104,105] It is recommended that NMR be initiated as early as possible in the rehabilitative process.[102] The goals of NMR are:

- To decrease pain and spasm by reducing the tone
- To restore mobility and control along the functional kinetic chain
- To restore force couple mechanisms to optimal efficiency
- To restore functional movements away from the base of support
- To restore functional movements against gravity

Neuromuscular control is governed by the central nervous system via the integration of information from the vestibular, vision, and somatosensory systems (refer to Chapter 5). Functional tasks require different types of balance control, including static and dynamic balance and automatic postural reactions, all of which are required to keep the center of gravity (COG) of an individual (see Chapter 4) over the base of support or to bring the center of gravity back to that position after perturbation. Weight-shifting exercises are ideal for this. For example, the following weight-shifting exercises may be used for the upper extremity:

- Standing and leaning against a treatment table or object
- In the quadruped position, rocking forward and backward with the hands on the floor or on an unstable object
- Quadruped in the three-point position (a Body Blade® can be added to this exercise to increase the difficulty)

- Kneeling in the two-point position
- Weight shifting on a Fitter® while in a kneeling position
- Weight shifting on a Swiss ball with the feet on a chair, in the push-up position
- Slide board exercises in the quadruped position moving hands forward and backward, in opposite diagonals and in opposite directions

The Swiss/Stability Ball

One of the advantages of using the stability ball is that it creates an unstable base, which challenges the postural stabilizer muscles more than using a stable base.

Ball Inflation and Sizing

It is important to choose the correct and appropriate size of ball, which is dependent upon patient size:

45 cm ball: shorter than 5'
55 cm ball: 5' to 5' 8"
65 cm ball: 5' 9" to 6'3"
75 cm ball: taller than 6'3"

With the patient sitting on the ball with both feet firmly planted on the ground, the patient's thigh should be parallel to the floor (the knee may be slightly above the hips).

- Pumping up the ball increases the level of difficulty in any given exercise.
- The further away the ball is from the support points, the greater the demand for core stability.
- Decreasing the number of support points increases the difficulty of the exercise.

Improving Coordination

Taber's Cyclopedic Medical Dictionary defines coordination as "the working together of various muscles for the production of a certain movement." Coordination involves an intricate and complex sequence of activities, which include:

- Reacting to sensory input
- Choosing and processing the proper motor program from learned skills
- Executing the action
- Predicting, evaluating, and adjusting

There are three main stages in coordination refinement:

- *Crude coordination:* Heavy reliance on visual and auditory input systems.
- *Fine coordination:* More reliance on proprioceptors and dynamic and static joint receptors.
- *Superfine coordination:* The final stage of motor learning that allows the effective execution of the desired movement under a variety of conditions.

Coordination demands vary from individual to individual—from the world-class athlete to the patient recovering from a stroke. Thus, the type and focus of the coordination training depend on the presenting condition. **Table 12-5** and **Table 12-6** give some examples of commonly employed coordination exercises for the trunk, lower extremities, and the upper extremities.

TABLE 12-5 Trunk and Lower Extremity Coordination Exercises

Task	Description	Modifications
Simple dynamic movements	The patient reaches in a variety of directions and a variety of distances to a pre-arranged target.	Increase the height of the center of gravity.
	The patient draws an imaginary circle or figure-eight pattern in the air with the upper extremity.	Increase the complexity of the dynamic movements.
Alternate heel-to-knee touching and heel-to-toe touching	From a supine position, the patient is asked to touch the knee and great toe alternately with the heel of the opposite extremity.	Change the speed of movement and/or the amount of weight.

TABLE
12-6

Coordination Exercises for the Upper Extremities

Task	Description	Modifications
Alternate nose to finger	The patient alternately touches the tip of his nose, and the tip of the clinician's finger with the index finger. The position of the clinician's finger may be altered during testing to assess the patient's ability to change distance, direction, and the force of movement.	Increase the speed of movement
Drawing a circle	The patient draws an imaginary circle or figure-eight pattern in the air with the upper extremity.	Have the patient draw smaller circles or tighter figure-eight patterns
Finger to finger	Both shoulders are abducted to 90°. With the elbows extended, the patient is asked to bring both hands to midline and approximate the index fingers from the opposing hands.	Change speed
Finger to nose	The shoulder is abducted to 90° with the elbows extended. The patient is asked to bring the tip of the index finger to the tip of the nose.	Make alterations to the starting position to test the different planes of motion Add weights to the wrist. Increase the speed of the movement
Finger opposition	The patient touches the tip of the thumb to the tip of each finger in sequence.	Change the frequency of movement Change the target
Finger to clinician's finger	The patient and clinician sit opposite each other. The clinician's index finger is held in front of the patient, and the patient is asked to touch the tip of their index finger to the tip of the clinician's index finger.	Change the frequency or speed of movement Alter the position of the index finger
Mass grasp	The patient is asked to alternatively open and close the fist.	Increase the frequency/speed
Pointing and past pointing	The clinician and the patient are positioned opposite each other (standing or sitting). Both have their shoulders at 90° of flexion, the elbows extended and the index fingers touching. The patient is asked to flex the shoulder to 180°, then return to the starting position. The patient is asked to move the arm to 0° of shoulder flexion.	Use cuff weights Increase the frequency/speed Progress from sitting to standing
Alternating movements: Pronation/supination	This test is done with the elbows flexed 90°, with the shoulders in neutral shoulder rotation. The patient is asked to supinate and pronate the forearm.	Measure the level of frequency of movement when ataxia is first observed
Alternating movements: Flexion/extension	The patient is asked to flex/extend the shoulder, elbow, or wrist.	Increase the speed of movement Add cuff weights
Tapping	The patient is positioned with the elbow flexed to 90°, the forearm pronated, and the hand resting on the knee. The patient is asked to repeatedly tap the hand against the knee.	Change the position. Increase the speed

1. What type of contraction occurs when there is tension produced in the muscle without any appreciable change in muscle length or joint movement?

2. What type of contraction occurs when a muscle slowly lengthens as it gives in to an external force that is greater than the contractile force it is exerting?

3. Of the three types of muscle actions, isometric, concentric, and eccentric, which one is capable of developing the most force?

4. What are the four biomechanical properties that human skeletal muscle possesses?

5. True or false: Rapid lengthening contractions generate less force than do slow ones (slower lengthening contractions).

6. Give two disadvantages of isometric exercise.

7. What is the best way to first exercise the postural (or extensor) musculature when it is extremely weak to facilitate muscle control?
   a. Eccentric exercises
   b. Isometric exercises
   c. Isokinetic exercises
   d. Electrical stimulation

8. What are the four parameters of exercise?

9. What is the best gauge of exercise intensity in a healthy individual?
   a. Blood pressure
   b. Heart rate
   c. Rating of perceived exertion
   d. Rate of perspiration

10. You ask a patient to assess his level of exertion using the Borg Rating of Perceived Exertion Scale (RPE). The patient rates the level of exertion as 9 on the 6–19 scale. A rating of 9 corresponds to which of the following?
    a. Very, very light
    b. Hard
    c. Very light
    d. Somewhat hard

11. The optimal exercise prescription to improve fast movement speeds and enhance endurance (improving fast-twitch fiber function) is:
    a. Low-intensity workloads for short durations
    b. High-intensity workloads for short durations
    c. Low-intensity workloads for long durations
    d. High-intensity workloads for long durations

12. You have been asked to prepare an exercise plan for a pregnant woman. The strengthening of which of the following muscles should be the focus to maintain a strong pelvic floor?
    a. Rectus abdominis, iliococcygeus, and piriformis
    b. Piriformis, obturator internus, and pubococcygeus
    c. Iliococcygeus, pubococcygeus, and coccygeus
    d. Obturator internus, piriformis, and external obliques

13. You are treating a 35-year-old with a prescription to improve aerobic conditioning. Which of the following is not a benefit of aerobic exercise?
    a. Improved cardiovascular fitness
    b. Increased high-density lipoprotein (HDL) cholesterol
    c. Improved flexibility
    d. Improved state of mind

14. You are treating a 15-year-old male soccer player who sustained a grade II inversion ankle sprain 2 weeks ago and who is now in the early subacute phase of rehabilitation. Which of the following interventions should the patient be performing?
    a. Closed-chain lower extremity strengthening, proprioceptive exercises, and an orthosis
    b. Weaning off crutches to a cane
    c. Protection, rest, ice, compression, and elevation (PRICE)
    d. Open-chain lower-extremity exercises only

15. You are treating a 73-year-old inpatient who received a cemented total hip replacement 2 days ago. Your focus should be on:
    a. Patient education regarding positions and movements to avoid
    b. Active range of motion exercises and early ambulation using a walker
    c. Passive ROM exercises
    d. Tilt table

16. You are treating a patient with a stable humeral neck fracture sustained a week ago. What would be the most appropriate exercise to begin with?
    a. Pendulum exercises
    b. Shoulder isometrics
    c. Manual PNF
    d. Modalities to control pain

17. You are treating a patient who has been referred to physical therapy to be set up on an exercise program to assist in weight loss. Which type of exercise program promotes weight loss?

18. You have decided to implement PNF exercises with a patient recovering from impingement syndrome of the shoulder. What is the best PNF diagonal pattern to improve function of the shoulder?
    a. D1 flexion
    b. D1 extension
    c. D2 flexion
    d. D2 extension

19. You are treating a patient with acute rotator cuff tendonitis and subacromial bursitis. The PT examination revealed that passive and active glenohumeral motions increased the patient's pain. Which of the following would you expect to be in the PT's POC?
    a. Modalities to reduce pain and inflammation
    b. Rotator cuff strengthening exercises
    c. Exercises to correct any muscle imbalances
    d. Shoulder isometrics

20. You have been asked to teach a class at a local gym for a group of geriatric athletes. Which of the following is not a general guideline for exercise prescription in this patient population?
    a. Use machines for strength training rather than free weights
    b. Always warm up prior to exercise
    c. "No pain, no gain"
    d. Try to incorporate both aerobic and anaerobic exercises

21. You are assisting a patient in improving anterior stability of the knee joint using exercises to strengthen muscle groups that will assist the anterior cruciate ligament. Which of the following muscle groups provides the most amount of active restraint?
    a. Gastrocnemius
    b. Hamstrings
    c. Quadriceps
    d. Hip adductors

22. You decide to use a contract-relax technique to improve a patient's active straight leg raise. Which of the following muscle groups should you emphasize the contraction of?
    a. Hip abductors and hip flexors
    b. Hamstrings and hip extensors
    c. Quadriceps and hip flexors
    d. Hip abductors and quadriceps

23. Which of the following exercises is indicated to enhance coordination?
    a. Codman exercises
    b. McKenzie exercises
    c. Frenkel exercises
    d. Williams exercises

24. You have been referred a patient with a prescription that reads *Knee strengthening and open-chain exercises only*. Which of the following is not an open-chain exercise?
    a. Knee extension
    b. Hamstring curls
    c. Squat
    d. Straight leg raise

25. A high school coach asks you which is the best type of exercise to improve an athlete's vertical jump. Which of the following exercise types would be the best to achieve this goal?
    a. Closed chain
    b. Open chain
    c. Plyometrics
    d. DeLorme's

26. You have been asked to supervise an exercise program for an obese patient who is 74 pounds overweight and is recovering from a mild myocardial infarction. The most appropriate exercise prescription for this patient is:
    a. Walking at an intensity of 50% of the patient's maximum heart rate
    b. Jogging at an intensity of 60% of the patient's maximum heart rate
    c. Swimming at an intensity of 75% of the patient's maximum heart rate
    d. No exercise with a focus on diet

27. You have been asked to supervise an exercise program for a 46-year-old individual who has limited endurance as a result of a sedentary lifestyle. There is no history of cardiorespiratory problems. An appropriate initial exercise intensity for this individual would be:
    a. 30% to 60% of the maximum heart rate
    b. 60% to 90% of the maximum heart rate
    c. 10% to 30% of the maximum heart rate
    d. 0% to 30% of the maximum heart rate

References

1. Tonkonogi M, Sahlin K: Physical exercise and mitochondrial function in human skeletal muscle. Exerc Sport Sci Rev 30:129–137, 2002
2. Sahlin K, Tonkonogi M, Soderlund K: Energy supply and muscle fatigue in humans. Acta Physiol Scand 162:261–266, 1998
3. Sahlin K, Ren JM: Relationship of contraction capacity to metabolic changes during recovery from a fatiguing contraction. J Appl Physiol 67:648–654, 1989

4. McMahon S, Jenkins D: Factors affecting the rate of phosphocreatine resynthesis following intense exercise. Sports Med 32:761–784, 2002

5. Walter G, Vandenborne K, McCully KK, et al: Noninvasive measurement of phosphocreatine recovery kinetics in single human muscles. Am J Physiol 272:C525–C534, 1997

6. Bangsbo J: Muscle oxygen uptake in humans at onset and during intense exercise. Acta Physiol Scand 168:457–464, 2000

7. Borg GAV: Psychophysical basis of perceived exertion. Med Sci Sports Exerc 14:377–381, 1992

8. Borg GAV: Perceived exertion as an indicator of somatic stress. Scand J Rehabil Med 2:92–98, 1970

9. Brooke MH, Kaiser KK: The use and abuse of muscle histochemistry. Ann N Y Acad Sci 228:121, 1974

10. Jull GA, Janda V: Muscle and Motor control in low back pain, in Twomey LT, Taylor JR (eds): Physical Therapy of the Low Back: Clinics in Physical Therapy. New York, Churchill Livingstone, 1987, pp 258

11. Hall SJ: The biomechanics of human skeletal muscle, in Hall SJ (ed): Basic Biomechanics. New York, McGraw-Hill, 1999, pp 146–185

12. Desmendt JE, Godaux E: Fast motor units are not preferentially activated in rapid voluntary contractions in man. Nature 267:717, 1977

13. Gans C: Fiber architecture and muscle function. Exerc Sport Sci Rev 10:160, 1982

14. Brown DA: Muscle: The ultimate force generator in the body, in Neumann DA (ed): Kinesiology of the musculoskeletal system: Foundations for physical rehabilitation. St. Louis, Mosby, 2002, pp 41–55

15. Kisner C, Colby LA: Resistance exercise for impaired muscle performance, in Kisner C, Colby LA (eds): Therapeutic Exercise. Foundations and Techniques (ed 5). Philadelphia, FA Davis, 2002, pp 147

16. Boeckmann RR, Ellenbecker TS: Biomechanics, in Ellenbecker TS (ed): Knee Ligament Rehabilitation. Philadelphia, Churchill Livingstone, 2000, pp 16–23

17. Brownstein B, Noyes FR, Mangine RE, et al: Anatomy and biomechanics, in Mangine RE (ed): Physical Therapy of the Knee. New York, Churchill Livingstone, 1988, pp 1–30

18. Deudsinger RH: Biomechanics in clinical practice. Phys Ther 64:1860–1868, 1984

19. Lakomy HKA: The biomechanics of human movement, in Maughan RJ (ed): Basic and Applied Sciences for Sports Medicine. Woburn, MA, Butterworth-Heinemann, 1999, pp 124–125

20. Jackson-Manfield P, Neumann DA: Structure and function of skeletal muscle, in Jackson-Manfield P, Neumann DA (eds): Essentials of Kinesiology for the Physical Therapist Assistant. St. Louis, MO, Mosby Elsevier, 2009, pp 35–49

21. McArdle W, et al: Exercise Physiology: Energy, Nutrition, and Human Performance. Philadelphia, Lea and Febiger, 1991

22. Astrand PO, Rodahl K: The Muscle and Its Contraction: Textbook of Work Physiology. New York, McGraw-Hill, 1986

23. Matsen FA III, Lippitt SB, Sidles JA, et al: Strength, in Matsen FA III, Lippitt SB, Sidles JA, et al (eds): Practical Evaluation and Management of the Shoulder. Philadelphia, W. B. Saunders, 1994, pp 111–150

24. Komi PV: Strength and Power in Sport. London, Blackwell Scientific Publications, 1992

25. Kisner C, Colby LA: Therapeutic Exercise. Foundations and Techniques. Philadelphia, F. A. Davis, 1997

26. Astrand PO, Rodahl K: Physical Training: Textbook of Work Physiology. New York, McGraw-Hill, 1986

27. DeLorme T, Watkins A: Techniques of Progressive Resistance Exercise. New York, Appleton-Century, 1951

28. Soest A, Bobbert M: The role of muscle properties in control of explosive movements. Biol Cybern 69:195–204, 1993

29. Komi PV: The stretch-shortening cycle and human power output, in Jones NL, McCartney N, McComas AJ (eds): Human Muscle Power. Champlain, IL, Human Kinetics, 1986, pp 27

30. Bandy W, Lovelace-Chandler V, Bandy B, et al: Adaptation of skeletal muscle to resistance training. J Orthop Sports Phys Ther 12:248–255, 1990

31. Connelly DM, Vandervoort AA: Effects of detraining on knee extensor strength and functional mobility in a group of elderly women. J Orthop Sports Phys Ther 26:340–346, 1997

32. Behm DG, Faigenbaum AD, Falk B, et al: Canadian Society for Exercise Physiology position paper: resistance training in children and adolescents. Appl Physiol Nutr Metab 33:547–561, 2008

33. Albert MS: Principles of exercise progression, in Greenfield B (ed): Rehabilitation of the knee: A Problem Solving Approach. Philadelphia, F. A. Davis, 1993

34. Albert M: Concepts of muscle training, in Wadsworth C (ed): Orthopaedic Physical Therapy: Topic —Strength and Conditioning Applications in Orthopaedics—Home Study Course 98A. La Crosse, WI, Orthopaedic Section, APTA, 1998

35. Clark MA: Integrated Training for the New Millenium. Thousand Oaks, CA, National Academy of Sports Medicine, 2001

36. Lange GW, Hintermeister RA, Schlegel T, et al: Electromyographic and kinematic analysis of graded treadmill walking and the implications for knee rehabilitation. J Orthop Sports Phys Ther 23:294–301, 1996

37. Worrell TW, Perrin DH, Gansneder B, et al: Comparison of isokinetic strength and flexibility measures between hamstring injured and non-injured athletes. J Orthop Sports Phys Ther 13:118–125, 1991

38. Anderson MA, Gieck JH, Perrin D, et al: The relationship among isokinetic, isotonic, and isokinetic concentric and eccentric quadriceps and hamstrings force and three components of athletic performance. J Orthop Sports Phys Ther 14:114–120, 1991

39. Steadman JR, Forster RS, Silfverskold JP: Rehabilitation of the knee. Clin Sports Med 8:605–627, 1989

40. Montgomery JB, Steadman JR: Rehabilitation of the injured knee. Clin Sports Med 4:333–343, 1985

41. Delsman PA, Losee GM: Isokinetic shear forces and their effect on the quadriceps active drawer. Med Sci Sports Exerc 16:151, 1984

42. Engle RP, Canner GC: Proprioceptive neuromuscular facilitation (PNF) and modified procedures for anterior cruciate ligament (ACL) instability. J Orthop Sports Phys Ther 11:230, 1989

43. Manske RC, Reiman MP: Muscle weakness, in Cameron MH, Monroe LG (eds): Physical Rehabilitation:

Evidence-Based Examination, Evaluation, and Intervention. St. Louis, MO, Saunders/Elsevier, 2007, pp 64–86

44. Grimsby O, Power B: Manual therapy approach to knee ligament rehabilitation, in Ellenbecker TS (ed): Knee Ligament Rehabilitation. Philadelphia, Churchill Livingstone, 2000, pp 236–251

45. American College of Sports Medicine: Guidelines for Exercise Testing and Prescription (ed 4). Philadelphia, Lea & Febiger, 1991

46. Cyriax J: Textbook of Orthopaedic Medicine, Diagnosis of Soft Tissue Lesions (ed 8). London, Bailliere Tindall, 1982

47. Hasson S, Barnes W, Hunter M, et al: Therapeutic effect of high speed voluntary muscle contractions on muscle soreness and muscle performance. J Orthop Sports Phys Ther 10:499, 1989

48. Davies GJ: Compendium of Isokinetics in Clinical Usage and Rehabilitation Techniques (ed 4). Onalaska, WI, S & S Publishers, 1992

49. Marino M: Current concepts of rehabilitation in sports medicine, in Nicholas JA, Herschman EB (eds): The lower extremity and spine in sports medicine. St. Louis, Mosby, 1986, pp 117–195

50. Grimes K: Heart disease, in O'Sullivan SB, Schmitz TJ (eds): Physical Rehabilitation (ed 5). Philadelphia, F. A. Davis, 2007, pp 589–641

51. Malone T, Nitz AJ, Kuperstein J, et al: Neuromuscular concepts, in Ellenbecker TS (ed): Knee Ligament Rehabilitation. Philadelphia, Churchill Livingstone, 2000, pp 399–411

52. Voight ML, Draovitch P, Tippett SR: Plyometrics, in Albert MS (ed): Eccentric Muscle Training in Sports and Orthopedics. New York, Churchill Livingstone, 1995

53. Assmussen E, Bonde-Peterson F: Storage of elastic energy in skeltal muscle in man. Acta Physiol Scand 91:385–392, 1974

54. Bosco C, Komi PV: Potentiation of the mechanical behavior of the human skeletal muscle through prestretching. Acta Physiol Scand 106:467–472, 1979

55. Cavagna GA, Saibene FP, Margaria R: Effect of negative work on the amount of positive work performed by an isolated muscle. J Appl Physiol 20:157, 1965

56. Cavagna GA, Disman B, Margarai R: Positive work done by a previously stretched muscle. J Appl Physiol 24:21–32, 1968

57. Wilk KE, Voight ML, Keirns MA, et al: Stretch-shortening drills for the upper extremities: theory and clinical application. J Orthop Sports Phys Ther 17:225–239, 1993

58. Wathen D: Literature review: Explosive/plyometric exercises. NSCA J 15:16–19, 1993

59. Janda V: Muscle Function Testing. London, Butterworths, 1983

60. Lentell G, Hetherington T, Eagan J, et al: The use of thermal agents to influence the effectiveness of a lowload of prolonged stretch. J Orthop Sports Phys Ther 16:200–207, 1992

61. Yoder E: Physical therapy management of nonsurgical hip problems in adults, in Echternach JL (ed): Physical Therapy of the Hip. New York, Churchill Livingstone, 1990, pp 103–137

62. Zachazewski JE: Flexibility for sports, in Sanders B (ed): Sports Physical Therapy. Norwalk, CT, Appleton and Lange, 1990, pp 201–238

63. Wallman HW: Stretching and flexibility, in Wilmarth MA (ed): Orthopaedic Physical Therapy: Topic —Strength and Conditioning—Independent Study Course 15.3. La Crosse, WI, Orthopaedic Section, APTA, 2005

64. Walker SM: Delay of twitch relaxation induced by stress and stress relaxation. J Appl Physiol 16:801–806, 1961

65. Bandy WD, Irion JM, Briggler M: The effect of time and frequency of static stretching on flexibility of the hamstring muscles. Phys Ther 77:1090–1096, 1997

66. Cipriani D, Abel B, Pirrwitz D: A comparison of two stretching protocols on hip range of motion: implications for total daily stretch duration. J Strength Cond Res 17:274–278, 2003

67. de Weijer VC, Gorniak GC, Shamus E: The effect of static stretch and warm-up exercise on hamstring length over the course of 24 hours. J Orthop Sports Phys Ther 33:727–733, 2003

68. Madding SW, Wong JG, Hallum A, et al: Effect of duration of passive stretch on hip abduction range of motion. J Orthop Sports Phys Ther 8:409–416, 1987

69. Willy RW, Kyle BA, Moore SA, et al: Effect of cessation and resumption of static hamstring muscle stretching on joint range of motion. J Orthop Sports Phys Ther 31:138–144, 2001

70. Godges JJ, MacRae H, Longdon C, et al: The effects of two stretching procedures on hip range of motion and gait economy. J Orthop Sports Phys Ther 10:350, 1989

71. Murphy P: Warming up before stretching advised. Phys Sports Med 14:45, 1986

72. Shellock F, Prentice WE: Warm-up and stretching for improved physical performance and prevention of sport-related injury. Sports Med 2:267–278, 1985

73. Worrell TW, Perrin DH: Hamstring muscle injury: The influence of strength, flexibility, warm-up, and fatigue. J Orthop Sports Phys Ther 16:12–18, 1992

74. Sutton G: Hamstrung by hamstring strains: A review of the literature. J Orthop Sports Phys Ther 5:184–195, 1984

75. Gleim GW, McHugh MP: Flexibility and its effects on sports injury and performance. Sports Med 24:289–299, 1997

76. Worrell TW: Factors associated with hamstring injuries: An approach to treatment and preventative measures. Sports Med 17:338–345, 1994

77. Jonhagen S, Nemeth G, Eriksson E: Hamstring injuries in sprinters: the role of concentric and eccentric hamstring strength and flexibility. Am J Sports Med 22:262–266, 1994

78. Cornelius WL, Hagemann RW, Jr., Jackson AW: A study on placement of stretching within a workout. J Sports Med Phys Fitness 28:234–236, 1988

79. Kisner C, Colby LA: Stretching for impaired mobility, in Kisner C, Colby LA (eds): Therapeutic Exercise. Foundations and Techniques (ed 5). Philadelphia, F. A. Davis, 2002, pp 65–108

80. DeVries HA: Evaluation of static stretching procedures for improvement of flexibility. Res Quart 33:222–229, 1962

81. Logan GA, Egstrom GH: Effects of slow and fast stretching on sacrofemoral angle. J Assoc Phys Ment Rehabil 15:85–89, 1961

82. Davies CT, White MJ: Muscle weakness following eccentric work in man. Pflugers Arch 392:168–171, 1981

83. Friden J, Sjostrom M, Ekblom B: A morphological study of delayed muscle soreness. Experientia 37:506–507, 1981

84. Hardy L: Improving active range of hip flexion. Res Q Exerc Sport 56:111–114, 1985

85. Cornelius WL, Hinson MM: The relationship between isometric contractions of hip extensors and subsequent flexibility in males. J Sports Med Phys Fitness 20:75–80, 1980

86. Markos PD: Ipsilateral and contralateral effects of proprioceptive neuromuscular facilitation techniques on hip motion and electromyographic activity. Phys Ther 59:1366, 1979

87. Holt LE, Travis TM, Okita T: Comparative study of three stretching techniques. Percep Motor Skills 31:611–616, 1970

88. Tanigawa MC: Comparison of hold-relax procedure and passive mobilization on increasing muscle length. Phys Ther 52:725–735, 1972

89. Sady SP, Wortman MA, Blanke D: Flexibility training: Ballistic, static or proprioceptive neuromuscular facilitation? Arch Phys Med Rehab 63:261–263, 1982

90. Prentice WE: A comparison of static stretching and PNF stretching for improving hip joint flexibility. Athl Train 18:56–59, 1983

91. Pollard H, Ward G: A study of two stretching techniques for improving hip flexion range of motion. J Man Physiol Ther 20:443–447, 1997

92. Chaitow L: An introduction to muscle energy techniques, in Chaitow L (ed): Muscle Energy Techniques (ed 2). London, Churchill Livingstone, 2001, pp 1–18

93. Mitchell FL, Jr.: Elements of muscle energy techniques, in Basmajian JV, Nyberg R (eds): Rational Manual Therapies. Baltimore, Williams & Wilkins, 1993, pp 285–321

94. Liebenson C: Active muscular relaxation techniques (part 1). J Manipulative Physiol Ther 12:446–451, 1989

95. Lewit K: Manipulative Therapy in Rehabilitation of the Motor System (ed 3). London, Butterworths, 1999

96. Lewit K, Simons DG: Myofascial pain: Relief by post-isometric relaxation. Arch Phys Med Rehab 65:452–456, 1984

97. Janda V: Muscles, motor regulation and back problems, in Korr IM (ed): The Neurological Mechanisms in Manipulative Therapy. New York, Plenum, 1978, p 27

98. Janda V: Muscle strength in relation to muscle length, pain and muscle imbalance, in Harms-Ringdahl K (ed): Muscle Strength. New York, Churchill Livingstone, 1993, p 83

99. Greenman PE: Principles of Manual Medicine (ed 2). Baltimore, Williams & Wilkins, 1996

100. Kloos AD, Givens-Heiss D: Exercise for impaired balance, in Kisner C, Colby LA (eds): Therapeutic Exercise. Foundations and Techniques (ed 5). Philadelphia, F. A. Davis, 2002, pp 251–272

101. Nashner LM: Sensory, neuromuscular, and biomechanical contributions to human balance., Balance: Proceedings of the American Physical Therapy Association Forum. Nashville, TN, June 13–15, 1989

102. Voight M, Blackburn T: Proprioception and balance training and testing following injury, in Ellenbecker TS (ed): Knee Ligament Rehabilitation. Philadelphia, Churchill Livingstone, 2000, pp 361–385

103. Risberg MA, Mork M, Krogstad-Jenssen H, et al: Design and implementation of a neuromuscular training program following anterior cruciate ligament reconstruction. J Orthop Sports Phys Ther 31:620 631, 2001

104. Lephart SM, Borsa PA: Functional rehabilitation of knee injuries, in Fu FH, Harner C (eds): Knee Surgery. Baltimore, MD, Williams & Wilkins, 1993

105. Lephart SM, Henry TJ: Functional rehabilitation for the upper and lower extremity. Orthop Clin North Am 26:579–592, 1995

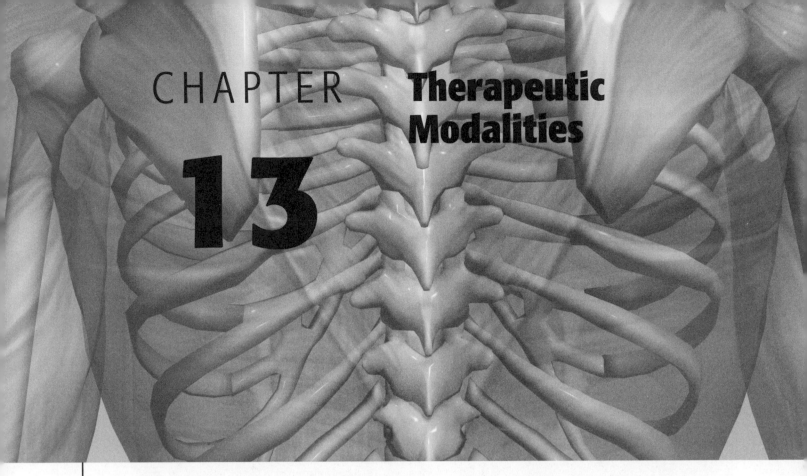

A number of modalities are used in physical therapy, the uses of which are determined by the goals of the intervention (**Table 13-1** and **Table 13-2**). The three recognized categories of modalities are physical agents, electrotherapeutic modalities, and mechanical modalities.

> ● **Key Point** According to the APTA policy statement on Direction and Supervision of the Physical Therapist Assistant, "regardless of the setting in which the service is provided, the determination to utilize physical therapist assistants for selected interventions requires the education, expertise and professional judgment of a physical therapist as described by the Standards of Practice, Guide to Professional Conduct and Code of Ethics."

If an intervention is delegated to a PTA based on the physical therapist's plan of care, the PTA must:

- Adhere to the relevant state practice acts, the practice setting, and any other regulatory agency.
- Assess and note the component of the patient's physical therapy plan that is being addressed by the use of a modality to determine whether use of the modality is still warranted.
- Ensure that any equipment to be used is correctly functioning, and calibrated, and that safety inspections of the device have been performed as per the clinic's policies and procedures.
- Adjust or modify an intervention within the established plan of care in response to data collection and patient clinical indications.
- Notify the physical therapist of any changing clinical condition that warrants a modification or termination of a particular intervention.
- Provide the patient with information about the procedure in addition to describing what the patient may feel during the application of the agent or modality.

TABLE 13-1 Electrotherapeutic and Thermal Modalities

Modality	Physiologic Responses
Cryotherapy (cold packs, ice)	Decreased blood flow (vasoconstriction) Analgesia Reduced inflammation Reduced muscle guarding/spasm
Thermotherapy (hot packs, whirlpool, paraffin wax)	Increased blood flow (vasodilation) Analgesia Reduced muscle guarding/spasm Increased metabolic activity
Ultrasound	Increased connective tissue extensibility Deep heat Increased circulation Reduced inflammation (pulsed) Reduced muscle spasm
Shortwave diathermy and microwave diathermy	Increased deep circulation Increased metabolic activity Reduced muscle guarding/spasm Reduced inflammation Facilitated wound healing Analgesia Increased tissue temperatures over a large area
Electrical stimulating currents (high voltage)	Pain modulation Muscle reeducation Muscle pumping contractions (retarded atrophy) Fracture and wound healing
Electrical stimulating currents (low voltage)	Wound healing Fracture healing
Electrical stimulating currents (interferential)	Pain modulation Muscle reeducation Muscle pumping contractions Fracture healing
Electrical stimulating currents (Russian)	Muscle strengthening
Electrical stimulating currents (microelectrical nerve stimulation [MENS])	Fracture healing Wound healing

- Perform the standard pretreatment checks (e.g., skin and sensory integrity, review of contraindications).
- Provide the patient with a call bell if he or she is to be left unattended.

● **Key Point** Temperature conversions:

Fahrenheit = (Temperature in Celsius × 9/5) + 32 *or* (Temperature in Celsius × 1.8) + 32

Celsius = (Temperature in Fahrenheit − 32) × 5/9 *or* (Temperature in Fahrenheit − 32) × 0.55

TABLE 13-2 — Clinical Decision Making on the Use of Various Therapeutic Modalities During the Various Stages of Healing

Clinical Presentation	Possible Modalities Used	Examples and Parameters (where applicable)
Acute—erythema (rubor), swelling (tumor), elevated tissue temperature (calor), and pain (dolor) Swelling subsides, warm to touch, discoloration, pain to touch, pain on motion	Cryotherapy Electrical stimulation Nonthermal ultrasound	Ice packs, ice massage, cold whirlpool (15°–20°C)
Subacute—pain to touch, pain on motion, swollen	Cryo/thermotherapy Electrical stimulation Ultrasound	Contrast baths, hot packs, paraffin wax, fluidotherapy, etc. (41°–45°C)
Chronic—no more pain to touch, decreasing pain on motion	Thermotherapy Electrical stimulation Ultrasound	

Physical Agents

Thermal modalities generally involve the transfer of thermal energy. Five types of thermal energy transfer are recognized (**Table 13-3**). Thermal agents can either increase tissue temperature or lower tissue temperature.

Cryotherapy

Traditionally, cryotherapy has been applied immediately to acute soft tissue injuries and for the first 24 to 48 hours post injury.

Indications

Cryotherapy is indicated for:

- Acute or chronic pain
- Myofascial pain syndrome
- Muscle spasm
- Bursitis
- Acute or subacute inflammation
- Musculoskeletal trauma (sprains, strains, contusions)
- Tendonitis

TABLE 13-3 — Types of Thermal Energy Transfer

Type	Description	Example
Evaporation	A change in state of a liquid to a gas with resultant cooling.	Vapocoolant sprays (Fluori-Methane)
Conduction	The transfer of heat from a warmer object to a cooler object through direct molecular interaction of objects in physical contact.	Cold pack, ice pack, ice massage, cold bath Paraffin bath
Convection	Occurs when particles (air or water) move across the body, creating a temperature variation.	Whirlpool
Radiation	The transfer of heat from a warmer source to a cooler source through a conducting medium, such as air.	Infrared lamp
Conversion	The transfer of heat when nonthermal energy (mechanical, electrical) is absorbed into tissue and transformed into heat.	Ultrasound Diathermy

Data from Bell GW, Prentice WE: Infrared modalities, in Prentice WE (ed): Therapeutic Modalities for Allied Health Professionals. New York, McGraw-Hill, 1998, pp 201–262

Contraindications

Cryotherapy is contraindicated for:

- Areas of compromised circulation
- Peripheral vascular disease
- Ischemic tissue
- Cold hypersensitivity
- Raynaud's phenomenon
- Cold urticaria
- Hypertension
- Infection
- Cryoglobulinemia

> ● **Key Point** Increased heart rate and blood pressure are associated with cold application to large areas of the body.[1] Conditioned patients should not have a problem with dizziness after cold applications, but care should be taken when transferring any patient from the whirlpool area.

Physiologic Effects

Cryotherapy causes the following physiologic effects:

- A decrease in muscle and intra-articular temperature. This decrease in muscle temperature[2] and intra-articular structures[3–5] occurs because of a decrease in local blood flow[6–10] and appears to be most marked between the temperatures of 40°C and 25°C (104°F and 77°F).[11] Temperatures below 25°C (77°F), which typically occur after 30 minutes of cooling therapy, actually result in an increase blood flow (*hunting effect*),[11] with a consequent detrimental increase in hemorrhage and an exaggerated acute inflammatory response.[12]
- Local analgesia.[9,10,13–17] The stages of analgesia achieved by cryotherapy are outlined in the next section.[18] It is worth remembering that the timing of the stages depends on the depth of penetration and varying thickness of adipose tissue.[19]
- Decreased muscle spasm.[13,20–23]
- Decrease in swelling.[13,24,25]
- Decrease in nerve conduction velocity.[26]

Application

Before the first application, the PTA performs an assessment of skin and sensory integrity, including temperature, and observes for any lesions in the area compared with findings during the initial evaluation. After the first 5 minutes of treatment the PTA visually observes the patient's skin for any adverse effects (e.g., urticaria, facial flush, anaphylaxis [medical emergency]). The normal response for a cold application, which typically lasts from 10 to 20 minutes, involves an overlapping sequence of cold, burning, aching, and numbness (CBAN). The stages of analgesia associated with cryotherapy are as follows:

- Cold sensation (0–3 minutes)
- Burning or aching (2–7 minutes)
- Local numbness or analgesia (5–12 minutes)
- Deep tissue vasodilation without increase in metabolism (12–15 minutes)

The patient should be advised as to these various stages, especially in light of the fact that the burning or aching phase occurs before the therapeutic phases. The patient is given a call bell and instructed to alert the clinician if there are any sensory changes.

Commercial Cold Packs

Commercial cold packs typically contain silica gel and are available in a variety of shapes and sizes. A cold pack requires a temperature of 23°F (−5°C). A towel is dampened with warm water and the excessive water wrung out. The cold pack is taken out of the refrigeration unit, wrapped in the moistened towel, and placed securely on the patient with elastic bandages or towels. One to three dry towels are placed over the cold pack to retard warming. The treatment time is typically 10 to 20 minutes. Cold packs must not maintain uniform contact with the body, so the PTA must observe the skin every 10 minutes. The patient should be kept warm throughout the treatment.

Ice Packs

An ice pack consists of crushed ice folded in a moist towel or placed in a plastic bag covered by a moist towel. The method of application, patient preparation, and treatment time is the same as for the cold packs.

> ● **Key Point** The various methods of applying cryotherapy (ice chips in toweling, cold gel packs, and ice bags) have been examined in different studies. The use of ice chips in toweling has been shown to be more effective in decreasing skin temperature than ice chips in plastic bags or cold gel packs.[5,27]

Ice Massage

Ice massage is recommended for small and contoured areas, allows for observation, and is inexpensive. Ice massage is typically performed by freezing water in a paper cup that can be torn away to expose the ice block, which is applied directly to the area in small, circular motions for 10 to 15 minutes before and after activity, up to six times a day. Ice massage has been shown to reduce tissue temperature faster than using a cold pack (17.9 minutes on average versus 28.2 minutes).[28]

Cryokinetics

Cryokinetics is a rehabilitation technique that involves the application of ice followed by progressive active exercises used for the treatment of strains and sprains.[9] The technique involves an initial application of cold for 20 minutes followed by a 3-minute bout of active exercise involving the injured area. This is followed by a 5-minute application of cold. The whole sequence of 3-minute exercise and 5-minute cold applications is repeated four times.

Cryostretching

Cryostretching is a rehabilitation technique that has been advocated to increase flexibility during healing.[9] The technique involves a 20-minute cold application followed by alternating periods of progressive passive stretching with isometric contractions and renumbing for a total of three cycles.

Cold Bath

A cold bath, using a basin or whirlpool, is commonly used for the immersion of the distal extremities. The temperature for a cold whirlpool used for acute conditions is in the range of 55°F to 64°F (13°C to 18°C).[1] Typically, the body part is immersed for 5 to 15 minutes, depending on the desired therapeutic effect.

Vapocoolant Spray

Vapocoolant sprays (Spray and Stretch, which has replaced the non-ozone-layer-friendly Fluori-Methane) are often used in conjunction with passive stretching and in the treatment of muscle spasms, trigger points, and myofascial referred pain.[29] The depth of cooling is superficial with this modality. Physiologically, the relief is accomplished through the theoretical gate control method of pain control (see Chapter 5).[29] Once the area to be treated has been identified, the clinician makes two to five sweeps with the spray in the direction of the muscle fibers, keeping the spray 12 to 18 inches from the skin. The sweeps are applied from the proximal to the distal aspect of the muscle attachments. Stretching should begin while applying the spray and continued after the spray is applied, using steady tension. The spray should be moved at approximately 4 inches per second across the skin, spraying the skin at an acute angle (approximately 30°) rather than at a perpendicular angle.[29] The liquid is allowed to evaporate completely before applying the next sweep. The entire treatment area should be covered using the spray, starting at the pain site and moving to the area of referred pain.[29] The length of treatment varies according to body segment. It is important to remember that vapocoolant sprays are dangerous if inhaled, they are inflammable, and they should not be used near the eyes and face or on large areas of damaged skin, puncture wounds, or other wounds.

Thermotherapy

Thermotherapy is the therapeutic application of heat. Thermal modalities generally involve the transfer of thermal energy (refer to Table 13-3). Thermotherapy is used in the later stages of healing, because the deep heating of structures during the acute inflammatory stage may destroy collagen fibers and accelerate the inflammatory process.[30] However, in the later stages of healing, an increase in blood flow to the injured area is beneficial.

Indications

Thermotherapy is indicated for:

- Pain control
- Chronic inflammatory conditions
- Trigger points
- Tissue healing
- Muscle spasm
- Decreased range of motion
- Desensitization

Contraindications

Thermotherapy is contraindicated for:

- Circulatory impairment
- Areas of malignancy; heat can increase the metabolic activity of a tumor and thereby increase the rate of growth[31]
- Acute musculoskeletal trauma
- Bleeding or hemorrhage, including hemophilia
- Sensory impairment; it is important to assess the patient's sensitivity to temperature, pain, and circulation status prior to the use of thermotherapy (see Chapter 3)
- Thrombophlebitis
- Arterial disease
- Pregnancy; the application of heat is contraindicated over the abdominal, pelvic, or low back regions of pregnant women due to the potential risk to the development and growth of the fetus[31]

● **Key Point** Application of a superficial hot pack over an area with significant subcutaneous fat results in decreased heating of deeper structures.

Physiologic Effects

The physiologic effects of a local heat application include:[7,32–35]

- Dissipation of body heat. This effect occurs through selective vasodilation and shunting of blood via reflexes in the microcirculation, and regional blood flow.[36]
- Decreased muscle spasm.[12,16,36,37] The muscle relaxation probably results from a decrease in neural excitability on the sensory nerves, and hence gamma input.
- Increased capillary permeability, cell metabolism, and cellular activity, which have the potential to increase the delivery of oxygen and chemical nutrients to the area while decreasing venous stagnation.[33,38]
- Increased analgesia through hyperstimulation of the cutaneous nerve receptors.
- Increased tissue extensibility.[36] This effect has obvious implications for the application of stretching techniques. The best results are obtained if heat is applied during the stretch, and if the stretch is maintained until cooling occurs after the heat has been removed.

> **● Key Point** For a heat application to have a therapeutic effect, the amount of thermal energy transferred to the tissue must be sufficient to stimulate normal function, without causing damage to the tissue.[39]

Although the human body functions optimally between 36°C and 38°C (98.6° and 100.4°F), an applied temperature of 40°C and 45°C (104°F and 113°F) is considered effective for a heat intervention.

> **● Key Point** Wet heat produces a greater rise in local tissue temperature compared with dry heat at a similar temperature.[40] However, at higher temperatures, wet heat is not tolerated as well as dry heat.

Superficial Heating Agents

The area to be treated should be positioned in such a way as to be easily observed, and to prevent a dependent position of the area, or any areas of the body distal to the treatment site. All clothing and jewelry should be removed from the treatment area. Before the first application, the PTA performs an assessment of skin and sensory integrity, including temperature, and observes for any lesions in the area compared with findings during the initial evaluation. If any are found, the PT should be notified.

> **● Key Point** Prior to the application of heat, the area to be treated should be assessed for protective sensation to avoid burning the patient.

The modality should be positioned correctly and the patient monitored during the application. The patient is given a call bell and instructed to alert the clinician if there are any sensory changes.

Heating Packs

Heating packs are made of a hydrophilic silicate gel encased in a canvas or nylon cover, which is immersed in a thermostatically controlled water unit (hydrocollator) that is typically 158°F to 167°F (70°C to 75°C). The hot packs are made in various sizes and shapes designed to fit different body areas. The moist heat pack causes an increase in the local tissue temperature, reaching its highest point about 8 minutes after the application.[41] The depth of penetration for traditional heating pads (and cold packs) is about 1 to 2 centimeters. These heating pads lead to changes in the cutaneous blood vessels and the cutaneous nerve receptors.[5] Before applying the hot pack, layers of terry cloth toweling (approximately six to eight, depending on the length of treatment and patient comfort) are placed between the skin and the hot pack. Having the patient lie on the pack is not recommended because this position may increase heat transfer beyond therapeutic levels and increase the risk of burn. The skin should be inspected every 5 minutes, and the patient should be provided with a call device to notify the clinician of any discomfort.

> **● Key Point** The skin normally looks pink or red with the application of heat. A dark red or mottled (a red area with white areas) appearance indicates that too much heat has been applied and that the treatment should cease. In such cases, a cold wet towel should be applied to the area and the supervising PT should be notified immediately.

Treatment times vary from 15 to 20 minutes, depending on the goal established by the evaluating PT. It is important that in every clinic some form of daily monitoring system for the water levels and temperature of the hot pack storage units is in place.

> **● Key Point** A daily temperature log for hot pack units is now required by The Joint Commission (TJC).

Paraffin Bath

Liquid paraffin, heated in a thermostatically controlled paraffin bath unit, is used to provide superficial heat to the hands and feet. Paraffin baths are a commonly used modality for stiff or painful joints and arthritis of the hands and feet, due to the ability of the wax to conform to irregularly contoured areas. It is, however, contraindicated when there is evidence of an allergic rash, open wounds, recent scars and sutures, or a skin infection. In addition, the contraindications of paraffin are essentially the same as for hot packs.

> ● **Key Point** Parraffin treatments provide six times the amount of heat available in water because the mineral oil in the paraffin lowers the melting point of the paraffin.[1] This provides the paraffin with a lower specific heat* than water, allowing for a slower exchange of heat to the skin.
>
> *Specific heat is the amount of heat per unit mass required to raise the temperature by 1°C. The specific heat of water is 1 calorie/gram °C = 4.186 joule/gram °C, which is approximately four times higher than air. Paraffin has a specific heat capacity of 2.14 to 2.9 joule/gram °C.

For clinical use, the wax used is a mixture of paraffin wax and mineral oil (approximately 2 lbs. wax/1 gallon of oil). Paraffin melts rapidly at 118°F to 130°F (48°C to 54°C) and self-sterilizes at 175°F to 200°F (79°C to 93°C).[42,43] The typical paraffin bath unit maintains a temperature of 113°F to 126°F (45°C to 52°C). The patient is asked to remove all jewelry (if jewelry cannot be removed, it is covered with several layers of gauze) and to wash and dry the area to be treated. The clinician inspects the area for infection and open areas. Due to the nature of the paraffin treatment, the treated area cannot easily be accessed for observation, so the PTA must periodically check the status of the patient and, if the patient is to be left unattended, he or she must be provided with a call bell. Three different procedures are commonly utilized:

- *Dip-wrap (glove) method:* When dipping into the paraffin, the first layer of wax should be the highest on the body segment and each successive layer lower than the previous one. This is to prevent subsequent layers from getting between the first layer and the skin and burning the patient.[1] With the fingers/toes apart, the patient is asked to dip the involved part (hand or foot) in the wax bath as far as possible and tolerable, while avoiding touching the sides or bottom of the wax bath to prevent burns. After a few seconds, the patient is asked to remove the hand/foot without moving the fingers/toes

to avoid cracks forming in the wax. The layer of paraffin hardens (becomes opaque). The patient repeats the process five more times. After the paraffin has solidified, the part is then wrapped in a plastic bag, wax paper, or treatment table paper and then in a towel or insulating glove to conserve the heat, thereby slowing down the rate of cooling of the paraffin. The involved extremity is elevated and the paraffin remains on for 15 to 20 minutes, until it cools, after which the clinician peels off the paraffin.

- *Paint:* As its name implies, for this method a brush is used to paint the treatment area with six to 10 layers of paraffin. The area is then covered, and the wax remains on for approximately 20 minutes.

- *Dip and immersion:* This method is similar to the dip-wrap method, except that patient's extremity remains comfortably in the bath after the final dip. Extra caution must be taken with this method compared with the other two due to the potential for greater heat exchange to occur.

Fluidotherapy

Fluidotherapy involves use of a container that circulates warm air (111°F to 125°F/44°C to 52°C) and small cellulose particles at varying degrees of agitation based on patient comfort. The extremity to be treated is placed into the container, and the dry heat is generated through the energy transferred by forced convection for a period of 20 minutes. Unlike a heating pack and paraffin bath, fluidotherapy allows for active movement during treatment and a constant treatment temperature. However, the treatment setup may require the extremity to be placed in a dependent position.

Infrared Lamp

The infrared lamp produces superficial heating of tissue through radiant heat with a depth of penetration of less than 1 to 3 millimeters. The patient is positioned approximately 20 inches from the source, and a moist towel is placed over the treatment area. The standard parameter for treatment indicates 20 inches in distance should equal 20 minutes of treatment. If the distance decreases, the intensity will increase, and the time of total treatment should decrease. The advantages of infrared are that direct contact with the skin is not required and that the area being treated can be easily observed. However, due to the limited depth of penetration, the dehydrating effects on wounds, and the risk of burns during treatment, the use of infrared is declining.

Deep Heating Agents

Ultrasound

Ultrasound can be used to deliver heat to either superficial or deep musculoskeletal tissues, such as tendon, muscle, and joint structures. The effects of ultrasound are chemical and thermal. The ultrasonic waves are delivered through the transducer, which has a metal faceplate with a piezoelectric crystal cemented between two electrodes. This crystal can vibrate very rapidly, converting electrical energy to acoustical energy. This energy leaves the transducer in a straight line.

Indications

Ultrasound is indicated for:

- Soft tissue repair
- Contracture
- Bone fracture healing
- Trigger point
- Dermal ulcer
- Scar tissue
- Pain
- Muscle spasm
- Plantar wart

Contraindications

Ultrasound is contraindicated in these instances:

- Over pregnant uterus
- Over cemented prosthetic joint
- Over cardiac pacemakers
- Over vital areas such as the brain, ear, eyes, heart, cervical ganglia, carotid sinuses, reproductive organs, or spinal cord[44]
- Over epiphyseal areas in children
- Over malignancy
- With impaired circulation
- With thrombophlebitis
- With impaired pain or temperature sensory deficits
- With infection

Physiologic Effects

As the energy travels further from the transducer, the waves begin to diverge. The depth of penetration depends on the absorption and scattering of the beam.

> **● Key Point** The specific effects and depth of penetration when using ultrasound are affected by the ultrasound wavelength or frequency (1 MHz or 3 MHz), the intensity (W/m²), contact quality of the transducer, treatment surface, and tissue type (e.g., muscle, skin, fat).[45,46] Scar tissue, tendon, and ligament demonstrate the highest absorption. Tissues that demonstrate poor absorption include bone, tendinous and aponeurotic attachments of skeletal muscle, cartilaginous covering of joint surfaces, and peripheral nerves lying close to bone.[47]

The portion of the sound head that produces the sound wave is referred to as the effective radiating area (ERA). The ERA, which is always smaller than the transducer, can be found on all transducers, allowing the PTA to determine appropriate treatment time.

Frequency

The depth of penetration of the ultrasound is roughly inversely related to its frequency.[48,49] A frequency of 3 megahertz (MHz) is more superficial, reaching a depth of approximately 2 centimeters, whereas 1 MHz is effective to a depth of 4 or 5 centimeters.[50]

Duty Cycle

A duty cycle refers to the percentage of time (the "on" time divided by the "on" time plus the "off" time multiplied by 100) that the ultrasound energy is being transmitted with a pulsed waveform to achieve the proposed associated nonthermal effects. Duty cycles less than 100% are usually termed *pulsed ultrasound*, whereas a 100% duty cycle is referred to as *continuous ultrasound*. Continuous mode ultrasound produces a thermal effect. Pulsed ultrasound with duty cycles of less than 20% have no thermal effect, whereas duty cycles above 20% have a thermal effect.

Acoustic Cavitation

Acoustic cavitation occurs as a result of the acoustic energy generated by ultrasound that develops into microscopic bubbles causing cavities that surround soft tissues. Two types of cavitation can occur:

- *Stable:* The microscopic bubbles increase and decrease in size but do not burst. Stable cavitation produces micro streaming, which is the minute flow of fluid that takes place around the vapor-filled bubbles that oscillate and pulsate.
- *Transient (unstable):* The microscopic bubbles increase in size over multiple cycles and implode, causing brief moments of local temperature and pressure increases in the area surrounding the bubbles. However, this process should not occur during therapeutic ultrasound as the intensities required are much higher than 3 W/cm².

The Beam Nonuniformity Ratio

The beam nonuniformity ratio (BNR) of ultrasound is the maximal/average intensity (W/cm²) found in the ultrasound field. BNR value should range between 2:1 and 6:1 (most devices often fall in the 5:1 or 6:1 range). The BNR of a particular unit is required to be listed on the device for consumer education and awareness. Each transducer produces sound waves in response to the vibration of the crystal. This vibration has different intensities at points on the transducer head, having peaks and valleys of intensity. The higher the quality of the transducer, the lower the BNR. The greater ratio difference in the BNR, the more likely the transducer will have *hot spots*. Hot spots are areas of high intensity and increase the likelihood of patient discomfort. High intensities have been shown to cause unstable cavitational effects and to retard tissue repair.[51,52]

Application

A pretreatment and posttreatment assessment of skin and sensory integrity should be completed and any unexpected changes be reported to the supervising PT. Ultrasound can be applied directly or indirectly:[44]

- Direct contact (transducer-skin interface): Used on relatively flat areas.
  - The clinician applies generous amounts of coupling medium (gel/cream) to the treatment area. If a hot spot is encountered, the PTA should apply more coupling agent or decrease the intensity.
  - The clinician selects an appropriate sound head size (ERA should be one-half the size of the treatment area).
  - Placing the sound head at right angles to the skin surface and using relatively light pressure (approximately 1 pound, or 450 grams), the clinician maintains the intensity at the desired level while moving the sound head slowly (approximately 1.75 inches/second, or 4 centimeters/second) in overlapping circles or longitudinal strokes and maintaining the sound head–body surface angle. Periosteal pain occurring during treatment may be due to any of the following: high intensity, momentary slowing, or cessation of the moving head.
  - The area covered should not be greater than two to three times the size of the ERA for 5 minutes of treatment. Areas larger than the aforementioned will require a separate application of ultrasound or another form of heat.
  - Intensity of continuous ultrasound is normally set between .5 to 2 W/cm^2 for thermal effects. Pulsed ultrasound for nonthermal effects is normally sent between 0.5 and 0.75 W/cm^2 with a 20% duty cycle.

  - The treatment time varies depending on the target tissue (muscle, tendon, and other soft tissues), the size of the area, intensity, condition, and frequency.
- *Indirect contact (water immersion):* The application of ultrasound over irregularly shaped body parts.
  - The clinician fills a container with water high enough to cover the treatment area. Ideally, a plastic container should be used because it reflects less acoustic energy than a metal one.
  - The body part to be treated is immersed in the water.
  - The sound head is placed in the water, keeping it 1/2 to 1 inch from the skin surface and at right angles to the body part being treated.
  - The clinician moves the sound head slowly, as in the direct contact method, while turning up the intensity to the desired level. If a stationary technique is being applied, the clinician should reduce the intensity or use pulsed ultrasound.
- *Indirect contact (fluid-filled bag):* An alternative technique to the immersion technique, but not commonly used. In this method, an ultrasound gel pad, a thin-walled bag such as a balloon, or a surgical glove is needed.
  - The bag is placed around the side of the sound head, squeezing out fluid until all the air is removed and the sound head is immersed in water.
  - The clinician applies a coupling agent on the skin and then places the bag over the treatment area.
  - While maintaining the sound head within the bag and increasing the intensity to the desired level, the clinician moves the head slowly while keeping a right angle between the sound head and the treatment area. The bag should not slide on the skin.

Phonophoresis

The indications and contraindications for phonophoresis are the same as for ultrasound, except the clinician needs to be aware of potential allergic reactions to the medications used.

Physiologic Effects

Phonophoresis refers to a specific type of ultrasound application in which pharmacologic agents, such as corticosteroids, local anesthetics, and salicylates, are introduced.[53–60] Phonophoresis has been used clinically since the early 1960s in attempts to drive these drugs transdermally into subcutaneous tissues. Both the thermal and nonthermal (mechanical) properties of ultrasound have been cited as possible mechanisms for the transdermal penetration of the pharmacologic agents. Increases in cell permeability and local vasodilation accompanied by the acoustic pressure wave may result in increased diffusion of the topical agent.[54,55,60]

> ● **Key Point** Recent papers have argued that many of the commonly used cream-based preparations do not allow adequate transmission of the acoustic wave.[45,46,61] Gel-based preparations appear to be superior with respect to the transmissivity of ultrasound. Consequently, gel-based corticosteroid compounds might be expected to be superior for phonophoresis applications.

Application

A pretreatment and posttreatment assessment of skin and sensory integrity should be completed and any unexpected changes be reported to the supervising PT. It is important that the PTA understands the specific indications and desired effects of the pharmacologic agents being used and that the patient status is monitored to determine the effectiveness of the treatment after every session.

Diathermy

Diathermy, which includes both shortwave (SW) and microwave (MW), is a thermal agent that produces therapeutic effects through conversion.

Indications

Diathermy is indicated:

- For wound care
- To decrease pain and edema
- To increase oxygen to the tissue through vasodilation
- To increase temperature
- To increase metabolic rate
- To decrease nerve conduction latency
- To increase collagen extensibility
- To increase muscle, bone, and nerve tissue repair by stimulation of protein synthesis at the cell membrane level
- To treat chronic inflammation

Contraindications

Diathermy is contraindicated in these instances:

- For patients with implanted deep brain stimulators
- For patients with internal or external metal implants

- For patients with cardiac pacemakers
- In the presence of malignancy
- During pregnancy
- Over the eyes, epiphysis of growing bone, or testes
- For patients with acute inflammation

Physiologic Effects

As with ultrasound, diathermy offers both thermal and nonthermal effects through the application of continuous or pulsed modes.

Application

The patient needs to be monitored often during treatment because the treated area is not visible. Any conductive material must be removed. This includes jewelry, clothes with zippers, synthetic fabrics, electronic devices, and metal-containing or magnetic equipment. A pretreatment and posttreatment assessment of skin and sensory integrity should be completed and any unexpected changes reported to the supervising PT.

> ● **Key Point** To avoid any potential exposure to hazardous levels of electromagnetic energy, the operator of the diathermy unit must stand behind the unit console.

- *Shortwave:* Applicators include inductive coil applicators or capacitive plates. SW delivers a thermal or pulsed electromagnetic field. The most common SW frequency used is 27.12 MHz. In the electrical circuit method, the area to be treated is placed between two conducting electrodes for 15 to 30 minutes. In the inductive field method, the treated area is placed into a magnetic field formed by electrodes, and the current is induced within the patient's body tissues, with the tissue resistance to the current producing an increase in temperature of the deep body tissues. Inductive coil applicators utilize a coil that generates alternating electric current, creates a magnetic field perpendicular to the coil, and produces eddy currents within the tissues. As the eddy currents cause an oscillation of ions, tissue temperature is increased.
- *Microwave:* Is applied using electromagnetic radiation directed through a coaxial cable to an antenna mounted in the treatment applicator. Treatment time is typically 15 to 30 minutes. Caution must be used when energy is reflected at fat/muscle and muscle/bone interfaces because it can increase superficial tissue temperatures (skin or fat).

Hydrotherapy

Physical Properties of Water

Water has several physical properties:

- *Buoyancy:* The upward force of buoyancy somewhat counteracts the effects of gravity. According to the Archimedes principle, any object submerged or floating in water is buoyed upward by a counterforce that helps support the submerged or partially submerged object against the downward pull of gravity, resulting in an apparent loss of weight. The center of buoyancy is the reference point of an immersed object on which the buoyant (vertical) forces of a fluid predictably act. In the vertical position, the human center of buoyancy is located at the sternum. Buoyancy can provide the patient with relative weightlessness and joint unloading, allowing performance of active motion and increased ease.[62] In addition, buoyancy allows the clinician three-dimensional access to the patient.
- *Hydrostatic pressure:* The pressure exerted on immersed objects. The pressure exerted by fluid on an immersed object is equal on all surfaces of the object (Pascal's law). Therefore, as the density of water and depth of immersion increase, so does hydrostatic pressure. From a clinical perspective, the proportionality of depth allows patients to perform exercise more easily when closer to the surface. It is important to remember that hydrostatic pressure can result in a number of cardiovascular shifts, including decreased peripheral blood flow and vital capacity, increased heart volume, increased stroke volume, and increased cardiac output, as well as a corresponding decrease or no change in the heart rate.
- *Viscosity:* Friction that occurs between molecules of liquid resulting in resistance to flow. From a clinical perspective, increasing the velocity of movement increases the resistance.

In addition, increasing the surface area while moving through the water increases the resistance.

- *Specific gravity:* Any object with a specific gravity less than that of water will float. The buoyant values of different body parts vary according to two factors:
  - Bone to muscle weight.
  - Amount and distribution of fat.
- *Specific heat:* The amount of heat per unit mass required to raise the temperature by 1°C. The specific heat of water is higher than that of any other common substance, and as a result, water plays a very important role in temperature regulation.
  - Water can store four times the heat as compared with air.
  - Water's thermal conductivity is approximately 25 times faster than air at the same temperature.
- *Surface tension:* Formed by the water molecules loosely binding together, whereby the attraction of surface molecules is parallel to the surface. From a clinical perspective, an extremity that moves through the surface performs more work than if it is kept under the water.
- *Drag force:* A factor of the shape of an object and its speed of movement. Objects that are more streamlined (thus minimizing the surface area at the front of the object) produce less drag force.

Physiologic Effects

Water has varying physiologic effects depending on its temperature. Various temperatures can be used depending on the desired goal:

- Very hot (104°F/40°C): Used for short exposures of 7 to 10 minutes to increase superficial temperature.
- Hot (99°F to 104°F/37°C to 40°C): Used to increase superficial temperature.
- Warm (96°F to 99°F/35.5°C to 37°C): Used to increase superficial temperature where a prolonged exposure is wanted, such as to decrease spasticity of a muscle in conjunction with passive exercise.
- Neutral (92°F to 96°F/33.5°C to 35.5°C): Used with patients that have an unstable core body temperature.
- Tepid (80°F to 92°F/27°C to 33.5°C): May be used in conduction with less vigorous exercise.

- Cool (67°F to 80°F/19°C to 27°C): May be used in conduction with vigorous exercise.
- Cold (55°F to 67°F/13°C to 19°C): Used for longer exposures of 10 to 15 minutes to decrease superficial temperature.
- Very cold (32°F to 55°F/0°C to 13°C): Used for short exposures of 1 to 5 minutes to decrease superficial temperature.

Whirlpool

Whirlpool therapies involve partial or total immersion of a body or body part in an immersion bath, in which the water is agitated and mixed with air so that it can be directed against, or around, the involved part. Whirlpool tanks come in various sizes:

- High boy (for upper extremities)
- Low boy (for lower extremities)
- Hubbard tank (for full body immersion)

A turbine, consisting of a motor secured to the side, pumps a combination of air and water throughout the tank. The water/air jet can be directed in the desired direction and height to increase stimulation, help control pain, or clean an area.[1] If the area is hypersensitive, the pressure can be directed away from it.

> **● Key Point** A *ground fault interrupter* (GFI) is a safety device that constantly compares the amount of electricity flowing from the wall outlet to the clinical unit with the amount returning to the outlet. If there is any leakage in the current flow detected, the GFI unit automatically shuts off current flow to reduce the chances of electrical shock. A GFI should be installed at the circuit breaker at the receptacle of all whirlpools and Hubbard tanks, and the unit should be checked periodically for leakage.

Application

The tank is filled to the desired level and appropriate temperature. Whirlpool liners may be used for patients with burns, wounds, or who are infected with blood-borne pathogens. If an antimicrobial is to be used, it should be added to the water during this time according to the following dilutions:

- Sodium hypochlorite (bleach): 200 parts per million (ppm)
- Povidone-iodine: 4 ppm
- Chloramine-T: 100 to 200 ppm

The patient is asked to uncover the treatment area adequately (as appropriate, any wound dressing is removed), and the skin is tested for thermal sensitivity. The checking of vital signs prior to and during immersion may also be appropriate based on

patient history. Patient comfort is ensured by avoiding pressure of the limb on the edge of the whirlpool (which may also compromise circulation); any pressure points should be padded. Once the patient is comfortable, the turbine direction is adjusted and then turned on. The force, direction, and depth of the jet/agitator are adjusted appropriately. During the treatment, the body part may be exercised. The patient should be accompanied throughout the treatment session and the vital signs monitored as appropriate. Whirlpool treatments can provide a sedative effect, and depending on the temperature of the water, they can cause fluctuations in blood pressure.[63]

Once the treatment is completed, the patient is asked to remove the body part from the water, and the area is dried and inspected. If appropriate, a clean dressing is applied. The whirlpool is drained, cleaned, and rinsed. Cleaning procedures vary according to clinical setting. In general, the inside of the tank, the outside of the agitator, the thermometer, and the drains are washed with disinfectant diluted in water. The disinfectant is allowed to stand for at least 1 minute. The agitator is placed in a bucket filled with water and disinfectant so that all openings are covered with the solution. The agitator is turned on for about 20 to 30 seconds, after which the motor is turned off and the agitator is removed from the bucket. The entire tank and all the equipment are then rinsed until the entire residue is removed. The tank is then drained.

Contrast Bath

Contrast baths use an alternating cycle (10 minutes warmth; 1 minute cold; 4 minutes cold) of warm (96°F to 99°F/35.5°C to 37°C) and cold (55°F to 67°F/13°C to 19°C) whirlpools that create a cycle of alternating vasoconstriction and vasodilation over a period of 30 minutes. Contrast baths are used most often in the management of extremity injuries to reduce swelling around injuries or to aid recovery from exercise.[64,65] The technique provides good contact over irregularly shaped areas, allows for movement during treatment, and assists with pain management. Disadvantages include potential intolerance to cold and dependent positioning. Contraindications for this modality include those for both thermotherapy and cryotherapy.

Aquatic Therapy

In the past decade, widespread interest has developed in aquatic therapy as a tool for rehabilitation. Among the psychological benefits, water motivates movement, because painful joints and muscles can be moved more easily and painlessly in water.

Indications
The indications for aquatic therapy include:

- Instances when partial weight-bearing ambulation is necessary
- To increase range of motion
- To improve standing balance
- To improve endurance/aerobic capacity
- To increase muscle strength via active-assisted, gravity-assisted, active, or resisted exercise[66]

The exact proportion and quantity of both land and water activity are determined by the needs and response of the patient.

Contraindications
Contraindications to aquatic therapy include:[66]

- Incontinence
- Urinary tract infections
- Unprotected open wounds/menstruation
- Autonomic dysreflexia
- Heat intolerance
- Severe epilepsy/uncontrolled seizures
- Uncontrolled diabetes
- Unstable blood pressure
- Severe cardiac and/or pulmonary dysfunction

Once any contraindications have been ruled out, the patient's water safety skills and swimming ability should be evaluated, as well as his or her general level of comfort in the water. The following strategies/techniques can be used:[67]

- *Position and direction of movement:* A three-part progression moving from buoyancy-assisted exercises, to buoyancy-supported exercises, and finally to buoyancy-resisted exercises. As with gravity, patient position and direction of movement can greatly alter the amount of assistance or resistance.
  - *Buoyancy-assisted exercises:* Involve movements toward the surface of the water and are similar to gravity-assisted exercises on land. For example, in the standing position, shoulder abduction and flexion, as well as the ascent phase of the squat, are considered buoyancy-assisted exercises. In the prone position, hip extension can be buoyancy assisted.
  - *Buoyancy-supported exercises:* Involve movements that are parallel to the bottom of the pool and are similar to gravity-minimized positions on land. For example, in the standing position, horizontal shoulder abduction/adduction is an example of such activity, as are hip and shoulder abduction in the supine position.
  - *Buoyancy-resisted exercises:* Involve movements toward the bottom of the pool. For example, in the supine position, shoulder and hip extension and the descent phase of the squat are considered buoyancy-resisted activities.
- *Depth of water:* Less support is provided by buoyancy in shallow water than in deeper water. In addition, modifications can be made by adding buoyant equipment or resisted equipment. A study by Harrison and Bulstrode[68] measured static weight bearing in a pool using a population of healthy adults.[69] Results indicated that weight bearing during immersion was reduced to less than land-based weight.
  - Immersion to C7 levels reduced weight to 5.9% to 10% of normal weight.
  - Immersion to the xiphosternum reduced weight to 25% to 37% of normal.
  - Immersion to the level of the anterior superior iliac spine (ASIS) reduced weight to 40% to 56% of normal.

  A follow-up study by Harrison and colleagues[70] compared weight bearing during immersed standing and slow and fast walking.[69] During slow walking, subjects had to be immersed to the ASIS before weight bearing was reduced to 75% of normal. Immersion to the clavicle during slow walking reduced weight bearing up to 50% of normal values, and immersion above the clavicle resulted in weight bearing 25% of normal or less. During fast walking, mid-trunk immersion produced weight bearing up to 75% of actual weight. Subjects had to be immersed deeper than the xiphosternum in order for weight bearing to be less than 50% and deeper than C7 for weight bearing to be less than 25% of normal values.
- *Lever arm length:* As with land-based exercises, the lever arm length can be adjusted to change the amount of assistance or resistance. For example, performing buoyancy-assisted shoulder flexion in a standing position is easier with the elbow straight (i.e., long lever) than with the elbow flexed (i.e., short lever). Conversely, buoyancy-resisted shoulder abduction is more

difficult with the elbow extended because of the long lever arm.

- *Buoyant equipment:* To further increase the amount of assistance (support for individuals in certain positions) or resistance, buoyant equipment can be added to the lever arm. As the buoyancy of the equipment increases, the resistance also increases. Equipment designed to assist with patient positioning can be applied to the neck, extremities, or trunk.

- *Viscosity:* The viscous quality of water allows it to be used effectively as a resistive medium. When moving through the water, the body experiences a frontal resistance proportional to the presenting surface area. This resistance can be increased by enlarging the surface area or by increasing the velocity of movement.

- *Water temperature:* Variable temperature control for the water should be available and the ambient air temperature should be 3°C higher than the water temperature for patient comfort. The body's ability to regulate temperature during immersion exercise differs from that during land exercise. Water conducts temperature 25 times faster than air, and water retains heat 1000 times more than air. With immersion there is less skin exposed to air, resulting in less opportunity to dissipate heat through normal sweating mechanisms. The following water temperatures are recommended based on activity:
  - ❑ 26°C to 33°C (78.8°F to 91.4°F) for aquatic exercises, including flexibility, strengthening, gait training, and relaxation. Therapeutic exercise performed in warm water (33°C/91.4°F) may be beneficial for patients with painful musculoskeletal areas.
  - ❑ 26°C to 28°C (78.8°F to 82.4°F) for cardiovascular training and aerobic exercise (active swimming).
  - ❑ 22°C to 26°C (71.6°F to 78.8°F) for intense and aerobic training.

It is important that the patient enters the water slowly so that all systems have an opportunity to gradually accommodate to the environment.

A variety of aquatic therapy techniques exist (**Table 13-4**). A sample program follows for a patient with low back pain: In waist-deep water at the side of the pool, the patient is asked to sit in an imaginary chair so that the back is against the pool wall, the thighs are parallel to the bottom of the pool, and the knees are aligned over the ankles. The back remains against the pool wall throughout the exercise. Arms are at the sides with palms facing backward, and shoulders are relaxed. The head faces straight ahead. The patient is asked to begin pumping the arms forward and back about 6 inches while inhaling for five counts and exhaling for five counts.

Design and Special Equipment

Certain characteristics of the pool should be taken into consideration if it is to be used for rehabilitation purposes:

- The pool should not be smaller than 3.04 m by 3.66 m (10 by 12 ft.).
- The pool should have both a shallow (1.25 m/2.5 ft.) and a deep (2.5 m/5 ft.-plus) area to allow for standing exercises and swimming or nonstanding exercise.
- The pool bottom should be flat and the depth gradations clearly marked.
- Rescue tubes, inner tubes, and wet vests should be purchased to assist in flotation activities. Aqua shoes will help prevent slipping on the bottom of the pool.
- Hand paddles, webbed gloves, and pull-buoys can be used for strengthening the upper extremities.
- Buoyant dumbbells (swim bars), which are available in short and long lengths, can be used for supporting the upper body or trunk in the upright position, and the lower extremities in the supine or prone positions.
- Kick boards, boots, and fins are useful for strengthening the lower extremities.

Advantages

The advantages of aquatic therapy include:

- The buoyancy of the water allows active exercise while providing a sense of security and causing little discomfort. Early in the rehabilitation process, aquatic therapy is useful in restoring range of motion and flexibility using a combination of the water's buoyancy, resistance, and warmth.
- The buoyancy provides support.
- The slow-motion effect of moving in water provides extra time to control movement and to react.
- The water provides tactile stimulation and feedback.
- Water exercise allows a gradual transition from non–weight-bearing to full weight-bearing exercises by adjusting the amount the body is submerged.

TABLE 13-4	Aquatic Specialty Techniques

Specialty Technique	Description
Ai Chi	A form of active aquatic therapy or fitness modeled after the principles of T'ai Chi and yogic breathing techniques. Ai Chi is typically provided in a hands-off manner (the clinician stands on the pool side to allow visual imaging of complex patterns by the patient). The patient stands in chest-deep water and is verbally and visually instructed by the clinician to perform a slow, rhythmic combination of therapeutic movements and deep breathing.
Aquatic proprioceptive neuromuscular facilitation (PNF)	A form of active aquatic therapy modeled after the principles and movement patterns of PNF. Aquatic PNF can be provided in either a hands-on or hands-off manner by the clinician. The patient is verbally, visually and/or tactilely instructed in a series of functional, spiral, and diagonal mass movement patterns while standing, sitting, kneeling, or lying in the water. The patterns may be performed actively or with assistance or resistance provided by specialized aquatic equipment or the clinician.
Bad Ragaz Ring Method	A form of active or passive aquatic therapy modeled after the principles and movement patterns of Knupfer exercises and PNF. Bad Ragaz is always performed in a hands-on manner by the clinician. The patient is verbally, visually, and/or tactilely instructed in a series of movement or relaxation patterns while positioned horizontally and supported by rings or floats in the water. The patterns may be performed passively (for flexibility and relaxation), actively, or with assistance or resistance provided by a clinician.
Fluid Moves® (Aquatic Feldenkrais®)	A form of active or passive aquatic therapy modeled after the Feldenkrais Method. Fluid Moves may be provided in either a hands-on or hands-off manner by the clinician. During active Fluid Moves the student, in a guided exploratory process, follows a sequence of movements based on the early developmental stages of the infant. The patient stands in chest-deep water, typically with his or her back to the pool wall, and is verbally and visually instructed by the clinician to perform a slow, rhythmic combination of therapeutic movements and deep breathing. The passive, hands-on component to Fluid Moves is modeled after the "Functional Integration" component of the Feldenkrais Method.
Halliwick Method	A form of adapted aquatics that can be modified into active aquatic therapy. Halliwick is almost always performed in a hands-on manner by the clinician and is typically done through the use of games within groups of patient-clinician pairs. The patient is usually held or cradled in the water while the clinician systematically and progressively destabilizes him or her in order to teach balance and postural control. The clinician progresses the patient through a series of activities that require more sophisticated rotational control in an attempt to teach the patient to swim (for adapted aquatics patients) or in an attempt to teach control over movement (for aquatic therapy patients). The patient is continuously required to react to, and eventually to predict, the demands of an unstable environment. The Halliwick Method combines the unique qualities of the water with rotational control patterns.
Swim Stroke Training and Modification	A form of active aquatic therapy that makes use of swim stroke training and modification with the intent to rehabilitate, not to teach swimming skills or to promote swim stroke efficiency. Swim Stroke Training and Modification may be provided in either a hands-on or hands-off manner by the clinician. The patient is positioned horizontally and is verbally, visually, and/or tactilely instructed in order to modify and execute various swim strokes.
Task-Type Training Approach	A set of principles that guide clinicians as they design treatment programs for reducing patients' disabilities. Task Type Training Approach (TTTA) was first described as a way to teach functional activities to patients who had sustained a stroke. The principles can be extended to include treatment of all patient disorders, particularly those involving neurologic dysfunction. The TTTA is best described as a task-oriented approach because it emphasizes functional skills performed in functional positions. Patients are encouraged to be active participants in their skill development, an important characteristic of task-oriented rehabilitation.
Watsu®	A form of passive aquatic therapy modeled after the principles of Zen Shiatsu (massage). Watsu is always performed in a hands-on manner by the clinician. The patient is usually held or cradled in warm water while the clinician stabilizes or moves one segment of the body, resulting in a stretch of another segment due to the drag effect. The patient remains completely passive while the clinician combines the unique qualities of the water with rhythmic flow patterns.

- The intensity of exercise can be controlled by manipulating the body's position or through the addition of exercise equipment.

Disadvantages

The disadvantages of aquatic therapy include:

- Costs of building and maintenance.
- Need for training and staffing appropriately.
- Difficulty treating patients with an inherent fear of water.
- Inability to treat patients that have open wounds, fever, urinary tract infections, allergies to the pool chemicals, cardiac problems, uncontrolled seizures, contagious skin diseases, or sores.
- Difficulty reproducing lower-extremity eccentric muscle contractions.

Electrotherapeutic Modalities

Indications

Electrotherapeutic modalities are used:

- To provide pain relief.
- To assist with wound care. The clinician should always use universal precautions when treating a patient with an open wound or lesion, and wear gloves, waterproof gown, goggles, and a mask, particularly when working with the possibility of splashing.
- To assist with burn care.
- To facilitate the resorption of effusion (edema control).
- To improve range of motion.
- To improve sprain/strain healing.
- The traditional uses of electrical stimulation are listed in **Table 13-5**.

Precautions

Use electrotherapy modalities cautiously in these instances:

- In cases of allergies to tapes and gels.
- In areas of absent or diminished sensation.
- In electrically sensitive patients.
- In placing an electrode over an area of significant adipose tissue, near the stellate ganglion, over the temporal and orbital region, or over damaged skin.

Contraindications

Electrotherapy modalities have the following contraindications:

- Decreased temperature sensation
- Impaired cognition

TABLE 13-5	Traditional Uses of Electrical Stimulation				
Use	Method	Frequency (Hz)	Pulses per Second	Time (minutes)
Pain relief	• High-frequency stimulation (80–120 Hz) and short duration should be used to stimulate the smallest unmyelinated nerve (C and delta) fibers in order to reduce pain (gate control theory). • Low-frequency (longer duration) stimulation, which stimulates the larger myelinated (alpha) fibers, should be used when producing muscle contractions is the goal. • Ultra-low frequencies can lead to increased endorphin production through initiation of the descending inhibition mechanisms (opiate pain control theory).	>100 (TENS, hi-volt galvanic stimulation [HVGS], and interferential current [IFC])	70–100	20–60
Reduction of edema	Electrical stimulation: • Produces a muscle pump action that increases the lymph and venous flow toward the heart. • Increases ion flow by attracting specific ions to a desired direction, as edema is believed to be slightly negatively charged (DC or high-volt).	100–150 (HVGS, IFC)	120 (negative polarity)	20

| TABLE 13-5 | Traditional Uses of Electrical Stimulation (continued) | | | |

Use	Method	Frequency (Hz)	Pulses per Second	Time (minutes)
Wound healing	• Healing is effected through modification of the local inflammatory response (+ polarity produces an increase in inflammation), increasing circulation (− polarity). • Pulsed currents (monophasic, biphasic, or polyphasic) with interrupted modulations can increase circulation and thus hasten metabolic waste disposal. • Electrical stimulation leads to restoration of electrical cell charges through the use of monophasic currents (low-volt continuous modulations and high-volt pulsed currents). It may also have a bactericidal effect (cathode) by producing disruption of DNA or RNA synthesis or the cell transport system of microorganisms. • Low-intensity continuous (non-pulsed and low-volt) direct current and high-volt pulsed current can be applied for wound healing (by use of ionic effects).	>100 or 1	Varies but typically 70–100	20
Muscle reeducation	Electrical stimulation is used to bring motor nerves and muscle fibers closer to the threshold for depolarization. Muscles are reeducated to respond appropriately using volitional effort by: • Providing proprioceptive feedback. • Assisting with active exercise to help produce a contraction (active-assisted). • Assisting in the coordination of muscle movement. Current intensity must be adequate for muscle contraction, and pulse duration should be set as close as possible to the duration needed for chronaxie of the tissue to be stimulated. The pulses per second (pps) should be high enough to give a titanic contraction (20–40 pps).	50–60	1–20	Fatigue (1–15)

Data from Riker DK: Assessment: Efficacy of transcutaneous electric nerve stimulation in the treatment of pain in neurologic disorders (an evidence-based review): Utility of transcutaneous electrical nerve stimulation in neurologic pain disorders. Neurology 74:1748–1749, 2010; Cheng JS, Yang YR, Cheng SJ, et al: Effects of combining electric stimulation with active ankle dorsiflexion while standing on a rocker board: A pilot study for subjects with spastic foot after stroke. Arch Phys Med Rehabil 91:505–512, 2010; Dubinsky RM, Miyasaki J: Assessment: Efficacy of transcutaneous electric nerve stimulation in the treatment of pain in neurologic disorders (an evidence-based review): Report of the Therapeutics and Technology Assessment Subcommittee of the American Academy of Neurology. Neurology 74:173–176, 2010; Meade CS, Lukas SE, McDonald LJ, et al: A randomized trial of transcutaneous electric acupoint stimulation as adjunctive treatment for opioid detoxification. J Subst Abuse Treat 38:12–21, 2010; Chan MK, Tong RK, Chung KY: Bilateral upper limb training with functional electric stimulation in patients with chronic stroke. Neurorehabil Neural Repair 23:357–365, 2009; and Kumaravel S, Sundaram S: Fracture healing by electric stimulation: Biomed 2009. Biomed Sci Instrum 45:191–196, 2009

- Recent skin graft
- Incontinence
- Confusion/disorientation
- Deconditioned state
- Bleeding

- Wound maceration
- Cardiac instability
- Profound epilepsy

The key points to remember when using electrical modalities are listed in **Table 13-6.**

TABLE 13-6	Key Points to Remember When Using Electrotherapeutic Modalities

The introduction of electricity to a patient can bring about one or more physiological changes.

The physical condition of the patient must be considered before introducing an electrical current.

The effect of the electrical current is produced in the electrically active tissue, such as muscles and nerves.

An energy delivered at a specific amplitude has a beneficial effect whilst the same energy at a lower amplitude may have no demonstrable effect.

Electrical current changes muscle fiber recruitment—type II muscle fibers are affected at lower density levels than type I muscle fibers.

The current is sensed more by the skin, due to the local resistance and ion concentrations in the local areas around the electrodes.

Data from Dutton M: McGraw-Hill's NPTE (National Physical Therapy Examination). New York: McGraw-Hill, 2009

Terminology

Note the following terminology associated with electrical modalities:

- *Electricity* is the force created by an imbalance in the number of electrons at two points:
  - *Negative pole:* An area of high electron concentration (cathode)
  - *Positive pole:* An area of low electron concentration (anode)
- *Charge:* An imbalance in energy. The charge of a solution has significance when attempting to "drive" medicinal drugs topically via iontophoresis and in attempting to artificially "fire" a denervated muscle. Cell membranes rest at a "resting potential," which is an electrical balance of charges. This balance must be disrupted to achieve muscle firing. Muscle depolarization is difficult to achieve with physical therapy modalities, whereas nerve depolarization occurs very easily with PT modalities.
- *Coulomb's law:* Like charges repel, unlike charges attract.
- *Watt:* A measure of electrical power (watts = volts × amperes)
- *Volt:* The electromotive force that must be applied to produce a movement of electrons; a measure of electrical power. Two modality classifications include high volt (greater than 100–150 V) and low volt (less than 100–150 V).
- *Amp:* A measure of electrical charge/current. Electrons move along a conducting medium as an electrical current. *Amplitude* refers to the magnitude of current and is associated with the depth of penetration; the deeper the penetration, the more muscle fiber recruitment is possible.

- *Resistance:* The opposition to flow of current. Factors affecting resistance include material composition (see "Physiologic Effects"), length (greater length yields greater resistance), and temperature (increased temperature leads to increased resistance). Preheating the treatment area may increase patient comfort, but it also increases resistance and the need for higher output intensities. To minimize resistance, the PTA can:
  - Reduce the skin-electrode resistance
  - Minimize the air-electrode interface
  - Keep the electrode and skin clean of oils
  - Use the shortest pathway for energy flow
  - Use the largest electrode that will selectively stimulate the target tissues

> **● Key Point** Ohm's law expresses the relationship between current flow (I), voltage (V), and resistance (R)—(I = V/R). The current flow is directly proportional to the voltage and inversely proportional to the resistance. Therefore:
> - When resistance decreases, current increases.
> - When resistance increases, current decreases; more voltage will be needed to get the same current flow.
> - When voltage increases, current increases.
> - When voltage decreases, current decreases.
> - When voltage is 0, current is 0.

- *Pulse duration (also known as the pulse width):* The length of time the electrical flow is "on." It represents the time for one cycle to occur (both phases in a biphasic current). Phase duration is an important factor in determining which tissue is stimulated; if the duration is too short, there will be no action potential.
- *Accommodation:* The increased threshold of excitable tissue when a slowly rising stimulus is

used. Both nerve and muscle tissues are capable of accommodating to an electrical stimulus, with nerve tissue accommodating more rapidly than muscle tissue. The quicker the rise time, the less the nerve can accommodate to the impulse.

- *Pulse rise time:* The time to peak intensity of the pulse (ramp):
  - ❑ Ramping is used to reduce the shock of the current.
  - ❑ Rapidly rising pulses cause nerve depolarization.
  - ❑ Slow-rising pulses allow the nerve to accommodate to the stimulus, and an action potential is not elicited. Use of slow-rising pulses is good for muscle reeducation when used with assisted contraction.
- *Pulse frequency (Hz):* Represents the number of pulses that occur in a unit of time:
  - ❑ *Low frequency:* 1K Hz and below (MENS 1 to 1K Hz)
  - ❑ *Medium frequency:* 1K to 100K Hz (interferential, Russian stimulation LVGS)
  - ❑ *High frequency:* Above 100K Hz (TENS, HVGS, diathermies)
- *Strength duration curve:* A graphic representation of the relationship between the intensity of an electric stimulus at the motor point of a muscle and the length of time it must flow to elicit a minimal contraction.
- *Rheobase:* Minimum intensity of an electrical stimulus that will elicit a minimal contraction.
- *Chronaxie:* The minimum time over which an electric current double the strength of the rheobase needs to be applied.

> ● **Key Point** Two mnemonic hints can be used to help differentiate between rheobase and chronaxie:
>
> 1. The root word *rheo* means "current" and *base* means "foundation": thus the rheobase is the foundation, or minimum, current (stimulus strength) that will produce a response.
> 2. The root word *chron* means "time" and *axie* means "axis:" chronaxie, then, is measured along the time axis and, thus, is a duration that gives a response when the nerve is stimulated at twice the rheobase strength.

- *Duty cycles:* On-off time. May also be called *interpulse interval*, which is the time between pulses:
  - ❑ A 1:1 ratio fatigues muscle rapidly.
  - ❑ A 1:5 ratio produces less fatigue.
  - ❑ A 1:7 ratio produces no fatigue (passive muscle exercise).

- *Current density:* The amount of charge per unit area; this is usually relative to the size of the electrode. Density will be greater with a small electrode, but the small electrode offers more resistance.

> ● **Key Point** Law of DuBois Reymond:
> - The amplitude of the individual stimulus must be high enough so that depolarization of the membrane will occur.
> - The rate of change of voltage must be sufficiently rapid so that accommodation does not occur.
> - The duration of the individual stimulus must be long enough so that the time course of the latent period (capacitance), action potential, and recovery can take place.

- *Fasciculation:* Involuntary motor unit firing. The clinician may see skin move, but no joint motion.
- *Fibrillation:* Involuntary firing of a single muscle fiber; indicative of denervation.
- *Frequency:* Represents the number of cycles or pulses per second (rate of oscillation). Frequency is normally described in Hertz (Hz) units.

Physiologic Effects

Electrical current that passes through tissue forces nerves to depolarize. Electrotherapeutic devices generate three different types of current: alternating (AC) or biphasic, direct (DC) or monophasic, or pulsed or polyphasic.

- *Alternating current (biphasic):* The energy travels in both a positive and negative direction. The wave form that occurs will be replicated on both sides of the isoelectric line. Alternating current is used in muscle retraining, spasticity, and stimulation of denervated muscle.
- *Direct current (DC):* Unidirectional current, sometimes called *galvanic*. The energy travels only in the positive or only in the negative direction. Direct current produces polar effects. It is important to remember that intact skin cannot tolerate a current density greater than $1mA/cm^2$.[71] Iontophoresis uses direct current.

Electrotherapeutic devices generate three different types of current:

- *Monophasic or direct (galvanic):* A unidirectional flow of electrons toward the positive pole.
- *Biphasic or alternating:* A flow of electrons that constantly changes direction or, stated differently, reverses its polarity.

- *Pulsed:* Usually contains three or more pulses grouped together, which are interrupted for short periods of time and repeat themselves at regular intervals; can be monophasic or biphasic.

Electrical current tends to choose the path of the least resistance to flow. Electricity has an effect on each cell and tissue that it passes through. The type and extent of the response are dependent on the type of tissue and its response characteristics. Typically, tissue that is highest in water content and consequently highest in ion content is the best conductor of electricity.

Good conductors within the body include:

- *Blood:* Blood is composed largely of water and ions and is consequently the best electrical conductor of all tissues.
- *Muscle:* Muscle is composed of about 75% water and is therefore a relatively good conductor.
- *Nerves:* The type of nerve and the rate at which the fiber is depolarized will determine the physiologic and, therefore, therapeutic effect achieved.[72,73] Nerves with larger diameters are depolarized before nerves with smaller diameters.

> ● **Key Point** No definitive studies have been done to support the use of electrical muscle stimulation to prevent muscle degeneration. If the nerve does not regenerate in time to reinnervate the muscle, there is no need to stimulate the muscle. With reinnervated muscle, it is theoretically possible to use alternating current stimulation. However, it is necessary to have a large number of reinnervated muscle fibers to stimulate the muscle with alternating current.

Poor conductors include:

- *Skin:* Offers the primary resistance to current flow; considered an insulator. The greater the impedance (resistance to current) of the skin, the higher the voltage of the electrical current required to stimulate underlying nerve and muscle.
- *Tendons:* Denser than muscle and contain relatively little water; poor conductors.
- *Fat:* Only about 14% water; poor conductor.
- *Bone:* Extremely dense, contains only about 5% water; the poorest biological conductor.

As electricity moves through the body, changes in physiologic functioning occur at the various levels of the system:

- Cellular level:
  - Excitation of nerve cells
  - Changes in cell membrane permeability

- Protein synthesis (with DC)
- Stimulation of fibroblasts, osteoblasts (with DC)
- Modification of microcirculation
- Tissue level:
  - Skeletal muscle contraction
  - Smooth muscle contraction
  - Tissue regeneration
- Muscle and joint level:
  - Modification of joint mobility
  - Muscle-pumping action to change circulation and lymphatic activity
  - An alteration of the microvascular system not associated with muscle pumping
  - An increased movement of charged proteins into the lymphatic channels with subsequent oncotic force bringing increases in fluid to the lymph system
  - Transcutaneous electrical stimulation cannot directly stimulate lymph, smooth muscle, or the autonomic nervous system without also stimulating a motor nerve
- Systematic:
  - Analgesic effects as endogenous pain suppressors are released and act at different levels to control pain
  - Analgesic effects from the stimulation of certain neurotransmitters control neural activity in the presence of pain stimuli.

> ● **Key Point** The limited studies on postsurgical or acutely injured patients seem to indicate that electrical muscle stimulation is either as effective as, or more effective than, isometric exercises at increasing muscle strength and bulk,[74–78] in both atrophied[79] and normal muscles.[80,81]

According to Taylor and colleagues,[82] the present regimens being used (i.e., one intervention per day or three times per week) may be insufficiently aggressive to provide benefit.

Electrodes and Their Placement

Electrodes are used in the therapeutic application of current:

- At least two electrodes are required to complete the circuit.
- The patient's body becomes the conductor.
- The strongest stimulation is where the current exits the body.
- Electrodes placed close together will give a superficial stimulation and be of high density.
- Electrodes spaced far apart will penetrate more deeply with less current density (interferential).

TABLE 13-7	Safety Considerations When Using Electrical Devices

The two-pronged plug has only two leads, both of which carry some voltage; consequently, the electrical device has no true ground (connected to the earth) and relies instead on the chassis or casing of the power source to act as a ground. This increases the potential for electrical shock.

The third prong of a three-pronged plug is designed to be grounded directly to the earth. However, never assume that all three-pronged wall outlets are automatically grounded. Although three-pronged plugs generally work well in dry environments, they may not provide sufficient protection from electrical shock in a wet or damp area. In such instances, it is mandated that any equipment used in a wet or damp environment should be fitted with a ground fault interrupter (GFI).

Equipment should be visually inspected before each use to check for frayed cords or other potential hazards.

The entire electrical system of the clinic should be designed or routinely evaluated by a qualified electrician.

Equipment should be reevaluated on an annual basis and any defective equipment should be removal from service immediately.

Plugs should not be jerked out of the wall by pulling on the cable.

Extension cords or multiple adapters should never be used.

- When stimulating a muscle, electrode orientation should be placed parallel to the muscle fibers along the line of pull of the muscle group.
- Generally, the larger the electrode, the less current density. If a large "dispersive" pad is creating muscle contractions, there may be areas of high current concentration and other areas that are relatively inactive, thus functionally reducing the total size of the electrode.
  - *Large electrodes:* Provide decreased current density, decreased impedance, and increased current flow.
  - *Small electrodes:* Provide increased current density, increased impedance, and decreased current flow.

Electrodes may be placed on or around the painful area. The configuration of the electrodes depends on the intent of the intervention:

- *Monopolar:* Requires one negative electrode and one positive electrode. The stimulating or active electrode is placed over the target area (e.g., motor point). A second dispersive electrode is placed at another site away from the target area. This technique is used with wounds, iontophoresis, and in the treatment of edema.
- *Bipolar:* Two active electrodes of equal size are placed over the target area. This technique is used for muscle weakness, neuromuscular facilitation, and spasms, as well as to increase range of motion.

- *Quadripolar:* Two electrodes from two separate stimulating circuits are positioned so that the individual currents intersect with each other.

Electrical Equipment Care and Maintenance

Electrical safety in the clinical setting should be of maximal concern to the clinician. The typical electrical circuit consists of a source producing electric power, a conductor that carries the power to a resistor or series of given elements, and a conductor that carries the power back to the power source. Safety considerations when using electrical equipment include those listed in **Table 13-7**.

Transdermal Iontophoresis

Indications

Transdermal iontophoresis has the following indications:

- To decrease inflammation
- To decrease pain
- To decrease calcium deposits
- To facilitate wound healing
- To decrease edema

Contraindications

Transdermal iontophoresis has the following contraindications:

- Cardiac pacemakers or other electrically sensitive implanted devices
- Known sensitivity to the drugs to be administered

- Known adverse reactions to the application of electrical current
- Damaged skin or recent scar tissue
- Across the temporal regions or for the treatment of the orbital region

Physiologic Effects

Transdermal iontophoresis is the application (by physical therapy) of selected ionic therapeutic agents through the skin utilizing a low-level electrical current. The principle behind iontophoresis is that an electrical potential difference will actively cause ions in solution to migrate according to their electrical charge; negatively charged ions are repelled from a negative electrode and attracted toward the positive electrode. In contrast, the positive ions are repelled from the positive electrode and attracted toward the negative electrode.[83,84] Ionized medications or chemicals do not ordinarily penetrate tissues, and if they do, it is not normally at a rate rapid enough to achieve therapeutic levels.[83] This problem is solved by providing a direct current energy source that provides penetration and transport.[83,84] Iontophoresis has proved to be valuable in the intervention of musculoskeletal disorders because it causes an increased penetration of drugs and other compounds into tissues by the use of an applied current. Iontophoresis has, therefore, been used for the transdermal delivery of systemic drugs in a controlled fashion.[85] The factors affecting transdermal iontophoretic transport include pH; intensity of the current, or current density, at the active electrode; ionic strength; concentration of drug; molecular size; and duration of the current flow (continuous or pulse current). The proposed mechanisms by which iontophoresis increases drug penetration are as follows:

- The electrical potential gradient induces changes in the arrangement of the lipid, protein, and water molecules.[86]
- Pore formation occurs in the stratum corneum (SC), the outermost layer of the skin.[87] The exact pathway by which ionized drugs transit the SC has not been elucidated. The impermeability of the stratum corneum is the main barrier to cutaneous or transcutaneous drug delivery. If the integrity of the SC is disrupted, the barrier to molecular transit may be greatly reduced.
- Hair follicles, sweat glands, and sweat ducts act as diffusion shunts with reduced resistance for ion transport.[88] Skin and fat are poor conductors of electrical current and offer greater resistance to current flow.

TABLE 13-8	Various Ions Used in Iontophoresis	
Ion	Polarity	Purpose/Condition
Acetate	–	Calcium deposits
Atropine sulfate	+	Hyperhidrosis
Calcium	+	Myopathy, muscle spasm
Chlorine	–	Scar tissue, adhesions
Copper	+	Fungus infection
Dexamethasone	+	Tendonitis, bursitis
Lidocaine	+	Trigeminal neuralgia
Hyaluronidase	+	Edema
Iodine	–	Adhesions, scar tissue
Magnesium	+	Muscle relaxant, bursitis
Mecholyl	+	Muscle relaxant
Potassium iodide	–	Scar tissue
Salicylate	–	Myalgia, scar tissue
Tap water	+/–	Hyperhidrosis

+, positive; –, negative.

Data from Chen UW, Banga AK: Iontophorestic (transdermal) delivery of drugs: Overview of historical development. J Pharm Sciences 78:353–354, 1989

Iontophoresis can be performed using a wide variety of chemicals (**Table 13-8**). For a chemical to be successful in iontophoresis, it must solubilize into ionic components.

Following the basic law of physics that *like poles repel*, the positively charged ions are placed under the positive electrode, while the negatively charged ions are placed under the negative electrode. If the ionic source is in an aqueous solution, it is recommended that a low concentration be used (2% to 4%) to aid in the dissociation.[89] Although electrons flow from negative to positive, regardless of electrode size, having a larger negative pad than a positive one will help shape the direction of flow.

Current intensity is recommended to be at 5 mA or less for all interventions. The duration of the treatment may vary from 15 to 20 minutes. Longer durations have been shown to produce a decrease in the skin impedance, thus increasing the likelihood of burns from an accumulation of ions under the electrodes.[90] The patient is thus monitored during and after the treatment to ensure that the skin is not burned under the electrode. Research has been focused on the development of iontophoretic patches for the systemic delivery of drugs. The iontophoretic patch has the option to monitor and control the power supplied during use, thus permitting safer and more reliable operation. The system can also detect the number of times the patch has been used and records the date and time of use, and its microprocessor can detect when the medication is exhausted. Furthermore, the controller can be rendered unusable to avoid abuse once the drug is exhausted.

Transcutaneous Electrical Nerve Stimulation

Transcutaneous electrical nerve stimulation (TENS) has been used effectively as a safe, noninvasive, drug-free method of treatment for various chronic and acute pain syndromes for many years. Depending on the parameters of electrical stimuli applied, there are several modes of therapy, resulting in different contributions of hyperaemic, muscle-relaxing, and analgesic components of TENS. TENS has been shown to be effective in providing pain relief in the early stages of healing following surgery[75,91–95] and in the remodeling phase.[96–99]

> **● Key Point** The percentage of patients who benefit from short-term TENS pain intervention has been reported to range from 50% to 80%, and good long-term results with TENS have been observed in 6% to 44% of patients.[96,98,100,101] However, most of the TENS studies rely solely on subjects' pain reports to establish efficacy and rarely on other outcome measures, such as activity, socialization, or medication use.

TENS units typically deliver symmetric or balanced asymmetric biphasic waves of 100- to 500-millisecond pulse duration, with zero net current to minimize skin irritation,[102] and they may be applied for extended periods (**Table 13-9**). The three modes of action that are theorized for the pain-relieving quality of this modality—gate control mechanism, endogenous opiate control, and central biasing—are described in Chapter 3. There are several guidelines when using TENS:

1. Electrodes may be placed close to the spinal cord segment that innervates a painful area.
2. Placing electrodes over sites where the nerve becomes superficial and can be stimulated easily may stimulate peripheral nerves that innervate a painful area.
3. Vascular structures contain neural tissue as well as ionic fluids that would transmit electrical stimulating current and may be most easily stimulated by electrode placement over superficial vascular structures.
4. Electrodes can be placed over trigger point and acupuncture locations.
5. Electrodes may be placed over specific dermatomes, myotomes, or sclerotomes that correspond to the painful area.

Russian Current or Medium-Frequency Alternating Current

The medium-frequency alternating current (MFAC) is more comfortable than other frequencies, especially if the current is delivered in bursts or if an interburst interval is used. Because medium-frequency stimulation is capable and effective in stimulating deep and superficial tissues, Russian current, a type of neuromuscular electrical stimulation (NMES) or functional elecetrical stimualtion (FES) is believed to augment muscle strengthening via polarizing both sensory and motor nerve fibers, resulting in tetanic contractions that are painless and stronger than those made voluntarily by the patient.

Interferential Current

Interferential current combines two high-frequency alternating waveforms that are biphasic. By using

TABLE 13-9	TENS Parameters and Effects			
Type	Frequency (Hz)	Duration (microseconds)	Amplitude (mA)	Muscle Contraction
Conventional	50–150	20–100	10–30	Yes
Low frequency (acupuncture)	1–4	100–200	30–80	Yes
Burst	70–100/burst	40–75	30–60	Yes
Brief intense (high intensity)	70–100/burst	15–200	30–60	No

overall shorter pulse widths and higher frequencies of each waveform, interferential current can penetrate deeper. Interferential current can be used for:[103]

- Muscle contraction (20 to 50 pps) together with the overall shorter pulse widths (100 to 200 microseconds).
- Pain management, using a frequency of 50 to 120 pps and a pulse width of 50 to 150 microseconds.
- Acustim pain relief, using a frequency of 1 pps.

Biofeedback

Biofeedback is a modality that is widely used in musculoskeletal rehabilitation. The clinical conditions for which biofeedback is most commonly used include muscle reeducation, which involves regaining neuromuscular control and/or increasing strength of a muscle, relaxation of muscle spasm or muscle guarding, and pain reduction. The biofeedback units most commonly used in physical therapy measure electromyographic (EMG) activity through skin surface electrodes, indicating the amount of electrical activity during muscle contraction. Specifically, the EMG measures the change in potential difference or voltage associated with depolarization. The biofeedback units provide auditory or visual feedback to give the patient information on timing of recruitment and intensity of muscle contractions. In addition, using biofeedback can help the patient regain function of a muscle that may have been lost or forgotten following injury. It is important to remember that there is no universally accepted standardized measurement scale used by the various EMG biofeedback units— different brands may give different readings for the same degree of muscle contraction. Consequently, EMG readings can be compared only when the same equipment is used for all readings. EMG skin surface electrodes come in a variety of sizes, and prior to attachment of the surface electrodes, the skin must be appropriately prepared by removing oil and dead skin, along with excessive hair, to reduce skin impedance. The electrodes are placed as near to the muscle being monitored as possible so that they are parallel to the direction of the muscle fibers, thereby reducing extraneous electrical activity. Three electrodes are typically used: two active electrodes and one reference or ground electrode.

The electrodes are placed in a bipolar arrangement. The active electrodes are placed in close proximity to one another, while the reference electrode is placed between the two active electrodes. As the active electrodes pick up electrical activity, the information is passed into a *differential amplifier*, which basically subtracts the signal from one active electrode from that of the other active electrode, thereby amplifying the difference between the signals. The ability of the differential amplifier to eliminate the common noise between the active electrodes is called the *common mode rejection ratio*. The external noise can be further reduced by using filters built into the unit. Signal sensitivity or signal gain can be set by the clinician on many units. If a high gain is chosen, the unit will have a high sensitivity for the muscle activity signal. This setting is typically used during relaxation training. Lower sensitivity levels are used more in muscle reeducation. Biofeedback units generally provide either visual and/or auditory feedback relative to the quantity of electrical activity.

Muscle Reeducation

Biofeedback for muscle reeducation is useful in patients who perform poorly on manual muscle tests—that is, those who can only elicit a fair, trace, or zero grade. The sensitivity setting is chosen by having the patient perform a maximum isometric contraction of the target muscle for 6 to 10 seconds. The gain is then adjusted so that the patient will be able to achieve the maximum on about two-thirds of the muscle contraction. The patient should be advised to look at the muscle when trying to contract it. Sometimes it may be necessary to move the active electrodes to the contralateral limb so that the patient can practice the muscle contraction. Between each contraction, the patient should be instructed to relax the muscle completely so that the feedback mode returns to baseline or zero prior to initiating another contraction. Ideally, a period of 5 to 10 minutes working with a single muscle or muscle group is most desirable to prevent fatigue.

Muscle Relaxation

In the muscle relaxation approach, the patient attempts to reduce the visual/auditory feedback from a biofeedback machine to zero. During relaxation training, the patient should be given verbal cues that will enhance relaxation of either individual muscles, muscle groups, or body segments. For example, biofeedback for relaxation is commonly used at the temporomandibular joint where monitoring of the frontal, temporal, and master muscles is used. As relaxation progresses, the spacing between the electrodes is increased and the sensitivity setting is adjusted from low to high. Both of these changes require the patient to relax more muscles, thus achieving greater relaxation.

Mechanical Modalities

Continuous Passive Motion

Continuous passive motion (CPM) refers to passive motion performed by a mechanical device that moves the joint slowly and continuously through a controlled ROM.[104] CPM machines have been designed for many body parts, including the hip, knee (most common), ankle, shoulder, elbow, wrist, and hand. For years, surgeons have debated the usefulness of CPM device use following surgery.

> **Key Point** CPM protocols vary significantly, ranging from 24 hours a day for as long as one month, to as little as 6 hours a day after surgery. The CPM machine is calibrated in degrees of motion and cycles per minute.

Typically, a low arc of 20° to 30° is used initially, progressing to 10° to 15° per day as tolerated. The rate of motion is typically one cycle per 45 seconds or 2 minutes. The patient is monitored during the first few minutes to ensure correct fit and patient comfort. Treatment duration varies from one hour three times a day to 24 hours a day. The use of a CPM device has been promoted as a means to facilitate a more rapid recovery by improving ROM, decreasing length of hospital stay, and lowering the amount of narcotic use.[105-115] However, studies have shown that the effect of CPM devices on analgesia consumption, ROM, hospital stay, and complications has been variable:

- Data support the use of CPM to decrease the rate of manipulation for poor ROM after total knee arthroplasty (TKA).
- The use of CPM has not been shown to result in more long-term increases in ROM than other methods of early movement and positioning.
- Although it appears that the use of a CPM device does help regain knee flexion quicker post TKA, it is not as effective in the enhancement of knee extension.
- Knee impairments and disability are not reduced with the use of a CPM at discharge from hospital.
- Because of standardized inpatient hospital clinical pathways, the length of hospital stay is not decreased by the use of a CPM device, but depending on the hospital involved, the overall cost is not increased.
- Wound complications probably are not increased with the use of CPM, provided that good technique is used in wound closure.

> **Key Point** It is still not clear whether ROM is achieved faster and whether the prevalence of deep vein thrombosis (DVT) and analgesics use are decreased with CPM.

Indications

CPM has the following indications:

- To decrease soft tissue stiffness
- To increase short-term ROM, which may result in early discharge from the hospital
- To promote healing of the joint surfaces (which promotes cartilage growth) and soft tissue
- To prevent adhesions and contractures and thus joint stiffness
- To decrease postoperative pain

Contraindications

CPM has the following contraindications:

- Nonstable fracture sites
- Excessive edema
- Patient intolerance

Mechanical Spinal Traction

Indications

Mechanical spinal traction has the following indications:

- Nerve impingement
- Herniated or protruding disc
- Subacute joint inflammation
- Joint hypomobility
- Degenerative joint disease
- Paraspinal muscle spasm

Contraindications

Mechanical spinal traction has the following contraindications:

- Joint instability or when motion is contraindicated
- Pregnancy (lumbar traction)
- Acute inflammatory response
- Acute sprain
- Osteoporosis
- Fracture
- Impaired cognitive function
- Central spinal stenosis

Physiologic Effects

Mechanical spinal traction involves the use of a distraction force applied to the cervical or lumbar spine to separate or attempt to separate the articular surfaces between the zygapophysial joints and the vertebral bodies. A number of methods can be employed to apply a distraction, including positional, gravity-assisted, and inversion techniques, but these sections will focus on the use of mechanical traction, which can be continuous or intermittent, as these are the most common methods. A call bell or cutoff switch is issued to the patient, and the patient should be closely monitored for any adverse reaction. Treatment time varies based on diagnosis and therapeutic goals and falls between 5 and 20 minutes.

Cervical Traction

Cervical traction can be applied with the patient in sitting or supine, although the supine position is generally preferred as it removes the weight of the patient's head and allows the patient to relax more. With intermittent traction, a duty cycle of either 1:1 or 3:1 is used. The treatment time varies according to condition: 5 to 10 minutes is recommended for acute conditions and disc protrusion, 15 to 30 minutes is recommended for other conditions.[116–118] Two methods of cervical traction can be used: the halter method or the use of the sliding device (Saunders). The halter device should not be used with patients with TMJ dysfunction or with patients who suffer from claustrophobia. The traction force used is determined by the treatment goals and by patient tolerance:

Acute Phase

Approximately 10 to 15 pounds of pull should be used initially, with progression up to 7% of the patient's body weight as tolerated. This is recommended to treat disc protrusions and muscle spasm, and to elongate soft tissue.[116–118] Joint distraction requires about 20 to 30 pounds of force.[116–118]

Halter Method

The head halter is placed under the occiput and the mandible and is then attached to the traction cord directly, or to the traction unit through a spreader bar. Generally, a starting position of approximately 20° to 30° of neck flexion is used (a pillow may be used).[116–118] The PT may decide to apply traction more specifically by varying the angle of neck flexion:[116–118]

- To increase the intervertebral space at the C1 to C5 levels, approximately 0° to 5° should be used.
- To increase the intervertebral space at the C5 through C7 levels, 25° to 30° of flexion is recommended.
- 15° of flexion is recommended for zygapophysial joint separation.[119]
- 0° of flexion is recommended for disc dysfunction.

Supine cervical traction has been found to be more efficacious than seated traction in the treatment of "cervical spine disorders."[117] The clinician should ensure that the traction force is applied to the occipital region and not to the mandible.

Saunders Device

The clinician places the patient's head on a padded headrest, in 20° to 30° of neck flexion. The clinician adjusts the neck yoke so that it fits firmly just below the mastoid processes. A head strap is typically used across the forehead to secure the head in place.

● **Key Point** The total treatment times to be used in cervical traction are only partially research based and can range from 5 to 30 minutes.

Lumbar Traction

A split table or other mechanism to eliminate friction between body segments and the table surface is a prerequisite to effective lumbar traction. In addition, a non-slip traction harness is needed to transfer the traction force comfortably to the patient and to stabilize the trunk while the lumbar spine is placed under traction. The patient should be suitably disrobed as clothing between the harness and the skin will also promote slipping.

The harness is applied when the patient is standing next to the traction table:

- The pelvic harness is applied so that the contact pads and upper belt are at or just above the level of the iliac crest.
- The contact pads are adjusted so that the harness loops provide the required direction of pull, encouraging either lumbar flexion or extension.
- The rib belt is then applied similarly with the rib pads positioned over the lower rib cage in a comfortable manner. The rib belt is then fitted snugly.

The patient is then asked to lie on the table:

- For disc protrusions (posterior or posterior lateral) the patient is positioned in the prone position with a normal to slightly flattened lumbar lordosis.
- For lateral spinal stenosis, the neutral spine position allows for the largest intervertebral foramen opening.

● **Key Point** In the supine position, the hip position can affect vertebral separation. As hip flexion increases from 0° to 90°, the traction produces a greater posterior intervertebral and facet joint separation.

Overall, patient positioning should be determined by patient needs and comfort.

As per the PT's instruction, a continuous or intermittent mode is used. The total treatment times to be used in lumbar traction are only partially research based and can range from 5 to 30 minutes.[120–122] The force of the lumbar traction pull is dependent on the goals of treatment and should be set with a force of less than half of the body weight for the initial treatment. Following the treatment session, the patient is reexamined. Any changes in symptoms are noted so that the results can be used to determine the parameters for the next session, or whether traction should be discontinued.

Intermittent Mechanical Compression

Two distinct kinds of tissue swelling are associated with injury:

- *Joint swelling:* Locked by the presence of blood and joint fluid accumulated within the joint capsule, which occurs immediately following injury to a joint.
- *Lymphedema (also known as lymphatic obstruction):* Swelling in the subcutaneous tissues that results from an excessive accumulation of lymph and usually occurs over several hours following injury.

Intermittent compression units are designed to keep venous and lymphatic flow from pooling into the interstitial space by applying a rhythmic external pressure. This type of external compression is designed to move lymph along and spread the intracellular edema over a larger area, enabling more lymph capillaries to become involved in removing the plasma proteins and water.[123] The most common treatments for lymphedema are a combination of the use of intermittent sequential gradient pumps, lymphatic massage, compression garments, or bandaging. Complex decongestive physiotherapy is an empiric system of lymphatic massage, skin care, and compressive garments.

Indications
Intermittent mechanical compression has the following indications:

- To control peripheral edema
- To shape a residual limb following amputation
- To manage scar formation
- To improve lymphatic and venous return
- To prevent deep vein thrombosis
- To prevent stasis ulcers

Contraindications
Intermitten mechanical compression has the following contraindications:

- Malignancy of treated area
- Presence of deep vein thrombosis
- Obstructed lymphatic channel
- Unstable or acute fracture
- Heart failure
- Infection of treated area
- Acute pulmonary edema
- Kidney or cardiac insufficiency
- Patients who are very young, or elderly and frail

Method of Application
The patient is asked to remove all jewelry on the extremity. The clinician checks the patient's blood pressure, measures the extremity, and records the data in the patient's chart. The patient is draped appropriately and is placed in a comfortable position with the limb elevated approximately 45° and abducted 20° to 70°. Pretreatment girth measures are taken. A stockinet is placed over the extremity to ensure that all wrinkles are removed. An appropriate-sized compression appliance is fitted on the extremity. The compression sleeves come as half-leg, full-leg, full-arm, or half arm. The deflated compression sleeve is connected to the compression unit via a rubber hose and connecting valve.

Once the machine has been turned on, there are three parameters available for adjustment with most intermittent pressure devices:[123]

- *Inflation pressure:* Pressure settings have been loosely correlated with blood pressure (somewhere around the patient's diastolic blood pressure and based on patient comfort).
- *On-off sequence or inflation/deflation ratio:* This is usually set to approximately 3:1, but it can be highly variable, with some protocols calling for a sequence of 30 seconds on, 30 seconds off; 1 minute on, 2 minutes off; 4 minutes on, 1 minute off. Patient comfort should be the primary deciding factor. As a general guideline, for edema reduction, a sequence of 45 to 90 seconds on/15 to 30 seconds off is used.
- *Total treatment time:* Treatment time varies. Most of the protocols for primary lymphedema call for 3- to 4-hour treatments, traumatic edema calls for 2-hour treatments, and residual limb reduction calls for 1- to 3-hour sessions. The average treatment for other conditions can be much shorter, lasting between 20 and 30 minutes.

The patient is given a call bell and should be monitored for comfort and blood pressure readings throughout the treatment. At the completion of the treatment, the unit is turned off and the stockinet and appliance removed. The extremity is then measured to see if the desired results have been achieved. If the edema is not reduced, another treatment may be needed after a short recovery time. The part should be wrapped with elastic compression wraps to help maintain the reduction. If not contraindicated, weight bearing should be encouraged to stimulate the venous pump.

CryoCuff and Cryopress

The AirCast CryoCuff® combines the therapeutic benefits of controlled compression to minimize hemarthrosis, edema hematoma, swelling, and pain. The cuff is anatomically designed to completely fit a number of different joints and body parts providing maximum cryotherapy. The cryopress is a sequential cryocompression unit. Studies have shown that cold therapy and compression combined have a better effect than compression or cryotherapy alone.[6,124]

Summary

Electrotherapeutic modalities, physical agents, and mechanical modalities are best used as adjuncts to other forms of therapeutic exercise. Decisions on how a particular modality may best be used are established by both theoretical knowledge and practical experience, and, for the PTA, they are based on the plan of care. For example, electrical stimulating currents may be used to stimulate sensory nerves to modulate pain, stimulate motor nerves to elicit a muscle contraction, introduce chemical ions into superficial tissues for medicinal purposes, and create an electrical field in the tissues to stimulate or alter the healing process. The modality used in the initial acute injury phase should be directed at reducing the amount of inflammation and swelling that occurs. During the later stages, the goal is to increase blood flow to the area and increase connective tissue extensibility and strength.

REVIEW Questions

1. In comparing the use of cold pack and hot pack treatments, which of the following statements is false?
   a. Cold packs penetrate more deeply than hot packs.
   b. Cold packs and hot packs can both cause skin burns.

   c. Cold decreases spasm by decreasing sensitivity to muscle spindles, and heat decreases spasm by decreasing nerve conduction velocity.
   d. None of the above.

2. As part of your weekly inspection, you test the temperature of the water in your hydrocullator to make sure it is appropriate to avoid a burn to the patient. What is the ideal temperature range?

3. Give three contraindications for aquatic exercise.

4. What should the temperature of the water be for water exercise?

5. What is the function of the transducer in an ultrasound machine?
   a. To change ultrasound waves into heat
   b. To change electricity into ultrasound waves
   c. To change ultrasound into sonic waves

6. Which of the following waves are not found on the electromagnetic spectrum?
   a. Ultraviolet
   b. Infrared
   c. Ultrasound

7. What units are used to measure electrical current?

8. All of the following are ions with a positive charge and may be introduced into tissue with the positive pole of a direct current except:
   a. Copper
   b. Zinc
   c. Histamine
   d. Salicylic acid

9. An example of the transmission of heat by conduction is:
   a. Ultrasound
   b. Hot pack
   c. Diathermy
   d. None of the above

10. Which of the following apply to positive ions?
    a. Attracted to the anode
    b. Produced by ionization of acids
    c. Attracted to the cathode
    d. None of the above

11. Which of the following show the best conductivity of all tissues to electrical current?
    a. Skin
    b. Tendon
    c. Bone
    d. Muscle

12. In stimulating denervated muscle, which of the following factors must be considered?
    a. Intensity
    b. Frequency

c. Duration

d. All of the above

13. The unit of power is represented by the:
a. Ohm
b. Volt
c. Watt
d. Ampere

14. Ultrasound waves cause the greatest rise in temperature in tissues with
a. Adipose (fat)
b. Cartilage
c. Tendon
d. Protein

15. Ultrasound has what theoretical effect on membrane permeability?
a. It increases it.
b. It decreases it.
c. It effects no change.
d. It alternately increases and decreases it.

16. The minimal amount of current necessary to elicit a threshold contraction of muscle is:
a. Chronaxie
b. Rheobase
c. Threshold
d. None of the above

17. In a strength-duration curve, the variable factors are:
a. Rheobase
b. Waveform
c. Both A and B
d. Neither A nor B

18. Local effects of a heat application include:
a. Local analgesia
b. Decreased blood flow in the area
c. Decreased tissue metabolism
d. None of the above

19. Local effects of cold applications include:
a. Vasoconstriction
b. Increased local circulation
c. Increased leukocytic migration
d. None of the above

20. You are treating a patient who demonstrates mild swelling on the dorsum of the hand and limited flexion of the metacarpophalangeal joints in all digits following a post open reduction of a Colles fracture 6 weeks ago. Which of the following would be the most appropriate heating agent to use?
a. Hot pack
b. Ultrasound

c. Paraffin bath
d. Massage

21. You have decided to use electrical stimulation on a patient rehabilitating from a patella tendon rupture. Which of the following types of current has the lowest total average current?
a. Russian
b. Interferential
c. High volt
d. Low volt

22. A 60-year-old patient with a left transfemoral amputation complains that his left foot is itching. Your best choice of intervention is:
a. Hot packs and ultrasound to the residual limb
b. Icing and vigorous massage to the residual limb
c. Iontophoresis to the residual limb
d. A psych consult

23. You are treating a patient with complaints of pain and muscle spasm in the cervical region. Past medical history reveals chronic heart disease and a demand-type pacemaker. Which of the following modalities should you avoid in this case?
a. Hot pack
b. TENS
c. Mechanical traction
d. Ultrasound

24. You are performing an in-service on the use of electrical equipment in the physical therapy department. Which of the following safety precautions would you stress to increase safety to the patient and therapist?
a. Never use an extension cord.
b. Never place the unit in close proximity to water pipes while treating the patient.
c. When using a device close to water, check that it is fitted with a ground fault interrupter.
d. All of the above should be stressed.

References

1. Bell GW, Prentice WE: Infrared modalities, in Prentice WE (ed): Therapeutic modalities for allied health professionals. New York, McGraw-Hill, 1998, pp 201–262
2. Johnson DJ, Moore S, Moore J, et al: Effect of cold submersion on intramuscular temperature of the gastrocnemius muscle. Phys Ther 59:1238–1242, 1979
3. Cobbold AF, Lewis OJ: Blood flow to the knee joint of the dog: Effect of heating, cooling and adrenaline. J Physiol 132:379–383, 1956

4. Wakim KG, Porter AN, Krusen FH: Influence of physical agents and certain drugs on intra-articular temperature. Arch Phys Med Rehab 32:714–721, 1951

5. Oosterveld FGJ, Rasker JJ, Jacobs JWG, et al: The effect of local heat and cold therapy on the intraarticular and skin surface temperature of the knee. Arthritis Rheum 35:146–151, 1992

6. Merrick MA, Knight KL, Ingersoll CD, et al: The effects of ice and compression wraps on intramuscular temperatures at various depths. J Athl Training 28:236–245, 1993

7. Abramson DI, Bell B, Tuck S: Changes in blood flow, oxygen uptake and tissue temperatures produced by therapeutic physical agents: Effect of indirect or reflex vasodilation. Am J Phys Med 40:5–13, 1961

8. Knight KL, Londeree BR: Comparison of blood flow in the ankle of uninjured subjects during therapeutic applications of heat, cold, and exercise. Med Sci Sports Exerc 12:76–80, 1980

9. Knight KL: Cryotherapy in Sports Injury Management. Champaign, IL, Human Kinetics, 1995

10. Knight KL: Cryotherapy: Theory, Technique, and Physiology. Chattanooga, TN, Chattanooga Corp, 1985

11. Pappenheimer SL, Eversole SL, Soto-Rivera A: Vascular responses to temperature in the isolated perfused hindlimb of a cat. Am J Physiol 155:458–451, 1948

12. Kalenak A, Medlar CE, Fleagle SB, et al: Athletic injuries: Heat vs cold. Am Fam Phys 12:131–134, 1975

13. McMaster WC, Liddle S, Waugh TR: Laboratory evaluation of various cold therapy modalities. Am J Sports Med 6:291–294, 1978

14. Daniel DM, Stone ML, Arendt DL: The effect of cold therapy on pain, swelling, and range of motion after anterior cruciate ligament reconstructive surgery. Arthroscopy 10:530–533, 1994

15. Konrath GA, Lock T, Goitz HT, et al: The use of cold therapy after anterior cruciate ligament reconstruction: A prospective randomized study and literature review. Am J Sports Med 24:629–633, 1996

16. Michlovitz SL: The use of heat and cold in the management of rheumatic diseases, in Michlovitz SL (ed): Thermal Agents in Rehabilitation. Philadelphia, F. A. Davis, 1990

17. Speer KP, R.F. Warren, and L. Horowitz: The efficacy of cryotherapy in the postoperative shoulder. J Shoulder Elbow Surg 5:62–68, 1996

18. Hocutt JE, Jaffee R, Rylander R, et al: Cryotherapy in ankle sprains. Am J Sports Med 10:316–319, 1982

19. Kellett J: Acute soft tissue injuries: A review of the literature. Med Sci Sports Exerc 18:5, 1986

20. McMaster WC: A literary review on ice therapy in injuries. Am J Sports Med 5:124–126, 1977

21. Hartviksen K: Ice therapy in spasticity. Acta Neurol Scand 3(Suppl):79–84, 1962

22. Basset SW, Lake BM: Use of cold applications in the management of spasticity. Phys Ther Rev 38:333–334, 1958

23. Starkey JA: Treatment of ankle sprains by simultaneous use of intermittent compression and ice packs. Am J Sports Med 4:142–143, 1976

24. Lamboni P, Harris B: The use of ice, air splints, and high voltage galvanic stimulation in effusion reduction. Athl Training 18:23–25, 1983

25. McMaster WC: Cryotherapy. Phys Sports Med 10:112–119, 1982

26. Waylonis GW: The physiological effects of ice massage. Arch Phys Med Rehab 48:42–47, 1967

27. Belitsky RB, Odam SJ, Hubley-Kozey C: Evaluation of the effectiveness of wet ice, dry ice, and cryogen packs in reducing skin temperature. Phys Ther 67:1080–1084, 1987

28. Zemke JE, Andersen JC, Guion WK, et al: Intramuscular temperature responses in the human leg to two forms of cryotherapy: Ice massage and ice bag. J Orthop Sports Phys Ther 27:301–307, 1998

29. Travell JG, Simons DG: Myofascial Pain and Dysfunction: The Trigger Point Manual. Baltimore, Williams & Wilkins, 1983

30. Feibel A, Fast A: Deep heating of joints: A reconsideration. Arch Phys Med Rehab 57, 1976

31. Cwynar DA, McNerney T: A primer on physical therapy. Lippincott's Primary Care Practice 3:451–459, 1999

32. Clark D, Stelmach G: Muscle fatigue and recovery curve parameters at various temperatures. Res Q 37:468–479, 1966

33. Baker R, Bell G: The effect of therapeutic modalities on blood flow in the human calf. J Orthop Sports Phys Ther 13:23, 1991

34. Knight KL, Aquino J, Johannes SM, et al: A re-examination of Lewis' cold induced vasodilation in the finger and ankle. Athl Training 15:248–250, 1980

35. Zankel H: Effect of physical agents on motor conduction velocity of the ulnar nerve. Arch Phys Med Rehab 47:197–199, 1994

36. Frizzell LA, Dunn F: Biophysics of ultrasound, in Lehman JF (ed): Therapeutic Heat and Cold (ed 3). Baltimore, Williams & Wilkins, 1982, pp 353–385

37. Lehman JF, Masock AJ, Warren CG, et al: Effect of therapeutic temperatures on tendon extensibility. Arch Phys Med Rehabil 51:481–487, 1970

38. Barcroft H, Edholm OS: The effect of temperature on blood flow and deep temperature in the human forearm. J Physiol 102:5–20, 1943

39. Griffin JG: Physiological effects of ultrasonic energy as it is used clinically. J Am Phys Ther Assoc 46:18, 1966

40. Abramson DI, Tuck S, Lee SW, et al: Comparison of wet and dry heat in raising temperature of tissues. Arch Phys Med Rehabil 48:654, 1967

41. Lehmann JF, Silverman DR, et al: Temperature distributions in the human thigh produced by infrared, hot pack and microwave applications. Arch Phys Med Rehabil 47:291, 1966

42. Sandqvist G, Akesson A, Eklund M: Evaluation of paraffin bath treatment in patients with systemic sclerosis. Disabil Rehabil 26:981–7, 2004

43. Stimson CW, Rose GB, Nelson PA: Paraffin bath as thermotherapy: An evaluation. Arch Phys Med Rehabil. 39:219–27, 1958

44. Draper DO, Prentice WE: Therapeutic ultrasound, in Prentice WE (ed): Therapeutic modalities for allied health professionals. New York, McGraw-Hill, 1998, pp 263–309

45. Benson HAE, McElnay JC: Transmission of ultrasound energy through topical pharmaceutical products. Physiotherapy 74:587–589, 1988

46. Cameron MH, Monroe LG: Relative transmission of ultrasound by media customarily used for phonophoresis. Phys Ther 72:142–148, 1992

47. Dyson M: Mechanisms involved in therapeutic ultrasound. Physiotherapy 73:116–120, 1987

48. Lehman JF, deLateur BJ, Stonebridge JB, et al: Therapeutic temperature distribution produced by ultrasound as modified by dosage and volume of tissue exposed. Arch Phys Med Rehabil 48:662–666, 1967

49. Lehman JF, deLateur BJ, Warren CG, et al: Heating of joint structures by ultrasound. Arch Phys Med Rehabil 49:28–30, 1968

50. Goldman DE, Heuter TF: Tabulator data on velocity and absorption of high frequency sound in mammalian tissues. J Acoust Soc Am 28:35, 1956

51. Dyson M, Pond JB: The effect of pulsed ultrasound on tissue regeneration. Physiotherapy 56:136, 1970

52. Dyson M, Suckling J: Stimulation of tissue repair by therapeutic ultrasound: A survey of the mechanisms involved. Physiotherapy 64:105–108, 1978

53. Antich TJ: Phonophoresis: The principles of the ultrasonic driving force and efficacy in treatment of common orthopedic diagnoses. J Orthop Sports Phys Ther 4:99–102, 1982

54. Bommannan D, Menon GK, Okuyama H, et al: Sonophoresis II: Examination of the mechanism(s) of ultrasound-enhanced transdermal drug delivery. Pharm Res 9:1043–1047, 1992

55. Bommannan D, Okuyama H, Stauffer P, et al: Sonophoresis. I: The use of high-frequency ultrasound to enhance transdermal drug delivery. Pharm Res 9:559–564, 1992

56. Byl NN: The use of ultrasound as an enhancer for transcutaneous drug delivery: Phonophoresis. Phys Ther 75:539–553, 1995

57. Byl NN, Mckenzie A, Haliday B, et al: The effects of phonophoresis with corticosteroids: a controlled pilot study. J Orthop Sports Phys Ther 18:590–600, 1993

58. Ciccone CD, Leggin BG, Callamaro JJ: Effects of ultrasound and trolamine salicylate phonophoresis on delayedonset muscle soreness. Phys Ther 71:39–51, 1991

59. Davick JP, Martin RK, Albright JP: Distribution and deposition of tritiated cortisol using phonophoresis. Phys. Ther 68:1672–1675, 1988

60. Dinno MA, Crum LA, Wu J: The effect of therapeutic ultrasound on the electrophysiologic parameters of frog skin. Med Biol 25:461–470, 1989

61. Ter Haar GR, Stratford IJ: Evidence for a non-thermal effect of ultrasound. Br J Cancer 45:172–175, 1982

62. Schrepfer R: Aquatic exercise, in Kisner C, Colby LA (eds): Therapeutic Exercise. Foundations and Techniques (ed 5). Philadelphia, F. A. Davis, 2002, pp 273–293

63. Downey JA: Physiological effects of heat and cold. Phys Ther 44:713–717, 1964

64. Cox JS: The diagnosis and management of ankle ligament injuries in the athlete. Athl Training 18:192–196, 1982

65. Marino M: Principles of therapeutic modalities: implications for sports medicine, in Nicholas JA, Hershman EB (eds): The Lower Extremity and Spine in Sports Medicine. St Louis, C. V. Mosby, 1986, pp 195–244

66. Martin G: Aquatic therapy in rehabilitation, in Prentice WE, Voight ML (eds): Techniques in Musculoskeletal Rehabilitation. New York, McGraw-Hill, 2001, pp 279–287

67. Thein-Brody L: Aquatic physical therapy, in Hall C, Thein-Brody L (eds): Therapeutic Exercise: Moving Toward Function (ed 2). Baltimore, MD, Lippincott Williams & Wilkins, 2005, pp 330–347

68. Harrison RA, Bulstrode S: Percentage weight bearing during partial immersion in the hydrotherapy pool. Physiother Practice 3:60–63, 1987

69. Americans with Disabilities Act of 1989: 104 Stat 327.101–336, 42 USC 12101 s2 (a) (8), 1989

70. Harrison RA, Hillma M, Bulstrode S: Loading of the lower limb when walking partially immersed: Implications for clinical practice. Physiotherapy 78:164–166, 1992

71. Pociask FD, Kahn J, Galloway K: Iontophoresis, ultrasound, and phonophoresis, in Placzek JD, Boyce DA (eds): Orthopaedic Physical Therapy Secrets. Philadelphia, Hanley & Belfus, Inc, 2001, pp 74–80

72. Scott O: Stimulative effects, in Kitchen S, Bazin S (eds): Clayton's Electrotherapy. London, W. B. Saunders, 1996

73. Low J, Reed A: Electrotherapy Explained: Principles and Practice. Oxford, Butterworth-Heinemann, 2000

74. Delitto A, Rose SJ, McKowen JM, et al: Electrical stimulation versus voluntary exercise in strengthening thigh musculature after anterior cruciate ligament surgery. Phys Ther 68:660–663, 1988

75. Goth RS, et al: Electrical stimulation effect on extensor lag and length of hospital stay after total knee arthroplasty. Arch Phys Med Rehab 75:957, 1994

76. Laughman RK, Youdas JW, Garrett TR, et al: Strength changes in the normal quadriceps femoris muscle as a result of electrical stimulation. Phys Ther 63:494–499, 1983

77. McMiken DF, Todd-Smith M, Thompson C: Strengthening of human quadriceps muscles by cutaneous electrical stimulation. Scand J Rehabil Med 15:25–28, 1983

78. Snyder-Mackler L, Delitto A, Bailey SL, et al: Strength of the quadriceps femoris muscle and functional recovery after reconstruction of the anterior cruciate ligament: A prospective, randomized clinical trial of electrical stimulation. J Bone Joint Surg Am 77:1166–1173, 1995

79. Gould N, Donnermeyer BS, Pope M, et al: Transcutaneous muscle stimulation as a method to retard disuse atrophy. Clin Orthop 164:215–220, 1982

80. Selkowitz DM: Improvement in isometric strength of quadriceps femoris muscle after training with electrical stimulation. Phys Ther 65:186–196, 1985

81. Currier DP, Mann R: Muscular strength development by electrical stimulation in healthy individuals. Phys Ther 63:915–921, 1983

82. Taylor K, Fish DR, Mendel FR, et al: Effect of a single 30 minute treatment of high voltage pulsed current on edema formation in frog hind limbs. Phys Ther 72:63–68, 1992

83. Gangarosa LP: Iontophoresis in dental practice. Chicago, Quintessence, 1982

84. Coy RE: Anthology of Craniomandibular Orthopedics. Seattle, International College of Craniomandibular Orthopedics, 1993

85. Burnette RR: Iontophoresis, in Hadgraft J, Guy RH (eds): Transdermal Drug Delivery: Developmental Issues and

Research Initiatives. New York, Marcel Dekker, 1989, pp 247–291

86. Chien YW, Siddiqui O, Shi M, et al: Direct current iontophoretic transdermal delivery of peptide and protein drugs. J Pharm Sci 78:376–384, 1989

87. Grimnes S: Pathways of ionic flow through human skin in vivo. Acta Dermatol Venereol 64:93–98, 1984

88. Lee RD, White HS, Scott ER: Visualization of iontophoretic transport paths in cultured and animal skin models. J Pharm Sci 85:1186–1190, 1996

89. O'Malley E, Oester Y: Influence of some physical chemical factors on iontophoresis using radioisotopes. Arch Phys Med Rehabil 36:310–313, 1955

90. Zeltzer L, Regalado M, Nichter LS, et al: Iontophoresis versus subcutaneous injection: A comparison of two methods of local anesthesia delivery in children. Pain 44:73–78, 1991

91. Smith MJ: Electrical stimulation for the relief of musculoskeletal pain. Phys Sports Med 11:47–55, 1983

92. Magora F, Aladjemoff L, Tannenbaum J, et al: Treatment of pain by transcutaneous electrical stimulation. Acta Anaesthesiol Scand 22:589–592, 1978

93. Mannheimer JS, Lampe GN: Clinical Transcutaneous Electrical Nerve Stimulation. Philadelphia, F. A. Davis, 1984, pp 440–445

94. Woolf CF: Segmental afferent fiber-induced analgesia: Transcutaneous electrical nerve stimulation (TENS) and vibration, in Wall PD, Melzack R (eds): Textbook of Pain. New York, Churchill Livingstone, 1989, pp 884–896

95. Smith MJ, Hutchins RC, Hehenberger D: Transcutaneous neural stimulation use in post-operative knee rehabilitation. Am J Sports Med 11:75–82, 1983

96. Long DM: Fifteen years of transcutaneous electrical stimulation for pain control. Stereotact Funct Neurosurg 56:2–19, 1991

97. Fried T, Johnson R, McCracken W: Transcutaneous electrical nerve stimulation: Its role in the control of chronic pain. Arch Phys Med Rehabil 65:228–231, 1984

98. Eriksson MBE, Sjölund BH, Nielzen S: Long-term results of peripheral conditioning stimulation as an analgesic measure in chronic pain. Pain 6:335–347, 1979

99. Fishbain DA, Chabal C, Abbott A, et al: Transcutaneous electrical nerve stimulation (TENS) treatment outcome in long term users. Clin J Pain 12:201–214, 1996

100. Ishimaru K, Kawakita K, Sakita M: Analgesic effects induced by TENS and electroacupuncture with different types of stimulating electrodes on deep tissues in human subjects. Pain 63:181–187, 1995

101. Eriksson MBE, Sjölund BH, Sundbärg G: Pain relief from peripheral conditioning stimulation in patients with chronic facial pain. J Neurosurg 61:149–155, 1984

102. Murphy GJ: Utilization of transcutaneous electrical nerve stimulation in managing craniofacial pain. Clin J Pain 6:64–69, 1990

103. Hooker DN: Electrical stimulating currents, in Prentice WE (ed): Therapeutic Modalities for Allied Health Professionals. New York, McGraw-Hill, 1998, pp 73–133

104. Kisner C, Colby LA: Range of motion, in Kisner C, Colby LA (eds): Therapeutic Exercise. Foundations and Techniques (ed 5). Philadelphia, F. A. Davis, 2002, pp 43–64

105. Johnson DP: The effect of continuous passive motion on wound-healing and joint mobility after knee arthroplasty. J Bone Joint Surg 72A:421–426, 1990

106. Basso M, Knapp L: Comparison of two continuous passive motion protocols for patients with total knee implants. Phys Ther 67:360–363, 1987

107. Colwell J, C.W, Morris BA: The influence of continuous passive motion on the results of total knee arthroplasty. Clin Orthop 276:225–228, 1992

108. Coutts RD: Continuous passive motion in the rehabilitation of the total knee patient: Its role and effect. Orthop Rev 15:27, 1986

109. Coutts RD, Toth C, Kaita JH: The role of continuous passive motion in the postoperative rehabilitation of the total knee patient, in Hungerford DS (ed): Total Knee Arthroplasty: A Comprehensive Approach. Baltimore, Williams & Williams, 1984, pp 126–132

110. Jordan LR, Siegel JL, Olivo JL: Early flexion routine, an alternative method of continuous passive motion. Clin Orthop 315:231–233, 1995

111. Maloney WJ, Schurman DJ, Hangen D, et al: The influence of continuous passive motion on outcome in total knee arthroplasty. Clin Orthop 256:162–168, 1990

112. Vince KG, Kelly MA, Beck J, et al: Continuous passive motion after total knee arthroplasty. J Arthroplasty 2:281–284, 1987

113. Wasilewski SA, Woods LC, Torgerson J, W.R, et al: Value of continuous passive motion in total knee arthroplasty. Orthopedics 13:291–295, 1990

114. Walker RH, Morris BA, Angulo DL, et al: Postoperative use of continuous passive motion, transcutaneous electrical nerve stimulation, and continuous cooling pad following total knee arthroplasty. J Arthroplasty 6:151–156, 1991

115. McInnes J, Larson MG, Daltroy LH, et al: A controlled evaluation of continuous passive motion in patients undergoing total knee arthroplasty. JAMA 268:1423–1428, 1992

116. Colachis SC, Strohm BR: Cervical traction: Relationship of traction time to varied tractive force with constant angle of pull. Arch Phys Med Rehabil 46:815–819, 1965

117. Deets D, Hands KL, Hopp SS: Cervical traction: A comparison of sitting and supine positions. Phys Ther 57:255–261, 1977

118. Harris PR: Cervical traction: Review of literature and treatment guidelines. Phys Ther 57:910–914, 1977

119. Wong AMK, Leong CP, Chen C: The traction angle and cervical intervertebral separation. Spine 17:136–138, 1992

120. Austin R: Lumbar traction a valid option. Aust J Physiother 44:280, 1998

121. Lee RY, Evans JH: Loads in the lumbar spine during traction therapy. Aust J Physiother 47:102–108, 2001

122. Pellecchia GL: Lumbar traction: A review of the literature. J Orthop Sports Phys Ther. 20:262–267, 1994

123. Hooker DN: Intermittent compression devices, in Prentice WE (ed): Therapeutic modalities for allied health professionals. New York, McGraw-Hill, 1998, pp 392–407

124. Aduayom I, Campbell PG, Denizeau F, et al: Different transport mechanisms for cadmium and mercury in Caco-2 cells: Inhibition of Cd uptake by Hg without evidence for reciprocal effects. Toxicol Appl Pharmacol 189:56–67, 2003

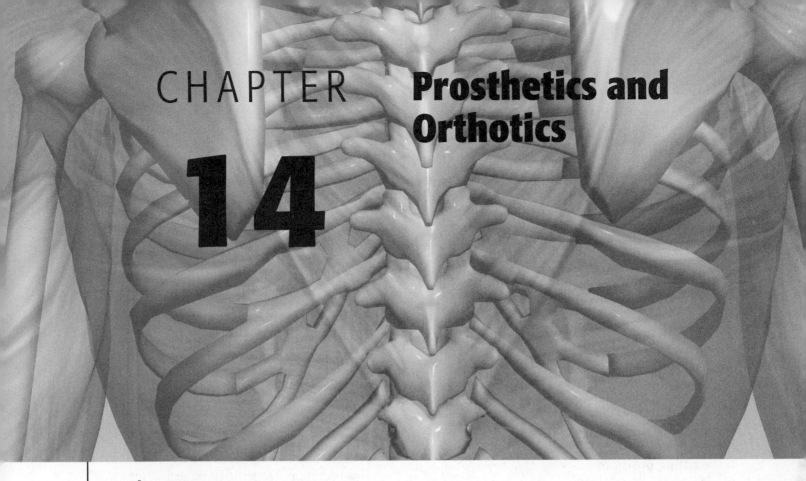

Amputation

The major reasons for amputation include disease (diabetes, peripheral vascular disease), infection (post joint replacement, osteomyelitis), tumor, trauma, and fracture (non-union).

> **● Key Point** *Amputation* refers to the cutting of a limb along the long bones axis. *Disarticulation* refers to the cutting of a limb through the joint.

Levels of Amputation[1]

The surgeon tries to maintain the greatest bone length and save all possible joints whatever the level of amputation:[2]

- *Partial toe:* Excision of any part of one or more toes.
- *Toe disarticulation:* Disarticulation of one or more toes at the metatarsophalangeal joint.
- *Partial foot/ray resection:* Resection of the third, fourth, and fifth metatarsals and digits.
- *Tarsometatarsal (LisFranc) disarticulation:* The disarticulation of all five metatarsals and the digits.
- *Transmetatarsal (Chopart):* Amputation through the midsection of all metatarsals, leaving only the calcaneus and talus.
- *Syme's:* Ankle disarticulation that may include removal of malleoli and distal tibial/fibular flares to create a smooth bony distal end with the attachment of the heel pad to the distal end of the tibia.

- *Long transtibial (below knee):* More than 50% of tibial length.
- *Transtibial (below knee):* Between 20% and 50% of tibial length.
- *Short transtibial (below knee):* Less than 20% of tibial length.
- *Knee disarticulation:* Amputation through the knee joint with shaping of the distal femur, squaring the condyles for an even weight-bearing surface. The knee disarticulation is most often used in children and young adults, but it is nearly always avoided in the elderly and patients with ischemic disease. Several advantages of the knee disarticulation include:
  - ❑ A large distal end covered by skin and soft tissues that is naturally suited for weight bearing.
  - ❑ A long lever arm controlled by strong muscles.
  - ❑ Increased stability of the patient's prosthesis.

   A main disadvantage of the knee disarticulation is cosmetic. The patient's prosthetic leg will have a knee that extends far beyond his or her own knee in the sitting position.

- *Long transfemoral (above knee):* More than 60% of femoral length.
- *Transfemoral (above knee):* Between 35% and 60% of femoral length.
- *Short transfemoral (above knee):* Less than 35% of femoral length.
- *Hip disarticulation:* An amputation through the hip joint capsule, removing the entire lower extremity, with closure of the remaining musculature over the exposed acetabulum. Hip disarticulation is generally performed as a result of failed vascular procedures following multiple lower-level amputations, or for massive trauma with crush injuries to the lower extremity.
- *Hemipelvectomy (HP):* Generally, in an HP operation, the leg, hip joint, and half of the pelvis are removed, and the remaining gluteal muscles are brought around and attached to the oblique abdominal muscles. The most common reason for HP is a rare form of connective tissue cancer known as sarcoma. There are various types of sarcomas, such as fibrosarcoma, osteosarcoma, and chondrosarcoma.
- *Hemicorporectomy:* Involves removal of the bony pelvis below the L4–L5 level, both lower limbs, the external genitalia, the bladder, rectum, and anus. Necessary life functions are maintained in the upper torso.

Hemicorporectomy has been performed for a variety of indications, including locally invasive pelvic cancer without metastatic spread, benign spinal tumors, intractable decubitus ulcers with malignant change, paraplegia in association with intractable pelvic osteomyelitis and decubitus ulceration, and crushing trauma to the pelvis. Given the high mortality following this procedure, especially when performed for visceral malignancy, the indications for its use are very restrictive.

Postoperative Dressings
Soft Dressings
Types of soft dressings include:

- *Elastic wrap:* An elastic compression bandage with a sterile dressing is commonly used during the immediate postoperative stage in cases of local infection to provide edema control, soft tissue support, and protection of the operative site. The elastic compression bandage and sterile dressing is generally removed and reapplied a minimum of three times per day following the immediate postoperative stage and removal of all surgical clips and sutures. Except for reapplication, the elastic compression bandage is normally kept in place at all times except during bathing. The patient is taught how to apply compression wrapping with elastic bandages or the use of an elastic shrinker (discussed later).

● **Key Point** Wrapping should be performed using either a diagonal or angular pattern, but not a circular pattern. Pressure should be applied distally to enhance shaping, and there should be no signs of wrinkles in the wrapping. Rewrapping should occur several times a day to maintain adequate pressure. Note the following guidelines:

- For transtibial amputations, use 3- to 4-inch wrap and ensure that the anchor wrap is applied above the knee.
- For transfemoral amputations, use 6-inch wrap and ensure the anchor wrap is applied around the pelvis.
- Full hip extension must be promoted following transfemoral amputations.

Rigid Dressings
A rigid dressing, the *immediate postoperative prosthesis* (IPOP) is sometimes used during the immediate postoperative stage in place of an elastic compression bandage for edema control and protection of the operative site.

- The advantages are that it allows early ambulation with a pylon and earlier fitting of the permanent prosthesis, promotes circulation and healing, and stimulates proprioception.

- The disadvantages are that because this dressing is not removable, and it does not permit wound inspections or daily dressing changes.

Semirigid Dressings

The classic compression treatment has been the Unna paste bandage impregnated with zinc oxide, glycerin, gelatin, and perhaps calamine, which dries to form a semirigid cast. This cast generally is changed once or twice weekly, depending on drainage and edema. The semirigid cast is useful in the initial phases of treatment for severe edema and to provide protection and soft tissue support. However, after the edema decreases, the semirigid cast is limited in its ability to accommodate limb volume changes and its inability to absorb drainage from highly exudative wounds.

Elastic Shrinker

The use of a shrinker (prosthetic compression sock) is not generally recommended until the incision line is adequately healed and there are no areas of open drainage. This is to avoid soft tissue trauma to the distal incision line while pulling compression socks into place. Shrinkers do provide a certain degree of independence with those individuals able to properly don them, especially if they are not able to properly wrap the residual limb. Currently available transfemoral shrinkers incorporate a hip spica, which provides good suspension except with obese individuals.

Postoperative Physical Therapy

Goals

Postoperative physical therapy has the following goals:

- To relieve post-op stump pain
- To promote healing of the residual limb
- To maintain or improve strength and range of motion
- To prevent contractures
- To train the patient to perform activities of daily living
- To maintain stump hygiene
- To prepare the stump for prosthetic fitting
- To provide appropriate follow-up care

Desensitization

The residual stumps are frequently highly sensitive post surgery and must become tolerant to touch and pressure. Typically, the clinician uses a progression of contact with soft materials such as cotton or lamb's wool, progressing to burlap-type materials. Rubbing, tapping, and performing resistive exercises with the stump also assist in preparing the limb for prosthetic fitting. The traditional toughening techniques (beating the stump with a towel-wrapped bottle, for example) are not recommended.

Range of Motion Exercises

Stretching and ROM exercises are extremely important postsurgically to prevent contractures.

Positioning

Contractures can develop as a result of muscle imbalance or fascial tightness, from a protective withdrawal reflex into hip and knee flexion, from loss of plantar stimulation in extension, or as a result of faulty positioning, such as prolonged sitting or placing the residual limb on a pillow.[2]

- *Above-knee amputee:* Prevent hip flexion, abduction, and external rotation contractures
- *Below-knee amputee:* Prevent hip flexion, abduction, and external rotation, and knee flexion contractures

Strength Training

Selected and specific strengthening exercises must be performed to increase the strength of the residual musculature. The hip extensors and abductors, as well as the knee extensors and flexors, are particularly important for prosthetic ambulation. Strengthening exercises are initiated with isometrics, progressing to isotonics with cuff weights. As strength improves, simple adaptations with traditional weight machines may be made.

- *Above-knee amputee:* Hip extension, abduction, adduction, pelvic tilt exercises
- *Below-knee amputee:* Hip extension, abduction, knee extension, and knee flexion exercises

Function

Medicare and Medicaid categorize patients with unilateral transfemoral transtibial amputations according to the following functional levels:[3]

- *Level 0:* Patient lacks ability or potential to transfer safely with or without assistance, and a prosthesis does not enhance quality of life or mobility. Not a prosthetic candidate, no prosthesis allowed, no components can be used.
- *Level 1:* Patient has ability or potential to use a prosthesis for transfer or ambulation on a level surface at a fixed cadence. Typical of limited and unlimited household ambulator.
- *Level 2:* Patient has ability or potential for ambulation with the ability to traverse lower-level environmental barriers such as curbs, stairs, or uneven surfaces. Typical of the limited community ambulator.
- *Level 3:* Patient has ability or potential for ambulation with variable cadence. Typical of the community ambulator who has the ability to traverse most environmental barriers and may have vocational, therapeutic, or exercise activity that demands prosthetic utilization beyond simple locomotion.
- *Level 4:* Patient has ability or potential for prosthetic utilization that exceeds basic ambulation skills, exhibiting high impact, stress, or energy levels. Typical of the prosthetic demands of the child, active adult, or athlete.

Patient Education

Patient education should focus on the following:

- The disease process, the physiological effects of the symptoms, and lifestyle changes to reduce risk factors.
- Methods of edema control.
- Benefits of exercise.
- Hygiene and skin care. The residual limb is kept clean and dry. Care must be taken to avoid abrasions, cuts, and other skin problems.
- Limb inspection. The patient is told to inspect the residual limb with a mirror each night to make sure there are no sores or impending

problems, especially in areas not readily visible. This inspection is particularly important if the person has diminished sensation.
- Residual limb wrapping.

Lower Limb Prosthetic Designs

A prosthesis is an artificial replacement for a body part. Prosthetic components have advanced tremendously over the years and now provide the amputee more comfortable and responsive prosthetic choices. A primary aim of the postsurgical period is to determine the individual's suitability for prosthetic replacement. Not all people with amputations are candidates for a prosthesis, regardless of personal desire.[2]

Partial Foot Amputations

Prosthetic devices for partial foot amputations include:

- Custom molded insole with toe filler. This is a simple foam filler with a plastic insert for the transverse arch of the foot and a heel counter for rear foot stability.
- Rigid plate. This is used to prevent the potential equinas deformity that can occur in the absence of the foot and the shortening of the gastrocnemius and soleus muscles.
- Slipper-type elastomer prosthesis. This provides a more cosmetic approach, where semiflexible urethane elastomers are modeled to provide a foot-shaped prosthesis with a soft socket that conforms to the residual foot.
- Syme ankle:
  - ❑ Veterans Administration prosthetic center Syme prosthesis: A media window or cutout of the distal end of the socket provides an opening for ease of donning of the bulbous end pad created by the anatomical heel pad.
  - ❑ Miami Syme prosthesis: The inelastic inner liner is an expandable wall that permits the bulbous distal end of the stump to pass down and sit snugly within the socket.

Phalangeal Amputations

Typically, a prosthesis is not necessary unless the foot is at risk for deformity or further injury.

Transphalangeal (Toe Disarticulation)

If one to three toes are involved, not including the first ray, a simple toe filler can be placed in the shoe. When the first digital great toe is involved, a steel shank spring can be used in the sole of the shoe to assist the push-off, in addition to the toe filler, if needed.

Transtibial (Below the Knee)

The lower leg has four muscle compartments: the anterior, lateral, deep posterior, and superficial posterior. The choice of which muscle compartment to use is based on the amount of padding each can afford. Most surgeons use the superficial posterior compartment—the gastrocnemius and soleus—as the main sources of padding, and they use the posterior flap procedure when approximately 20% to 50% of the tibial length is retained. In this procedure, the gastrocnemius and soleus muscles are wrapped around the distal end of the limb and sutured anteriorly.

> ● **Key Point** The surgeon's goal is to retain as much of the useful remaining nerve function in the residual limb as possible while also carefully minimizing nerve scarring and painful neuromas.

Transfemoral (Above the Knee)

Ideally, 35% to 60% of the femoral length is spared with the transfemoral amputation. The higher the level of lower limb amputation, the greater the energy expenditure required for walking.[4,5] A person with a transfemoral amputation usually walks more slowly than before but expends more energy over a longer time because it takes a greater effort to walk with an amputation in the thigh. For those who have undergone transfemoral amputations, the energy required is 50% to 65% greater than that required for those who have not undergone amputations. Complications associated with this procedure include:

- Balance and stability problems. Problems like stumbling and falling, while difficult to measure, are probably related to both physical and mental energy and balance.
- The need for a more complicated prosthetic device.
- Difficulty rising from a seated position.
- Prosthetic comfort while sitting.

Hip Disarticulation

Function following a hip disarticulation with a modern prosthesis is acceptable. Patients are ambulatory at approximately 6 months with the use of one cane.

Hemipelvectomy

For a high-level amputee, the energy requirements to use a prosthesis have been reported to be as much as 200% of normal ambulation. Consequently, only a small percentage of people become long-term wearers. These patients present a particularly challenging array of clinical issues, including deconditioning, pain management, altered gait mechanics, altered sexual functioning, and edema/lymphedema management.

Hemicorporectomy

Rehabilitation following a hemicorporectomy focuses on the development of a total contact bucket prosthesis that permits an upright sitting posture in a wheelchair and releases the upper limbs for other functions. The prosthesis is adjusted to accommodate the stoma sites and to reduce pressure on the terminal lumbar spine. Discomfort from heat buildup limits use of the bucket for some patients.

Upper limb strengthening, vocational training, psychological counseling, sex hormone replacement, education, and dietary advice to avoid obesity are all further aspects of what is a lengthy process of readjustment. Patients must, in addition, learn the importance of lifelong careful fluid balance, given the reduced ability of the autonomic system to autoregulate circulating blood volume.

Prosthetic Components

The following sections generically describe the components and socket designs, as there are literally hundreds of specific components, variations, and combinations of prosthetic designs.

Shanks

The area between the knee and the foot is commonly referred to as the shank. There are two basic structural designs at the shank that determine the general structural classification of a prosthesis:

- *Exoskeletal design:* The exterior of the structure provides the required support for the weight of the body. Thermosetting plastic and wood are the common materials used for fabrication.
- *Endoskeletal design:* An internal skeleton or pylon (a narrow vertical support typically made of metal or plastic tubing connecting the socket to the foot-ankle assembly) that supports the load with an outer covering, usually made of foam to give the shank a cosmetic shape.

Foot Socket Designs

Articulated Foot–Ankle Assemblies
Types of articulated foot–ankle assemblies include:

- *Single-axis foot:* The single-axis foot allows dorsiflexion (5° to 7°) and plantarflexion (15°), which are limited by rubber bumpers or spring systems. No medial/lateral or rotary motion is permitted, which makes this design suitable for flat and even surfaces.

- *Multiple-axis foot:* This type of foot allows lateral and rotary movements and is therefore more suitable for uneven terrain. However, due to the complexity of their design, some of these can be bulky and require frequent maintenance and adjustments.
- *Endolite multiflex ankle:* This design allows full range of motion, including inversion, eversion, and some rotation, in addition to plantar and dorsiflexion, which make it suitable to a wide variety of terrains.
- *Tru-step foot:* This design, which features a three-point weight transfer system and shock-absorbing heel, permits eight motions: plantar flexion, dorsiflexion, inversion, eversion, abduction, adduction, supination, and pronation. In addition, the three bumpers within the system can be changed to provide the correct resistance for a smooth gait.
- *Total concept foot:* This type of foot functions as a dynamic response system with a single carbon fiber deflector plate, and the single-axis angle has adjustable bumpers that control plantar and dorsiflexion. The design incorporates an innovative heel height adjustment of the ankle of up to 10 degrees of dorsiflexion for ascending, or 25 degrees of plantarflexion for descending ramps or hills.

Nonarticulated Foot–Ankle Assemblies
Types of nonarticulated foot–ankle assemblies include:

- *Solid-Ankle-Cushioned-Heel (SACH) Foot/Durometer:* This is perhaps the most prescribed prosthetic foot worldwide. The molded heel cushion, made of a high-density foam rubber, forms the foot and ankle into one component. At heel strike, the rubber heel wedge compresses to stimulate plantarflexion. There are no moving parts, and thus no maintenance and no noise. The limitations include limited adjustment of plantar/dorsiflexion, difficulty walking up inclines due to compression of the heel, and limited motion for active people.
- *Stationary Attachment Flexible Endoskeletal II (SAFE II) Foot:* This foot is designed to mimic the human subtalar joint and incorporates two fiber bands. The long plantar ligament band provides stability, while the plantar fascia band

is designed to tighten, providing a semi-rigid lever for a smooth transition at toe off.

- *Seattle Foot:* This foot is designed for the more active individual due to its ability to "store energy" during midstance to terminal stance and transfer that energy during toe-off. It also has the appearance of an anatomic foot due to its external foam covering, which is reinforced with Kevlar.
- *Carbon Copy II:* The Carbon Copy II is a solid ankle design with a heel made of a polyurethane foam cushion, which provides two-stage resistance at terminal stance based on whether the user is walking or running.
- *Flex Foot:* The Flex Foot uses the entire distance from the socket, not just the length of the keel to "store energy" within an anterior deflector plate, giving it the greatest energy return of the dynamic response feet. As a result, this design is popular with athletes.

Knee Socket Designs
There are two general classifications of sockets: the hard socket, where there is direct contact between the socket's inner surface and stump, and the soft socket, which incorporates the use of a liner as a cushion between the socket and stump, and in some cases provides suspension.

Patella Tendon-Bearing Sockets
Patella tendon-bearing sockets incorporate a total contact design, which creates a totally closed system around the skin at the distal end, and which offers a more intimate fit, thus avoiding skin lesion problems that can occur when the soft tissues are not completely supported.

- The anterior wall is high enough to encompass the distal half of the patella.
- The posterior wall rises slightly higher than the knee joint line and provides an anterior force to maintain the patella on the patella bar (a small bulge in the socket) as well as prevents excessive pressure on the hamstrings via a contoured socket.
- The medial and lateral walls are slightly higher than the anterior wall, adding stability, although for the most part stability in the mediolateral plane is provided by the amputee's own knee.

There are two main variations:

- *PTB-supracondylar:* Has higher medial and lateral walls to encompass both femoral condyles, thereby increasing medial and lateral stability of the knee.

- *PTB-supracondylar/suprapatellar:* Also has higher medial and lateral walls to encompass both femoral condyles, but this type also raises the anterior wall to cover all of the patella, with the suprapatellar area of the socket being contoured inward to create a "quadricep bar," which results in additional suspension and resistance to recurvatum in the case of very short stumps, or unstable knees, respectively.

Transtibial Amputee Suction Socket Designs

Many of today's sockets utilize a suction suspension, which creates a vacuum between a flexible roll on the sleeve and the skin, between the sleeve and the socket, or both, in order to hold the socket on the stump. The sleeves are made from silicon, urethane, or other composite gel materials. All of the sleeves are rolled on to the stump, creating a sealed airless environment to keep the sleeve on the limb. The socket is connected to the sleeve by a pin and lock system, or a one-way valve system.

- *Pin and lock system:* When the sleeve-covered limb is placed completely into the socket, a locking mechanism at the distal socket receives the pin, locking the sleeve securely to the socket. A release pin is found on the exterior of the socket, or the sleeve can be removed.
- *Valve system:* This design permits the expulsion of air out of the socket as the limb is inserted, but it does not permit air to return back into the socket. To seal the top of the socket, an external suspension sleeve that covers the socket is rolled over the thigh.

Benefits of the suction systems include:

- Secure suspension
- Reduced pistoning
- Reduced friction
- Reduced perspiration
- Elimination of straps, cups, or sleeves

Transtibial Amputee Suspension Systems

Frequently, more than one suspension system is necessary—for example, one for suspending the socket, and a secondary system to provide an added sense of security. Common suspension methods include the supracondylar cuff, thigh corset or thigh lacer, inverted Y-strap and waist belt, neoprene sleeve or latex sleeve, medial wedge, lateral wedge, suction, and removable medial brim.

Transfemoral Amputee Socket Designs

Quadrilateral Socket   The quadrilateral design is characterized by a series of reliefs or depressions in the socket designed to reduce pressure on relatively firm tissue, tendons, muscles, and bulges produced by a buildup of materials intended to press on soft areas to provide load sharing. The advantages of such a socket include:

- Muscular contractions are permitted, which reduces atrophy.
- Total contact is present between the socket and stump with a wider medial-lateral than anterior-or-posterior dimension.
- It provides the ability to customize different sizes and shapes caused by soft tissue and bony prominences.
- The anterior wall is 2.5 inches higher than the medial wall, with a prominent Scarpa's bulge, maintaining the ischial tuberosity on the ischial seat by providing counterpressure against the posterior wall.
- The socket does not press on the pubic ramus due to the fact that the medial brim is the same height as the posterior brim.

Ischial Containment Socket   This socket is characterized by:

- The encapsulation of the ischial tuberosity within the socket via a high posterior wall.
- Greater adduction of the femur, placing the muscles in an optimal length-tension position for better quality of muscular contraction.
- A narrow medial-lateral dimension within the socket that allows the pelvis and the socket to act as one for greater prosthetic control.
- The pocketing of the gluteus maximus within a gluteal channel, which applies a stretch to the hamstrings.
- A lateral wall that rises superiorly over greater trochanter with femoral adduction (10° to 15°), which is maintained via a force applied to the greater trochanter and the length of the shaft of the femur, with a counterforce applied at the ischial ramus.

Transfemoral Amputee Suspension Systems

For the most part, the suspension systems described for the transtibial sockets apply for the transfemoral sockets. One significant difference, used only with transfemoral amputees, is a technique referred to as partial suction, where stump socks are used but there is still a close fit, but where a secondary suspension system such as a Silesian bandage or pelvic belt must be incorporated into the design.

Prosthetic Knee Units

Knee Axis   There are two classifications of knee axes:

- *Single:* Works like a hinge joint to maintain a single stationary axis point that either end may move around; the most common type of axis used.
- *Polycentric:* Any knee unit with more than one axis. Traditionally referred to as the four-bar linkage system. The advantages of this system include:
  - ❑ An instantaneous center of rotation is created as the shank moves about the knee axis.
  - ❑ During sitting, the shank moves under the distal end of the socket, preventing the prosthetic knee from protruding too far in front of the contralateral anatomic knee.
  - ❑ During ambulation, as the shank moves posterior to the knee's center, greater toe clearance is permitted during swing.

Swing Phase Control Mechanisms   Three general classifications of swing phase control mechanisms are available:

- *Mechanical constant friction:* The swing resistance is generated by a friction system that creates a drag on the prosthetic shank or controls the speed of walking. However, these units do not have the ability to vary the speed of cadence. The advantages of this system include:
  - ❑ It is the simplest of the knee units and is therefore relatively low in cost.
  - ❑ The units are typically lightweight and durable, with few mechanical parts.
- *Pneumatic or air-controlled:* Air-filled cylinders that provide a cadence response using the spring action of a compressible medium, air.
  - ❑ When the knee is flexed, the piston rod compresses the air, storing energy.
  - ❑ As the knee moves into extension during late swing, the energy is returned, assisting with extension.
  - ❑ An adjustment screw controls resistance. The key advantage of this system is the cadence-responsive function.
- *Hydraulic or fluid controlled:* Liquid-filled cylinders that provide a cadence response using an essentially incompressible medium, oil.

When the knee flexes, a piston rod is pushed into an oil-filled cylinder, forcing the oil through one or more chambers, thus regulating the speed of movement. The degree of resistance can be controlled by an adjustment screw, which varies the cross-sectional area of the chamber(s):

- ❑ A greater cross-sectional area, which lowers the resistance, is desired if the amputee has a slow, weak gait.
- ❑ A smaller cross-sectional area, which increases the resistance, is desired with a faster walking speed.

● **Key Point**   The major advantages of hydraulic systems are a cadence-responsive function and the ability of most designs to withstand greater forces than the pneumatic units. The disadvantages include cost, weight, mechanical failure, and maintenance.

Extension Bias Assists   Although not technically a knee design classification, this unit design helps advance the limb or extend the knee during the swing phase. Two basic types are available:

- *Internal:* A spring provides assistance with extension once knee flexion is completed during ambulation. If the knee flexion is greater than 60 degrees, the knee will remain flexed as in sitting.
- *External:* An adjustable/nonadjustable elastic strap is attached to the socket anteriorly, descending to the anterior shank.
  - ❑ As the knee is flexed, the strap is stretched.
  - ❑ Once an extension force is initiated, the strap shortens.

Stance Phase Control Mechanisms   Stance control can be established individually or in combination through the following five major mechanisms:

- *Alignment:* The vast majority of knee units require that the trochanter-knee-ankle (TKA) or weight line pass anterior to the axis, creating an extension moment and, in turn, knee stability.
- *Manual locks:* This type of design prevents any knee motion once engaged. Manual locks are available with one of two basic lock systems:
  - ❑ Manually operated, where a small lever or ring and cable system is accessible to the amputee to engage or disengage as needed.
  - ❑ Spring-loaded, which engages automatically when the knee is extended.

- *Weight-activated friction knee:* With this type of knee, the unit functions as a constant friction knee during the swing phase; however, during weight bearing in the stance phase, a housing with a high coefficient of friction (which can be adjusted to the amputee's body weight) presses against the knee mechanism and prevents knee flexion.
- *Hydraulic Swing-N-Stance control units:* As weight is applied when the knee is in full extension, and up to 25 degrees of flexion, increased resistance is employed from the cylinder, as too rapid a fluid flow results in immediate closing of valves that stop fluid flow, preventing the knee from buckling and allowing the amputee to regain balance.
- *Polycentric axis knee unit:* One key advantage of the polycentric knee axis design in stance is that because there is no one center of rotation, a greater zone of stability exists.

Hip Joints

Hip Flexion Bias System
A coil spring is compressed during midstance and released during preswing, thrusting the prosthetic thigh forward, which eliminates excessive pelvic rocking.

Littig Hip Strut
A carbon composite strut in the shape of a band connects to the socket and the knee unit, so that as body weight is placed over the strut (the thickness and length of which can be adjusted according to the height and weight of the amputee), it deflects or bends. As the patient moves into swing, the strut recoils or thrusts the prosthetic limb forward, reducing the need for excessive pelvic motion.

Lower Limb Prosthetic Training

The development of specific anticipated goals and expected outcomes of the individual patient with an amputation is based on the following general goals:[2]

- To reduce (or prevent) postoperative edema and promote healing of the residual limb
- To prevent joint contractures, general debility, and integumentary disturbances
- To maintain or regain strength in the affected lower extremity
- To maintain or increase strength in the remaining extremity
- To demonstrate the ability to correctly perform a home exercise program
- To learn proper care of the remaining extremity

The patient must learn to walk with a prosthesis, apply and remove the prosthesis, care for the prosthesis, monitor skin and any pressure points, ambulate on difficult terrain, and use the commode at night.

Donning
Correct application of the prosthesis and frequent inspection of the amputated limb are very important, especially for the beginner and those with poor circulation.[6]

Proprioceptive Training
Proprioceptive training includes balance activities and mobility training. All patients must learn to balance on the amputated side. Parallel bars provide good support to both sides of the body, whereas a plinth or sturdy table offers the dual advantages of providing good support on only one side, ordinarily the contralateral side, and unidirectional control. A typical sequence is outlined below:

- Orientation to center the gravity and base of support. Various methods of proprioceptive and visual feedback may be employed to promote the amputee's ability to maximize the displacement of the center of mass over the base of support.
- The amputee must learn to displace the center of mass forward and backward as well as from side to side.
- Single limb standing. Single limb balance over the prosthetic limb, while advancing the sound limb, should be practiced in a controlled manner so that, when called on to do so in a dynamic situation such as walking, this skill can be employed with relatively little difficulty. The amputee's ability to control sound limb advancement is directly related to the ability to control prosthetic limb stance.
- Stool stepping. The amputee stands in the parallel bars with the sound limb in front of a 4- to 8-inch stool or block (depending on level of ability). The patient is asked to slowly step onto the stool with the sound limb while using bilateral upper extremity support on the parallel bars. A challenge can be added by asking the patient to remove the sound-side hand from the parallel bars, and eventually the other hand.
- Exercises to improve the control of the musculature of the stump side to maintain balance over the prosthesis.
- Exercises to enhance the patient's proprioception so as to be able to detect the available sensation within the stump/socket interface.

- Visualization. The amputee must be able to visualize the prosthetic foot and its relationship to the ground.

Gait Training[7]

Individuals who have undergone amputations often adapt a unique way of ambulating with a prosthesis, but these adaptations also bring about challenges in diagnosing problems with their gait. Several factors determine optimal gait: pelvic rotation, pelvic obliquity, lateral displacement of the body, knee flexion in the stance phase, and foot and ankle mechanism. The common gait deviations of transtibial and transfemoral prosthetic gait, are described in **Table 14-1** and **Table 14-2**. Gait training occurs on flat, even surfaces, initially within the parallel bars, then with an assisted device, and finally independently as appropriate.

- Gait training on stairs, curbs, uneven surfaces, ramps, and hills.
- Braiding.
- Falling and lowering oneself to the ground.
- Floor to standing techniques.
- Running skills as appropriate.

Upper Limb Prosthetic Devices

Levels of Upper Limb Amputation

Classification for upper limb amputees is based on the anatomic location of the amputation or surgical site. The acceptance of upper limb prosthetic devices varies depending on the age, activity level, and comfort level of the amputee.

Terminal Devices

Hooks

The most common terminal device used is the split-hook type, which allows the amputee to grasp objects between the fingers of the hook by opening and closing the hook in a pincer-type motion.

Voluntary Opening Hooks

The fingers of the hook are opened when the amputee exerts a force on the control cable of a voluntary opening hook against the force of the rubber bands, which act as a spring to close the fingers and provide prehension, or a pinch force.

Voluntary Closing Hooks

This type of hook permits the amputee more precise ability to close the device because the closing of the device is powered by the amputee using a cable control. This type of device is preferred for control of fine work without great exertion.

Hands

Although not as functional as the hook, the prosthetic hand is more cosmetically appealing to some amputees.

Voluntary Opening Hands

The operation of a voluntary opening hand is the same as that of the voluntary opening hook, except the fingers form the "three-jaw-chuck" pinch with the index and middle finger joining the thumb.

Passive or Cosmetic Hands

These units have no functional mechanism and are intended purely for cosmetic effect.

Wrist Units

Wrist units are used for attaching the terminal device to the forearm and to provide terminal device pronation/supination. Wrist units can be either constant-friction controlled or locking, and they are very practical affectations permitting easier control for midline activities such as eating, grooming, and dressing.

Transradial Sockets

Split Socket

Typically used with a very short transradial amputee, split sockets are used with stepped-up hinges because elbow flexion is often limited.

Munster (Self-Suspending) Socket

This type of socket, designed for the short transradial amputee, has an extremely narrow anterior-posterior dimension that suspends the socket on the residual limb.

Northwestern University Supracondylar Socket

This design has become the most popular self-suspending socket design because it very adequately suspends the unit without any loss of range of motion in the sagittal plane.

Hinges

Transradial hinges connect the socket to a triceps cuff or pad on the posterior upper arm and assist with suspension and stability.

Flexible Elbow Hinges

Constructed from flexible materials such as Dacron webbing fabric, leather, or lightweight metals, flexible elbow hinges assist with suspension of the forearm shell and permit rotational motion of the forearm in long transradial amputees and wrist disarticulations.

TABLE 14-1

Gait Deviations According to Prosthetic Causes and Amputee Causes

Deviation	Prosthetic Causes	Amputee Causes
Lateral bending of the trunk	Prosthesis too short Improperly shaped lateral wall Medial wall too high Prosthesis abducted	Poor balance Abduction contracture Short residual limb Weak hip abductors on prosthetic side Hypersensitive and painful residual limb
Abducted gait	Prosthesis too long High medial wall Improperly shaped lateral wall Prosthesis abducted Inadequate suspension Knee friction too high	Abduction contracture Adductor roll Weak hip flexors and adductors Pain over lateral residual limb
Circumducted gait (the foot returns to the proper position at heel strike)	Prosthesis too long Too much friction in the knee Socket too small Excessive plantar flexion of prosthetic foot	Abduction contracture Weak hip flexors Lacks confidence to flex the knee Painful anterior distal stump Inability to initiate prosthetic knee flexion
Excessive knee flexion during stance	Socket set anterior in relation to foot Foot set in excessive dorsiflexion Stiff heel Prosthesis too long	Knee flexion contracture Hip flexion contracture Anterior pain in residual limb Decrease in quadriceps strength Inadequate balance
Vaulting	Prosthesis too long Inadequate socket suspension Excessive alignment stability Foot too much plantar flexion	Residual limb discomfort Fear of stubbing toe Short residual limb Painful residual limb
Rotation of forefoot at heel strike (external rotation)	Excessive toe-out built-in Loose-fitting socket Inadequate suspension Rigid SACH heel cushion	Inadequate muscle control Weak internal rotators Short residual limb
Forward trunk flexion	Socket too large Poor suspension Knee instability	Hip flexion contracture Weak hip extensors Pain with ischial weight bearing Inability to initiate prosthetic knee flexion
Medial or lateral whip	Knee rotation to great Tight socket fit Valgus in the prosthetic knee Improper alignment of toe break	Weak hip rotators Knee instability
Foot drag	Inadequate suspension of the prosthesis Prosthesis too long	Weakness in the hip abductors or ankle plantarflexors on the contralateral side
Uneven arm swing	An improperly fitting socket causing limb discomfort	Inadequate balance Uneven timing

Data from Dutton M: McGraw-Hill's NPTE (National Physical Therapy Examination). New York, McGraw-Hill, 2009

TABLE 14-2	**Gait Problems of the Below Knee Amputee**	
Problem	**Cause**	**Solution**
Delayed, short, and limited knee flexion after heel strike	Heel wedge is too soft; foot is too far anterior	Stiffen heel wedge; move foot posterior
Toe remains off floor after heel strike	Heel wedge is too stiff; foot is too anterior; there is too much dorsiflexion	Soften heel wedge; move foot posterior; plantarflex foot
Knee remains extended throughout stance phase	Too much plantar flexion	Dorsiflex foot
"Hillclimbing" sensation near end of stance phase	Foot is too far anterior; too much plantar flexion	Move foot posterior; dorsiflex foot
Knee is too forcefully and rapidly flexed after heel strike. High pressure against anterior-distal tibia at heel strike	Heel wedge is too stiff; foot is too far dorsiflexed	Soften heel; move foot anterior; plantarflex foot
Hips level, but prosthesis appears short	Foot too far posterior; foot too dorsiflexed	Move foot anterior; plantarflex foot
Toe off floor as patient stands or knee flexed too much	Foot too dorsiflexed	Plantarflex foot
Uneven heel rise	Knee joint may have inadequate friction; there may be an inadequate extension aid	Adjust accordingly
Foot slap	Plantar flexion resistance is too low	Increase plantar flexion resistance

Data from Dutton M: McGraw-Hill's NPTE (National Physical Therapy Examination). New York, McGraw-Hill, 2009

Rigid Elbow Hinges

Constructed of more rigid metals and composite plastics, rigid hinges are used for midforearm to short transradial amputations with normal range of motion at the elbow.

Transradial Harness and Controls

The function of a harness is to suspend the prosthesis from the shoulder so that the socket is held firmly in place on the stump. Movement of the scapulothoracic region, scapula abduction or protraction, and shoulder flexion increase the pull on the control cable or create excursion, which in turn controls the terminal device or elbow joint as the amputee wishes.

Figure 8 Harness

This is the most commonly used harness. The axilla loop acts as a reaction point for the transmission of body forces to the terminal device.

Chest Strap Harness

This type of harness is used when the amputee cannot tolerate an axilla loop, or if greater suspension is required for heavy lifting. The chest strap harness is not appropriate for women because it has a tendency to rotate up on the chest when excessive forces are applied to the control cable.

Figure 9 Harness

This type of harness is typically employed with the self-suspending prosthesis and consists of an axilla loop and a control attachment strap, which provides greater freedom and comfort over conventional harnesses.

Elbow Units

External

These units are used with an elbow disarticulation prosthesis with an outside locking hinge system.

Internal

This type of unit is designed for a transhumeral amputee with at least 2 inches of the distal humerus removed. It is designed with the space required to accommodate an inside locking of the unit, which allows the user to lock the elbow in 11 different positions of flexion.

Use of the Prosthesis

At the earliest opportunity, the amputee must learn how to don and doff the prosthesis independently and to check the fit. Correct operation of the prosthesis can take some time and patience. Gross movements are typically taught initially, and as control of the prosthesis improves, finer motor movements are introduced. Use training emphasizes employing the prosthesis as an assistive device, complementing maneuvers of the sound hand. Skills to practice include:

- Washing the face
- Drinking from a cup
- Dressing, including practice with buttoning, using a zipper, and managing other garment fasteners
- Writing
- Dining
- Advanced activities as appropriate (driving, bicycling, playing a musical instrument)

Orthotics

An orthoses is an external appliance worn to restrict or assist motion or to transfer load from one area to another. Orthoses are designed to promote control, correction, stabilization, or dynamic movement.[8]

> **● Key Point** Note the following definitions:
> - *Splint:* An orthoses intended for temporary use.
> - *Orthotic:* An adjective, often used as a noun.
> - *Orthotist:* The healthcare professional who designs, fabricates, and fits orthoses of the limbs and trunk.
> - *Pedorthist:* The healthcare professional who designs, fabricates, and fits only shoes and foot orthoses.

Lower Limb Orthoses: Components/Terminology

Foot Orthoses

The primary goal of a foot orthoses is to get the subtalar joint to function around neutral position and to facilitate pronation during the initial part of stance and supination during the latter part of stance. In addition, foot orthoses can be used to treat specific symptoms or to alleviate symptoms by altering the mechanical function of the subtalar neutral position.

> **● Key Point** Foot orthoses can be classified into three general categories:
> - *Soft:* Flexible foam type materials provide cushioning, improve shock absorption, decrease shear forces, and are used to redistribute plantar pressures, affording comfort with limited joint control.
> - *Semirigid:* A combination of soft and rigid materials including cork, rubber, or plastics providing some flexibility and shock absorption; designed to balance or control the foot.
> - *Rigid:* Strong and durable materials such as plastics or metals are used to assist with transfer of weight, to stabilize flexible deformities, and to control abnormal motion.

Shoe Modifications

Shoe modifications can be either internal or external.

Internal Modifications

Internal modifications involve a corrective adaptation that is fixed inside the shoe. Three of the more common internal modifications include:

- *Medial longitudinal arch support (scaphoid pad):* A rubber or leather pad often used in conjunction with a medial longitudinal counter to prevent depression of the subtalar joint by posting the sustentaculum tali and the navicular tuberosity.
- *Metatarsal pad:* A rubber or semisoft pad that is placed at the apex of the metatarsal shafts, relieving the metatarsal heads from excessive pressure and supporting the collapsed transverse metatarsal arch.
- *Heel cushion:* A viscoelastic material placed in the heel cup of an orthosis directly into the shoe to accommodate for the inability to achieve a neutral position in the sagittal plane, to achieve shock attenuation, and to relieve calcaneal stress fractures or heel pain.

External Modifications

External modifications involve a corrective adaptation that is fixed outside of the shoe. External modifications include corrections to the heel or outsole:

Heel Corrections Types of heel corrections include:

- *Medial heel wedge:* A leather wedged insert incorporated into the heel; used to elevate and maintain the medial margin of the shoe to decrease hyperpronation and designed to shift the weight laterally.

- *Lateral heel wedge:* A leather wedged insert incorporated into the heel; used to elevate and maintain the lateral margin of the shoe to decrease supination and designed to shift the weight medially.
- *Thomas heel:* The heel of the shoe extends anteriorly 1 inch on the medial aspect to assist with balance, support the longitudinal arch, and assist in maintaining the subtalar joint in a neutral position. The Thomas heel is often coupled with medial heel wedges to assist with stability during ambulation.
- *Reverse Thomas heel:* The opposite of the Thomas heel, the reverse Thomas heel is extended 1 inch on the lateral aspect to assist with balance and subtalar joint alignment. It is used in conjunction with lateral heel wedges.
- *Heel flare:* Either a medial or lateral extension of the shoe heel that broadens the base of support for greater ability.

Outsole Corrections Types of outsole corrections include:

- *Medial sole wedge:* Used to correct forefoot eversion and promote inversion.
- *Lateral sole wedge:* Used to correct forefoot inversion and promote eversion.
- *Rocker bottom:* Positioned posterior to the metatarsal heads to redistribute body weight over the entire plantar surface, reduce stress to the forefoot, and assist in rollover during ambulation.
- *Metatarsal bar:* Positioned just posterior to the metatarsal heads to transfer the forces from the metatarsophalangeal joints to the metatarsal shafts.

Ankle–Foot Orthoses

Ankle–foot orthoses (AFO) are designed to control the rate and direction of tibial advancement and to maintain an adequate base of support while meeting the specific demands for functional gait. There are several designs of AFOs.

Shoe and Foot Attachments
Types of shoe and foot attachments include:

- *Stirrup (solid):* A one-piece attachment with a solid metal plate riveted to the sole of the shoe, creating a U-shaped frame that forms the medial and lateral upright.
- *Stirrup (split):* A two-piece attachment with a metal plate riveted to the sole of the shoe that has two channels to permit donning and doffing of the removable metal uprights.
- *Caliper:* Very similar to the split stirrup with a metal plate riveted to the sole of the shoe, except that the uprights are slightly lighter and round.
- *Molded shoe insert:* A plastic custom-formed plate that attaches directly to the metal uprights with a calf band for proximal support.

Ankle Joints and Controls
Types of ankle joints and controls include:

- *Plantar flexion stop:* A posterior stop restricting plantar flexion but allowing full dorsiflexion.
- *Dorsiflexion stop:* An anterior stop that restricts dorsiflexion but allows full plantar flexion.
- *Limited motion stop:* The ankle joint that limits motion in all directions.
- *Free motion joint:* Ankle joint that provides medial and lateral stability from the uprights while permitting full plantar/dorsiflexion. Plastic AFOs use lightweight joints that permit free motion.

Assists
Types of assists include:

- *Dorsiflexion assist:* A posterior spring assist with dorsiflexion that permits full plantar flexion, which compresses the spring during the early stance phase of gait.
- *Dorsiflexion, plantar flexion assist (dual channel) or bi-channel adjustable ankle locks (BiCAAL):* Joints with an anterior and posterior spring that assist with the plantar and dorsiflexion to varying degrees according to the adjusted settings of the springs.

Varus and Valgus Correction
Types of varus and valgus corrections include:

- *Medial T-strap:* A leather strap that arises from the shoe quarter covering the medial malleolus and buckles to the lateral upright, pushing laterally to correct a valgus (eversion) deformity.
- *Lateral T-strap:* A leather strap that arises from the shoe quarter covering the lateral malleolus and buckles to the medial upright, pushing medially to correct a varus (inversion) deformity.
- *Supramalleolus orthosis (SMO):* A low-profile supramalleolar design for subtalar joint control to limit varus or valgus. The ankle joint also assists with dorsiflexion during swing.

Knee-Ankle-Foot Orthoses

The primary purpose of most knee orthotic devices is to provide knee control in one or more planes. Types of knee joints include:

- *Single-axis joint:* Designed to behave like a hinge, preventing movement in the coronal plane, providing medial/lateral stability, while permitting movement in the sagittal plane.
- *Offset axis joint:* A single-axis joint design with the axis set further posterior from the weight line than the standard single-axis joint, promoting maximal knee extension during weight bearing without having to use a mechanical lock.
- *Polycentric axis joint:* Designed to mimic the instantaneous center of rotation present in the anatomic knee. The two-geared mechanical joint is still confined to a uniplanar path.

Knee-Locking Devices

Types of knee-locking devices include:

- *Drop ring locks:* The most common locking system. It has small rings that slide down over the proximal portion of a single axis knee joint to maintain full knee extension during standing. It may be raised manually to release for sitting or free knee flexion and extension.
- *Spring-loaded pull rod:* A spring system with a control rod that can be extended to a height of convenient reach to permit easier release of the locking mechanism. It is often prescribed for clients with poor balance or dexterity issues.
- *Pawl or bail locks:* Levers positioned posterior to the knee that provide easy release of the locking mechanism for sitting. Typically prescribed for patients with extreme balance disturbances or who cannot free their hands to operate a locking system while sitting.
- *Adjustable knee lock:* A variety of mechanisms are available to preset the knee-lock range of motion to a specific degree of flexion or extension.

Hip-Knee-Ankle-Foot Orthoses

Hip Joints

Types of hip joints include:

- *Single axis:* Most commonly, hip joints are single-axis joints permitting flexion and extension while restricting abduction, adduction, and rotation.

- *Double axis:* The double axis locks two planes of motion with an adjustable start to set limits as needed in each direction (flexion, extension, abduction, adduction).

Hip Locks

Types of hip locks include:

- *Drop locks:* Similar to the knee drop lock, a small ring slides down over the axis to lock the joint in extension while standing.
- *Two-position hip locks:* Designed to lock in full extension and 90 degrees of hip flexion, this locking system proves to be a great asset when poor sitting balance is present.

Pelvic Bands

Types of pelvic bands include:

- *Unilateral band:* Used when a single limb orthosis requires proximal stability. A rigid band can be incorporated that encircles the pelvis between the iliac crest and the greater trochanter, with a flexible belt that continues around the waist.
- *Bilateral band:* Most commonly the bilateral pelvic band is used for bilateral heel-knee-ankle-foot orthoses (HKAFOs) in which the padded metal band encompasses the pelvis just about the buttock with a posterior band positioned over the sacrum.
- *Double or pelvic girdle:* When maximal control is required, the entire proximal pelvis is encapsulated from the iliac crest to just proximal to the greater trochanter with varying support posteriorly depending on strength and pelvis stability.
- *Silesian belt:* A flexible strap that attaches to a proximal portion of the orthosis and encircles the pelvis, assisting in stabilizing the orthosis and providing suspension.

Reciprocal Gait Orthosis

The reciprocal gait orthosis (RGO) is designed to permit a reciprocal gait, as opposed to the traditional swing-through gait used with HKAFOs. The types of disabilities that can often benefit from these devices include spinal cord injury levels as high as C8 to T12–L1, myelodysplasia, osteogenesis imperfecta, spina bifida, paraplegia, muscular dystrophy (not the Duchenne type), and cerebral palsy. The reciprocal motion is facilitated by a variety of mechanisms:

- A cable system that couples the passive hip flexion and extension movements that advance the lower limbs in a reciprocal fashion.

- A bar balance system (isocentric system) located at the lumbosacral level of the orthoses, which provides the reciprocating hip flexion action.
- A low-profile push-pull cable system (ARGO) that not only provides a reciprocating motion at the hip but also assists with standing through a hip and knee extension assist mechanism.

Standing Frame and Swivel Walker

The standing frame, designed for children, consists of broad-based, posterior nonarticulated uprights extending from a flat base to a mid-torso chest band, and a posterior thoracolumbar band. The shoes are strapped to the base of the frame. A similar orthosis is the Swivel Walker, which is made in both child and adult sizes. The major difference is the base, which has two distal plates that rock slightly to enable a swiveling gait.

Parapodium

The parapodium differs from the standing frame by virtue of joints that permit the wearer to sit. Parapodiums permit the wearer to stand without crutch support, freeing the hands for play or vocational activities.

Thoracic, Lumbosacral Orthoses

There are two general classifications of thoracic, lumbosacral orthoses: flexible and rigid.

Flexible

Flexible types of orthoses include:

- *Sacroiliac corset (binder):* Encircles the waist from the iliac crest to the greater trochanter, extending anteriorly to the symphysis pubis to promote stability for patients with postpartum or sacroiliac instability.
- *Lumbosacral corset:* Primarily designed for patients with back pain.
- *Thoracolumbosacral corset:* Similar to the lumbosacral corset, but includes a shoulder strap to restrict spinal motion to the thoracic region as well as to the lumbar region.

Rigid

Rigid types of orthoses include:

- *Lumbosacral orthosis (Williams):* Incorporates a single three-point pressure system to limit trunk extension in the lumbar spine and to increase intra-abdominal pressure. Lordosis is decreased to limit lumbar extension, while the pelvic and thoracic bands resist the medial forces that tend to limit lateral trunk motions.

- *Thoracic-lumbosacral orthoses:*
  - *Taylor (flexion/extension control):* Designed with two three-point pressure systems, which limit both flexion and extension of the lumbar and thoracic spine.
  - *Jewett (flexion control):* Incorporates a three-point pressure system using two pads to promote hyperextension and thus restricting forward flexion.
  - *Plastic body jacket (flexion-extension-lateral-rotary control):* A well-fitted body jacket designed to restrict motion in all planes. Frequently used postsurgically or following an acute trauma.

Cervical Orthoses

Types of cervical orthoses include:

- *Soft collar:* Provides mechanical restraint for cervical flexion and extension and, to a lesser degree, side bending and rotation.
- *Hard collars (Philadelphia collar):* Provide more rigid stabilization of the cervical spine and typically offer some type of chin and occipital support.
- *Halo-cervical orthoses:* Provide the greatest reduction in cervical mobilization. A cranial ring is secured to the skull using four metal pins. The ring is attached by four metal bars to a plastic vest and is worn continuously.

Upper Limb Orthoses

The purpose of the majority of upper limb orthoses is to position the hand in the most functional position and/or to create usable prehension.

Hand and Wrist Orthoses

Types of hand and wrist orthoses include:

- *Basic or short opponens:* Designed to immobilize the first carpometacarpal (CMC) and metacarpophalangeal (MCP) joints and position the thumb in opposition and abduction to maintain the webspace and the architecture of the hand for future procedures.
- *Long opponens splint (volar forearm wrist orthosis):* Designed to immobilize the first carpometacarpal (CMC) and metacarpophalangeal (MCP) joints and position the thumb in extension and opposition, preserving the webspace.
- *Volar forearm static wrist hand orthosis (resting hand splint):* Designed to place the hand and wrist in a neutral, functional, or lumbrical

position, with the MCP joints flexed to 60 to 90 degrees, and the IP and PIP joints flexed to 0 to 45 degrees. The wrist is in slight extension to neutral.

- *Wrist-driven prehension (tenodesis) orthosis:* Designed specifically for patients with spinal cord injury at the C6 to C7 level and who have the 3-/5 to 3+/5 extensor carpi radialis muscle strength.

Elbow Orthoses
Types of elbow orthoses include:

- *Static orthosis:* Designed to restrict motion and promote tissue healing.
- *Dynamic orthosis:* Provides a low load with a prolonged stretch. Often used for patients with burns and elbow contractures.
- *Shoulder-elbow-wrist (airplane) orthosis:* Used to protect the soft tissues of the shoulder and prevent contractures. The shoulder is abducted 70 to 90 degrees, with the majority of body weight borne on the iliac crest and lateral trunk.

Summary

The use of orthotics and prosthetics, as well as the fabrication and custom fitting of artificial limbs and orthopedic braces, continues to emerge as an important adjunct to physical therapy interventions. The correct prescription of an orthotic or prosthetic can help amputees and individuals with musculoskeletal disabilities and injuries improve their quality of life and regain their self-confidence.

REVIEW Questions

1. What is the difference between an amputation and a disarticulation?
2. The primary benefit of residual limb wrapping following lower extremity amputation is to:
   a. Prevent lymphedema
   b. Prevent contractures
   c. Prepare the limb for the prosthesis
   d. None of the above
3. In terms of the length of the prosthesis, what would cause the vaulting phenomena in a patient with an above-knee prosthesis?
4. Which of the following advantages does the valve have in the anteromedial inferior

aspect of the thigh portion in an above-knee prosthesis?
   a. It eliminates air during the swing phase.
   b. It eliminates air during the stance phase.
   c. It gains air during the swing phase.
   d. It gains air during the stance phase.
5. A patient with a transfemoral amputation and an above-knee prosthesis demonstrates knee instability while standing. His knee buckles easily when he shifts his weight. What could be the cause of his problem?
   a. The prosthetic knee is set too far anterior to the TKA line.
   b. The prosthetic knee is set too far posterior to the TKA line.
   c. It is a problem of phantom sensation.
   d. None of the above.
6. In order to increase the knee stability of an above-knee prosthesis wearer, should you move the TKA line posterior to the knee joint or anterior to it?
7. You have been asked to fit a 62-year-old patient with a transfemoral amputation with a temporary prosthesis containing a SACH prosthetic foot. This prosthetic foot:
   a. Allows full sagittal and frontal plane motion
   b. Permits sagittal plane motion only
   c. Allows limited sagittal plane motion with a small amount of mediolateral motion
   d. Allows no motion
8. Which of the following statements does not describe the characteristics of the wall design of a quadrilateral socket?
   a. The anterior and lateral walls are 2½ to 3 inches higher than the posterior and medial walls.
   b. The posterior and lateral walls are 2 inches higher than the medial and anterior walls.
   c. The medial wall is 2½ inches higher than the posterior wall, and the anterior and lateral walls are the same height.
   d. The height of the posterior wall is 2 inches lower than all the other walls.
9. You are assessing the functional level of a patient with a unilateral transfemoral transtibial amputation using the Medicare and Medicaid classification. The patient demonstrates the ability or potential to use a prosthesis for transfer or ambulation on a level surface at a fixed cadence. What functional level does this correspond with?

10. A common above-knee amputee gait deviation is lateral trunk bending. Which of the following is not a cause?
   a. Weak hip abductor
   b. Weak hip adductor
   c. Pain of the stump
   d. Abducted socket

11. A common above-knee amputee deviation is circumduction. Which of the following is not a cause of this deviation?
   a. Insufficient knee flexion
   b. Socket is too large
   c. Excessive plantar flexion
   d. Inadequate suspension

12. A common above-knee amputee gait deviation is wide base walking. Which of the following is not a cause of this deviation?
   a. The prosthesis is too short.
   b. The mechanical hip joint is set in abduction.
   c. The patient has pain in the groin area.
   d. None of the above.

13. The SACH prosthesis is defined as:
   a. Solid ankle cork heel
   b. Solid ankle cushioned heel
   c. Soft ankle cushioned heel
   d. Soft ankle custom heel

14. Upon assessing a patient's gait using her prosthetic device, you notice that the socket has a poor fit and appears to have a weak suspension system with the knee friction being too soft. Which of the following gait deviations would you likely observe?
   a. Lateral whip
   b. Pistoning of the socket
   c. Circumduction
   d. None of the above

15. You have been asked to teach a patient in a wheelchair how to descend from a curb. Which is the safest method?
   a. Tilt the trunk backward and go down backward
   b. Tilt the trunk backward and go down forward
   c. Tilt the trunk forward and go down forward
   d. Tilt the trunk forward and go down backward

16. You are treating a patient with right hemiplegia. The most appropriate feature you would expect to find on the wheelchair would be:
   a. Detachable arm rests
   b. Elevating leg rests
   c. A 17-inch seat height
   d. A feeding tray

References

1. Gailey RS: Considerations in treating amputees, in Prentice WE, Voight ML (eds): Techniques in Musculoskeletal Rehabilitation. New York, McGraw-Hill, 2001, pp 715–743
2. May BJ: Amputation, in O'Sullivan SB, Schmitz TJ (eds): Physical Rehabilitation (ed 5). Philadelphia, F. A. Davis, 2007, pp 1031–1055
3. White SC: Health Care Financing Administration Common Procedure Coding System. Washington, DC, US Government Printing Office, 2001
4. Wu YJ, Chen SY, Lin MC, et al: Energy expenditure of wheeling and walking during prosthetic rehabilitation in a woman with bilateral transfemoral amputations. Arch Phys Med Rehabil. 82:265–269, 2001
5. Traugh GH, Corcoran PJ, Reyes RL: Energy expenditure of ambulation in patients with above-knee amputations. Arch Phys Med Rehabil. 56:67–71, 1975
6. Edelstein JE: Prosthetics, in O'Sullivan SB, Schmitz TJ (eds): Physical Rehabilitation (ed 5). Philadelphia, F. A. Davis, 2007, pp 1251–1286
7. Ellis W, Kishner S: Gait analysis after amputation, Available at: http://www.emedicine.com/orthoped/topic633.htm, 2004
8. Gailey RS: Orthotics in Rehabilitation, in Prentice WE, Voight ML (eds): Techniques in Musculoskeletal Rehabilitation. New York, McGraw-Hill, 2001, pp 325–346

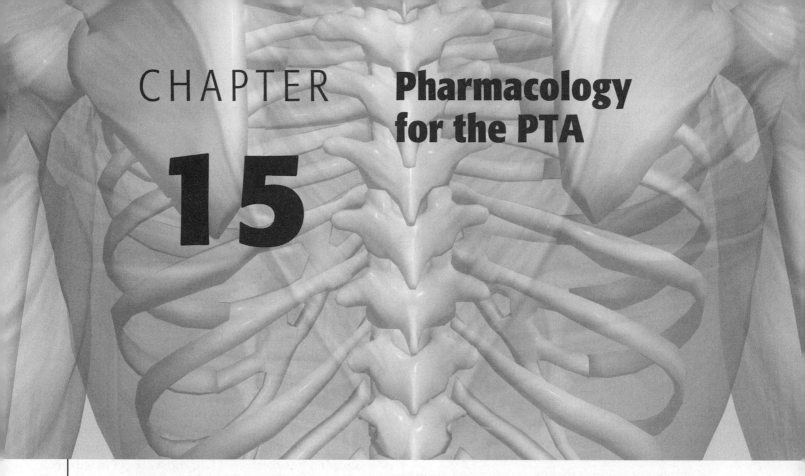

Pharmacology for the PTA

15

Pharmacology is defined as the study of how chemical substances affect living tissue. A drug is any substance that can be used to modify a chemical process or processes in the body—for example, to treat an illness, relieve a symptom, enhance a performance or ability, or alter states of mind.

> **● Key Point** Note the following terminology:
> - *Drug:* Any substance that can be used to modify a chemical process or processes in the body—for example, to treat an illness, relieve a symptom, enhance a performance or ability, or alter states of mind.
> - *Pharmacology:* The science of studying both the mechanisms and the actions of drugs, usually in animal models of disease, to evaluate their potential therapeutic value.
> - *Pharmacy:* The mixing and dispensing of drugs, and the monitoring of drug prescriptions for appropriateness and the monitoring of patients for adverse drug interactions.
> - *Pharmacotherapeutics:* The use of chemical agents to prevent, diagnose, and cure disease.
> - *Pharmacokinetics:* The study of how the body absorbs, distributes, metabolizes, and eliminates a drug.
> - *Pharmacodynamics:* The study of the biochemical and physiologic effects of drugs and their mechanisms of action at the cellular or organ level.
> - *Pharmacotherapy:* The treatment of a disease or condition with drugs.
> - *Pharmacogenetics:* The study of how variation in human genes leads to variations in our response to drugs and helps direct therapeutics according to a person's genotype.
> - *Toxicology:* The study of the negative effects of chemicals on living things, including cells, plants, animals, and humans.

Pharmacotherapy

Although physical therapists and assistants are not permitted by law to prescribe or dispense prescription drugs, an understanding of the potential effects of certain types of drugs commonly encountered during the rehabilitation process is essential.[1] Drug therapy is one of the mainstays of modern treatments, and PTAs often encounter patients who are taking various medications.

These medications may be administered to treat pre-existing conditions that are not directly related to the condition being treated with physical therapy but can nonetheless have an impact on the patient's response to rehabilitation.[2] As PTAs monitor the effects of their interventions, they must also understand the effects and potential interactions of all available resources, including pharmacological interventions, offered by other members of the healthcare team. Controlled substances are drugs classified according to their potential for abuse. A black box warning (also sometimes called a *black label warning* or *boxed warning*), named for the black border that usually surrounds the text of the warning, appears on the package insert for prescription drugs that carry a significant risk of serious or even life-threatening adverse effects. The U.S. Food and Drug Administration (FDA) can require a pharmaceutical company to place a black box warning on the labeling of a prescription drug or in literature describing it. It is the strongest warning that the FDA requires. It is important for the PTA to have a working knowledge of pharmacology because of the number of drugs currently on the market and the number of physical therapy patients that are likely to have been prescribed medications. Some beneficial effects of the drugs may be enhanced by physical therapy interventions, but in other cases the interventions may have negative consequences.

● **Key Point** In the absence of data supporting a therapeutic benefit for a drug, toxicity associated with any drug, including herbal supplements, can still occur.

Musculoskeletal Pharmacology

The following discussion emphasizes drugs that are prescribed to control pain and/or inflammation.

Narcotic/Opioid Analgesics

The term *narcotic* specifically refers to any substance that induces sleep. Most of the narcotics used in medicine are referred to as *opioids*, as they are derived directly from opium or are synthetic opiates. Opioids decrease the perception of pain rather than eliminate or reduce the painful stimulus. Inducing slight euphoria, opioid agonists reduce the sensitivity to exogenous stimuli. Opioid toxicity characteristically presents with a depressed level of consciousness. Opiate toxicity should be suspected when the clinical triad of central nervous system depression, respiratory depression, and pupillary constriction is present. Drowsiness, red and swollen eyes, and euphoria are frequently seen. Other important presenting signs are ventricular arrhythmias, acute mental status changes, and seizures.

Non-Opioid Analgesics

Cyclooxygenase (COX) is an enzyme that is responsible for formation of important biological mediators called *prostanoids*, including prostaglandins, prostacyclin, and thromboxane. Pharmacological inhibition of COX can provide relief from the symptoms of inflammation and pain. The main COX inhibitors are the nonsteroidal anti-inflammatory drugs (NSAIDs), including ibuprofen, Voltaren, and many others.

● **Key Point** Different tissues express varying levels of COX-1 and COX-2. Although both enzymes act basically in the same fashion, selective inhibition can make a difference in terms of side effects.

The NSAIDs are not selective and inhibit all types of COX. The resulting inhibition of prostaglandin and thromboxane synthesis has the effect of reduced inflammation as well as antipyretic, antithrombotic, and analgesic effects. The most frequent adverse effects of this class of medication are an irritation of the gastric mucosa—a direct effect of inhibition of prostaglandin synthesis, which normally has a protective role in the gastrointestinal tract.

● **Key Point** NSAIDs currently are the medication of choice to help control the inflammatory process at initial presentation. It has not been proven that these agents have a specific effect on fibroblast function or on connective tissue healing.[3,4] However, the analgesic effects of the anti-inflammatory medications make it easier to rehabilitate injured structures, as well as the muscles in the surrounding kinematic chain, and can help curb further inflammatory response as patients increase their activity level.[5,6]

NSAIDs also may alter kidney blood flow by interfering with the synthesis of prostaglandins in the kidney involved in the autoregulation of blood flow and glomerular filtration.[7]

Because COX-2 is usually specific to inflamed tissue, there is much less gastric irritation associated with COX-2 inhibitors, with a decreased risk of peptic ulceration. The selectivity of COX-2 does not seem to negate other side effects of NSAIDs, most notably an increased risk of renal failure, and there is evidence that indicates an increase in the risk for heart attack, thrombosis, and stroke through an increase of thromboxane unbalanced by prostacyclin (which is reduced by COX-2 inhibition).

Corticosteroids

Corticosteroids are natural anti-inflammatory hormones produced by the adrenal glands under the control of the hypothalamus. The injection of corticosteroids can be used to decrease the pain at the site of inflammation, at least temporarily. Synthetic corticosteroids (cortisone, dexamethasone) are commonly used to treat a wide range of immunological and inflammatory musculoskeletal conditions. Corticosteroids exert their anti-inflammatory effects by binding to a high-affinity intracellular cytoplasmic receptor present in all human cells.[8] As a result, these agents are capable of producing undesirable and sometimes severe systemic adverse effects that may offset clinical gains in many patients. The side effects of corticosteroids emulate from exogenous hypercortisolism, which is similar to the clinical syndrome of Cushing disease (see Chapter 9).

Muscle Relaxants

Muscle relaxants are thought to decrease muscle tone without impairment in motor function by acting centrally to depress polysynaptic reflexes. As muscle guarding and spasm accompany many musculoskeletal injuries, it was originally thought that these drugs, by eliminating the spasm and guarding, would facilitate the progression of a rehabilitation program. However, other drugs with sedative properties, such as barbiturates, also depress polysynaptic reflexes, making it difficult to assess if centrally acting skeletal muscle relaxants actually are muscle relaxants as opposed to nonspecific sedatives.[10]

Neurologic System Pharmacology

Anti-Anxiety Medications

Selective Serotonin Reuptake Inhibitors

Selective serotonin reuptake inhibitors (SSRIs) are commonly prescribed psychotherapeutic agents. The most serious drug-related adverse effect of SSRIs is the potential to produce serotonin syndrome (SS), which is characterized by mental status changes, neuromuscular dysfunction, and autonomic instability, and is thought to be secondary to excessive serotonin activity in the spinal cord and brain. Symptoms attributed to serotonin excess may include the following:

- Restlessness
- Hallucinations
- Shivering
- Diaphoresis
- Nausea
- Diarrhea
- Headache

Monoamine Oxidase Inhibitors

Neurotransmitters are generally monoamines. When released into the synaptic space, neurotransmitters are either reabsorbed into the proximal nerve or destroyed by monoamine oxidase (MAO) in the synaptic cleft. Circulating monoamines, such as epinephrine, norepinephrine, and dopamine, are inactivated when they pass through the liver. Monoamine oxidase inhibitors (MAOIs) indirectly degrade the monamines and inhibit breakdown of the neurotransmitters norepinephrine, serotonin, and dopamine, resulting in hypertension, tachycardia, tremors, seizures, and hyperthermia.

Benzodiazepines

Benzodiazepines (BZDs) are sedative-hypnotic agents that are used for a variety of situations, including seizure control, anxiety, alcohol withdrawal, insomnia, drug-associated agitation, and as muscle relaxants (antispasticity agents) and preanesthetic agents. They also are frequently combined with other medications for conscious sedation before procedures or interventions. BZDs exert their action by potentiating the activity of GABA, the major inhibitory neurotransmitter in the CNS. Enhanced GABA neurotransmission results in sedation, striated muscle relaxation, anxiolysis, and anticonvulsant effects. Stimulation of peripheral nervous system (PNS) GABA receptors may cause decreased cardiac contractility, vasodilation, and enhanced perfusion.

Sedative-Hypnotics

Sedative-hypnotics are a group of drugs that cause CNS depression. Benzodiazepines (see previous section) and barbiturates are the most commonly used agents in this class. Most sedative-hypnotics stimulate the activity of GABA, the principal inhibitory neurotransmitter in the CNS. Mild toxicity resembles ethanol intoxication. Moderate poisoning leads to respiratory depression and hyporeflexia. Severe poisoning leads to flaccid areflexic coma, apnea, and hypotension.

Antidepressants

Tricyclic Antidepressants

Tricyclic antidepressants (TCAs) are used in the treatment of depression, chronic pain, and enuresis (involuntary discharge of urine, especially while asleep). Patients with depression and those with chronic pain are at high risk for abuse, misuse, and overdosing of these drugs. TCAs affect the cardiovascular, central nervous, pulmonary, and gastrointestinal systems. The toxic effects on the myocardium result in a slower myocardium depolarization that leads to arrhythmia, myocardial depression, and hypotension. CNS toxicity manifests as confusion, hallucinations, ataxia, seizures, and coma. The effects on the pulmonary system include pulmonary edema, adult respiratory distress syndrome, and aspiration pneumonitis. Finally, TCAs cause a slowing of the gastrointestinal (GI) system, which results in delayed gastric emptying, decreased motility, and prolonged transit time.

Antiepileptic Drugs

Many structures and processes are involved in the development of a seizure, including neurons, ion channels, receptors, glia, and inhibitory and excitatory synapses. Antiepileptic drugs (AEDs) are designed to modify these processes to favor inhibition over excitation in order to stop or prevent seizure activity. AEDs can produce dose-related adverse effects, which include dizziness, diplopia, nausea, ataxia, and blurred vision.

Neuroleptics (Antipsychotics)

The term *neuroleptic* refers to the effects on cognition and behavior of antipsychotic drugs that reduce confusion, delusions, hallucinations, and psychomotor agitation in patients with psychoses. Neuroleptics also are used as sedatives, for their antiemetic properties, to control hiccups, to treat migraine headaches, as antidotes for drug-induced psychosis, and in conjunction with opioid analgesia. Any of the acute adverse effects of neuroleptics may occur in these settings. Neuroleptics are also utilized in conjunction with antidepressants, as mood stabilizers when psychotic symptoms are present, or to enhance the effect of other medications when attempting to control mania. Generally, all neuroleptic medications are capable of causing the following symptoms:

- *Hypotension:* Phenothiazines are potent alpha-adrenergic blockers that result in significant orthostatic hypotension, even in therapeutic doses for some patients. In overdose, hypotension may be severe.
- *Anticholinergic effects:* Neuroleptic agent toxicity can result in tachycardia, hyperthermia, urinary retention, ileus, mydriasis, toxic psychosis, and hot, dry, flushed skin.
- *Extrapyramidal symptoms:* Alteration in the normal balance between central acetylcholine and dopamine transmission can produce dystonia, torticollis, acute parkinsonism, akathisia, and other movement disorders.
- *Neuroleptic malignant syndrome:* All of the major tranquilizers have been implicated in the development of neuroleptic malignant syndrome (NMS), a life-threatening derangement that affects multiple organ systems and results in significant mortality.
- *Seizures:* Most major tranquilizers lower the seizure threshold and can result in seizures at high doses and in susceptible individuals.
- *Hypothermia:* Certain major tranquilizers prevent shivering, limiting the body's ability to generate heat.
- *Cardiac effects:* Prolongation of the QT interval and QRS can result in arrhythmias.
- *Respiratory depression:* Hypoxia and aspiration of gastric contents can occur in children and in mixed overdose.

Spasticity

The use of oral medications for the treatment of spasticity[11] may be very effective. At high dosages, however, oral medications can cause unwanted adverse effects that include sedation as well as changes in mood and cognition. These adverse effects preclude their extensive use in children, since the intellectual function of the majority of children with spasticity is at best precarious, and sedation inevitably results in some degree of impaired learning or school performance.

- *Benzodiazepines (diazepam and clonazepam):* These drugs may improve passive range of motion and reduce hyperreflexia, painful spasms, and anxiety. Sedation, weakness, hypotension, adverse gastrointestinal effects, memory impairment, incoordination, confusion, depression, and ataxia may occur. Tolerance and dependency can occur, and withdrawal phenomena, notably seizures, have been associated with abrupt cessation of therapy.

- *Baclofen (oral and intrathecal pump):* Studies show that baclofen improves clonus, flexor spasm frequency, and joint range of motion, resulting in improved functional status. Adverse effects include sedation, ataxia, weakness, and fatigue.
- *Dantrolene sodium:* Dantrolene sodium is useful for spasticity of supraspinal origin, particularly in patients with cerebral palsy or traumatic brain injury. It decreases muscle tone, clonus, and muscle spasm. Adverse effects include generalized weakness, including weakness of the respiratory muscles, drowsiness, dizziness, weakness, fatigue, and diarrhea.
- *Tizanidine:* The antispasticity effects of tizanidine are the probable result of inhibition of the H-reflex. Dry mouth, somnolence, asthenia, and dizziness are the most common adverse events associated with tizanidine.

Cardiovascular System Pharmacology
Refer to **Table 15-1**.

Pulmonary System Pharmacology
The delivery of a drug to the lungs allows the medication to interact directly with the diseased tissue and reduces the risk of adverse effects, specifically systemic reactions, and allows for the reduction of dose compared with oral administration. Most of the inhaled drugs are administered through a pressurized metered-dose inhaler. Dry pounder inhalers or breath-activated devices are delivery devices that scatter a fine powder into the lungs by means of a brisk inhalation. The other major drug delivery system for pulmonary problems is the nebulizer, a device that dispenses liquid medications as a mist of extremely fine particles in oxygen or room air that is inhaled.

Bacterial Infections
Bacteria are unicellular organisms that consist of a cell wall, sometimes a membrane, DNA without a nuclear envelope, and protoplasm containing metabolites and enzymes. Drugs that affect these microorganisms are called *antibacterial* drugs and are relatively specific for bacteria only. Most antibacterial drugs have five major sites of action as follows:

1. Inhibition of synthesis and/or damage to the bacterial cell wall.
2. Inhibition of synthesis and/or damage to the cytoplasmic membrane.
3. Modification of synthesis and/or metabolism of microbial nucleic acids.
4. Inhibition or modification of microbial protein synthesis by disrupting ribosomal function.
5. Inhibition or modification of microbial cell metabolism.

Antibacterials/antibiotics are among the most frequently prescribed medications in modern medicine. Although there are well over 100 antibiotics, the majority come from only a few types of drugs. The main classes of antibiotics are outlined in **Table 15-2**. In orthopedics, antibiotics are commonly used to treat general bone (e.g., osteomyelitis) and joint infections (e.g., septic arthritis), for preoperative surgical prophylaxis, and for fracture management with internal fixation.

> ● **Key Point** Despite excellent antibiotics and preventative treatments, patients who undergo a joint replacement can develop an infection, which will often require removal of the implanted joint in order to treat the infection effectively.

In general, antibacterial drugs can cause nausea, vomiting, allergic reactions, and superinfections.

> ● **Key Point** Healthcare professionals have been shown to be a primary source of spreading infections. These are referred to as *nosocomial infections*. It is recommended that healthcare providers wear gloves, wash hands with soap for at least 15 to 30 seconds, and use disinfective solutions to minimize the spread of infection.

Vitamins
Vitamins are organic substances that must be provided in small quantities in the diet for the synthesis of co-factors, which are essential for metabolic function and cannot be manufactured by the body. Populations at risk for vitamin deficiency include:

- Infants and preschoolers
- Pregnant and lactating women

TABLE 15-1

The Most Common Cardiac Drugs, Their Indications, Mechanisms of Action, and Their Implications for Physical Therapy

Drug	Indications	Mechanism of Action	Implication
Angiotensin-converting enzyme (ACE) inhibitors	Hypertension Congestive heart failure Diabetic nephropathy Migraine headaches	Inhibit ACE, which causes less stimulation of angiotensin receptors, blood vessel dilation, and a fall in blood pressure.	Advise the patient to change positions and get up slowly because orthostatic hypotension may occur. Notify the physician if the patient complains about a sore throat (early warning sign of agranulocytosis).
α agonists	Nasal congestion Allergic conditions Bronchoconstriction	Stimulate α agonist receptors, resulting in constriction of blood vessels (with increased peripheral resistance and increased blood pressure), and prevent urinary outflow.	Some of these drugs are available over the counter (OTC), and patients often assume that OTC drugs are safe. Advise older men that use of OTC α agonists can lead to urinary hesitancy or even retention in the presence of benign prostatic hyperplasia. Inquire about the use of OTC medications that contain α agonists if you notice that blood pressure has increased in a patient.
α blockers	Hypertension Benign prostatic hyperplasia	Block α agonist receptors, resulting in dilation of blood vessels (with decreased peripheral resistance and decreased blood pressure), and increase urinary outflow.	Advise the patient to change positions and get up slowly because orthostatic hypotension may occur. Monitor patients after strenuous exercise because of risk of hypotensive episode.
Antiarrhythmic drugs	Arrhythmias/dysrhythmias	Can affect the movement of electrical and muscular activity of the heart. There are four major classes: • Sodium channel blockers • β blockers • Drugs that slow the efflux of potassium • Calcium channel blockers	Advise patients to strictly adhere to the prescribed dosing and avoid caffeine. Monitor patient for peripheral edema or dyspnea. Advise the patient to change positions and get up slowly because orthostatic hypotension may occur.
Anticholinergics	Arrhythmias Peptic ulcer and irritable bowel syndrome Urinary bladder hypermotility Asthma Parkinson disease	Inhibit muscarinic (M) cholinergic receptors, thereby reducing the action of acetylcholine, resulting in increased heart rate and contractility, dilation of bronchial muscles, and decreased gut and bladder activity.	Expect some increases in heart rate in all patients and some mental confusion in older patients. Keep the exercise environment cool; these patients have a decreased ability to sweat and lose heat.

Data from Vogel W: Introduction to pharmacology, in Sueki D, Brechter J (eds): Orthopedic Rehabilitation Clinical Advisor. St Louis, Mosby, 2010, pp 873–922

TABLE 15-2 Classes of Antibiotics

Type	Action	Examples	Implications for Physical Therapy
Penicillin	Bactericidal agent; acts by inhibiting cell membrane synthesis.	Penicillin and amoxicillin	Advise patients to follow prescription schedule strictly and to continue taking drugs even if clinical signs or symptoms have subsided.
Cephalosporin	Bactericidal agent; mainly used to counter staphylococcal organisms	Cephalexin (Keflex)	
Aminoglycosides	Bactericidal agent; generally effective against aerobic gram-negative bacteria (*Klebsiella, Pseudomonas, Escherichia coli*)		Adhere to drug warnings that tetracyclines and quinolones must be taken as prescribed because their use with food or antacids can render them ineffective.
Macrolide	Bacteriostatic agent; inhibits organism replication and is used to counter organisms such as *Chlamydia, Clostridium, Staphylococcus aureus*, and *Bacteroides*	Erythromycin (E-Mycin), clarithromycin (Biaxin), and azithromycin (Zithromax)	Notify supervising PT if patient exhibits an unexplained rash or abdominal discomfort. Advise the patient to avoid exposure to sunlight because these drugs can cause photosensitization.
Quinolone	Bacteriostatic agent; broadly effective against all gram-negative rods (e.g., *E. coli*, salmonella, and *Pseudomonas*)	Ciprofloxacin (Cipro), levofloxacin (Levaquin), and ofloxacin (Floxin)	
Sulfonamide	Bacteriostatic agent; prescribed for the treatment of certain urinary tract infections but also for other (nonorthopedic-related) infections	Co-trimoxazole (Bactrim) and trimethoprim (Proloprim)	
Tetracycline	Bacteriostatic agent; rarely used in the treatment of orthopedic infections	Tetracycline (Sumycin, Panmycin) and doxycycline (Vibramycin)	

- The elderly
- People of a low socioeconomic status
- People with chronic disease states

Fat-Soluble Vitamins

The fat-soluble vitamins are A, D, E, and K. After being absorbed by the intestinal tract, these vitamins are stored in the liver and fatty tissues. Fat-soluble vitamins require protein carriers to move through body fluids, and excesses of these vitamins are stored in the body. Because these vitamins are not water soluble, it is possible for them to reach toxic levels.

Vitamin A

Vitamin A helps prevent retardation of growth and protect skin integrity. It is essential to the eyes, epithelial tissue, and reproductive functions. Common food sources include green, orange, and yellow vegetables, liver, butter, egg yolks, and fortified margarine.

Signs and symptoms of vitamin A deficiency include:

- Keratomalacia (softening and subsequent ulceration and perforation of the cornea)
- Xerophthalmia (dryness and ulceration of the conjunctiva and cornea)
- Nyctalopia (night blindness)
- Growth failure
- Rough and dry skin

Signs and symptoms of vitamin A toxicity include:

- Appetite loss
- Hair loss
- Enlarged liver and spleen

Vitamin D

Vitamin D stimulates calcium absorption from the small intestine. It also increases the blood flow levels of minerals such as phosphorus. Common food sources include fortified milk, fish oils, and fortified margarine.

Signs and symptoms of vitamin D deficiency include:

- Rickets (in children of underdeveloped countries)
- Impaired growth
- Skeletal abnormalities
- Osteomalacia
- Spontaneous fractures
- Muscular tetany

Signs and symptoms of vitamin D toxicity include:

- Calcification of soft tissues
- Other forms of hypercalcemia

Vitamin E
Vitamin D functions as in antioxidant, with exact mechanisms not clearly defined, but it is said to stabilize cell membranes and preserve red blood cells, especially those that are constantly exposed to high levels of oxygen such as the lungs. Common food sources include vegetable oils, wheat germ, nuts, and fish.

Signs and symptoms of vitamin E deficiency include:

- Abnormal red blood cell hemolysis (breakdown)
- Edema

Signs and symptoms of vitamin E toxicity include:

- Decreased thyroid hormone levels
- Increased triglycerides

Vitamin K
Vitamin K is necessary for the synthesis of at least two of the proteins involved in blood clotting. Common food sources include dark green leafy vegetables, cheese, egg yolks, and liver.

Signs and symptoms of vitamin K deficiency include:

- Hemorrhage
- Defective blood clotting

No signs and symptoms of vitamin K toxicity have been reported.

Water-Soluble Vitamins
Water-soluble vitamins include the B complex, vitamin C, biotin, choline, and folacin (folic acid).

Water-soluble vitamins are not stored in the body in any significant amount, which significantly reduces the incidences of toxicity but requires that they be included in the diet on a daily basis.

Thiamine
Thiamine (B_1) metabolizes carbohydrates and has been found to prevent beriberi and diseases of the nervous system. Common food sources include grains, meat, and yeast.

Signs and symptoms of thiamine deficiency include:

- Neurological symptoms
- Cardiovascular symptoms
- Beriberi (in underdeveloped countries)

Riboflavin
Riboflavin (B_2) facilitates selected enzymes involved in carbohydrate, protein, and fat metabolism. Common food sources include milk, green leafy vegetables, eggs, and peanuts.

Signs and symptoms of riboflavin deficiency include:

- Angular stomatitis (inflammation at the corners of the mouth, associated with a wrinkled or fissured epithelium that does not involve the mucosa)
- Inflammation of the tongue
- Photophobia with lacrimation
- Scaling of the skin

Niacin
Niacin (B_3) facilitates several enzymes that regulate energy metabolism. Common food sources include meats, whole grains, and white flour.

Signs and symptoms of niacin deficiency include:

- Pellagra
- Diarrhea
- Dementia
- Dermatitis

Pantothenic Acid
Pantothenic acid (B_5) is found in living tissue, and it is essential for the metabolism of fatty acids and for the growth of some animals. Common food sources include liver, eggs, and whole grains.

Signs and symptoms of pantothenic acid deficiency include:

- Headache
- Fatigue

- Poor muscle coordination
- Burning feet syndrome

Pyridoxine

Pyridoxine (B_6) is essential in the metabolism of proteins, amino acids, carbohydrates, and fat. Common food sources include liver, red meats, whole grains, and potatoes.

Signs and symptoms of pyrodoxine deficiency include:

- Peripheral neuropathy
- Convulsions
- Hyperirritability
- Depression

Cyanocobalamin

Cyanocobalamin (B_{12}) is essential for the functioning of all cells and aids in hemoglobin synthesis. Common food sources include meats, whole eggs, and egg yolks.

Signs and symptoms of cyanocobalamin deficiency include:

- Pernicious anemia
- Various psychological disorders

Ascorbic Acid

Ascorbic acid (vitamin C) performs many functions:

- It assists the body to combat infections.
- It facilitates wound healing.
- It is necessary for the development and maintenance of bones, cartilage, connective tissue, and blood vessels.

Common food sources include citrus fruits, tomatoes, and cantaloupe.

Signs and symptoms of ascorbic acid deficiency include:

- Anemia
- Scurvy (spongy gums, loosening of the teeth, and bleeding into the skin and mucous membranes)

Biotin

Biotin is necessary for the action of many enzyme systems. Common food sources include liver, meats, and milk.

Signs and symptoms of biotin deficiency include:

- Anemia
- Depression
- Muscle pain

- Anorexia
- Dermatitis

Choline

Choline is a soluble ammonia derivative (amine) that is found in animal and plant tissue and is synthesized from methionine, which is an amino acid. Choline is an important component of compounds necessary for nerve function, and it helps to prevent fat from being deposited in the liver.

Folacin

Folacin (folic acid) is involved in the formation of red blood cells and in the functioning of the gastrointestinal tract. Common food sources include yeast, dark-green leafy vegetables, and whole grains.

Signs and symptoms of folacin deficiency include:

- Impaired cell division
- Alteration of protein synthesis

Minerals

Minerals, like vitamins, are important nutrients found in foods. The main difference is that vitamins are organic substances (meaning that they contain the element carbon), while minerals are inorganic substances. There are two groups of minerals: major minerals and trace minerals (**Table 15-3** and **Table 15-4**).

Dietary and Nutritional Supplements

Vitamin C

In addition to those roles mentioned in the "Vitamins" section, vitamin C is vital for the formation of collagen. Vitamin C activates the enzymes that convert proline and lysine into hydroxyproline and hydroxylysine, respectively, both of which are needed to give collagen its correct three-dimensional structure.

Chondroitin Sulfate

Chondroitin sulphate is a sulfur-containing polysaccharide found naturally in the body, and which is reportedly essential for joint cartilage health. Glucosamine is an amino-acid-containing monosaccharide, concentrated in joint cartilage, which is used to synthesize cartilage glycosaminoglycan (GAG for short). GAGs are large molecules composing long-branched chains of sugars and smaller nitrogen-containing molecules known as amino-sugars. The action of orally administered chondroitin sulfate has yet to be clarified. Possible actions include promotion and maintenance of the structure and function of cartilage (referred to as chondroprotection), pain relief of osteoarthritic joints, and anti-inflammatory activity.

TABLE
15-3

Minerals: Sources and Functions

Mineral	Function	Common Food Sources
Summary of Major Minerals		
Calcium (Ca)	Aids in formation of bones and teeth, normal blood clotting, muscle contraction and relaxation, heart, and nerve function.	Milk and other dairy products, greens broccoli, salmon, sardines, legumes
Phosphorus (P)	Aids in formation of bones and teeth. Regulates body energy. Helps transport fat in the body as a part of phospholipids. Helps maintain normal acid/base balance in the body.	Meat, fish, poultry, eggs, milk, cereal products
Magnesium (Mg)	Necessary for muscle contraction and nerve function.	Meat, seafood, nuts, legumes, dairy products, whole grains.
Sodium (Na)	Important component of body fluids.	Table salt, meat, seafood, milk, cheese, eggs, baking soda, baking powder, bread, vegetables, processed foods
Potassium (K)	Important component of body fluids.	Potatoes, melons, citrus fruit, banana, and most fruits and vegetables; meat; milk; legumes
Summary of Some Trace Minerals		
Iron (FE)	Located in hemoglobin and myoglobin in muscle cells. Needed to carry oxygen.	Liver, meats, egg yolks, nuts, enriched or whole grains, legumes
Iodine (I)	Part of thyroid hormones (thyroxin and triiodothyronine).	Seafood, iodized salt
Selenium (SE)	Acts as an antioxidant.	Grains, meat, poultry, fish, dairy products
Zinc (Zn)	Part of important enzyme systems. Found in the hormone insulin.	Meat, seafood, whole grains
Chromium (Cr)	Helps body use insulin.	Liver, brewer's yeast, whole grains, nuts, cheeses
Copper (Cu)	Part of many enzymes.	Legumes, grains, nuts, seeds, organ meat
Fluoride (Fl)	Part of teeth and bone. Helps prevent cavities in teeth.	Fluoridated drinking water, fish, tea

Data from Dutton M: McGraw-Hill's NPTE (National Physical Therapy Examination). New York, McGraw-Hill, 2009

TABLE
15-4

Minerals Supplied by Food Groups

Food Group	Minerals Supplied
Milk	Calcium, phosphorus, and potassium
Meats	Iron, copper, zinc, chromium, phosphorus, and sulfur
Fruits	Magnesium, manganese, potassium, and iron
Vegetables	Potassium, magnesium, iodine, and selenium
Bread, cereals, and grains	Iron, copper, zinc, manganese, magnesium, molybdenum, chromium, and phosphorus

Data from Dutton M: McGraw-Hill's NPTE (National Physical Therapy Examination). New York, McGraw-Hill, 2009

Glucosamine Sulphate

Glucosamine is used in the manufacture of very large molecules found in cartilage called proteoglycans. These are large linear chains of repeating polysaccharide units (GAGs), which radiate out from a protein core like the bristles of a bottle brush and can attract and hold water like a sponge. When compressed, this bound water helps to absorb force and distribute it equally, which explains the ability of cartilage to protect the joints under load and during movement. In the body, these GAG chains are synthesized from glucose, the amino acid glutamine, and sulphate, but there is plenty of evidence that additional supplementation not only increases GAG significantly but can also relieve the pain and inflammation associated with osteoarthritis.

REVIEW Questions

1. Which federally regulated agency directs the drug development process and gives approval for the marketing of a new drug?

2. What is the study of how the body absorbs, distributes, metabolizes, and eliminates a drug called?

3. Which of the two NSAID types, Cox-1 or Cox-2, is safer to use in patients who are predisposed to gastric or kidney malfunctions?

4. You are treating a 72-year-old woman with a diagnosis of Parkinson disease. You notice that the patient performs well on certain days and poorly on others. Which of the following ways can you possibly improve the patient's performance on the days when she performs poorly?
   a. Schedule the patient's sessions so that there are fewer sessions on the days she usually performs poorly.
   b. Call the physician and recommend another medication.
   c. Encourage the patient to decrease her daily dosage of medication to 400 mg/day on the days she usually performs poorly.
   d. None of the above.

5. You are examining a 58-year-old man with Parkinson disease. The patient reports that he is taking a medication for the disease but cannot remember its name. Which of the following medications is the patient probably taking?
   a. Levodopa
   b. Cortisone

   c. Beta blocker
   d. Glutamate blocker

6. A patient asks you to explain the function of his medication Cardizem (a calcium channel blocker). Which of the following points should be included in your explanation?
   a. Cardizem causes decreased contractility of the heart and vasodilation of the coronary arteries.
   b. Cardizem causes decreased contractility of the heart and vasoconstriction of the coronary arteries.
   c. Cardizem causes increased contractility of the heart and vasodilation of the coronary arteries.
   d. Cardizem causes increased contractility of the heart and vasoconstriction of the coronary arteries.

7. Following a myocardial infarction, a patient was placed on medications that included a beta-adrenergic blocking agent. When monitoring this patient's response to exercise, you would expect this drug to:
   a. Cause the heart rate to be low at rest, and to increase very little with exercise.
   b. Cause the heart rate to be low at rest, and to increase linearly with exercise intensity.
   c. Increase proportionally to changes in systolic blood pressure.
   d. Increase proportionally to changes in diastolic blood pressure.

8. True or false: Acetaminophen (paracetamol) is an NSAID.

9. True or false: NSAIDs are eliminated from the body via the liver.

10. True or false: Both iontophoresis and phonophoresis can be used to deliver corticosteroids.

11. Symptoms attributed to serotonin excess may include the following, except:
    a. Restlessness
    b. Nausea
    c. Diaphoresis
    d. All of the above

12. True or false: Monoamine oxidase inhibitors (MAOIs) are used to treat anxiety.

13. What class of drugs are sedative-hypnotic agents that are used for a variety of situations that include seizure control, anxiety, alcohol withdrawal, insomnia, control of drug-associated agitation, as muscle relaxants (antispasticity agents), and as preanesthetic agents?

14. A slowing myocardium depolarization that leads to arrhythmia, myocardial depression, and hypotension is a potential side effect of which drug type?

15. Diazepam and clonazepam are commonly used to treat what condition?

References

1. Dionne RA: Pharmacologic treatments for temporomandibular disorders. Surg Oral Medi Oral Pathol Oral Radiol Endod 83:134–142, 1997
2. Ciccone CD: Basic pharmacokinetics and the potential effect of physical therapy interventions on pharmacokinetic variables. Phys Ther 75:343–351, 1995
3. Nirschl RP: Prevention and treatment of elbow and shoulder injuries in the tennis player. Clin Sports Med 7:289–308, 1988
4. Teitz CC, Garrett WE Jr, Miniaci A, et al: Tendon problems in athletic individuals. J. Bone Joint Surg 79A:138–152, 1997
5. Pease BJ, Cortese M: Anterior knee pain: Differential diagnosis and physical therapy management, Orthopaedic Physical Therapy Home Study Course 92-1. La Crosse, Wisconsin, Orthopaedic Section, APTA, 1992
6. Sperling RL: NSAIDs. Home Healthcare Nurse 19:687–689, 2001
7. Clive DM, Stoff JS: Renal syndromes associated with nonsteroidal antiinflammatory drugs. N Engl J Med 310:563–572, 1984
8. Brattsand R, Linden M: Cytokine modulation by glucocorticoids: Mechanisms and actions in cellular studies. Aliment Pharmacol Ther 10(Suppl. 2):81–90; Discussion 1–2, 1996
9. Stetts DM: Patient Examination, in Wadsworth C (ed): Current Concepts of Orthopaedic Physical Therapy—Home study Course 11.2.2. La Crosse, WI, Orthopaedic Section, APTA, 2001
10. Elenbaas JK: Centrally acting oral skeletal muscle relaxants. Am J Hosp Pharm 37:1313–1323, 1980
11. Vanek ZF, Menkes JH: Spasticity, Available at: http://www.emedicine.com/neuro/topic706.htm, 2005

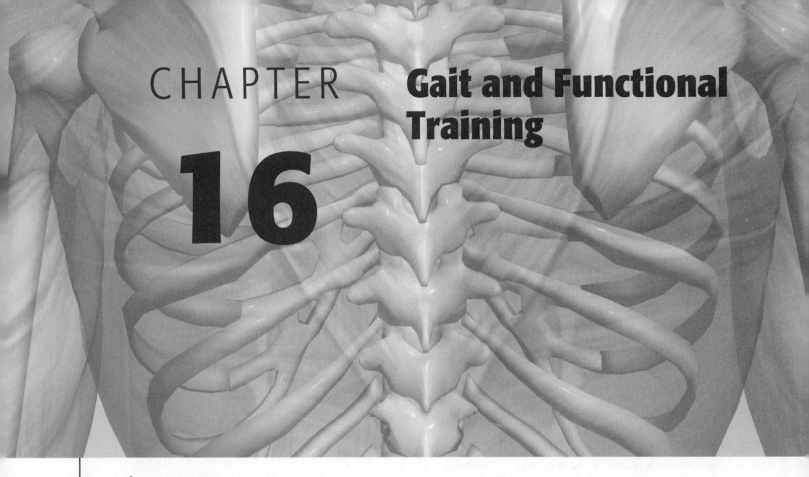

CHAPTER 16

Gait and Functional Training

Terminology

Base of Support

The base of support, defined as the distance between an individual's feet while standing and during ambulation, includes the part of the body in contact with the supporting surface and the intervening area.[1] The normal base of support is considered to be between 5 and 10 centimeters.

> ● **Key Point** Larger than normal bases of support are observed in individuals who have muscle imbalances of the lower limbs and trunk, as well as in those who have problems with overall static dynamic balance.[2]

Center of Gravity

The center of gravity (COG), which changes both vertically and horizontally during gait (see later), may be defined as the point at which the three planes of the body intersect each other. In the human, that point is approximately 2 inches (5 centimeters) anterior to the second sacral vertebra. As the COG moves forward with each step, it briefly passes beyond the anterior margin of the base of support, resulting in a temporary loss of balance.[1] This temporary loss of equilibrium is counteracted by the advancing foot at initial contact, which establishes a new base of support.

Temporal Parameters

Step Length

Step length is defined as the linear distance between the right and left foot during gait. Step length is measured as the distance between the same point of one foot on successive footprints (ipsilateral to the contralateral foot fall).

Stride Length

Stride length is the distance between successive points of foot-to-floor contact of the same foot. A stride is one full lower extremity cycle. Two step lengths added together make the stride length. Stride length can be estimated based on height (females: height × 0.413; males: height × 0.415). The average length of the female stride is 2 feet. The average length of the male stride is 2.5 feet.[3] Typically, the stride length does not vary more than a few inches between tall and short individuals.

Cadence

Cadence is defined as the number of separate steps taken in a certain time. Normal cadence is between 90 and 120 steps per minute.[4,5] The cadence of women is usually six to nine steps per minute slower than that of men.[4] Cadence also is affected by age, decreasing from the age of 4 to the age of 7 years, and then again in advancing years.[6]

Velocity is defined as the distance a body moves in a given time and is thus calculated by dividing the distance traveled by the time taken. Velocity is expressed in meters per second. Reductions in velocity correlate with joint impairments, amputation levels, and numerous acute pathologies due to pain.

Gait Cycle

Walking involves the alternating action of the two lower extremities. The walking pattern is studied as a gait cycle (Figure 16-1). The gait cycle consists of two periods (**Table 16-1**).

Stance Period

The stance period describes the entire time the foot is in contact with the ground and the limb is bearing weight. It begins with the initial contact of the foot on the ground and concludes when the ipsilateral foot leaves the ground. Within the stance period (60% of the gait cycle), two tasks and four intervals are recognized.[7-9] The two tasks are weight acceptance and single-limb support. According to the Rancho Los Amigos terminology, the four intervals are loading response, midstance, terminal stance, and preswing.[9] As the initial contact of one foot is occurring, the contralateral foot is preparing to come off the floor.

> ● **Key Point** For the stance phase, standard terminology uses the terms *heelstrike* (initial contact), *foot flat* (loading response), *midstance, heel-off* (terminal stance), and *toe-off* (preswing).

Weight Acceptance

The weight acceptance task occurs during the first 10% of the stance period. This consists of intervals of *initial contact* (when the heel first hits the ground) and *loading response*. The loading response interval begins as the foot comes flat with the floor and one limb bears weight while the other leg begins to go through its swing period. This interval may be referred to as the *initial double stance period* and consists of the first 0% to 10% of the gait cycle.[9]

Single Leg Support

The middle 40% of the stance period is divided equally into midstance and terminal stance. The midstance interval, representing the first half of the single-limb support task, begins as one foot is lifted and continues until the body weight is aligned over the forefoot.[9]

The terminal stance interval is the second half of the single-limb support task (Table 16-1). It begins when the heel of the weight-bearing foot lifts off the ground and continues until the contralateral foot strikes the ground. Terminal stance composes the 30% to 50% phase of the gait cycle.[9]

Limb Advancement

The preswing interval (*heel-off* in traditional terminology) represents the 50% to 60% phase of the gait cycle (Table 16-1). The preswing interval refers to the last 10% of the stance period. This interval begins with initial contact of the contralateral limb and ends with ipsilateral toe-off. Because both feet are on the floor at the same time during this interval, double support occurs for the second time in the gait cycle. This last portion of the stance period is, therefore, referred to as the *terminal double stance*.

Swing Period

The swing period constitutes 40% of the gait cycle. Gravity and momentum are the primary sources of motion for the swing period.[10] Within the swing period, one task and four intervals are recognized.[7-9] The task involves limb advancement.

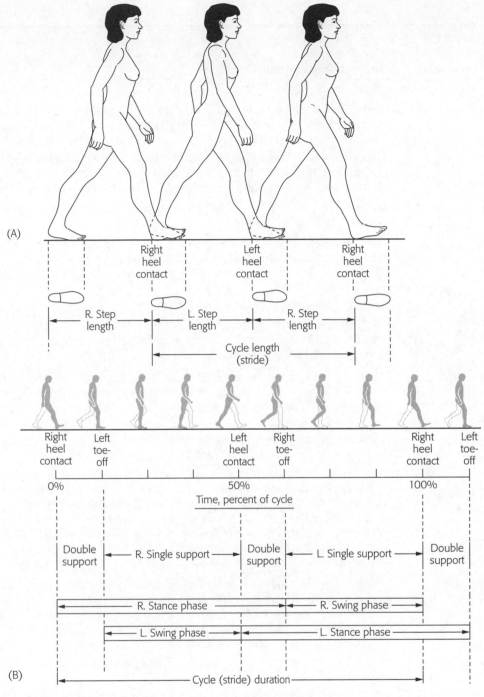

The gait cycle.

Source: Inman VT, Ralston H, Todd F: Human Walking. Baltimore, Lippincott, Williams & Wilkins, 1981.

● **Key Point** In addition to representing the final portion of the stance period and single-limb support task, the preswing interval is considered in some texts as part of the swing period.

Limb Advancement

The swing period involves the forward motion of the non-weight-bearing foot. According to the Rancho

Los Amigos terminology, the three intervals of the swing period include:[9]

1. *Initial swing:* This interval (referred to as *acceleration* in traditional terminology) begins with lifting of the foot from the floor and ends when the swinging foot is opposite the stance foot. It represents the 60% to 73% phase of the gait cycle.[9]

TABLE 16-1	The Gait Cycle	
Period	**Component**	**Biomechanics and Muscle Actions**
Stance phase	Initial contact	The center of gravity is at its lowest point.
		Ankle: The ankle is held in neutral dorsiflexion through isometric activation of the dorsiflexor muscles (e.g., tibialis anterior). As the ankle transitions toward the loading response, the dorsiflexor muscles are eccentrically active to lower the ankle into plantarflexion.
		Knee: The knee is slightly flexed as a way to absorb the shock of initial weight bearing. The quadriceps are eccentrically active to allow a slight give to the flexed knee and to prevent the knee from buckling as weight is transferred onto the stance limb.
		Hip: The hip is in about 30° of flexion, and as weight-bearing continues, the hip extensor muscles are isometrically active.
	Loading response	*Ankle:* The ankle has just rapidly moved into 5° to 10° of plantarflexion. This motion is controlled through eccentric activation of the dorsiflexor muscles. Immediately following this point, the ankle begins to move toward dorsiflexion as the lower leg advances forward over the fixed foot.
		Knee: The knee continues to flex to about 15°, acting as a shock-absorbing spring; the knee extensor muscles continue to be active eccentrically.
		Hip: The hip extensor muscles shift from isometric to slight concentric activation, guiding the hip toward extension.
	Midstance	*Ankle:* The ankle approaches about 5° of dorsiflexion, during which time the dorsiflexor muscles are inactive and the plantarflexor muscles are eccentrically active, controlling the rate at which the lower leg advances forward over the foot.
		Knee: The knee reaches near full extension. Because the line of gravity falls just anterior to the medial-lateral axis of rotation of the knee, the knee is mechanically locked into extension, requiring little activation from the quadriceps at this time.
		Hip: The hip approaches 0° of extension, and the hip extensors such as the gluteus maximus are only slightly active to help stabilize the hip as the body is propelled forward. This activation is minimal during slow walking on level surfaces, but it increases significantly with increasing speed and slope of the walking surface. During midstance, the stance leg is in single limb support as the other leg is freely swinging toward the next step. The hip abductor muscles (e.g., gluteus medius) of the stance leg therefore are active to stabilize the hip in the frontal plane, preventing the opposite side of the pelvis from dropping excessively.
	Preswing	*Ankle:* At the beginning of preswing, the heel breaks contact with the ground and the ankle continues to dorsiflex to about 10°, stretching the Achilles tendon, which prepares the calf muscles for propulsion. As the heel lift continues, the plantarflexor muscles switch their activation from eccentric (to control forward motion of the leg) to concentric. This concentric action produces plantarflexion for propulsion or push-off.
		Knee: The extended knee prepares to flex, often driven by a short burst of activity from the hamstring muscles.
		Hip: The hip continues to extend to about 10° of extension with eccentric activation of the hip flexors, in particular the iliopsoas, helping to control the rate and amount of extension. Tight ligaments of the hip or tight hip flexor muscles will reduce the amount of extension at this point in the gait cycle, thereby reducing stride length.
	Toe-off	*Ankle:* The ankle continues plantarflexing (to about 15°) through concentric activation of the plantarflexor muscles. The muscular force for push-off is typically shared between the plantarflexors and the hip extensor muscles. Activation of the gastrocnemius and soleus is usually minimal while walking on level surfaces and at slow speed, but it increases significantly with increasing speed and incline.
		Knee: The knee is flexed 30°.
		Hip: The slightly extended hip starts to flex due to concentric activation of the hip flexor muscles.

TABLE
16-1

Period	Component	Biomechanics and Muscle Actions
Swing phase	Initial swing	*Ankle:* The plantarflexed ankle begins to dorsiflex by concentric activation of the dorsiflexor muscles. The dorsiflexing ankle allows the foot to clear the ground as it is advanced forward.
		Knee: The knee continues to flex, largely driven by indirect action of the flexing hip.
		Hip: The hip flexor muscles continue to contract, pulling the extended thigh forward.
	Midswing	*Ankle:* The ankle is held in neutral dorsiflexion via isometric activation of the dorsiflexor muscles.
		Knee: The knee is flexed about 45° to 55°, which helps shorten the functional length of the lower limb to facilitate its advance.
		Hip: The hip approaches about 30° of flexion through concentric activation of the hip flexor muscles.
	Terminal swing	*Ankle:* The ankle dorsiflexors continue their isometric activation, holding the ankle in neutral dorsiflexion and preparing for initial contact.
		Knee: The knee has moved from a flexed position in midswing to almost full extension.
		Hip: The hip flexor muscles, which have powered the leg in to nearly 35° of hip flexion, become inactive in terminal swing, but the hip extensor muscles are active eccentrically to decelerate the forward progression of the thigh.

2. *Midswing:* This interval begins as the swinging limb is opposite the stance limb and ends when the swinging limb is forward and the tibia is vertical. It represents the 73% to 87% phase of the gait cycle.[9]

3. *Terminal swing:* This interval (referred to as *deceleration* in traditional terminology) begins with a vertical tibia of the swing leg with respect to the floor and ends the moment the foot strikes the floor. It represents the last 87% to 100% of the gait cycle.

● **Key Point** For the swing phase, standard terminology uses the following terms: *acceleration* (initial swing), *midswing*, and *deceleration* (terminal swing).

● **Key Point** The precise duration of the gait cycle intervals depends on a number of factors, including age, impairment, and the patient's walking velocity. As gait speed increases, it develops into jogging and then running, with changes in each of the intervals. For example, as speed increases, the stance period decreases and the terminal double stance phase disappears altogether. This produces a double unsupported phase.[11]

The Six Determinants of Gait

For gait to be efficient and to conserve energy, the center of gravity (COG) must undergo minimal displacement. To minimize the energy costs of walking, the body uses a number of biomechanical mechanisms:[12]

■ *Pelvic rotation:* The rotation of the pelvis normally occurs about a vertical axis in the transverse plane toward the weight-bearing limb. The total pelvic rotation is approximately 4 degrees to each side.[6] Forward rotation of the pelvis on the swing side prevents an excessive drop in the body's center of gravity. The pelvic rotation also results in a relative lengthening of the femur, and thus step length, during the termination of the swing period.[9] If the pelvis does not rotate, the COG's position is somewhat lower during periods of double-limb support, and the COG's total vertical amplitude is greater.

■ *Pelvic tilt:* Lateral pelvic tilting (dropping on the unsupported side) during midstance prevents an excessive rise in the body's center of gravity. If the pelvis does not drop, the COG's position is somewhat higher during midstance, and the COG's total vertical amplitude is greater.

● **Key Point** The amount of lateral tilting of the pelvis may be accentuated in the presence of a leg length discrepancy, or hip abductor weakness, the latter of which results in a Trendelenburg sign. The Trendelenburg sign is said to be positive if, when standing on one leg, the pelvis drops on the side opposite to the stance leg. The weakness is present on the side of the stance leg; the gluteus medius is not able to maintain the center of gravity on the side of the stance leg.

- *Displacement of the pelvis:* To avoid significant muscular and balancing demands, the pelvis shifts over the support point of the stance limb. If the lower extremities dropped directly vertical from the hip joint, the center of mass would be required to shift 3 to 4 inches to each side to be positioned effectively over the supporting foot. The combination of femoral varus and anatomical valgum at the knee permits a vertical tibial posture with both tibias in close proximity to each other. This narrows the walking base to 5 to 10 centimeters (2 to 4 inches) from heel center to heel center, thereby reducing the lateral shift required of the COG to 2.5 centimeters (1 inch) toward either side.

- *Knee flexion in stance:* Knee motion is intrinsically associated with foot and ankle motion. At initial contact before the ankle moves into a plantarflexed position and thus is relatively more elevated, the knee is in relative extension. Responding to a plantarflexed posture, the knee flexes. Midstance knee flexion prevents an excessive rise in the body's COG during that period of the gait cycle. If not for the midstance knee flexion, the COG's rise during midstance would be larger, as would its total vertical amplitude. Passing through midstance as the ankle remains stationary with the foot flat on the floor, the knee again reverses its direction to one of extension.

- *Knee motion:* As the heel comes off the floor in terminal stance, the ankle again is elevated, and the knee flexes. In preswing, as the forefoot rolls over the metatarsal heads, the ankle moves even higher in elevation as flexion of the knee increases.

> **● Key Point** The movements of the thigh and lower leg occur in conjunction with the rotation of the pelvis. The pelvis, thigh, and lower leg normally rotate toward the weight-bearing limb at the beginning of the swing period.[13] Hip motion occurs in all three planes during the gait cycle:
>
> • Hip rotation occurs in the transverse plane. The hip begins in internal rotation during the loading response. Maximum internal rotation is reached near midstance and then the hip externally rotates during the swing period, with maximal external rotation occurring in terminal swing.[14]
> • The hip flexes and extends once during the gait cycle, with the limit of flexion occurring at the middle of the swing period, and the limit of extension being achieved before the end of the stance period.
> • In the coronal plane, hip adduction occurs throughout early stance and reaches a maximum at 40% of the cycle.[15] Hip adduction occurs in the early swing period, which is followed by slight hip abduction at the end of the swing phase, especially if a long stride is taken.[14–16]

- *Ankle mechanism:* For normal foot function and human ambulation, the amount of ankle joint motion required is approximately 10 degrees of dorsiflexion and 20 degrees of plantarflexion. At initial contact, the foot is elevated due to the heel lever arm. This mechanism, controlled by the muscle action of the pretibial muscles and triceps surae, serves to lengthen the leg and smooth the pathway of the COG during the stance phase.

> **● Key Point** In normal walking, about 60 degrees of knee motion is required for adequate clearance of the foot in the swing period. A loss of knee extension, which can occur with a flexion deformity, results in the hip being unable to extend fully, which can alter the gait mechanics.

- *Foot mechanism:* The controlled lever arm of the forefoot at preswing is particularly helpful as it rounds out the sharp downward reversal of the COG. Thus, it does not reduce a peak displacement period of the COG as the earlier determinants did but rather smoothes the pathway.

> **● Key Point** An adaptively shortened gastrocnemius muscle may produce movement impairment by restricting normal dorsiflexion of the ankle from occurring during the midstance to heel raise portion of the gait cycle. This motion is compensated for by increased pronation of the subtalar joint, increased internal rotation of the tibia, and resultant stresses to the knee joint complex.

Abnormal Gait Syndromes

A summary of the common gait deviations and their causes are outlined in **Table 16-2**.[17]

Pre-Gait Activities

When progressing a patient toward gait (**Table 16-3**), the clinician must give thought to three factors:

- Body weight bearing (load acceptance). Patients that have not ambulated in over 3 months should have their body weight gradually introduced:
  - ❑ Sitting with the feet on the floor and bending forward over the feet.
  - ❑ Standing with both feet parallel.
  - ❑ Gradual placement of one lower extremity into a more forward position, placing more weight over the extremity that is more posterior (directly under the body's center of gravity).
- Muscle strength and control of the trunk, hips, and lower extremities.
  - ❑ Standing requires the ability to stabilize the trunk (co-contraction of the trunk muscles).

TABLE
16-2

Some Gait Deviations and Their Causes

Deviation	Possible Reasons
Slower speed than expected for person's age	Generalized weakness Poor endurance Pain Joint motion restrictions Poor voluntary motor control
Shorter stance phase on involved side and decreased swing phase on uninvolved side	Pain in lower limb and/or pelvic region Decreased joint motion
Stance phase longer on one side	Pain Lack of trunk and pelvic rotation Weakness of lower limb muscles Restrictions in lower limb joints Poor muscle control Increased muscle tone
Sideways trunk lean	Ipsilateral lean—hip abductor weakness (gluteus medius/Trendelenburg gait) Contralateral lean—decreased hip flexion in swing limb Painful hip Abnormal hip joint (due to congenital dysplasia, coxa vara, etc.) Wide walking base Unequal leg length
Anterior trunk leaning at initial contact	Weak or paralyzed knee extensors or gluteus maximus Decreased ankle dorsiflexion Hip flexion contracture
Posterior trunk leaning at initial contact	Weak or paralyzed hip extensors, especially gluteus maximus (gluteus maximus gait) Hip pain Hip flexion contracture Inadequate hip flexion in swing Decreased knee range of motion
Increased lumbar lordosis at end of stance	Inability to extend hip, usually due to flexion contracture or ankylosis
Pelvic drop during stance	Contralateral gluteus medius weakness Adaptive shortening of quadratus lumborum on swing side Contralateral hip adductor spasticity
Excessive pelvic rotation	Adaptively shortened/spasticity of hip flexors on same side Limited hip joint flexion
Circumducting hip	Functional leg-length discrepancy Arthrogenic stiff hip or knee
Hip hiking	Functional leg-length discrepancy Inadequate hip flexion, knee flexion, or ankle dorsiflexion Hamstring weakness Quadratus lumborum shortening
Vaulting	Functional leg-length discrepancy Vaulting occurs on shorter limb side

(continued)

TABLE 16-2 Some Gait Deviations and Their Causes (Continued)

Deviation	Possible Reasons
Abnormal internal hip rotation (toe-in)	Adaptive shortening of iliotibial band
	Weakness of hip external rotators
	Femoral anteversion
	Adaptive shortening of hip internal rotators
Abnormal external hip rotation (toe-out)	Adaptive shortening of hip external rotators
	Femoral retroversion
	Weakness of hip internal rotators
Increased hip adduction (scissors gait)	Spasticity or contracture of ipsilateral hip adductors
	Ipsilateral hip adductor weakness
	Coxa vara
Inadequate hip extension (mid- and late stance)/ excessive hip flexion (swing)	Hip flexion contracture
	Iliotibial band contracture
	Hip flexor spasticity
	Pain
	Arthrodesis (surgical or spontaneous ankylosis)
	Loss of ankle dorsiflexion
Inadequate hip flexion	Hip flexor weakness
	Hip joint arthrodesis
Decreased hip swing through (psoatic limp)	Legg–Calvé–Perthes disease
	Weakness or reflex inhibition of psoas major muscle
Excessive knee extension/inadequate knee flexion at initial contact and loading response: increased knee extension during stance, and decreased knee flexion during swing	Pain
	Anterior trunk deviation/bending
	Weakness of quadriceps; hyperextension is a compensation and places body weight vector anterior to knee
	Spasticity of the quadriceps; noted more during the loading response and during initial swing intervals
	Joint deformity
Excessive knee flexion/inadequate knee extension at initial contact or around midstance: increased knee flexion in early stance, decreased knee extension in midstance and terminal stance, and decreased knee extension during swing	Knee flexion contracture, resulting in decreased step length and decreased knee extension in stance
	Increased tone/spasticity of hamstrings or hip flexors
	Decreased range of motion of ankle dorsiflexion in swing period
	Weakness of plantarflexors, resulting in increased dorsiflexion in stance
	Lengthened limb
Inadequate dorsiflexion control ("foot slap") during initial contact to midstance Steppage gait during the acceleration through deceleration of the swing phase	Weak or paralyzed dorsiflexors
	Lack of lower limb proprioception
	Weak or paralyzed dorsiflexor muscles
	Functional leg-length discrepancy
Increased walking base (>20 cm)	Deformity such as hip abductor muscle contracture
	Genu valgus
	Fear of losing balance
	Leg-length discrepancy

TABLE
16-2

Some Gait Deviations and Their Causes (Continued)

Deviation	Possible Reasons
Decreased walking base (<10 cm)	Hip adductor muscle contracture
	Genu varum
Excessive eversion of calcaneus during initial contact through midstance	Excessive tibia vara (refers to frontal plane position of the distal one-third of leg as it relates to supporting surface)
	Forefoot varus
	Weakness of tibialis posterior
	Excessive lower extremity internal rotation (due to muscle imbalances, femoral anteversion)
Excessive pronation during midstance through terminal stance	Insufficient ankle dorsiflexion (<10°)
	Increased tibial varum
	Compensated forefoot or rearfoot varus deformity
	Uncompensated forefoot valgus deformity
	Pes planus
	Long limb
	Uncompensated medial rotation of tibia or femur
	Weak tibialis anterior
Excessive supination during initial contact through midstance	Limited calcaneal eversion
	Rigid forefoot valgus
	Pes cavus
	Uncompensated lateral rotation of tibia or femur
	Short limb
	Plantarflexed first ray
	Upper motor neuron muscle imbalance
Excessive dorsiflexion	Compensation for knee flexion contracture
	Inadequate plantarflexor strength
	Adaptive shortening of dorsiflexors
	Increased muscle tone of dorsiflexors
	Pes calcaneus deformity
Excessive plantarflexion	Increased plantarflexor activity
	Plantarflexor contracture
Excessive varus	Contracture
	Overactivity of muscles on medial aspect of foot
Excessive valgus	Weak invertors
	Foot hypermobility
Decreased or absence of propulsion (plantarflexor gait)	Inability of plantarflexors to perform function, resulting in a shorter step length on involved side

Data from Perry J: Hip gait deviations, in Perry J (ed): Gait Analysis: Normal and Pathological Function. Thorofare, NJ, Slack, 1992, pp 245–263; Perry J: Knee abnormal gait, in Perry J (ed): Gait Analysis: Normal and Pathological Function. Thorofare, NJ, Slack, 1992, pp 223–243; Perry J: Ankle and foot gait deviations, in Perry J (ed): Gait Analysis: Normal and Pathological Function. Thorofare, NJ, Slack, 1992, pp 185–220; Perry J: Pelvis and trunk pathological gait, in Perry J (ed): Gait Analysis: Normal and Pathological Function. Thorofare, NJ, Slack, 1992, pp 265–279; Perry J: Gait analysis: Normal and pathological dunction. Thorofare, NJ, Slack, 1992; and Levine D, Whittle M: Gait Analysis: The Lower Extremities. La Crosse, WI, Orthopaedic Section, APTA, 1992

TABLE 16-3 Body Position and Posture Progressions Used in Motor Development Training

Activities of Increasing Complexity			
Recumbent	Sitting	Crawling/Kneeling	Walking
Supine	Side sitting	Prone on elbows	Normal gait
Side lying	Sitting with bilateral upper-extremity support	Quadruped	1 step
Hook lying	Sitting with unilateral upper-extremity support	Tall-Kneeling	High step
Prone	Sitting with without upper-extremity support	Half-kneeling	Tandem walk
Prone on elbows		Sit to stand	Braiding
Bridging		Squat	4 × 4 beam walk
			Walk forward
			Walk backward
			Skipping

- Progressions include exercising the patient in sitting and applying challenges from all directions, initially using anterior-posterior challenges, advancing to lateral challenges and then to diagonal and rotary movements.
  - The quadruped position can be used to help develop strength and stability in three-dimensional planes and coordination of the co-contractors that maintain trunk stability.
- Hip stability and control.
  - Hip stability is required for the stance phase.
  - Controlled hip mobility is required for the swing phase.
- Knee stability and control.
  - Knee stability helps prevent genu recurvatum in the stance phase.
  - Controlled knee mobility is required for the swing phase.
- Ankle stability and control. Ankle stability/strength helps prevent foot drop (dorsiflexors) and provide propulsion (plantarflexors).
- Balance. The goal is to gradually raise the center of gravity of the body while maintaining the stability of the trunk:
  - The initial goal is to perfect static sitting balance without upper extremity support.
  - Initially both upper extremities are used to maintain balance.
  - This is progressed to one extremity and then no upper extremity support.

- Dynamic sitting balance.
  - Moving one and then two of the upper extremities to and from the body with increasing distances and speed.
  - Moving the whole body into and out of a stable position, such as scooting.
- The center of gravity can be raised in tall kneeling to provide a challenge for the structures that provide anterior-posterior stability (see Chapter 12).
  - The half-kneel position provides a challenge for the structures that provide lateral stability and assist with stability during diagonal movements.
- A Swiss/stability ball can also be employed to develop both balance and trunk strength as well as coordination.
- Standing. The progression for this is similar to that used to improve sitting balance: the initial focus is on static standing stability before advancing to movement of the extremities, and then to translations of the body in various directions.

Gait Training with Assistive Devices

Assistive devices, in order of the stability they provide, include a walker, crutches, walker cane (hemi-walker), quad cane, straight cane, and bent cane, with the walker providing the most stability. Correct fitting of an assistive device is important to ensure the safety of the patient and to allow for minimal energy expenditure. Once fitted, the patient should be taught the correct walking technique with the device. The fitting depends on the device chosen:

- *Walkers, hemiwalking canes, quad canes, and standard canes:* The height of the device handle should be adjusted to the level of the greater trochanter of the patient's hip and/or at the level of the ulnar styloid process with the elbow flexed 20 to 25 degrees.
- *Standard crutches:* A number of methods can be used for determining the correct crutch length for axillary crutches. The crutch tip should be vertical to the ground and positioned approximately 15 centimeters (6 inches) lateral and 5 centimeters (2 inches) anterior to the patient's foot. The handgrips of the crutch are adjusted to the height of the greater trochanter of the hip of the patient and/or at the level of the ulnar styloid process with the elbow flexed 20 to 25 degrees. There should be a 5- to 8-centimeter (2- to 3-inch) gap between the tops of the axillary pads and the patient's axilla. Bauer and colleagues[18] found that the best calculation of ideal crutch length was either 77% of the patient's height or the height minus 40.6 centimeters (16 inches).
- *Forearm/Loftstrand crutches:* The crutch is adjusted so that the handgrip is level with the greater trochanter of the patient's hip and the top of the forearm cuff 1 to 1.5 inches distal to the olecranon process, and/or at the level of the ulnar styloid process with the elbow flexed 20 to 25 degrees.

- *Canes:* Canes are used to provide support and protection, to reduce pain in the lower extremities, and to improve balance during ambulation.[19] It is common practice to instruct patients with lower extremity pain to use the cane in the hand contralateral to the symptomatic side.[20] The use of a cane in the contralateral hand helps preserve reciprocal motion and a more normal pathway for the COG.[21] Use of a cane can transmit 20% to 25% of body weight away from the lower extremities.[22,23] The cane also allows the subject to increase the effective base of support, thereby decreasing the hip abductor force exerted.

The clinician must always provide adequate physical support and instruction while working with a patient using an assistive gait device. The clinician positions himself or herself posterolaterally on the involved side of the patient, to be able to assist the patient on the side where the patient will most likely have difficulty. In addition, a gait belt should be fitted around the patient's waist to enable the clinician to assist the patient.

The selection of the proper gait pattern to instruct the patient is dependent on the patient's balance, strength, cardiovascular status, coordination, functional needs, and weight-bearing status (**Table 16-4**). In addition to observing the weight-bearing status, the patient may be prescribed an appropriate gait pattern. Several gait patterns are recognized.

Two-Point Pattern

The two-point gait pattern, which closely approximates the normal gait pattern, requires the use of

---

TABLE 16-4	Types of Weight-Bearing Status	
Weight-Bearing Status	**Description**
Non-weight bearing (NWB)	Patient not permitted to bear any weight through the injured limb.
Partial weight bearing (PWB)	Patient permitted to bear a portion (e.g., 25%, 50%) of his or her weight through the injured limb.
Touch-down weight-bearing (TDWB)/toe-touch weight-bearing (TTWB)	Patient permitted minimal contact of the injured limb with the ground for balance. The expression "as though walking on eggshells" can be used to help the patient understand.
Weight bearing as tolerated (WBAT)	The patient is permitted to bear as much weight through the injured limb as is comfortable.
Full weight bearing	Patient no longer medically requires an assistive device.

an assistive gait device (canes or crutches) on each side of the body. This pattern requires the patient to move the assistive gait device and the contralateral lower extremity at the same time (Figure 16-2). This pattern requires coordination and balance.

Two-Point Modified Pattern

The two-point modified pattern is the same as the two-point pattern except that it requires only one assistive device, positioned on the opposite side of the involved lower extremity. This pattern cannot be used if there are any weight-bearing restrictions (i.e., PWB, NWB), but it is appropriate for a patient with unilateral weakness or mild balance deficits. The patient is instructed to move the cane and the

involved leg simultaneously, and then the uninvolved leg (Figure 16-3).

Three-Point Gait Pattern

This pattern is used for non-weight bearing when the patient is permitted to bear weight through only one lower extremity. The three-point gait pattern involves the use of two crutches or a walker. It cannot be used with a cane or one crutch. The three-point gait pattern requires good upper body strength, good balance, and good cardiovascular endurance. The pattern is initiated with the forward movement of the assistive gait device (refer to Figure 16-2). Next, the involved lower extremity is advanced as the patient presses down on the assistive gait device

Ambulation Pattern with Assistive Aid

Two-point: Assistive aid *(crutch)* and opposite lower extremity *(foot)* advance *simultaneously;* bilateral canes, crutches, or reciprocal walker may be used.

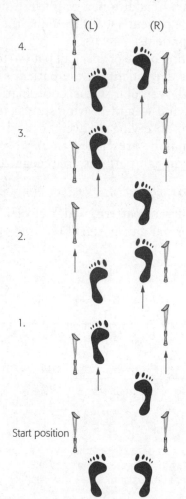

Figure 16-2 Two-point gait pattern.

Source: Adapted from Pierson FM, Fairchild SL: Principles and Techniques of Patient Care, Philadelphia, W.B. Saunders Company,1994.

Ambulation Pattern with Assistive Aid

Modified two-point: Only one assistive aid *(crutch)* is used; the assistive aid and the opposite lower extremity *(foot)* advance *simultaneously;* the assistive aid is held in the hand opposite the affected lower extremity; one cane or crutch may be used.

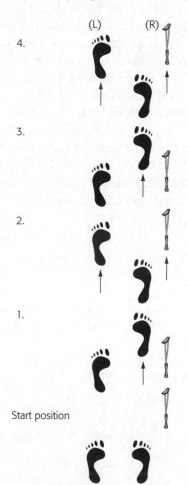

Figure 16-3 Two-point modified.

Source: Adapted from Pierson FM, Fairchild SL: Principles and Techniques of Patient Care, Philadelphia, W.B. Saunders Company,1994.

and advances the uninvolved lower extremity. Two methods of advancing the lower extremity can be used:

- *Swing to:* The uninvolved lower extremity is advanced to a point at which it is parallel to the involved lower extremity.
- *Swing through:* The involved lower extremity is advanced ahead of the uninvolved lower extremity.

Three-Point Modified or Three-Point One Pattern

A modification of the three-point gait pattern requires two crutches or a walker. This pattern is used when the patient can bear full weight with one lower extremity but is only allowed to partially bear weight on the involved lower extremity. In partial weight bearing, only part of the patient's weight is allowed to be transferred through the involved lower extremity. It must be remembered that most patients have difficulty replicating a prescribed weight-bearing restriction and will need constant reinforcement.[24]

The pattern is initiated with the forward movement of one of the assistive gait devices, and then the involved lower extremity is advanced forward (refer to Figure 16-3). The patient presses down on the assistive gait device and advances the uninvolved lower extremity, using either a "swing-to" or a "swing-through" pattern.

Four-Point Pattern

The four-point gait pattern, which requires the use of an assistive gait device (canes or crutches) on each side of the body, is used when the patient requires maximum assistance with balance and stability. The pattern is initiated with the forward movement of one of the assistive gait devices, and then the contralateral lower extremity, the other assistive gait device, and finally the opposite lower extremity (e.g., right crutch, then left foot; left crutch, then right foot).

Four-Point Modified Pattern

The four-point modified pattern is the same as the four-point except that it requires only one assistive device, positioned on the opposite side of the involved lower extremity. This pattern cannot be used if there are any weight-bearing restrictions (i.e., PWB, NWB), but it is appropriate for a patient with unilateral weakness or mild balance deficits. The patient is instructed to move the cane, then the involved leg, and then the uninvolved leg.

Stair Negotiation

Ascending Stairs

To ascend steps, the patient must first move to the front edge of the step. The walker will have to be turned toward the opposite side of the handrail or wall. Ascending more than two or three stairs with a walker is not recommended.

- To ascend stairs using a walker, the patient is instructed to grasp the stair handrail with one hand and to turn the walker sideways so that the two front legs of the walker are placed on the first step. When ready, the patient pushes down on the walker handgrip and the handrail and advances the uninvolved lower extremity onto the first step. The patient then advances the uninvolved lower extremity to the first step and moves the legs of the walker to the next step. This process is repeated as the patient moves up the steps.
- To ascend steps or stairs with crutches, the patient should grasp the stair handrail with one hand and grasp both crutches by the handgrips with the other hand. If the patient is unable to grasp both crutches with one hand, or if the handrail is not stable, then the patient should use both crutches only, although this is not recommended if there are more than two or three steps. When in the correct position at the front edge of the step, the patient pushes down on the crutches and handrail, if applicable, and advances the uninvolved lower extremity to the first step. The patient then advances the involved lower extremity, and finally the crutches. This process is repeated for the remaining steps.
- To ascend steps or stairs with one or two canes, the patient should use the handrail and the cane(s). If the handrail is not stable, then the patient should use the cane(s) only. The patient pushes down on the cane(s) or handrail, if applicable, and advances the uninvolved lower extremity to the first step. The patient then advances the involved lower extremity. This process is repeated for the remaining steps.

Descending Stairs

In order to descend steps, the patient must first move to the front edge of the top step. Descending more than two or three stairs with a walker is not recommended.

- To descend stairs using a walker, the walker is turned sideways so that the two front legs of the walker are placed on the lower step. One hand is placed on the rear handgrip, and the other hand grasps the stair handrail. When ready, the patient lowers the involved lower extremity down to the first step. Then the patient pushes down on the walker and handrail and advances the uninvolved lower extremity down the first step. This process is repeated as the patient moves down the steps.
- To descend steps or stairs with crutches, the patient should use one hand to grasp the stair handrail and the other to grasp both crutches and handrail. If the patient is unable to grasp both crutches with one hand, or if the handrail is not stable, then the patient should use both crutches only, although this is not recommended if there are more than two or three steps. When ready, the patient lowers the involved lower extremity down to the first step. Next, the patient pushes down on the crutches and handrail, if applicable, and advances the uninvolved lower extremity down to the first step. This process is repeated for the remaining steps.
- To descend steps or stairs with one or two canes, the patient should use the cane(s) and handrail. If the handrail is not stable, then the patient should use the cane(s) only. When ready, the patient lowers the involved lower extremity down to the first step. Next, the patient pushes down on the cane(s) and handrail, if applicable, and advances the uninvolved lower extremity down to the first step. This process is repeated for the remaining steps.

Instructions

Whichever gait pattern is chosen, it is important that the patient receive verbal and illustrated instructions for use of the assistive gait device to negotiate stairs, curbs, ramps, doors, and transfers. These instructions should include any weight-bearing precautions pertinent to the patient, the appropriate gait sequence, and a contact number at which to reach the clinician if questions arise.

Bed Mobility and Transfer Training

The most common types of patient training encountered by the PTA in the inpatient environment include bed mobility (e.g., pulling a patient up in bed) and transfer training (e.g., transferring a patient from the bed to another surface such as a chair or gurney).

Pulling Patient Up in Bed

The clinician and an assistant, standing on opposite sides of the bed, use a draw-sheet to slide the patient up in bed. Every attempt should be made to decrease the amount of friction to make this move more comfortable for the patient and to reduce the stress on the lifters. The head of the bed is lowered and the top of the bed is adjusted to waist or hip level of the shorter person. The two lifters grasp the draw-sheet, with palms up and elbows flexed, pointing one foot in the direction the patient is to be moved. The patient should be asked to bend the knees, push down with the feet, and pull up using a trapeze. The lifters lean in the direction of the move using the legs and body weight. On the count of three, the patient is lifted and pulled up the bed. This step is repeated as many times as needed.

Bed to Chair Transfer Training

Prior to performing a bed transfer, the clinician should consider the following:

- The patient's level of cognition and mobility. It is important to be able to communicate with the patient about the transfer details and his or her responsibility during the transfer.
- How much assistance the clinician requires. When in doubt, a second person should be utilized. Commands and counts are used to synchronize the actions of the participants. The various levels of physical assistance are outlined in **Table 16-5**.
- Equipment needs. The appropriate equipment should be arranged prior to the transfer.
- Correct positioning of both the patient and the clinician. The clinician should maintain a large base of support and use proper body mechanics throughout the transfer. Manual contacts can be used with the patient to direct his or her participation during the transfer.

Moving Patient Out of Bed to a Wheelchair

The steps of the move are explained to the patient, and the patient is told that he or she can rest when needed. The ability of the patient to help is assessed, and the clinician makes the determination as to whether further help is necessary. A transfer belt is recommended to provide a firm handhold. The clinician positions and locks the wheelchair close to the bed and helps the patient turn over and sit on/scoot to the edge of the bed. The clinician places

TABLE 16-5	Levels of Physical Assistance
Independent	The patient does not require any assistance to complete the task.
Supervision	The patient requires the clinician to observe throughout completion of the task.
Contact guard	The patient requires the clinician to maintain contact with the patient to complete the task. Contact guard is usually needed to assist if there is a loss of balance.
Minimal assist	The patient requires 25% assistance from the clinician to complete the task.
Moderate assist	The patient requires 50% assistance from the clinician to complete the task.
Maximal assist	The patient requires 75% assistance from the therapist to complete the task.
Dependent	The patient is unable to participate and the clinician must provide all of the effort to perform the task.

his or her arms around the patient's chest and clasps the hands behind the patient's back. Supporting the leg farther from the wheelchair between the legs, the clinician leans back, shifts his or her weight, and lifts. The patient pivots toward the chair if possible or is guided by the clinician. If the patient's legs are weak and appear to be buckling, the clinician can brace his or her knees against the patient's knees. Once correctly positioned, the patient bends toward the clinician, who bends the knees and lowers the patient into the back of the wheelchair.

Transfers on Level Surfaces (Bed to Gurney)
The clinician and an assistant stand on opposite sides of the bed, with the clinician on the side of the direction of the transfer. A large plastic garbage bag is placed between the sheet and the draw-sheet, beneath one edge of the patient's torso. The patient's legs are moved closer to the edge of the bed. Grasping the draw-sheet on both sides of the bed, on a count of three the clinician leans backward and shifts the weight, sliding the patient to the edge of the bed, while the assistant holds the sheet to keep it from slipping. The bed is raised so that it is slightly higher than the gurney, and the head of the bed is lowered. The patient's legs are moved onto the gurney, and the assistant kneels on the bed. On the count of three, the clinician and assistant grasp the draw-sheet and slide the patient onto the gurney. This may take several attempts.

Moving from Wheelchair to Toilet or Tub Seat
The wheelchair is positioned as close to the destination as possible. The clinician locks the wheelchair and fastens the transfer belt. The clinician helps the patient slide to the edge of the wheelchair and positions the patient's feet directly under his or her body. The clinician lifts the patient, grasping the back of the transfer belt, and helps the patient pivot around in front of the toilet, keeping the patient's knees between the clinician's legs. The patient grasps each of the safety rails as they are slowly and gently lowered down onto the toilet.

Dependent Transfers
Three-Person Carry/Lift Transfer
The three-person carry/lift is used to transfer a patient from a stretcher to a bed or treatment plinth. Three clinicians carry the patient in a supine position; one clinician supports the head and upper trunk, the second clinician supports the trunk, and the third supports the lower extremities. The clinician at the head of the bed is usually the one to initiate commands. The clinicians flex their elbows, positioned under the patient, and roll the patient on his or her side toward them. The clinicians then lift on command and move in a line to the destination surface, then lower and position the patient properly.

Two-Person Lift Transfer
The two-person lift is used to transfer a patient between two surfaces of different heights or when transferring a patient to the floor. Standing behind the patient, the first clinician should place the arms underneath the patient's axilla. The clinician should grasp the patient's left forearm with the right hand and grasp the patient's right forearm with the left hand. The second clinician places one arm under the mid to distal thighs and uses the other arm to support the lower legs. The clinician at the head usually initiates the command to lift and transfer the patient out of the chair to the destination surface.

Dependent Squat Pivot Transfer

The dependent squat pivot transfer is used to transfer a patient who cannot stand independently but can bear some weight through the trunk and lower extremities. The clinician should position the patient at a 45-degree angle to the destination surface. The patient places the upper extremities on the clinician's shoulders but should not be allowed to pull on the clinician's neck. The clinician should position the patient at the edge of the surface, hold the patient around the hips and under the buttocks, and block the patient's knees in order to avoid buckling while standing. The clinician should utilize momentum, straighten his or her legs, and raise the patient or allow the patient to remain in a squatting position. The clinician should then pivot and slowly lower the patient to the destination surface.

Hydraulic or Mechanical Lift Transfer

A hydraulic or mechanical lift is a device required for dependent transfers when a patient is obese, there is only one clinician available to assist for the transfer, a patient has a weight-bearing restriction on bilateral lower extremities, or a patient is totally dependent. A body sling is required for the lift transfer. Two primary types of sling exist: full body, which covers the posterior surface of the patient from the shoulders to the back of the thighs/knees, and a sling that has divided legs that cross between the patient's legs and support him or her on the posterior surface of the thighs. The hydraulic lift is locked in position before the transfer. The clinician positions the sling under the patient by rolling the patient from side to side, and then attaches the S-ring to the bars on the lift. The longer length of chain is attached at the lower end of the sling to encourage a seated position. Once all attachments are checked, the clinician should pump the handle on the device in order to elevate the patient. Once the patient is elevated, the clinician can navigate the lift with the patient to the destination surface. Once transferred, the chains should be removed; however, the webbed sling should remain in place in preparation for the return transfer.

Assisted Transfers

Sliding Board Transfer

A sliding board is used for a patient who has some sitting balance, has some upper extremity strength, and can adequately follow directions. The patient should be positioned at the edge of the wheelchair or bed and should lean to one side while placing one end of the sliding board sufficiently under the proximal thigh. The other end of the sliding board should be positioned on the destination surface. The patient should not hold on to the end of the sliding board in order to avoid pinching the fingers. The patient should place the lead hand 4 to 6 inches away from the sliding board and use both arms to initiate a push-up and scoot across the board. The clinician should guard in front of the patient and assist as needed while the patient performs a series of push-ups across the board.

Stand Pivot Transfer

A stand pivot transfer is used when a patient is able to stand and bear weight through one or both of the lower extremities. The patient must possess functional balance and the ability to pivot. Patients with unilateral weight-bearing restrictions or hemiplegia may utilize this transfer and lead with the uninvolved side. The transfer may also be used therapeutically, leading with the involved side for a patient post-cerebrovascular accident (CVA). The patient should be positioned at the edge of the wheelchair or bed to initiate the transfer. The clinician can assist the patient to keep the feet flat on the floor while bringing the head and trunk forward. The clinician should assist the patient as needed with his or her feet. The clinician must guard or assist the patient through the transfer and instruct the patient to reach back for the surface before he or she begins to sit down. Once the stand pivot is performed, the clinician should assist as needed to ensure control with lowering the patient to the destination surface.

Stand Step Transfer

The stand step transfer is used with a patient who has the necessary strength and balance to weight shift and step during the transfer. The patient requires guiding or supervision from the clinician and performs the transfer as a stand pivot transfer except that the patient actually takes a step to maneuver and reposition his or her feet instead of using a pivot.

Push-Up (Pop-Over) Transfer

The push-up transfer is used for a patient with good sitting balance who can lift the buttocks clear of a sitting surface (e.g., a patient with a complete C7 level spinal cord injury can be independent with this transfer without a sliding board). It can be used as a progression in transfer training from using a sliding board. The patient utilizes a head-hips relationship to successfully complete the transfer—movement of the head in one direction results in movement of the hips in the opposite direction toward the support surface being transferred to.

Wheelchairs

A wheelchair is a medical device that takes the form of a chair on wheels. It is used by people for whom walking is difficult or impossible due to illness or disability. Wheelchairs are available in a variety of sizes, styles, and classes:

- Indoor wheelchairs have a small wheelbase to allow maneuvering in confined spaces, but lack the ability or power to negotiate obstacles.
- Indoor/outdoor wheelchairs provide mobility for those who stay on finished services, such as sidewalks, driveways, and flooring.
- Active indoor/outdoor wheelchairs provide the ability to travel long distances, move fast, and drive over unstructured environments such as grass, gravel, and uneven terrain.

Wheelchair Measurements[25]

To get a properly fitted wheelchair, the patient ideally should have a seated examination on a simulator, a chair specifically designed for planar seated examinations. If a simulator is not available, the measurement can be done on a firm surface with the patient's hips, knees, and ankles positioned at 90 degrees (**Table 16-6**).

Wheelchair Components

Frame

Wheelchair users today have a choice of stainless steel, chrome, aluminum, airplane aluminum, steel tubing, an alloy of chrome and lightweight materials, titanium, and other lightweight composite materials (for example, sports chairs accommodate a tucked position, include leg straps, slanted drive wheels, and small push rims). The ultralight wheelchair is the highest-quality chair, designed specifically for active people.

> **● Key Point** In general, the lighter the weight of the frame, the greater the ease of use, but the lesser amount of structural strength provided.

The two most common types of frames currently available are:

- *Rigid frame:* The frame remains in one piece and the wheels are released for storage or travel. Advantages:

- ❑ It facilitates stroke efficiency.
- ❑ It increases distance/stroke.
- *Standard cross-brace frame:* The cross-brace enables the frame to collapse or fold for transport or storage. Advantages:
  - ❑ It facilitates mobility in the community.
  - ❑ The wheelchair is folded by first raising the footplates and then pulling up on the handles (located on either side of the seat), rather than pulling up on the middle of the upholstery, the latter of which can tear the upholstery.

Anti-Tipping Device

An anti-tipping device consists of posterior extensions attached to the low horizontal supports. These supports prevent the chair from tipping backward and limit the ability to go over curbs or over doorsills. A similar device is the Hill holder, which is a mechanical brake that allows the chair to go forward but automatically applies the brakes if the chair goes into reverse.

Seating System

Many wheelchairs come with a fabric or sling seat. The disadvantages of a sling seat are that the hips tend to slide forward, the thighs tend to adduct and internally rotate, and the patient sits asymmetrically, which reinforces poor pelvic position.

- *Insert or contour seats:* Create a stable, firm sitting surface, provide improved pelvic position (neutral), and reduce the tendency for the patient to slide forward or sit with a posterior pelvic tilt.
- *Seat cushions:* Function to distribute weight-bearing pressures, which assists in preventing decubitus ulcers in patients with decreased sensation and prolongs wheelchair sitting times (**Table 16-7**).
- *Suspension elements:* Reduce discomfort and various harmful physiological effects, such as chronic low back pain and disc degeneration, caused by extended exposure to the vibration sustained propelling a wheelchair in communities.

Backrest

The standard-height backrest provides support to the mid-scapula region.

- A lower back height may increase functional mobility—typically seen in sports chairs—but may also increase back strain.

TABLE 16-6	Standard Wheelchair Measurements	
Dimension	**Guidelines**	**Average Size**
Seat height/ leg length	Measurement taken from the user's heel to the popliteal fold. Two inches are added to this measurement to allow clearance of the footrest. Seat-to-floor height is important if the patient is going to propel the wheelchair using his or her feet. Seat-to-floor height can be adjusted down approximately 2 inches by using a "dual axle" wheelchair.	Standard seat-to-floor height for a wheelchair is 18 to 20 inches. Hemi is 17.5 to 18.5 inches depending on manufacturer. Anything lower is a "super" or "ultra" Hemi.
Seat depth	Measurement taken from the user's posterior buttock, along the lateral thigh to the popliteal fold. Should be slightly shorter (about 2 inches) than the femur length (taking into consideration functional issues such as foot propulsion/leg management; pressure distribution; knee range of motion; leg length discrepancies/leg alignment; and hanger angle of the leg rest).	Adult: 16 inches Narrow adult: 16 inches Slim adult: 16 inches Junior: 16 inches Child: 11.5 inches Tiny tot: 11.5 inches
Seat width	Measurement taken of the widest aspect of the user's buttocks, hips or thighs. Two inches is added to this measurement so as to provide space for bulky clothing, orthoses, or clearance of the trochanters from the armrest side panel.	• Transport wheelchair: seat width + 3 inches • Standard folding wheelchair: seat width + 8 inches • Reclining wheelchairs: seat width + 8 inches • Bariatric wheelchairs: seat width + 8 inches
Back height	Measurement taken from the seat of the chair to the floor of the axilla with the user's shoulder flexed to 90°. Four inches is subtracted from this measurement to allow the final height to be below the inferior angles of the scapulae. N.B.: This measurement will be affected if a seat cushion is to be used—the person should be measured while seated on the seat cushion, or the thickness of the cushion must be considered by adding that value to the actual measurement.	Adult: 16 to 16.5 inches. If the back height is too high, it can impair propulsion and scapular mobility, promote a kyphotic posture, and impair sitting balance. If the back height is too low, it can promote a kyphotic posture, impair sitting balance, and cause inappropriate placement of anterior support devices for the shoulder/chest.
Armrest height	Measurement taken from the seat of the chair to the olecranon process with the user's elbow flexed to 90°. One inch is added to this measurement. N.B.: This measurement will be affected if a seat cushion is to be used—the person should be measured while seated on the seat cushion, or the thickness of the cushion must be considered by adding that value to the actual measurement.	Adult: 9 inches above the chair seat. If the armrest is set too high, it can increase pressure/pain at the glenohumeral joint and increase difficulty maneuvering joystick. If the armrest is set too low, it can create kyphosis or scoliosis, increase ischial tuberosity pressure, and promote or worsen shoulder subluxation.

- Lateral trunk supports provide improved trunk alignment for patients with scoliosis or poor stability.
- Insert or contour backs improve trunk extension and overall upright alignment.
- A high back height may be necessary for patients with poor trunk stability or with extensor spasms.

Brakes

Brakes are an important safety feature. Most brakes consist of a lever system with a cam or a ratchet. Extensions may be added to increase the ease of both locking and unlocking. A wheelchair with a reclining back requires an additional brake. Brakes must be engaged for all transfers in and out of the chair.

TABLE 16-7	Types of Wheelchair Cushions		
Type of Cushion	**Advantages**		**Disadvantage**
Pressure-relieving air cushion	Lightweight		Expensive
	Accommodates moderate to severe postural deformity and improve pressure distribution		Base may be unstable for some patients
			Requires continuous maintenance
Pressure-relieving fluid/ gel or combination	Accommodates moderate to severe postural deformity		Requires some maintenance
	Makes it easy for caregivers to reposition the patient		Heavy
			Moderately expensive
Pressure-relieving contoured foam	Is designed to accommodate moderate to severe postural deformity		May interfere with slide board transfers
	Makes it easy for caregivers to reposition patient		

Wheels/Tires

Most wheelchairs use four wheels: two large wheels (standard spokes or spokeless) at the back (fitted with an outer rim that allows for hand grip and propulsion) and two smaller ones (casters) at the front. The tires used for the rear wheels may be narrow and hard rubber, pneumatic inflatable, semi-pneumatic, or radial tires.

● **Key Point** Pneumatic tires provide a smoother ride and increased shock absorption but require more maintenance than solid tires.

The standard size for the rear wheel is 24 inches. Smaller and larger wheel sizes are available.

- An outer rim enables the patient to propel him- or herself. For patients with only one functional arm, two outer rims can be fitted on one wheel so that arm drive achieves both forward and backward propulsion.
- Projections (vertical, oblique, or horizontal) may be attached to the rims to facilitate with propulsion in patients with poor handgrip. However, the horizontal and oblique extensions add to the overall width of the chair and may reduce maneuverability.
- Casters vary in size (ranging from 6 to 8 inches in diameter) and composition (pneumatic, solid rubber, plastic, or a combination of these). Caster locks can be added to facilitate wheelchair stability during transfers.

Leg Rests

Leg rests come in a variety of designs.

- *Swing away:* Feature detachable leg rests that facilitate the ease in transfers and a front approach to the wheelchair when ambulating.
- *Elevating:* Most frequently necessary when the patient is unable to flex the knee, for postural support, or when a dependent leg contributes to lower extremity edema. The length of the leg rest is adjustable to accommodate the full length of the patient's leg, and a padded calf support is provided. The position of the leg rest is adjusted by pushing down on a lever on the side of the chair. Elevating leg rests can be released from the wheelchair or pivoted to one side during transfers. Elevated leg rests are contraindicated for patients with hypertonicity or adaptive shortening of the hamstrings.
- *Fixed:* Fixed leg rests are, as the name suggests, leg rests that cannot be modified or removed.

Foot Rests

A footrest is standard equipment on a wheelchair. In rigid-frame chairs the footrests are usually incorporated into the frame of the chair as part of the design. Cross-brace folding chairs often have footrests that swivel, flip up, and/or can be removed.

- *Foot plates:* Can be adjusted to accommodate the patient's foot. They provide a resting base for the feet so that the feet are in neutral with a knee flexed to 90 degrees.
- *Heel loops:* Can be fitted to help maintain the foot position and prevent posterior sliding of the foot. Ankle and calf straps can be added to stabilize the feet on the foot plates.

- *Toe loops:* May also be used when the patient has difficulty maintaining the foot on the footplate in a forward direction.

Armrests

Adjustable armrests are available in several styles, including:

- Desk length (to allow the user closer access to desks and tables). Allows the patient to remove and reverse the armrest so that the higher part is closer to the front edge in order to aid in pushing to standing.
- Full length.
- Wraparound (space saver). Reduces the overall width of the chair by 1½". The height of the armrests can also be adjusted.

> ● **Key Point** Armrests can also be fitted with upper extremity support surface trays or troughs, which are helpful if the user has difficulty with upper body balance or decreased use of the upper extremities.

> ● **Key Point** Many lightweight manual chairs are designed without armrests, which makes it easier for the user to roll up to a desk or table and to perform transfers, in addition to providing a streamlined look.

Seat Belts

Seat belts can be used for safety or for positioning. Restraining belts are used to prevent patients from falling out of the wheelchair. Seat belts can be fitted to grasp over the pelvis at a 45-degree angle to the seat to help position the pelvis. The position can also be adjusted to provide lateral or medial support at the hip and knee to maintain alignment of the lower extremities and/or control spasticity.

Specialized Wheelchairs

Pediatric Wheelchairs

A pediatric wheelchair must have approximately 4 inches of available space in the frame to accommodate growth. In addition, the seating system should be flexible enough to accommodate tonal or postural changes. Examples of flexibility in the system involve the placement of laterals, which are often attached to tracks, or the backrest can include T-nuts placed throughout the back to allow easy hardware mounting. Pediatric chairs often employ linear seating systems (to accommodate the delicate balance between providing contours in the system and accommodating growth) versus molded seats, which are more difficult to increase in size. Similarly, a contoured

backrest is more accommodating and provides more contact surface and thus more comfort.

Reclining Wheelchairs

The purpose of the reclining wheelchair is to allow intermittent or constant reclined positioning. Reclining wheelchairs are designed with an extended back and typically with elevating leg rests. The angle of the back is adjusted by releasing knobs on the side of the wheelchair. A head support is required on a reclining wheelchair. A bar across the back of the reclining wheelchair provides support and stability. Reclining wheelchairs are indicated for patients who are unable to independently maintain an upright sitting position. The chairs can be controlled either manually or electrically (if the patient cannot do active push-ups or pressure relief maneuvers).

Hemi Chair

A hemi chair, with a seat height of approximately 17.5 inches, is designed to be low to the ground, allowing propulsion with the noninvolved upper and/or lower extremities.

Tilt in Space

A tilt-in-space chair is designed to allow for a reclining position without losing the required 90 degrees of hip flexion and 90 degrees of knee flexion. This type of chair is indicated for patients with extensor spasms that may throw the patient out of the chair, or for pressure relief.

One-Arm Drive

A chair with one-arm drive is designed with the drive mechanisms located on one wheel, usually with two outer rims (or a push lever). The patient is able to propel the wheelchair by pushing on both rims (or the lever) with one hand.

Amputee Chair

An amputee chair is modified so that the drive wheels are placed posterior (approximately 2 inches backwards) to the vertical back supports, thereby lengthening the base of support and enhancing posterior stability.

Powered Chairs

Powered chairs utilize a power source (such as a battery) that propels the wheelchair. Microprocessors allow the control of the wheelchair to be adapted to various controls (joystick, head, breath). This type of chair is usually prescribed for patients who are not capable of self-propulsion or who have very low endurance. Recent changes in the power bases have allowed for such innovations as power seat functions (power tilt, recline, elevating leg rest, seat elevator) and control interfaces (mini joysticks, head controls). Power wheelchair bases can be classified in one of three categories, based on the drive wheel location relative to the system's center of gravity:

- *Rear-wheel drive:* Drive wheels are located behind the user's center of gravity, and the casters are located in the front, providing predictable drive characteristics and stability.
- *Mid-wheel drive:* Drive wheels are directly below the user's center of gravity and generally have a set of casters or anti-tippers in the front and rear of the drive wheels. The advantage of this system is a smaller turning radius. The disadvantage is a tendency to rock or pitch forward, especially with sudden stops or fast turns.
- *Front-wheel drive:* Drive wheels are located in front of the user's center of gravity. This design provides stability and a tight turning radius, and the ability to climb obstacles or curbs more easily. One of the disadvantages of this design is its rearward center of gravity, which makes it difficult to drive in a straight line, especially on uneven surfaces.

Wheelchair Training[26]

A number of areas need to be addressed when training a patient on how to be as functionally independent as possible with a wheelchair.

Posture

It is important for the patient to maintain good posture in the wheelchair. He or she should be seated well back in the chair, with the lower extremities on the footrests or leg rests. The patient should be able to maintain a seated position when his or her balance is challenged.

Wheelchair Management

The various components of the wheelchair should be reviewed with the patient, and the patient should perform all of the necessary tasks while being supervised by the clinician. Wheelchair users are susceptible to muscle imbalances. Nearly every motion and or repetitive motion is forward, working such areas as the shoulder flexors (pectoralis major, and anterior deltoid) and shoulder internal rotators. These anterior muscles can become adaptively shortened, while the upper back muscles become weak and elongated. The typical posture of the wheelchair user is rounded shoulders with mild thoracic kyphosis and a forward head. This posture can result in impingement of the soft tissue structures of the acromiohumeral space.

Wheelchair Mobility

Depending on functional level, the patient is instructed on how to:

- Operate the wheel locks, foot supports, and armrests, and to use the mechanisms safely without tipping forward or sideways out of the chair seat.
- Transfer in and out of the chair with the least possible assistance. This may involve transfer training from the wheelchair to the car seat.
- Propel the wheelchair in all directions and around corners.
- Perform a wheelie. A wheelie is performed by balancing on the rear wheels of a wheelchair while the caster wheels are in the air. Wheelies are important for patients who need to go up and down curbs independently when there are no curb ramps. Initially, the clinician must be positioned behind the chair and move with the chair, with the hands held beneath the wheelchair handles, ready to catch the wheelchair if it tilts too far backward. The patient should be taught how to tuck the head into the chest if he or she falls backward to avoid hitting the back of the head while performing the maneuver without assistance. To perform a wheelie, the patient places the hands at 11:00 and 1:00 on the wheels, then leans forward and arches the back. At first the patient practices by bouncing the body off the back of the chair and leaning back while holding the hands still; the front of the chair is raised by pushing backward on the back of the chair. The patient practices until he or she can actually bounce the front end off the ground. By changing the center of gravity (by pushing the chair forward while the body is going backward) the patient will achieve a point of equilibrium.

Once the patient is able to bounce the front end off the ground and is able to find a point of equilibrium, he or she progresses to reaching back and placing the hands at about 10:00 on the wheels. From this point, the patient leans forward, arches the back, and then begins to push forward quickly while letting the body come back against the chair (when the back hits the chair, the hands should be in the 12:00 position). By continuing to lean back and while pushing the chair forward, the front end should start to leave the ground, and by the time the hands get to the 2:00 position, the front end should feel weightless, as the chair balances on the rear axle. To maintain equilibrium, the patient will need to be able to move the chair forward if the front end begins to fall down or backward if the chair begins to fall backward. This may be accomplished by sliding the hands back to about the 1:00 position, without taking the hands off the wheels. Once the chair is up and balanced, the patient will need to keep just a fraction of weight on the front end, so that if balance is lost the chair will fall forward, not backward.

- "Pop a wheelie" and move forward and backward in the wheelie position. Once the patient is ready to try a wheelie independently, a good place to begin practicing is on carpeting, grass, or sand.

REVIEW Questions

1. Define the gait cycle.
2. What are the functional tasks associated with normal gait?
3. What are the two periods of the gait cycle?
4. What are the four intervals of the stance phase called?
5. What are the four intervals of the swing phase called?
6. What are the three gait parameters that are the most meaningful to measure in the clinic?
7. What are the three primary determinants of gait velocity?
8. What is the average normal cadence in adults without pathology?
9. Where is the center of gravity (COG) of the body located?
10. True or false: During the gait cycle, the COG is displaced both vertically and posteriorly.
11. True or false: During the gait cycle the thoracic spine and the pelvis rotate in the same direction as each other to enhance stability and balance.
12. Describe the characteristics of a positive Trendelenburg.
13. Which of the following muscles is active throughout the entire gait cycle?
    a. Tibialis anterior
    b. Soleus

c. Hamstrings
d. Quadriceps

14. List three effects that a weak tibialis anterior could have on gait.
15. During the normal gait cycle, when do the hamstrings have their maximum activity?
16. Paralysis or marked weakness of the pretibial muscle group produces:
    a. Foot drop during swing phase
    b. Excessive foot eversion
    c. Excessive foot inversion
    d. None of the above
17. During the stance phase of gait:
    a. The calf muscles become active.
    b. The quadriceps are active.
    c. The hip abductors are active.
    d. All of the above.
18. A positive Trendelenburg sign results from paralysis of:
    a. Hip flexors
    b. Hip abductors
    c. Hip extensors
    d. Hip adductors
19. You are observing a patient ambulating. The patient lurches backward during the stance phase. What type of gait is the patient demonstrating?
    a. Wide-based gait
    b. Antalgic gait
    c. Gluteus medius gait
    d. Extensor gait
20. An individual demonstrates a steppage gait pattern during ambulation activities. Steppage gait is characterized by excessive:
    a. Knee and hip extension
    b. Knee and hip flexion
    c. Knee and ankle flexion
    d. Knee and ankle extension
21. At which point in the normal gait cycle is there maximum activity of the gluteus medius and minimus?
22. Weakness of which muscle can cause a Trendelenburg gait pattern?
23. While observing the gait of a 67-year-old man with arthritis of the left hip, you observe a left lateral trunk lean. Why does the patient present with this gait deviation?
    a. To increase the joint compression force of the involved hip by moving the weight toward it.
    b. To decrease the joint compression force by moving the weight toward the involved hip.

c. To bring the line of gravity closer to the involved hip joint.

d. Because his right leg is shorter.

24. You observe a patient demonstrating a significant posterior trunk lean at initial contact. Which is the most likely muscle that you will need to focus on during the exercise session in order to minimize this gait deviation?

25. Which three orthopaedic conditions could be associated with quadriceps avoidance?

26. A patient who has a recent fracture of the right tibia and fibula has developed foot drop of the right foot during gait. Which nerve is causing this loss of motor function?

27. Following a hip fracture that is now healed, your patient presents with weak hip flexors (2/5), with all other muscles within functional limits. During gait, which gait characteristic would you expect to see?

28. Which of the following assistive devices offers the most stability?

a. Cane

b. Walker

c. Crutches

d. Quad cane

29. When measuring a patient for crutches, where should the crutch tip be placed?

30. When measuring a patient for crutches, how large a gap should there be between the tops of the axillary pads and the patient's axilla?

a. 1 to 2 inches

b. 2 to 3 inches

c. 3 to 4 inches

d. No gap

31. You have just finished transferring a patient from a bed to a chair who required 25% assist from you to complete the task. How would you document in the chart the level of assistance required?

a. Contact guard

b. Minimal assist

c. Moderate assist

d. Maximal assist

32. You are measuring a patient to assess the seat depth for a wheelchair from the user's posterior buttock, along the lateral thigh to the popliteal fold. How many inches should you add/subtract from this measurement?

a. Add 2 inches

b. Subtract 2 inches

c. Add 1 inch

d. Subtract 1 inch

References

1. Luttgens K, Hamilton N: The Center of Gravity and Stability, in Luttgens K, Hamilton N (eds): Kinesiology: Scientific Basis of Human Motion (ed 9). Dubuque, IA, McGraw-Hill, 1997, pp 415–442

2. Epler M: Gait, in Richardson JK, Iglarsh ZA (eds): Clinical Orthopaedic Physical Therapy. Philadelphia, WB Saunders, 1994, pp 602–625

3. Perry J: Stride Analysis, in Perry J (ed): Gait Analysis: Normal and Pathological Function. Thorofare, NJ, Slack, 1992, pp 431–441

4. Perry J: Gait Analysis: Normal and Pathological Function. Thorofare, NJ, Slack, 1992

5. Rogers MM: Dynamic foot mechanics. J Orthop Sports Phys Ther 21:306–316, 1995

6. Gage JR, Deluca PA, Renshaw TS: Gait analysis: Principles and applications with emphasis on its use with cerebral palsy. Inst Course Lect 45:491–507, 1996

7. Scranton J, P.E., Rutkowski R, Brown TD: Support phase kinematics of the foot, in Bateman JE, Trott AW (eds): The Foot and Ankle. New York, BC Decker, 1980, pp 195–205

8. Mann RA, Hagy J: Biomechanics of walking, running, and sprinting. Am J Sports Med 8:345–350, 1980

9. Perry J: Gait Cycle, in Perry J (ed): Gait Analysis: Normal and Pathological Function. Thorofare, NJ, Slack, 1992, pp 3–7

10. Luttgens K, Hamilton N: Locomotion: Solid surface, in Luttgens K, Hamilton N (eds): Kinesiology: Scientific Basis of Human Motion (ed 9). Dubuque, IA, McGraw-Hill, 1997, pp 519–549

11. Mann RA, Moran GT, Dougherty SE: Comparative electromyography of the lower extremity in jogging, running and sprinting. Am J Sports Med 14:501–510, 1986

12. Whitehouse PA, Knight LA, Di Nicolantonio F, et al: Heterogeneity of chemosensitivity of colorectal adenocarcinoma determined by a modified ex vivo ATP-tumor chemosensitivity assay (ATP-TCA). Anticancer Drugs 14:369–375, 2003

13. Richardson JK, Iglarsh ZA: Gait, in Richardson JK, Iglarsh ZA (eds): Clinical Orthopaedic Physical Therapy. Philadelphia, Saunders, 1994, pp 602–625

14. Giannini S, Catani F, Benedetti MG, et al: Terminology, parameterization and normalization in gait analysis, Gait Analysis: Methodologies and Clinical Applications. Washington, DC, IOS Press, 1994, pp 65–88

15. Oatis CA: Role of the hip in posture and gait, in Echternach J (ed): Clinics in Physical Therapy: Physical Therapy of the Hip. New York, Churchill Livingstone, 1983, pp 165–179

16. Perry J: The hip, Gait Analysis: Normal and Pathological Function. Thorofare, NJ, Slack, 1992, pp 111–129

17. Rengachary SS: Gait and Station; examination of coordination, in Wilkins RH, Rengachary SS (eds): Neurosurgery (ed 2). New York, McGraw-Hill, 1996, pp 133–137

18. Bauer DM, Finch DC, McGough KP, et al: A comparative analysis of several crutch length estimation techniques. Phys Ther 71:294–300, 1991

19. Joyce BM, Kirby RL: Canes, crutches and walkers. Am Fam Phys 43:535–542, 1991

20. Deaver GG: What every physician should know about the teaching of crutch walking. JAMA 142:470–472, 1950

21. Baxter ML, Allington RO, Koepke GH: Weight-distribution variables in the use of crutches and canes. Phys Ther 49:360–365, 1969

22. Jebsen RH: Use and abuse of ambulation aids. JAMA 199:5–10, 1967

23. Kumar R, Roe MC, Scremin OU: Methods for estimating the proper length of a cane. Arch Phys Med Rehabil 76:1173–1175, 1995

24. Li S, Armstrong CW, Cipriani D: Three-point gait crutch walking: Variability in ground reaction force during weight bearing. Arch Phys Med Rehab 82:86-92, 2001

25. Edelstein JE: Prosthetics, in O'Sullivan SB, Schmitz TJ (eds): Physical Rehabilitation (ed 5). Philadelphia, FA Davis, 2007, pp 1251–1286

26. Dutton M: McGraw-Hill's NPTE (National Physical Therapy Examination). New York, McGraw-Hill, 2009, pp 1014–1015.

Guide for Conduct of the Physical Therapist Assistant

A. Purpose

1. This Guide for Conduct of the Physical Therapist Assistant (Guide) is intended to serve physical therapist assistants in interpreting The Standards of Ethical Conduct for a Physical Therapist Assistant (Standards) of the American Physical Therapy Association (APTA). The Guide provides guidelines by which physical therapist assistants may determine the propriety of their conduct. It also is intended to guide the development of physical therapist assistant students. The Standards and Guide apply to all physical therapist assistants. These guides are subject to change as the dynamics of the profession change and as new patterns of healthcare delivery are developed and accepted by the professional community and the public. This Guide is subject to monitoring and timely revision by the Ethics and Judicial Committee of the Association.

B. Interpreting Standards

1. The interpretations expressed in this Guide reflect the opinions, decisions, and advice of the Ethics and Judicial Committee. These interpretations are intended to guide a physical therapist assistant in applying general ethical principles to specific situations. They should not be considered inclusive of all situations at a physical therapist assistant may encounter.

Standard 1

1. A physical therapist assistant shall respect the rights and dignity of all individuals and shall provide compassionate care.
   a. Attitude of a physical therapist assistant
      1. A physical therapist assistant shall recognize, respect, and respond to individual and cultural difference with compassion and sensitivity.
      2. A physical therapist assistant shall be guided at all times by concern for the physical and psychological welfare of patients/clients.
      3. A physical therapist assistant shall not harass, abuse, or discriminate against others.

Standard 2

1. A physical therapist assistant shall act in a trustworthy manner towards patients/clients.
   a. Trustworthiness
      1. A physical therapist assistant shall always place the patient's/client's interest(s) above those of the physical therapist assistant. Working in the patients/client's best interests requires sensitivity to the patient's/client's vulnerability and an effective working relationship between a physical therapist and a physical therapist assistant.
      2. A physical therapist assistant shall not exploit any aspect of the physical therapist assistant—patient/client relationship.
      3. A physical therapist assistant shall clearly identify him/herself as a physical therapist assistant to patients/clients.
      4. A physical therapist assistant shall conduct him/herself in a manner that supports the physical therapist—patient/client relationship.
      5. A physical therapist assistant shall not engage in any sexual relationship or activity, whether consensual or nonconsensual, with any patient/client entrusted to his/her care.
      6. A physical therapist assistant shall not invite, accept, or offer gifts or other considerations that affect or give an appearance of affecting his/her provision of physical therapy interventions.
   b. Exploitation of patients
      1. A physical therapist assistant shall not participate in any arrangements in which patients/clients are exploited. Such arrangements include situations where referring sources enhance their personal incomes by referring to or recommending physical therapy services.
   c. Truthfulness
      1. A physical therapist assistant shall not make statements that he/she knows or should know are false, deceptive, fraudulent, or misleading.
      2. Although it cannot be considered unethical for a physical therapist assistant to own or have a financial interest in the production, sale, or distribution of products/services, he/she must act in accordance with law and make full disclosure of his/her interest to patients/clients.
   d. Confidential information
      1. Information relating to the patient/client is confidential and shall not be communicated to a third party not involved in that patient's/client's care without the prior consent of the patient/client, subject to applicable law.
      2. A physical therapist assistant shall refer all requests for release of confidential information to the supervising physical therapist.

Standard 3

1. A physical therapist assistant shall provide selected physical therapy interventions only under the supervision and direction of a physical therapist.
   a. Supervisory relationship
      1. A physical therapist assistant shall provide interventions only under the supervision and direction of a physical therapist.
      2. A physical therapist assistant shall provide only those interventions that have been selected by the physical therapist.
      3. A physical therapist assistant shall not provide any interventions that are outside his/her education, training, experience, or skill,

and shall notify the responsible physical therapist of his/her inability to carry out the intervention.

4. A physical therapist assistant may modify specific interventions within the plan of care established by the physical therapist in response to changes in the patient's/client's status.

5. A physical therapist assistant shall not perform examinations and evaluations, determine diagnoses and prognoses, or establish or change a plan of care.

6. Consistent with a physical therapist assistant's education, training, knowledge, and experience, he/she may respond to the patient's/client's inquiries regarding interventions that are within the established plan of care.

7. A physical therapist assistant shall have regular and ongoing communication with a physical therapist regarding the patient's/client's status.

Standard 4

1. A physical therapist assistant shall comply with laws and regulations governing physical therapy.
   a. Supervision
      1. A physical therapist assistant shall know and comply with applicable law. Regardless of the content of any law, a physical therapist assistant shall provide services only under the supervision and direction of a physical therapist.
   b. Representation
      1. A physical therapist assistant shall not hold him/herself out as a physical therapist.

Standard 5

1. A physical therapist assistant shall achieve and maintain competence in the provision of selected physical therapy interventions.
   a. Competence
      1. A physical therapist assistant shall provide interventions consistent with his/her level of education, training, experience, and skill.

   b. Self-assessment
      1. A physical therapist assistant shall engage in self-assessment in order to maintain competence.
   c. Development
      1. A physical therapist assistant shall participate in educational activities that enhance his/her basic knowledge and skills.

Standard 6

1. A physical therapist assistant shall make judgments that are commensurate with their educational and legal qualifications as a physical therapist assistant.
   a. Patient safety
      1. A physical therapist assistant shall discontinue immediately any intervention(s) that, in his/her judgment, may be harmful to the patient/client and shall discuss his/her concerns with the physical therapist.
      2. A physical therapist assistant shall not provide any interventions that are outside his/her education, training, experience, or skill and shall notify the responsible physical therapist of his/her inability to carry out the intervention.
      3. A physical therapist assistant shall not perform interventions while his/her ability to do so safely is impaired.
   b. Judgments of patient/client status
      1. If in a judgment of the physical therapist assistant, there is a change in the patient/client status he/she shall report this to the responsible physical therapist.
   c. Gifts and other considerations
      1. A physical therapist assistant shall not invite, accept, or offer gifts, monetary incentives, or other consideration that affect or give an appearance of affecting his/her provision of physical therapy interventions.

Standard 7

1. A physical therapist assistant shall protect the public and the confession from unethical, incompetent, and illegal acts.

a. Consumer protection
   1. A physical therapist assistant shall report any conduct that appears to be unethical or illegal.
b. Organizational employment
   1. A physical therapist assistant shall inform his/her employer(s) and/or appropriate physical therapist of any employer practice that causes him or her to be in conflict with the Standards of Ethical Conduct of the Physical Therapist Assistant.

2. A physical therapist assistant shall not engage in any activity that puts him or her in conflict with the Standards of Ethical Conduct for the Physical Therapist Assistant, regardless of directives from a physical therapist or employer.

From Guide to physical therapist practice: Phys Ther 81:S13–S95, 2001. Courtesy of the American Physical Therapist Association.

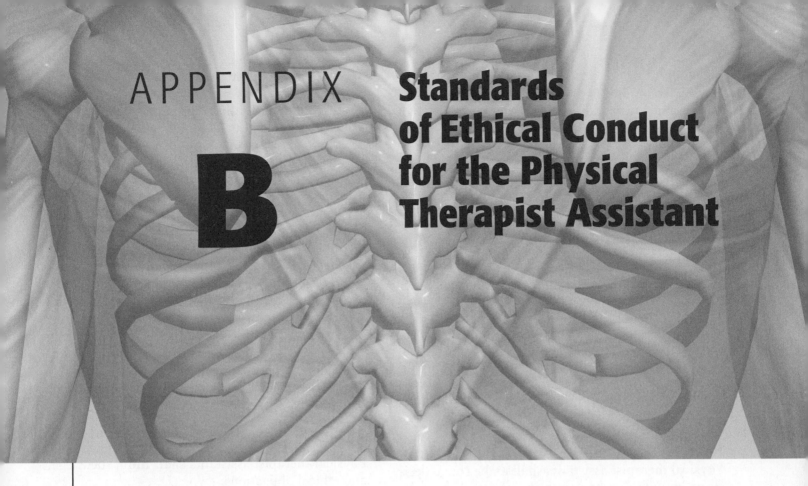

APPENDIX B

Standards of Ethical Conduct for the Physical Therapist Assistant

Preamble

The Standards of Ethical Conduct delineate the ethical obligations of all physical therapist assistants as determined by the House of Delegates of the American Physical Therapy Association (APTA). The Standards of Ethical Conduct provide a foundation for conduct to which all physical therapist assistants shall adhere. Fundamental to the Standards of Ethical Conduct is the special obligation of physical therapist assistants to enable patients/clients to achieve greater independence, health and wellness, and enhanced quality of life. No document that delineates ethical standards can address every situation. Physical therapist assistants are encouraged to seek additional advice or consultation in instances where the guidance of the Standards of Ethical Conduct may not be definitive.

Standards

Standard 1

Physical therapist assistants shall respect the inherent dignity, and rights, of all individuals.

1A. Physical therapist assistants shall act in a respectful manner toward each person regardless of age, gender, race, nationality, religion, ethnicity, social or economic status, sexual orientation, health condition, or disability.

1B. Physical therapist assistants shall recognize their personal biases and shall not discriminate against others in the provision of physical therapy services.

Standard 2

Physical therapist assistants shall be trustworthy and compassionate in addressing the rights and needs of patients/clients.

2A. Physical therapist assistants shall act in the best interests of patients/clients over the interests of the physical therapist assistant.

2B. Physical therapist assistants shall provide physical therapy interventions with compassionate and caring behaviors that incorporate the individual and cultural differences of patients/clients.

2C. Physical therapist assistants shall provide patients/clients with information regarding the interventions they provide.

2D. Physical therapist assistants shall protect confidential patient/client information and, in collaboration with the physical therapist, may disclose confidential information to appropriate authorities only when allowed or as required by law.

Standard 3

Physical therapist assistants shall make sound decisions in collaboration with the physical therapist and within the boundaries established by laws and regulations.

3A. Physical therapist assistants shall make objective decisions in the patient's/client's best interest in all practice settings.

3B. Physical therapist assistants shall be guided by information about best practice regarding physical therapy interventions.

3C. Physical therapist assistants shall make decisions based upon their level of competence and consistent with patient/client values.

3D. Physical therapist assistants shall not engage in conflicts of interest that interfere with making sound decisions.

3E. Physical therapist assistants shall provide physical therapy services under the direction and supervision of a physical therapist and shall communicate with the physical therapist when patient/client status requires modifications to the established plan of care.

Standard 4

Physical therapist assistants shall demonstrate integrity in their relationships with patients/clients, families, colleagues, students, other healthcare providers, employers, payers, and the public.

4A. Physical therapist assistants shall provide truthful, accurate, and relevant information and shall not make misleading representations.

4B. Physical therapist assistants shall not exploit persons over whom they have supervisory, evaluative or other authority (e.g., patients/clients, students, supervisees, research participants, employees).

4C. Physical therapist assistants shall discourage misconduct by health care professionals and report illegal or unethical acts to the relevant authority, when appropriate.

4D. Physical therapist assistants shall report suspected cases of abuse involving children or vulnerable adults to the supervising physical therapist and the appropriate authority, subject to law.

4E. Physical therapist assistants shall not engage in any sexual relationship with any of their patients/clients, supervisees, or students.

4F. Physical therapist assistants shall not harass anyone verbally, physically, emotionally, or sexually.

Standard 5

Physical therapist assistants shall fulfill their legal and ethical obligations.

5A. Physical therapist assistants shall comply with applicable local, state, and federal laws and regulations.

5B. Physical therapist assistants shall support the supervisory role of the physical therapist to ensure quality care and promote patient/client safety.

5C. Physical therapist assistants involved in research shall abide by accepted standards governing protection of research participants.

5D. Physical therapist assistants shall encourage colleagues with physical, psychological, or substance-related impairments that may adversely impact their professional responsibilities to seek assistance or counsel.

5E. Physical therapist assistants who have knowledge that a colleague is unable to perform their professional responsibilities with reasonable skill and safety shall report this information to the appropriate authority.

Standard 6

Physical therapist assistants shall enhance their competence through the lifelong acquisition and refinement of knowledge, skills, and abilities.

6A. Physical therapist assistants shall achieve and maintain clinical competence.

6B. Physical therapist assistants shall engage in lifelong learning consistent with changes in their roles and responsibilities and advances in the practice of physical therapy.

6C. Physical therapist assistants shall support practice environments that support career development and lifelong learning.

Standard 7

Physical therapist assistants shall support organizational behaviors and business practices that benefit patients/clients and society.

7A. Physical therapist assistants shall promote work environments that support ethical and accountable decision-making.

7B. Physical therapist assistants shall not accept gifts or other considerations that influence or give an appearance of influencing their decisions.

7C. Physical therapist assistants shall fully disclose any financial interest they have in products or services that they recommend to patients/clients.

7D. Physical therapist assistants shall ensure that documentation for their interventions accurately reflects the nature and extent of the services provided.

7E. Physical therapist assistants shall refrain from employment arrangements, or other arrangements, that prevent physical therapist assistants from fulfilling ethical obligations to patients/clients.

Standard 8

Physical therapist assistants shall participate in efforts to meet the health needs of people locally, nationally, or globally.

8A. Physical therapist assistants shall support organizations that meet the health needs of people who are economically disadvantaged, uninsured, and underinsured.

8B. Physical therapist assistants shall advocate for people with impairments, activity limitations, participation restrictions, and disabilities in order to promote their participation in community and society.

8C. Physical therapist assistants shall be responsible stewards of health care resources by collaborating with physical therapists in order to avoid overutilization or underutilization of physical therapy services.

8D. Physical therapist assistants shall educate members of the public about the benefits of physical therapy.

Proviso: The Standards of Ethical Conduct for the Physical Therapist Assistant as substituted will take effect July 1, 2010, to allow for education of APTA members and nonmembers.

From Standards of Ethical Conduct for the Physical Therapist Assistant. HOD S06-09-20-18 [Amended HOD S06-00-13-24; HOD 06-91-06-07; Initial HOD 06-82-04-08] [Standard]. Courtesy of the American Physical Therapist Association.

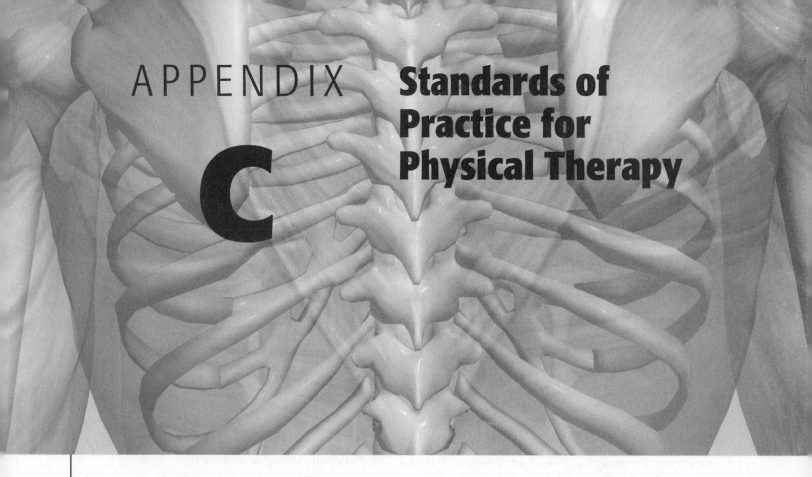

APPENDIX C

Standards of Practice for Physical Therapy

The APTA Criteria for standards of practice for physical therapy (HOD S06-03-09-10 [Amended HOD 06-03-09-10; HOD 06-99-18-22; HOD 06-96-16-31; HOD 06-91-21-25; HOD 06-85-30-56; Initial HOD 06-80-04-04; HOD 06-80-03-03]) is outlined next.

> **● Key Point** BOD P00-00-00-00 stands for Board of Directors/month/year/page/vote in the Board of Directors Minutes; the "P" indicates that it is a position (see below). For example, BOD P11-97-06-18 means that this position can be found in the November 1997 Board of Directors minutes on Page 6 and that it was Vote 18.
>
> P: Position | S: Standard | G: Guideline | Y: Policy | R: Procedure

Preamble

The physical therapy profession's commitment to society is to promote optimal health and functioning in individuals by pursuing excellence in practice. The American Physical Therapy Association attests to this commitment by adopting and promoting the following Standards of Practice for Physical Therapy. These Standards are the profession's statement of conditions and performances that are essential for provision of high quality professional service to society, and provide a foundation for assessment of physical therapist practice.

I. Ethical/Legal Considerations

A. Ethical Considerations

The physical therapist practices according to the Code of Ethics of the American Physical Therapy Association.

The physical therapist assistant complies with the Standards of Ethical Conduct for the Physical Therapist Assistant of the American Physical Therapy Association.

B. Legal Considerations

The physical therapist complies with all the legal requirements of jurisdictions regulating the practice of physical therapy.

The physical therapist assistant complies with all the legal requirements of jurisdictions regulating the work of the assistant.

II. Administration of the Physical Therapy Service

A. Statement of Mission, Purposes, and Goals

The physical therapy service has a statement of mission, purposes, and goals that reflects the needs and interests of the patients/clients served, the physical therapy personnel affiliated with the service, and the community.

B. Organizational Plan

The physical therapy service has a written organizational plan.

C. Policies and Procedures

The physical therapy service has written policies and procedures that reflect the operation, mission, purposes, and goals of the service, and are consistent with the Association's standards, policies, positions, guidelines, and Code of Ethics.

D. Administration

A physical therapist is responsible for the direction of the physical therapy service.

E. Fiscal Management

The director of the physical therapy service, in consultation with physical therapy staff and appropriate administrative personnel, participates in the planning for and allocation of resources. Fiscal planning and management of the service is based on sound accounting principles.

F. Improvement of Quality of Care and Performance

The physical therapy service has a written plan for continuous improvement of quality of care and performance of services.

G. Staffing

The physical therapy personnel affiliated with the physical therapy service have demonstrated competence and are sufficient to achieve the mission, purposes, and goals of the service.

H. Staff Development

The physical therapy service has a written plan that provides for appropriate and ongoing staff development.

I. Physical Setting

The physical setting is designed to provide a safe and accessible environment that facilitates fulfillment of the mission, purposes, and goals of the physical therapy service. The equipment is safe and sufficient to achieve the purposes and goals of physical therapy.

J. Collaboration

The physical therapy service collaborates with all disciplines as appropriate.

III. Patient/Client Management

A. Patient/Client Collaboration

Within the patient/client management process, the physical therapist and the patient/client establish and maintain an ongoing collaborative process of decision making that exists throughout the provision of services.

B. Initial Examination/Evaluation/ Diagnosis/Prognosis

The physical therapist performs an initial examination and evaluation to establish a diagnosis and prognosis prior to intervention.

C. Plan of Care

The physical therapist establishes a plan of care and manages the needs of the patient/client based on the examination, evaluation, diagnosis, prognosis, goals, and outcomes of the planned interventions for identified impairments, functional limitations, and disabilities.

The physical therapist involves the patient/client and appropriate others in the planning, implementation, and assessment of the plan of care.

The physical therapist, in consultation with appropriate disciplines, plans for discharge of the patient/client taking into consideration achievement of anticipated goals and expected outcomes, and provides for appropriate follow-up or referral.

D. Intervention

The physical therapist provides or directs and supervises the physical therapy intervention consistent with the results of the examination, evaluation, diagnosis, prognosis, and plan of care.

E. Reexamination

The physical therapist reexamines the patient/client as necessary during an episode of care to evaluate progress or change in patient/client status and modifies the plan of care accordingly or discontinues physical therapy services.

F. Discharge/Discontinuation of Intervention

The physical therapist discharges the patient/client from physical therapy services when the anticipated goals or expected outcomes for the patient/client have been achieved. The physical therapist discontinues intervention when the patient/client is unable to continue to progress toward goals or when the physical therapist determines that the patient/client will no longer benefit from physical therapy.

G. Communication/Coordination/ Documentation

The physical therapist communicates, coordinates, and documents all aspects of patient/client management including the results of the initial examination and evaluation, diagnosis, prognosis, plan of care, interventions, response to interventions, changes in patient/client status relative to the interventions, reexamination, and discharge/discontinuation of intervention and other patient/client management activities.

IV. Education

The physical therapist is responsible for individual professional development. The physical therapist assistant is responsible for individual career development.

The physical therapist and the physical therapist assistant, under the direction and supervision of the physical therapist, participate in the education of students.

The physical therapist educates and provides consultation to consumers and the general public regarding the purposes and benefits of physical therapy.

The physical therapist educates and provides consultation to consumers and the general public regarding the roles of the physical therapist and the physical therapist assistant.

V. Research

The physical therapist applies research findings to practice and encourages, participates in, and promotes activities that establish the outcomes of patient/client management provided by the physical therapist.

VI. Community Responsibility

The physical therapist demonstrates community responsibility by participating in community and community agency activities, educating the public, formulating public policy, or providing pro bono physical therapy services.

Relationship to Vision 2020: Professionalism; (Practice Department, ext 3176)

[Document updated: 12/14/2009]

From Standards of Practice for Physical Therapy. HOD S06-03-09-10 [Amended HOD 06-03-09-10; HOD 06-99-18-22; HOD 06-96-16-31; HOD 06-91-21-25; HOD 06-85-30-56; Initial HOD 06-80-04-04; HOD 06-80-03-03]. Courtesy of the American Physical Therapist Association.

D

Regular Time	Military Time	Regular Time	Military Time
Midnight	0000	Noon	1200
1:00 A.M.	0100	1:00 P.M.	1300
2:00 A.M.	0200	2:00 P.M.	1400
3:00 A.M.	0300	3:00 P.M.	1500
4:00 A.M.	0400	4:00 P.M.	1600
5:00 A.M.	0500	5:00 P.M.	1700
6:00 A.M.	0600	6:00 P.M.	1800
7:00 A.M.	0700	7:00 P.M.	1900
8:00 A.M.	0800	8:00 P.M.	2000
9:00 A.M.	0900	9:00 P.M.	2100
10:00 A.M.	1000	10:00 P.M.	2200
11:00 A.M.	1100	11:00 P.M.	2300

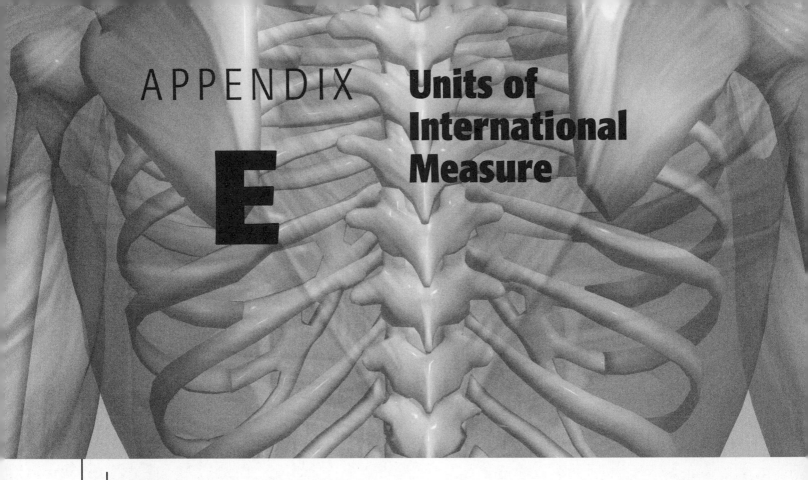

APPENDIX E Units of International Measure

Length

Unit	Inches	Feet	Yards	Miles	Centimeters	Meters
1 inch	1	0.8333333	0.02777778	0.00001578283	2.54	0.0254
1 foot	12	1	0.3333333	0.0001893939	30.48	0.3048
1 yard	36	3	1	0.0005681818	91.44	0.9144
1 mile	63,360	5280	1760	1	160,934.4	1609.344
1 centimeter	0.3937008	0.03280840	0.01093613	0.000006213712	1	0.01
1 meter	39.37008	3.280840	1.093613	0.0006213712	100	1

Temperature

0°C (freezing point)	32°F
100°C (boiling point)	212°F

To convert Celsius to Fahrenheit: (degrees centigrade × 9/5) + 32

To convert Fahrenheit to Celsius: (degrees Fahrenheit − 32) × 5/9

Weight

1 ounce (oz.)	0.0625 pounds (lb.)	28.35 grams (g)	0.028 kilograms (kg)
1 pound	16 oz.	454 g	0.454 kg
1 g	0.035 oz.	0.0022 lb.	0.001 kg
1 kg	35.27 oz.	2.2 lb.	1000 g

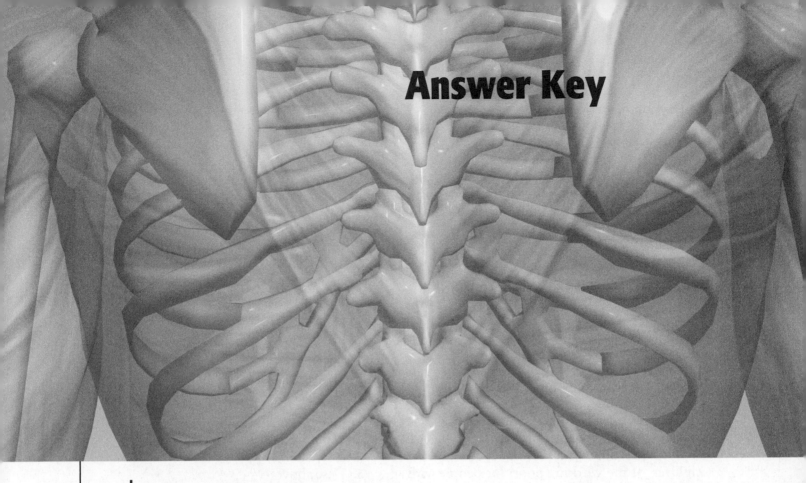

Answer Key

Chapter 1: Fundamentals

1. b. *The Guide to Physical Therapist Practice*
2. True
3. b. To make autonomous decisions concerning the accreditation status of continuing education programs for the physical therapists and physical therapist assistants
4. d. a and c
5. a. Impairment
6. c. Examination
7. a. To allow the clinician to evaluate progress and modify interventions as appropriate
8. b. Observation
9. a. Measurable physiological characteristics, including height and weight
10. d. None of the above
11. c. Prognosis
12. d. All of the above
13. c. Intervention
14. A patient has a diagnosed impairment or functional limitation, whereas a client is not necessarily diagnosed with impairments or functional limitations, but seeks services for prevention or promotion of health, wellness, and fitness.
15. Subjective, objective, assessment, and plan
16. False
17. d. Race
18. b. Physical therapy director
19. True
20. b. Cleaning the whirlpool

21. e. All of the above
22. b. To perform all aspects of treatment using correct body mechanics
23. c. Allow a patient to increase in frequency from 2 times/week to 3 times/week
24. b. Certified Outpatient Rehabilitation Facility
25. b. To inform the patient that it would be inappropriate for him or her to comment on the lab results before the physician has assessed the lab results and spoken to the patient
26. a. Subjective
27. True. The essential data collection skills are outlined in Table 1-1.

Chapter 2: Healthcare Administration

1. Health maintenance organization
2. The primary care physician (PCP)
3. True
4. False. It is funded by payroll tax, under the Federal Insurance Contributions Act (FICA).
5. A program that provides insurance coverage for children of the working poor, for people with full-time jobs, which do not offer employment-based insurance, and for those who earn too much for Medicaid but not enough to afford private insurance.
6. Uninsured individuals with HIV/AIDS
7. To regulate major capital expenditures, which may adversely impact the cost of healthcare services, to prevent the unnecessary expansion of healthcare facilities, and encourage the appropriate allocation of resources for healthcare purposes.
8. A written instruction, such as a living will or a durable power of attorney for health care, that provides instructions for the provision of medical treatment *in anticipation* of those times when the individual executing the document no longer has decision-making capacity.
9. The Americans with Disabilities Act (ADA)
10. The Commission on Accreditation of Rehabilitation Facilities (CARF)
11. Every 3 years
12. Medicare Part A is only for inpatient treatment.
13. Part B
14. The Balanced Budget Act of 1997
15. To provide a mechanism to spread the risk of unforeseen medical expenditures across a broad base to protect the individual from personal expenditures.

16. True
17. Consumer-driven healthcare plans
18. A failure to exercise an accepted degree of professional skill or learning by one rendering professional that results in injury, loss, or damage.
19. True
20. Every 12 months
21. Medicaid
22. CPT and Common Procedural Coding System procedure codes
23. True: The informed consent should include a description of the proposed intervention, as well as the risks, benefits, and concerns of the proposed intervention.

Chapter 3: Research and Evidence-Based Practice

1. A population is the totality of all subjects possessing certain common characteristics that are being studied.
2. Inferential
3. Descriptive
4. Ratio-level
5. c. Colors of theraband in a PT department
6. a. Water temperatures of three whirlpools in the PT department
7. Random, systematic, stratified, and cluster
8. Systematic
9. True
10. Discrete
11. Nominal
12. Mode
13. 320
14. 30
15. The square root of the variance is the standard deviation.
16. False
17. Many variables are normally distributed, and the distribution can be used to describe these variables.
18. 1, or 100%
19. 50% of the area lies below the mean, and 50% of the area lies above the mean.
20. 68%
21. The validity of the study was threatened with the introduction of sampling bias.
22. a. A statement ensuring the subject's commitment to participate for the duration of the study.
23. d. Stratified random sample

24. a. Leg isokinetic exercises are highly correlated with RPE, while arm isokinetic exercises are only moderately correlated.

Chapter 4: Musculoskeletal Physical Therapy

1. A shoulder dislocation is a true separation between the head of the humerus and the glenoid. A shoulder separation involves a disruption of the acromioclavicular joint.
2. The complex consists of the central fibrocartilage articular disk, palmar and dorsal radioulnar ligament, ulnar collateral ligament, and a sheath from the extensor carpi ulnaris. It attaches to the ulna board of the radius and the distal ulna.
3. In the direction of hip extension, adduction, and internal rotation.
4. a. The anterior tibialis, the posterior tibialis, and the fibularis (peroneus) longus
5. The sternoclavicular joint
6. Supraspinatus, infraspinatus, teres minor, pectoralis major
7. The obturator internus
8. The acromioclavicular joint
9. Extension
10. Maximum dorsiflexion
11. Sartorius, gracilis, and semitendinosis
12. Popliteus
13. A fracture of the radius and the ulna
14. A fracture of the distal tibia and fibula
15. Radial nerve damage
16. Elbow extension and forearm supination
17. 70° of elbow flexion and 10° of forearm supination
18. 70° of elbow flexion and 35° of forearm supination
19. The scaphoid
20. Avascular necrosis
21. The anterior tibial artery
22. The anterior talofibular ligament
23. The medial meniscus
24. To prevent posterior displacement of the tibia on the femur
25. Hamstrings
26. 12- to 18-year-old females
27. Vastus medialis obliquus
28. Posterior drawer and the sag test
29. Extension, internal rotation, abduction
30. Ober test
31. Transverse ligament
32. The lateral pterygoid

33. Sternoclavicular, acromioclavicular, glenohumeral, scapulothoracic
34. The acromioclavicular ligament and the coracoclavicular ligament
35. Supination of the forearm
36. MCP flexion and IP extension
37. The atlantoaxial joint
38. Three
39. Anteriorly
40. Infraspinatus, teres minor, posterior deltoid
41. Sartorius, rectus femoris
42. c. Rotation
43. The calcaneus bone and the talus
44. The distal interphalangeal joints
45. The plantar calcaneonavicular ligament
46. b. Hamstrings
47. d. The navicular tuberosity
48. a. Scaphoid and capitate
49. c. Anterior cruciate ligament
50. a. An increase in the angle of inclination between the neck of the femur and the shaft.
51. c. Operative sectioning of a bone
52. c. Is a systemic disease
53. a. The median nerve
54. b. Median
55. c. Median nerve
56. c. Anterior cruciate ligament
57. d. Rhomboid major
58. c. Drop-arm test
59. c. Pectoralis minor
60. b. Thomas
61. d. Latissimus dorsi and lower trapezius
62. c. Serratus anterior
63. d. Abductor pollicus longus
64. d. Extensor digitorum communis
65. c. Contracted iliotibial band
66. b. Varus stress
67. a. Cold/intermittent compression combination followed by elevation.
68. c. Gastrocnemius
69. b. The disc
70. a. Stretching the iliopsoas and iliotibial (IT) band; strengthening the abdominals

Chapter 5: Neuromuscular Physical Therapy

1. c. Bowel and bladder control
2. c. Adductor magnus
3. a. Sartorius
4. c. Loss of pain sensation
5. Increase

6. b. Tingling in the radial side of the hand and pain in the hand at night
7. c. Coma
8. a. They are mostly venous in origin, involving the venous dural sinuses.
9. d. Myoneural junction block
10. b. Pneumococcus
11. Cranial nerves III and IV
12. Cranial nerves V through VIII
13. b. 31
14. C1–4
15. C5–T1
16. Ophthalmic, maxillary, and mandibular
17. The spinal accessory nerve (XI) and the vagus nerve (X)
18. The hypothalamus
19. Sympathetic
20. Hypoglossal
21. Spinal accessory
22. Lateral cord
23. Long thoracic nerve
24. Axillary nerve and radial nerve
25. Posterior
26. Coracobrachialis, brachialis, biceps brachii
27. The ulnar nerve
28. The deep fibular (peroneal) nerve
29. The obturator and tibial division of the sciatic
30. The radial nerve
31. The median nerve
32. The median nerve
33. The ulnar nerve
34. The median nerve
35. Phalen test and Tinel test
36. Supraspinatus and infraspinatus
37. Long thoracic nerve
38. Thoracodorsal nerve
39. Gluteus medius and minimus, tensor fascia lata
40. C7
41. Wrist extensors
42. c. Medial heads of flexor digitorum profundus
43. Median nerve
44. a. Lateral cutaneous (femoral) nerve of the thigh
45. d. Femoral
46. e. Adjacent dorsal surfaces of the first and second toes
47. e. Serratus anterior
48. b. Flexor carpi ulnaris
49. Flexor pollicis longus and pronator quadratus
50. Klumpke paralysis
51. Coracobrachialis

52. The third ventricle
53. The anterior cerebral arteries
54. The circle of Willis
55. The understanding of language
56. The corpus callosum
57. The trigeminal nerve
58. The ulnar nerve
59. Impairments of circulation, integumentary integrity, muscle performance, posture; functional limitations in self-care, home management, work
60. *Arousal:* The physiological readiness of the human system for activity; *Attention:* Selected awareness of the environment or responsiveness to a stimulus or task without being distracted by other stimuli; *Orientation:* The patient's awareness of time, person, and place; *Cognition:* The process of knowing and includes both awareness and judgment.
61. c. The increased conduction velocity as the action potential jumps from node to node of Ranvier.
62. d. All the different tactile receptors
63. It is monosynaptic
64. d. They are innervated by one very large, type Ia fiber that serves both fiber types.
65. True
66. d. Kinesthesia
67. c. The vestibular apparatus
68. d. Flexor withdrawal reflex
69. d. The vomiting reflex
70. c. Telencephalon
71. Occipital lobe
72. Parietal lobe
73. Temporal lobe
74. Hypothalamus
75. d. The corpus callosum
76. c. Control of the right side of the body
77. c. Blushing
78. True
79. True
80. d. Sweating and salivation
81. a. Facilitation of early movement in synergistic patterns followed quickly by movement patterns out of synergy
82. a. Bilateral KAFOs.
83. a. Involve the patient in decision making, emphasizing safety and independent performance.
84. a. Will likely be resistant to activity training if unfamiliar activities are used.
85. a. Serratus anterior

Chapter 6: Cardiovascular Physical Therapy

1. d. During one minute
2. To carry oxygen-deficient blood that has just returned from the body to the lungs, where carbon dioxide is exchanged for oxygen.
3. Hemoglobin
4. To delay the impulse from the SA node
5. The right side
6. The right and left coronary arteries
7. Right atrium
8. The AV valves closing
9. c. Do not have attachments to papillary muscles
10. c. Systole
11. d. Higher than normal cardiac output
12. d. Opening and closing of the four major heart valves
13. To prevent the valves from everting when the ventricles contract thereby stopping any back flow of blood.
14. True
15. b. Right atrium, left atrium, ventricles
16. During diastole
17. d. No appreciable change in mean pressure
18. d. Chemoreceptors
19. d. Cardiac function
20. The reflex decreases the sympathetic input and heart rate on those occasions when the heart is beating too rapidly.
21. d. Decreased peristalsis
22. d. Excess fluid in the intercellular space
23. d. All of the above
24. a. Aortic stenosis
25. b. Dyspnea
26. d. Stenosis of the aortic valves
27. a. Pulmonary edema
28. c. Left ventricle
29. b. Atherosclerosis
30. b. Atrial depolarization
31. c. Ventricular repolarization
32. c. Buerger disease
33. d. All of the above
34. b. Left ventricular pressure exceeds left atrial pressure
35. d. Dyspnea with exertion
36. Systolic blood pressure <120 mm Hg and diastolic blood pressure <80 mm Hg
37. Venous stasis, vascular damage, and hypercoaguability
38. The calf veins
39. 50% occur within the first 24 hours; 85% occur within the first four days.
40. Pulmonary embolism
41. Early ambulation, extremity elevation, range of motion exercises, graduated elastic stockings, intermittent pneumatic compression stockings, and anticoagulation measures
42. The clinical presentation may be variable, but most often patients have dyspnea, pleuritic chest pain, hypoxemia, and tachypnea.

Chapter 7: Pulmonary Physical Therapy

1. c. The alveoli
2. The left
3. Ventilation
4. Apex
5. The right lung
6. Diaphragm
7. True
8. b. Ability to lower the surface tension of the water molecules on the alveolar surface.
9. Pleural cavity
10. b. Area occupied by the conducting airways that does not permit gas exchange.
11. The total volume of gas that is not involved in gas exchange.
12. c. Expiratory reserve volume
13. d. Vital capacity
14. Tidal volume
15. b. Functional residual capacity
16. e. Residual volume
17. True
18. d. The P_{CO_2} levels of the blood
19. d. In the reticular substance of the medulla and pons
20. Carbon dioxide
21. In the carotid and aortic bodies
22. 7.36–7.44
23. b. Total lung capacity
24. b. Tidal volume
25. c. Residual volume
26. False. High breathing frequencies are commonly observed in patients with restrictive lung disease.
27. True
28. 1
29. d. Bronchial asthma
30. c. Chronic bronchitis
31. b. Decreased resonance to percussion over the lung fields

32. Bronchiectasis
33. d. Emphysema
34. c. Acute bronchitis

Chapter 8: Integumentary Physical Therapy

1. True
2. Any five from the following: Provides protection against injury or invasion; secretes oils that lubricate the skin; provides insulation; maintains homeostasis (fluid balance, regulation of body temperature, excretion of excess water, urea, and salt via sweat); maintains body shape; provides cosmetic appearance and identity; synthesizes vitamin D, stores nutrients, provides cutaneous sensation via receptors in the dermis.
3. Stratum basale
4. Stratum corneum
5. Dermis
6. c. The skin and mucous membranes
7. Moisture, temperature, texture, turgor, and mobility
8. Patch
9. Plaque
10. Bulla
11. Granulation tissue nourishes the macrophages and fibroblasts that have migrated into the wound and, as healing continues, provides a substrate for the migration of epidermal cells.
12. An overgrowth of dense fibrous tissue that usually develops after healing of a skin injury.
13. Athlete's foot
14. Psoriasis
15. Bony prominences of the hip, sacrum, and heel
16. d. Systemic lupus erythematosus
17. False. It is benign.
18. Karposi sarcoma
19. Asymmetry, Border irregularity, Color variegation, Diameter, Evolving
20. b. Second degree
21. Cardiac arrhythmias, ventricular fibrillation, renal failure, spinal cord damage, and respiratory arrest
22. d. Thymus
23. d. Fever
24. d. Pallor
25. d. All of the above
26. Stage IV
27. Flexion contractures
28. Occlusion dressing
29. Moist dressings
30. A topical treatment used as an adjunct to wound healing to facilitate wound closure in acute surgical wounds as well as with more challenging, slow-to-heal wounds.
31. Sharp debridement, enzymatic debridement, and autolytic debridement
32. Wet-to-dry dressings, wound irrigation, and hydrotherapy (whirlpool)

Chapter 9: Pathology

1. Any four from fungi (yeast and molds); helminths (e.g., tapeworms); mycobacteria; viruses; mycoplasmas; bacteria; rickettsiae; chlamydiae; protozoa; and prions
2. Small, gram-negative, obligate intracellular organisms that cause several diseases, including Rocky Mountain spotted fever and epidemic typhus.
3. Viruses
4. Prion
5. Infections that originate or occur in a hospital or hospital-like setting.
6. *Streptococcus pyogenes* (group A *Streptococcus*)
7. Hepatitis A, acute hepatitis B, and hepatitis E
8. Unprotected sexual contact, contaminated needles, and maternal–fetal transmission in utero or at delivery or through contaminated breast milk.
9. Influenza A
10. Phenols, halogens (chlorine, iodine, and bromine), and alcohol
11. False. Disinfection applies to the process of reducing the number of viable microorganisms present in a sample (sterilization is the killing of *all* microorganisms in a material or on the surface of an object).
12. c. It is contagious.
13. Any four from the following—unusual bleeding or discharge; a lump or thickening of any area (e.g., breast); a sore that does not heal; a change in bladder or bowel habits; hoarseness of voice or persistent cough; indigestion or difficulty in swallowing; unexplained weight loss; night pain not related to movement; and a change in the size or appearance of a wart or mole.
14. b. Endocrine tumors
15. d. Giant cell tumor
16. c. Osteomalacia
17. a. Retinoblastoma
18. b. An altered genome due to a mutation of one or more genes.

19. c. Tumor size, lymph node involvement, tumor metastasis
20. d. Neuroblastoma
21. Extracellular fluid (ECF)
22. Kidney
23. b. Liver
24. c. Lymphocyte
25. a. Hemangioma
26. d. All of the above
27. There is a delay in coagulation time.
28. Kegel exercises
29. True
30. Any four from the following-: Hyperglycemia (raised blood sugar), glycosuria (raised sugar in the urine), polyuria (excessive excretion of urine), polydipsia (excessive thirst), excessive hunger (polyphagia), weight loss, and fatigue.
31. A type of hyperthyroidism.
32. Hypofunction of the adrenal cortex
33. Relaxin
34. Postexertional malaise lasting more than 24 hours; tender lymph nodes; muscle pain; multiple arthralgias without swelling or redness; substantial impairment in short-term memory or concentration; headaches of a new type, pattern, or severity; sore throat; and unrefreshing sleep.
35. Paranoid
36. d. Psychotic disorders
37. b. The original affect for one object is transferred to another object.
38. a. The original affect for one object is transferred to another object.
39. b. It usually begins at about middle age.
40. Stocking-like distribution of anesthesia over an extremity.
41. Bulimia

Chapter 10: Pediatric Physical Therapy

1. To ensure that all children who have special needs will be supported in access to free and appropriate public education.
2. To meet the needs of the family as they relate to their child's development, as well as meet the needs of the child.
3. Motor control refers to processes of the brain and spinal cord that govern posture and movement
4. Motor development refers to the processes of change in motor behavior that occur over relatively extended time periods.

5. Born before 37 weeks of gestational age.
6. Three to 4 months.
7. Five to 6 months.
8. Eight to 9 months.
9. Twelve months.
10. c. Maintain pivot prone posture
11. Verbal, post response, augmented feedback about the response outcome
12. One hand supports the infant's head in midline, the other supports the back. The infant is raised to 45 degrees and the head is allowed to fall through 10 degrees. Mature response is abduction, then adduction, of the limbs.
13. Infant positioned in quadruped. Arm and head do the same thing, legs do the opposite (e.g., head is extended, arms extend, and legs flex).
14. Extension of extremities on face side, flexion of extremities on skull side.
15. Placing reaction.
16. Hip flexion, abduction, and external rotation; knee flexion; ankle dorsiflexion
17. c. The agonist is inhibited and the antagonist is facilitated.
18. Salty perspiration, decreased tolerance to exercise, clubbing of the fingernails, cyanosis, orthopnic posture (leaning forward), thin and small stature
19. b. Scoliosis
20. a. Talipes equinovarus
21. d. The tendency for fractures is more severe following puberty.
22. b. Hip
23. b. Femoral anteversion, femoral external rotation, foot pronation
24. d. All of the above
25. d. All of the above
26. c. Slipped capital femoral epiphysis
27. a. Pulled elbow
28. c. Acetabular dysplasia
29. c. Ankle
30. Spina bifida myelocele
31. Spina bifida occulta
32. Spina bifida syringomyelocele
33. a. The boy's most serious physical problems from the perspective of his parent/caretakers.
34. Torticollis
35. b. Navicular
36. b. Anorexia nervosa
37. b. Adapt a desk and wheelchair to provide adequate sitting balance.
38. d. Osgood–Schlatter disease

Chapter 11: Geriatric Physical Therapy

1. Gerontology
2. Weight-bearing joints.
3. b. Taking three prescription medications
4. c. Measuring serum 25-hydroxyvitamin D concentration
5. b. An exercise program
6. c. A single intervention that consists of education on risk factor modification
7. d. All of the above
8. c. Dislocated hip
9. b. Anterior cerebral artery
10. Any four of the following: smoking, obesity, lack of exercise, diet, and excess alcohol consumption.
11. a. Sidelying on the sound side with the affected upper extremity supported on a pillow with the shoulder protracted and elbow extended.
12. a. Hematuria and ecchymosis
13. d. Reduction of nerve conduction velocity
14. Middle cerebral artery
15. Posterior cerebral artery
16. Parkinson disease
17. Resting tremor, rigidity, and bradykinesia
18. The onset of chronic, insidious memory loss that is slowly progressive.
19. A durable power of attorney for health care, and a living will.
20. Informed consent

Chapter 12: Therapeutic Exercise

1. Isometric contraction
2. Eccentric
3. Eccentric
4. Extensibility, elasticity, irritability, and the ability to develop tension
5. False. More force.
6. The strength gains are developed at a specific point in the range of motion and not throughout the range; not all of a muscle's fibers are activated.
7. b. Isometric exercises
8. Type/mode of exercise, intensity, duration, and frequency
9. b. Heart rate
10. c. Very light
11. b. High-intensity workloads for short durations.
12. c. Iliococcygeus, pubococcygeus, and coccygeus
13. b. Increased high-density lipoprotein (HDL) cholesterol

14. a. Closed-chain lower extremity strengthening, proprioceptive exercises, and an orthosis
15. a. Patient education regarding positions and movements to avoid.
16. a. Pendulum exercises
17. Exercise of low intensity and long duration
18. c. D2 flexion
19. a. To use modalities to reduce pain and inflammation
20. c. No pain, no gain
21. b. Hamstrings
22. b. Hamstrings and hip extensors
23. c. Frenkel exercises
24. c. Squat
25. c. Plyometrics
26. a. Walking at an intensity of 50% of the patient's maximum heart rate
27. a. 30% to 60% of the maximum heart rate

Chapter 13: Therapeutic Modalities

1. c. Cold decreases spasm by decreasing sensitivity to muscle spindles and heat decreases spasm by decreasing nerve conduction velocity.
2. 165°F to 175°F (73.92°C to 79.4°C)
3. Any three of the following: incontinence, urinary tract infections, unprotected open wounds, heat intolerance, severe epilepsy, uncontrolled diabetes, unstable blood pressure or severe cardiac and/or pulmonary dysfunction
4. 92°F to 95°F
5. b. To change electricity into ultrasound waves
6. c. Ultrasound
7. Amps
8. d. Salicylic acid
9. b. Hot pack
10. c. Attracted to the cathode
11. d. Muscle
12. d. All of the above
13. c. Watt
14. d. Protein
15. a. It increases it.
16. b. Attracted to the cathode
17. b. Waveform
18. a. Local analgesia
19. a. Vasoconstriction
20. c. Paraffin bath
21. c. High volt
22. b. Icing and vigorous massage to the residual limb
23. b. TENS
24. d. All of the above

Chapter 14: Prosthetics and Orthotics

1. Amputation refers to the cutting of a limb along the long bones axis, whereas disarticulation refers to cutting of a limb through the joint.
2. a. Prevent lymphedema
3. A prosthesis that was too long
4. b. It eliminates air during the stance phase.
5. a. The prosthetic knee is set too far anterior to the TKA line.
6. Posterior
7. c. Allows limited sagittal plane motion with a small amount of mediolateral motion
8. a. The anterior and lateral walls are 2½ to 3 inches higher than the posterior and medial walls.
9. Level 1
10. b. Weak hip adductor
11. b. Socket is too large
12. a. The prosthesis is too short.
13. c. Soft ankle cushioned heel
14. b. Pistoning of the socket
15. c. Tilt the trunk backward and go down forward
16. c. A 17-inch seat height

Chapter 15: Pharmacology for the PTA

1. The Food and Drug Administration (FDA)
2. Pharmacokinetics
3. Cox-2
4. a. Schedule the patient's sessions so that there are fewer sessions on the days she usually performs poorly.
5. a. Levodopa
6. a. Cardizem causes decreased contractility of the heart and vasodilation of the coronary arteries.
7. a. Cause the heart rate to be low at rest, and to increase very little with exercise.
8. False
9. False. NSAIDS are eliminated from the body via the kidneys.
10. True
11. d. All of the above
12. True
13. Benzodiazepines
14. Tricyclic depressants
15. Spasticity

Chapter 16: Gait and Functional Training

1. The interval of time between any of the repetitive events of walking
2. Weight acceptance, single limb support, and swing limb advancement
3. Stance and swing
4. Loading response, mid stance, terminal stance and pre-swing.
5. Pre-swing, initial swing, mid-swing, and terminal swing.
6. Gait velocity, stride length, and cadence
7. The repetition rate (cadence), physical conditioning, and the length of the person's stride.
8. 113 steps/min
9. Approximately midline in the frontal plane and slightly anterior to the second sacral vertebra in the sagittal plane.
10. False. It is displaced vertically and laterally.
11. False. They move in opposite directions to each other.
12. A positive Trendelenburg sign is indicated when the pelvis lists toward the non-weight-bearing side during single-limb support.
13. a. Tibialis anterior
14. Foot slap immediately after initial contact; foot drop during swing; excessive hip and knee flexion during swing
15. During the end of the swing phase
16. a. Foot drop during swing phase
17. d. All of the above
18. b. Hip abductors
19. d. Extensor gait
20. b. Knee and hip flexion
21. Midstance
22. Gluteus medius
23. c. To bring the line of gravity closer to the involved hip joint.
24. Gluteus maximus
25. Quadriceps weakness (due to inhibition, swelling, or pain), patellofemoral pain, and anterior cruciate ligament deficiency
26. Deep fibular (peroneal)
27. Circumduction of the hip
28. b. Walker
29. The crutch tip should be vertical to the ground and positioned approximately 15-cm (6-inch) lateral and 5-cm (2-inch) anterior to the patient's foot.
30. a. 1–2 inches
31. b. Minimal assist
32. b. Subtract 2 inches

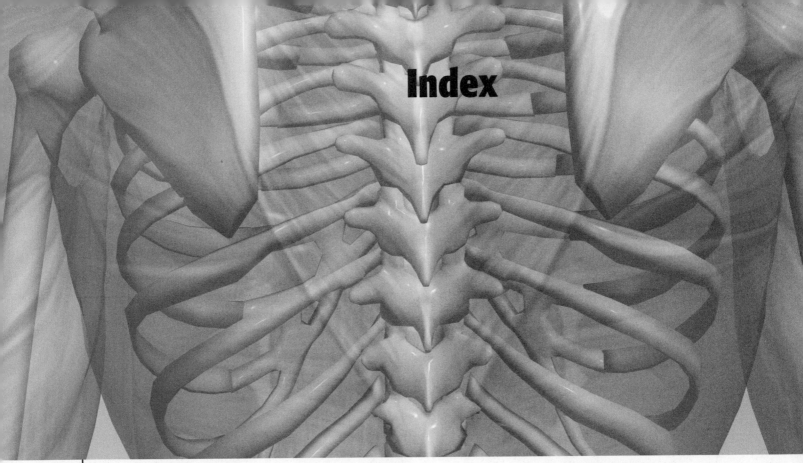

Index